Contemporary Topics in Women's Mental Health

Contemporary Topics in Women's Mental Health

Global perspectives in a changing society

Editors

Prabha S. Chandra
Department of Psychiatry, National Institute of Mental Health and Neurosciences, Bangalore, India

Helen Herrman
Orygen Youth Health Research Centre, The University of Melbourne, Melbourne, Australia

Jane Fisher
Key Centre for Women's Health in Society, The University of Melbourne, Melbourne, Australia

Marianne Kastrup
Psychiatric Department Rigshospitalet, Copenhagen, Denmark

Unaiza Niaz
The Psychiatric Clinic & Stress Research Center, Karachi, Pakistan; The University of Health Sciences, Lahore, Pakistan

Marta B. Rondón
Cayetano Heredia University, Lima, Peru

Ahmed Okasha
Institute of Psychiatry, Ains Shams University, Cairo, Egypt

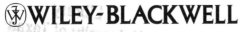

WILEY-BLACKWELL

A John Wiley & Sons, Ltd., Publication

Library of Congress Cataloging-in-Publication Data

Contemporary topics in women's mental health : global perspectives in a changing society / editors, Prabha S. Chandra ... [et al.].
    p. ; cm.
  Includes bibliographical references.
  ISBN 978-0-470-75411-5 (cloth)
  1. Women–Mental health. 2. Women–Mental health–Social aspects. 3. Mentally ill women. I. Chandra, Prabha S.
  [DNLM: 1. Mental Disorders. 2. Women's Health. 3. Interpersonal Relations. 4. Women's Health Services – ethics. WM 140 C7613 2009]
  RC451.4.W6C673 2009
  362.196′890082–dc22

                                            2009021622

ISBN 978-0-470-75411-5
A catalogue record for this book is available from the British Library.
Set in 10.5/12.5 Minion-Regular by Laserwords Private Ltd, Chennai, India.
Printed in Singapore by Markono Print Media Pte Ltd
First Impression 2009
Cover illustration and Art Work by Meghana S. Chandra

Contents

Foreword   xv
Preface   xvii
List of Contributors   xix

SECTION 1   Current themes in psychiatric disorders among
             women   1
             Ahmed Okasha and Prabha S. Chandra

1. Psychotic disorders and bipolar affective disorder   9
    Rangaswamy Thara and Ramachandran Padmavati

    1.1   Psychotic disorders in women   9
    1.2   Schizophrenia   10
    1.3   Bipolar disorder   17
    1.4   Other psychoses   25
    1.5   Special issues in women with severe mental illness   27

2. Depression and anxiety among women   37
    Nadia Kadri and Khadija Mchichi Alami

    2.1   Introduction   37
    2.2   Epidemiology   37
    2.3   Transcultural aspects of affective disturbances in sub-Saharan Africa   41
    2.4   Treatment effects   42
    2.5   Sex differences in depression and anxiety disorders: Biological
          determinants   44
    2.6   Sex differences in depression and anxiety disorders: Social factors   46
    2.7   Mood and anxiety disorders across lifespan in women   50
    2.8   Pregnancy   52
    2.9   Motherhood   53
    2.10 Conclusion   55

3. Somatisation and dissociation — 65

Santosh K. Chaturvedi and Ravi Philip Rajkumar

3.1 Introduction — 65
3.2 Somatisation – definitions and concept — 66
3.3 Dissociation – definitions and concept — 66
3.4 The diagnosis and classification of somatoform and dissociative disorders — 68
3.5 The neurobiology of somatisation and dissociation — 70
3.6 Psychosocial factors — 74
3.7 Conversion disorder — 81
3.8 Hypochondriasis — 83
3.9 Dissociative disorders — 85
3.10 Conclusions — 88

4. Eating disorders — 97

Sarvath Abbas and Robert L. Palmer

4.1 Introduction — 97
4.2 Risk factors and pathogenesis — 98
4.3 Distribution — 100
4.4 Presentation, assessment, diagnosis and engagement — 100
4.5 Treatment and management — 104
4.6 Conclusion — 111

5. Suicidality in women — 117

Gergö Hadlaczky and Danuta Wasserman

5.1 Definitions — 117
5.2 Epidemiology — 118
5.3 Suicidality and mental disorders and risk — 126
5.4 Suicide prevention — 129

6. Alcohol and substance abuse — 139

Florence Baingana

6.1 Introduction — 139
6.2 Genetics of alcohol and drug abuse — 140
6.3 Burden of the problem and patterns of drinking — 140
6.4 Alcohol and drug abuse, risky sexual behaviour and HIV vulnerability — 141
6.5 Stigma, women and alcohol and drug abuse — 143
6.6 Health consequences — 143
6.7 Social and economic consequences — 143
6.8 Interventions — 144
6.9 Challenges — 145

6.10 Research 145

6.11 Recommendations 145

6.12 Conclusions 146

7. **Psychiatric consequences of trauma in women** 149

   Elie G. Karam, Mariana M. Salamoun and Salim El-Sabbagh

   7.1 Introduction 149

   7.2 What types of traumata are more common among women? 150

   7.3 How do women respond to trauma? 154

   7.4 What are the trauma related risk factors? 156

   7.5 Which mental disorders are related to trauma? 159

   7.6 Future directions 164

8. **Voices of consumers – women with mental illness share their experiences** 169

   Shoba Raja

   8.1 'Ni Tagibebu' – 'I will change my lifestyle' 169

   8.2 Determined to go against the odds 173

   8.3 Brilliant madness – a narrative by a young woman from India who is recovering from mental illness 177

   8.4 From illness to purpose and recovery . . . 180

   8.5 Conclusions 186

SECTION 2   The interface between reproductive health and psychiatry 189

   Prabha S. Chandra

9. **Mental health aspects of pregnancy, childbirth and the postpartum period** 197

   Jane Fisher, Meena Cabral de Mello and Takashi Izutsu

   9.1 Mental health and maternal mortality 198

   9.2 Mental health and antenatal morbidity 200

   9.3 Depression in pregnancy 200

   9.4 Anxiety in pregnancy 201

   9.5 Cultural preferences and mental health in pregnancy 202

   9.6 Inflicted violence and mental health in pregnancy 203

   9.7 Mental health and postpartum morbidity 203

   9.8 Postpartum blues or mild transient mood disturbance 204

   9.9 Postpartum psychotic illness 204

   9.10 Postpartum depression 205

9.11   Psychosocial risk factors for postpartum depression   206
9.12   Infant factors and maternal mental health   208
9.13   Cultural specificity of postpartum mood disturbance   208
9.14   Maternal mental health, infant development and the
       mother-infant relationship   210
9.15   Prevention and treatment of maternal mental health problems   212
9.16   Summary   213

10. **Psychosocial issues and reproductive health conditions:
     An interface**   **227**

     Veena A. Satyanarayana, Geetha Desai and Prabha S. Chandra

10.1   Introduction   227
10.2   Infertility – a psychosocial appraisal   228
10.3   The psychological implications of hysterectomy   235
10.4   Gynaecological infections   238
10.5   Conclusions   245

11. **Menopause and women's mental health: The need for
     a multidimensional approach**   **259**

     Jill Astbury

11.1   Introduction   259
11.2   Social, cultural and contextual factors   260
11.3   Variation in symptoms and symptom patterns   260
11.4   The research evidence   264
11.5   Is menopause a time of increased risk for women's mental
       health?   264
11.6   The relationship between menopause and depression in
       midlife   264
11.7   The need for a life course perspective   267
11.8   Methodological difficulties   270
11.9   Therapeutic approaches in mid life   271
11.10 Conclusion   275

SECTION 3   Service delivery and ethics   **281**

     Marta B. Rondón

12. **Ethics in psychiatric research among women**   **287**

     Laura Roberts and Kristen Prentice

12.1   The scientific imperative to include women in psychiatric research 287
12.2   The ethical challenges of psychiatric research   289
12.3   Unique challenges of psychiatric research in women   291
12.4   Summary   295

13. Integrating mental health into women's health and primary healthcare: The case of Chile   **301**

Graciela Rojas and Enrique Jadresic

13.1   Introduction   301
13.2   Integrating mental health into primary healthcare   302
13.3   Integrating mental health into women's health   307

14. Gender sensitive psychiatric care for children and adolescents   **317**

Corina Benjet

14.1   Mental health services for children and adolescents   317
14.2   Barriers to service use   319
14.3   Recommendations for gender sensitive psychiatric care of children and adolescents   319

15. Gender sensitive care for adult women   **323**

Marta B. Rondón

15.1   Introduction   323
15.2   Gender sensitive and informed mental healthcare: Basic strategies   325
15.3   Principles of gender sensitive care   327
15.4   Characteristics of gender sensitive services   328

16. Psychopharmacology   **337**

Silvana Sarabia

16.1   History of psychopharmacology   337
16.2   Ethics   338
16.3   Sources and interpretation of data   340
16.4   Women in clinical trials   341
16.5   Pharmacodynamics and pharmacokinetics in women   342
16.6   Psychotropic treatments in women   343
16.7   Treatment of postpartum disorders   351

SECTION 4   Impact of violence, disasters, migration and work   **359**

Unaiza Niaz and Marianne Kastrup

17. Women and disasters   **369**

Unaiza Niaz

17.1   Wars and women's mental health   370
17.2   Natural disasters and women   377

18. Intimate partner violence interventions   **387**

Krishna Vaddiparti and Deepthi S. Varma

18.1 Mental health consequences of intimate partner violence on women   387
18.2 Victim focused interventions   388
18.3 Interventions with batterers of violence   391
18.4 Other intervention approaches   396
18.5 Conclusion   398

19. Migration and mental health in women: Mental health action plan as a tool to increase communication between clinicians and policy makers   **405**

Solvig Ekblad

19.1 Definitions: Mental health and health   405
19.2 Introduction   406
19.3 Risk factors   408
19.4 Resilience and coping   409
19.5 The impact of domestic violence on immigrant women's mental health   410
19.6 Access to mental healthcare services   411
19.7 The ADAPT model (Adaptation and Development after Persecution and Trauma)   412
19.8 The case of Mrs Aba, her family and the community   413
19.9 Theory of change logic: Mental health action planning   415

20. Work and women's mental health   **423**

Saida Douki

20.1 Introduction: A late but growing awareness   423
20.2 The job burnout   424
20.3 A higher risk for burnout   428
20.4 Work and women's mental health issues   434
20.5 Management issues   438
20.6 Conclusion   439

21. Globalisation and women's mental health: Cutting edge information   **443**

Unaiza Niaz

21.1 Concept and process of globalisation   443
21.2 Gendered effects of globalisation   444
21.3 The impact of globalisation and liberalisation on women's health   445
21.4 Education and empowerment in women   446
21.5 The United Nations' and World Bank's approach to women's education   447
21.6 The global and local intersection of feminism in muslim societies   448

21.7   Other impacts of globalisation   451
21.8   Internet addiction   455
21.9   Mental health issues related to the use of internet and mobile
       phones in the developing countries   456
21.10 Recommendations to counteract negative effects of globalisation   458

22.   The impact of culture on women's mental health   463

Marianne Kastrup and Unaiza Niaz

22.1   Introduction   463
22.2   Definitions   464
22.3   Epidemiological perspectives   466
22.4   Cultural aspects of stress   466
22.5   Diagnostic considerations   469
22.6   Cultural and social practices and their impact on mental health   473
22.7   Therapeutic issues   477
22.8   Perspectives   478

23.   Female mutilation   485

Amira Seif Eldin

23.1   Definition   485
23.2   Introduction   485
23.3   Historical background   486
23.4   Classification   487
23.5   Epidemiology of FGM   488
23.6   Physical complications of FGM   489
23.7   Psychological complications   490
23.8   Posttraumatic stress disorder and memory problems after FGM   491
23.9   Obstacles facing changing harmful social convention: Female
       genital mutilation/cutting   491
23.10 The basic concept for FGM elimination (The mental map for FGM)   494
23.11 Recommendations in countries where FGM is commonly practised   495

SECTION 5   Gender, social policy and implications for
             promoting women's mental health   499

Jane Fisher and Helen Herrman

24.   Women's mental health in the context of broad global
         policies   507

Takashi Izutsu

24.1   Introduction   507
24.2   Definitions of health and the right to health made by the United Nations   508

24.3   The Fourth World Conference on Women: Platform for Action (1995)   509
24.4   Conventions   510
24.5   Other international tools   512
24.6   New aid environment: Sector wide approaches and the poverty reduction
       strategy paper   513
24.7   Conclusion   514

25. **Families of origin as agents determining women's mental
     health**   **517**
     Wenhong Cheng
25.1   Introduction   517
25.2   The impact of the family of origin's perspectives about females on the
       growth of women   518
25.3   Impact of parenthood on women's mental health   519
25.4   Families, social change and women's mental health   521
25.5   Conclusion   522

26. **The unpaid workload: Gender discrimination in
     conceptualisation and its impact on maternal wellbeing**   **525**
     Jane Fisher
26.1   Introduction   525
26.2   Maternal desire   526
26.3   Disenfranchised grief and motherhood   526
26.4   Fantasies of motherhood   527
26.5   Fantasies about the workload   527
26.6   Workload of motherhood   528
26.7   Occupational fatigue as a determinant of maternal mood?   529
26.8   Recognition and valuing of work and occupational satisfaction   531
26.9   Training and education for mothering   532
26.10 Presumptions about the contributions of others to the workload   534
26.11 Collegial relationships   534
26.12 Honouring the work of motherhood in practice and policy   535
26.13 Conclusion   537

27. **Foundations of human development: Maternal care in the
     early years**   **539**
     Linda M. Richter and Tamsen Rochat
27.1   Child development and human culture   539
27.2   Interactions and relationships   541
27.3   Maternal mental health and children's development   542
27.4   Maternal care   543
27.5   Implications for mental healthcare   544

27.6   Increased choices for women   544

27.7   Conclusion   545

28.   The adverse impact of psychological aggression, coercion and violence in the intimate partner relationship on women's mental health   549

Toshiko Kamo

28.1   Introduction   549

28.2   Prevalence and nature of intimate partner violence   549

28.3   Impact of intimate partner violence on general health   551

28.4   Mental health problems among women affected by intimate partner violence   551

28.5   Intimate partner violence, children and intergenerational patterns of abuse   555

28.6   Conclusion   556

Index   559

Foreword

Women have more illness than men. Even in high income countries where women have longer life expectancy than men, they still suffer more from illness. This is especially true of mental illness, which, all too commonly the forgotten family member, is a major cause of suffering globally. Understanding mental illness in women, then, has great potential to improve population health and change clinical practice.

One approach to understanding mental illness in women is to examine biological causes, linked to endocrine control of the reproductive system, for example, or the activity of serotonin-specific neuronal systems. There are the obvious links between some mental illness and changes in reproductive function: the menstrual cycle, the postpartum period, and the peri-menopause. A quite different approach is to study the place of women in society and the role of social, economic, cultural and psychological causes of illness.

These two approaches should not be in opposition. It is highly relevant and important to understand the biological processes that underpin mental illness. Equally, not to focus on the social determinants of illness that arise from the way society is organised or, regrettably, disorganised is to fail to understand the causes of mental illness in the fullest sense.

Similarly, both cause of illness and its consequences are important. The wider society, the community and the family may all have a role to play in causing or exacerbating mental illness. In its turn, illness has a powerful effect on the functioning of family and community and affects the wider society.

Causative factors for illness rightly claim attention. Violence (whether social or interpersonal), poverty, disrupted family relations, discrimination and stigma, employment and working conditions, and early childhood influences may all be potent contributors to mental illness. It is important to remember there may be protective factors at work as well. Resilience of individuals, families and communities may all help protect from mental illness in the face of adversity.

Illness, then, is recognised, but what about treatment? Cognitive Behaviour Therapy has been emphasised as an alternative to pharmacotherapy; is this a luxury that only rich countries can afford? No, appears to be the answer from this book. It is quite possible to integrate treatment for mental illness with other treatment in resource-poor settings.

These were the perspectives taken by the WHO Commission on Social Determinants of Health. The Commission recognised the fundamental importance for health equity of mental illness: tackling its social causes as well as ensuring an appropriate response to illness when it occurs. I am therefore delighted to see this book with its depth of understanding and evidence. It has the potential to further the cause both of improving the status of women in society and responding to the major global burden of mental illness.

Sir Michael Marmot
Professor of Epidemiology and Public Health, UCL
Chair Commission on Social Determinants of Health

Preface

The World Psychiatric Association is instrumental in disseminating knowledge to mental health professionals in every part of the globe. The book is another contribution to this endeavour. It was inspired by the XIII World Congress of Psychiatry in Cairo 2006, chaired by Professor Ahmed Okasha. It brings knowledge in the field up to date and discusses psychiatric disorders among women in a manner that is relevant to clinical practice and considers cultural and social realities in perspective. The various sections acknowledge rapidly changing conditions, including better education and more working women in some countries, and the widespread effects of globalisation. The book also focuses on challenges such as migration, war and violence and their impact on the mental health of women. While we are conscious that women's mental health and psychiatric disorders cannot be divorced from social and cultural realities, the book also gives due attention to the current advances in neurobiology of psychiatric disorders among women.

Preparing the book was a journey undertaken by mental health researchers from several cultures and geographical zones working in unison for a common cause, which developed in discussion between publishers, section editors and the consumers. The chapter topics evolved as the book took shape, much like women's lives the world over, where creative solutions have to be found depending on where life leads.

The book is special in two respects. First, a deliberate attempt is made to ensure representation of prominent authors from several parts of the world. Second, topics that are important for women and adolescent girls in today's changing world are juxtaposed with discussion of the classic psychiatric syndromes in order to make the book relevant and contemporary for clinicians, researchers and policymakers in the field. The book has five sections, each featuring several chapters and concluding with a commentary from the section editors. The authors are prominent researchers in the field from 12 countries and all continents are represented.

The first section discusses important psychiatric disorders. The second focuses on reproductive health and its interface with women's mental health. The third section has chapters related to ethics and service delivery. The fourth section addresses culture, globalisation and social change, while the final section considers social policy and health promotion related to women's mental health.

Even though we cast our net wide in terms of topics, we acknowledge that there may be relevant areas that are not touched on or are dealt with insufficiently. Sometimes there is discussion of topics in more than one section and chapter: for example, violence as a risk factor for psychiatric problems and as an important consideration in interventions is raised by several authors. We retain these overlaps so that the chapters can be read independently and to note the various consequences for women's mental health and the range of responses required to a problem of this type.

We gratefully acknowledge the expert and dedicated work by the authors and the Wiley-Blackwell publishing and production teams. Thanks to Meghana S. Chandra for providing us with the illustrations and cover art. We also thank the lovely and brave women who share experiences of their mental health journey in Chapter 8 in Section 1. We hope that clinicians, researchers, students and policymakers in the field of women's mental health will enjoy reading and learning from this book as much as we enjoyed and learnt while bringing it together.

The Editors

List of Contributors

Sarvath Abbas
Leicestershire Eating Disorder
Service, Leicestershire Partnership
NHS Trust, Leicester, UK

Khadija Mchichi Alami
Ibn Rushd University Psychiatric
Centre, Casablanca, Morocco

Jill Astbury
School of Psychology, Victoria
University, Melbourne, Australia

Florence Baingana
Makerere University School of Public
Health, Kampala, Uganda

Corina Benjet
Instituto Nacional de Psiquiatrıa,
México DF, Mexico

Prabha S. Chandra
Department of Psychiatry, National
Institute of Mental Health and
Neurosciences, Bangalore, India

Santosh Kumar Chaturvedi
Department of Psychiatry, National
Institute of Mental Health and
Neurosciences, Bangalore, India

Wenhong Cheng
Department of Child and Adolescent
Psychiatry, Shanghai Mental Health
Centre, Medical School, Shanghai
Jiaotong University, Shanghai, China

Meena Cabral de Mello
Child and Adolescent Health and
Development, WHO, Geneva,
Switzerland

Geetha Desai
Department of Psychiatry, National
Institute of Mental Health and
Neurosciences, Bangalore, India

Saida Douki
Faculty of Medicine of Tunis, Razi
Hospital, Tunis, Tunisia

Solvig Ekblad
Stress Research Institute, Stockholm
University, and Karolinska Institutet,
Stockholm, Sweden

Amira Seif Eldin
Department of Community Medicine,
Faculty of Medicine, Alexandria
University, Alexandria, Egypt

Salim El-Sabbagh
Department of Psychiatry and Clinical
Psychology, Faculty of Medicine,
Balamand University, Beirut,
Lebanon

Jane Fisher
Key Centre for Women's Health in
Society, WHO Collaborating Centre in
Women's Health, University of
Melbourne, Melbourne, Australia

Gergö Hadlaczky
Karolinska Institutet, Stockholm,
Sweden

Helen Herrman
Orygen Youth Health Research
Centre, The University of Melbourne;
WHO Collaborating Centre in Mental
Health, Melbourne, Australia

Takashi Izutsu
United Nations Population Fund,
New York, USA

Enrique Jadresic
Sociedad de Neurologja, Psiquiatrja y
Neurociruga de Chile, Universidad de
Chile, Vitacura Santiago, Chile

Nadia Kadri
Ibn Rushd University Psychiatric
Centre, Casablanca, Morocco

Toshiko Kamo
Institute of Women's Health, Tokyo
Women's Medical University, Tokyo,
Japan

Elie G. Karam
Department of Psychiatry and Clinical
Psychology, St. Georges Hospital
University Medical Center, Beirut,
Lebanon

Marianne Kastrup
Transcultural Psychiatry, Psychiatric
Department, Rigshospitalet,
Copenhagen, Denmark

Unaiza Niaz
The Psychiatric Clinic & Stress
Research Centre, Karachi, Pakistan;
University of Health Sciences,
Lahore, Pakistan

Ahmed Okasha
WHO Collaborating Centre for
Training and Research in Mental
Health, Institute of Psychiatry, Ain
Shams University, Cairo, Egypt

Ramachandran Padmavati
Schizophrenia Research Foundation,
Chennai, India

Robert L. Palmer
Department of Health Sciences,
University of Leicester; Leicestershire
Eating Disorders Service,
Leicestershire Partnership NHS Trust,
Leicester, UK

Kristen Prentice
Maryland Psychiatric Research Centre,
University of Maryland School of
Medicine, Baltimore, USA

Shoba Raja
BasicNeeds, Bangalore, India

Ravi Philip Rajkumar
Department of Psychiatry, National
Institute of Mental Health and
Neurosciences, Bangalore, India

Linda M. Richter
Child, Youth, Family and Social
Development Programme, Human
Sciences Research Council, Durban,
South Africa

Laura Roberts
Department of Population Health,
Medical College of Wisconsin,
Milwaukee, USA

Tamsen Rochat
Child, Youth, Family and Social
Development Programme, Human
Sciences Research Council, Durban,
South Africa

Graciela Rojas
Departamento Psiquiatrja y Salud
Mental, Hospital Cljnico Universidad
de Chile, Santiago de Chile, Chile

Marta B. Rondón
Cayetano Heredia University, Lima,
Peru

Mariana M. Salamoun
Institute for Development Research
Advocacy and Applied Care (IDRAAC),
Beirut, Lebanon

Silvana Sarabia
Asociacion Psiquiatrica Peruana,
Lima, Peru

Veena A. Satyanarayana
Epidemiology and Prevention
Research Group, Department of
Psychiatry, Washington University
School of Medicine, St. Louis, USA

Rangaswamy Thara
Schizophrenia Research Foundation,
Chennai, India

Krishna Vaddiparti
Department of Psychiatric Social
Work, Institute of Human Behaviour
and Allied Sciences, Delhi, India

Deepthi S. Varma
Population Council, Golf Links, Delhi,
India

Danuta Wasserman
Karolinska Institutet, Stockholm,
Sweden

World Psychiatric Association Evidence and Experience in Psychiatry Series

Series Editor (2005 -) : Helen Herrman, WPA Secretary for Publications, University of Melbourne, Australia

The *Evidence & Experience in Psychiatry* series, launched in 1999, offers unique insights into both investigation and practice in mental health. Developed and commissioned by the World Psychiatric Association, the books address controversial issues in clinical psychiatry and integrate research evidence and clinical experience to provide a stimulating overview of the field.

Focused on common psychiatric disorders, each volume follows the same format: systematic review of the available research evidence followed by multiple commentaries written by clinicians of different orientations and from different countries. Each includes coverage of diagnosis, management, pharma and psycho- therapies, and social and economic issues. The series provides insights that will prove invaluable to psychiatrists, psychologists, mental health nurses and policy makers.

Depressive Disorders, 3e
Edited by Helen Herrman, Mario Maj and Norman Sartorius
ISBN: 9780470987209

Substance Abuse
Edited by Hamid Ghodse, Helen Herrman, Mario Maj and Norman Sartorius
ISBN: 9780470745106

Schizophrenia 2e
Edited by Mario Maj, Norman Sartorius
ISBN: 9780470849644

Dementia 2e
Edited by Mario Maj, Norman Sartorius
ISBN: 9780470849637

Obsessive-Compulsive Disorders 2e
Edited by Mario Maj, Norman Sartorius, Ahmed Okasha, Joseph Zohar
ISBN: 9780470849668

Bipolar Disorders
Edited by Mario Maj, Hagop S. Akiskal, Juan José López-Ibor, Norman Sartorius
ISBN: 9780471560371

Eating Disorders
Edited by Mario Maj, Kathrine Halmi, Juan José López-Ibor, Norman Sartorius
ISBN: 9780470848654

Phobias
Edited by Mario Maj, Hagop S. Akiskal, Juan José López-Ibor, Ahmed Okasha
ISBN: 9780470858332

Personality Disorders
Edited by Mario Maj, Hagop S. Akiskal, Juan E. Mezzich
ISBN: 9780470090367

Somatoform Disorders
Edited by Mario Maj, Hagop S. Akiskal, Juan E. Mezzich, Ahmed Okasha
ISBN: 9780470016121

Other World Psychiatric Association titles

WPA Secretary for Publications (2005 -) : Helen Herrman, University of Melbourne, Australia

Special Populations

The Mental Health of Children and Adolescents: an area of global neglect
Edited by Helmut Remschmidt, Barry Nurcombe, Myron L. Belfer, Norman Sartorius and Ahmed Okasha
ISBN: 9780470512456

Families and Mental Disorders
Edited by Norman Sartorius, Julian Leff, Juan José López-Ibor, Mario Maj, Ahmed Okasha
ISBN: 9780470023822

Disasters and Mental Health
Edited by Juan José López-Ibor, George Christodoulou, Mario Maj, Norman Sartorius, Ahmed Okasha
ISBN: 9780470021231

Approaches to Practice and Research

Psychiatric Diagnosis: challenges and prospects
Edited by Ihsan M. Salloum and Juan E. Mezzich
ISBN: 9780470725696

Recovery in Mental Health: reshaping scientific and clinical responsibilities
By Michaela Amering and Margit Schmolke
ISBN: 9780470997963

Handbook of Service User Involvement in Mental Health Research
Edited by Jan Wallcraft, Beate Schrank and Michaela Amering
ISBN: 9780470997956

Religion and Psychiatry: beyond boundaries
Edited by Peter J. Verhagen, Herman M. van Praag, Juan José López-Ibor, John Cox, Driss Moussaoui
ISBN: 9780470694718

Psychiatrists and Traditional Healers: unwitting partners in global mental health
Edited by Mario Incayawar, Ronald Wintrob and Lise Bouchard
ISBN: 9780470516836

Psychiatric Diagnosis and Classification
Edited by Mario Maj, Wolfgang Gaebel, Juan José López-Ibor, Norman Sartorius
ISBN: 9780471496816

Psychiatry in Society
Edited by Norman Sartorius, Wolfgang Gaebel, Juan José López-Ibor, Mario Maj
ISBN: 9780471496823

Psychiatry as a Neuroscience
Edited by Juan José López-Ibor, Mario Maj, Norman Sartorius
ISBN: 9780471496564

Early Detection and Management of Mental Disorders
Edited by Mario Maj, Juan José López-Ibor, Norman Sartorius, Mitsumoto Sato, Ahmed Okasha
ISBN: 9780470010839

Also available in electronic editions only, through Wiley Online Library:
WPA Anthology of Italian Language Psychiatric Texts
WPA Anthology of Spanish Language Psychiatric Texts
WPA Anthology of French Language Psychiatric Texts

SECTION 1

Current themes in psychiatric disorders in women

Ahmed Okasha[1] and Prabha S. Chandra[2]

[1]WHO Collaborating Center for Training and Research in Mental Health, Institute of Psychiatry, Ain Shams University, Cairo, Egypt
[2]Department of Psychiatry, National Institute of Mental Health and Neurosciences, Bangalore, India

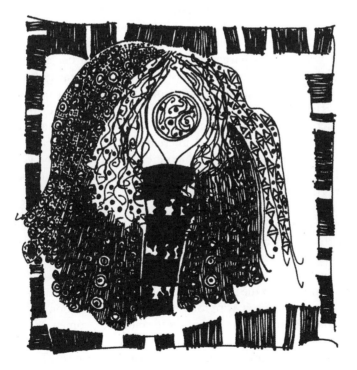

Contemporary Topics in Women's Mental Health   Edited by Chandra, Herrman, Fisher, Kastrup,
© 2009 John Wiley & Sons, Ltd   Niaz, Rondón and Okasha

Commentary

The section on psychiatric disorders among women is a tapestry of eight chapters woven together with threads of different hues and colours. The authors of each chapter in this section are authorities in their respective fields and have offered us a multidimensional pattern of different psychiatric disorders in the context of today's changing world for women across the world. The tapestry is complex, with many details and intricate design, much like the lives of women with psychiatric problems. The challenge for the authors has been to discuss each disorder in its social, cultural, biological dimensions, to look at links, to caution against overmedicalisation of emotional distress and finally to consider holistic treatment models.

In the context of today's fast changing world, viewing psychiatric illnesses needs a holistic worldview, a view that is de-centralised and which does not have a narrow perspective. The view is hence kaleidoscopic in that it is widened both physically and psychologically – where the disorder is viewed in a much larger context, and the multiple mirrors reflect images on each other. These images are those of the concepts of femininity and masculinity, of cultural and social realities, of violence and safety, of social networks and isolation and of motherhood and the nurturing roles of women. A kaleidoscopic view logically reflects the many multi-faceted identities, which women have today and which keep changing based on the interplay of lights and mirrors in the form of roles, relationships, the impact of biology and finally, the state of society.

The last two decades have seen major changes, particularly for women. The changes have been in role, relationships, ecosystems, safety, education and biological advances. In addition, information and technology has made life easier in some ways but challenging in others. Two of the major changes for humankind and one which has particularly influenced women in this decade are globalisation and the impact of wars and terror in different parts of the world.

In the contemporary world, psychiatric disorders have to be viewed in the context of all these changes rather than a narrow medical microscope which seldom gives the larger picture.

In this commentary, we will try to highlight at least one key message from each chapter, try to follow different threads in the tapestry to see where they link with each other, look at caveats in knowledge and research and identify a few future goals.

A unifying theme in several chapters, particularly the ones on somatisation and dissociation and that on the psychiatric aspects of trauma, is the complex nature of trauma related psychiatric symptoms in women. Somatisation and dissociation are among the most important responses to trauma in women. Multiple factors that may be individual, social or biological play a role in shaping the nature and severity of individual symptoms in response to a given stressor. The chronic and disabling nature of somatisation and the dramatic impact of dissociation, poses a significant burden to affected women, leading to impaired quality of life, high social and occupational disability and increased healthcare utilisation and costs.

The authors of these chapters emphasise that the symptoms of somatisation and dissociation may reflect a cry for help, a failure of existing coping mechanisms and a need for support and understanding from family, friends and professionals. These need to be understood and addressed recognising the unique cultural framework of each woman.

However, in keeping with the current research, the authors have tried to also focus on biological underpinnings of both somatisation and dissociation. They have described complex integrative models that attempt to explain the genesis of somatoform symptoms, conversion and dissociation which include the central effects of inflammatory and immune mediators and the role of female sex hormones as stress-immune system interactions.

The authors also focus on two important issues in the understanding of these disorders using different philosophies of medicine. Firstly, is the difficulty in entirely conceptualising dissociation in women using the Descartian mind–body dualistic approach. Secondly, they emphasise how traditional systems of medicine may offer interesting perspectives and solutions. In Eastern medical systems such as Ayurveda, all suffering is considered as a whole and the same holds good in most of traditional medicine where a sharp distinction between the 'mental' and the 'physical' does not occur. The authors have very wisely discussed that women from many non western cultures may hence not distinguish between the emotions of anxiety, irritability and depression because they tend to express distress in somatic terms or they may organise their concepts of dysphoria in ways different from western ones. The cultural basis of somatisation can change the hues of presentation including the frequency, form and content of somatic or dissociative symptoms, or by having specific effects on women that place them at risk for somatisation or dissociation [1].

Another important point in several of the chapters in this section is the intricate relationship between trauma, violence and most psychiatric disorders in women. In a society where women's experience of emotional and physical violence is common place, and discussing emotions related to it may have lost its meaning because of social acceptance of the subordinate role of women; somatisation and dissociation may reflect a 'cry for help' and a way of communication to the healthcare professionals that all is not well.

One of the criticisms in recent psychiatric literature is the lack of gender specific issues in therapy. Most therapy unfortunately is still gender neutral, despite acknowledging the complexities of women's lives in different parts of the world and in changing societies. The authors in the chapter on somatisation and dissociation have attempted to give some comprehensive guidelines about a biopsychosocial approach to complaints, in which the treating doctor examines the relative contributions of biological, individual psychological and social variables, and a stress-diathesis model are useful both in assessing patients and in communicating the diagnosis. Specific points that can be stressed initially include reversibility, emphasis on positive aspects, encouraging self-help and establishing an alliance with family members and other caregivers.

Halliburton [2] found that, in India, spirit possession was being replaced by complaints of 'psychological tension', perhaps reflecting changing explanatory models and mental health-related beliefs. It is important to understand these cultural variations, and the meanings attached to them by the patient and their community, in order to treat dissociation in such settings.

Kadri and Alami focus on the epidemiology of anxiety and depressive disorders in women and discuss the possible reasons for the major sex differences. Some important issues in the understanding of women and anxiety disorders have stemmed from the finding that women have a higher prevalence of anxiety disorders compared to men and the manner in which these disorders manifest may also be different. Several social and cultural issues appear to be important in the manifestation and consequences of conditions like agoraphobia, including specific socially defined roles in anxiety disorders among women. These roles, specially in some societies where women lack independence may account not only for the higher prevalence of agoraphobia but may also account for higher practised agoraphobia and the socioeconomic position and absence of women from the labour market [3, 4]. Several authors have since made a case for gender sensitive epidemiological research that takes into account several important variables while discussing incidence, prevalence and co morbidity of psychiatric disorders [5].

In addition, pre existing anxiety disorders may contribute to the higher prevalence of depressive disorders in women as pre existing anxiety appears to be a predictor of future depression and dysthymia [3, 5]. Some of the unanswered questions about anxiety disorders relate to their manifestation and recognition in cultures where women should not be heard, do not have too many independent roles and should not go out. Do anxiety disorders in these situations manifest differently? Does increasing employment among women lead to a decrease in phobic disorders? The concept of Gender Role Stress (GRS) that makes certain roles stressful for men and women (being in control and always being strong in men) as opposed to the need for women to be nurturing, relational, have socially appropriate body image and be dependent, needs more examination [6]. There is also a need to understand anxiety disorders using the masculinity/femininity dimensions of either gender.

The chapter also examines the role of biology and socio cultural factors in anxiety and depressive disorders in women including the important role of repro-ductive biology. They specifically discuss research in the context of Arab women and the societal issues that might contribute to mood and anxiety disorders such as forced marriages, polygamy, work related roles and female circumcision.

The authors mention that aetiological research, while important, should not overshadow gender focused treatment research, which is unfortunately still lacking despite major strides in treatment. A finding of some concern in anxiety research is the repeated finding of higher benzodiazepine prescriptions for women compared to men. More meta analysis of treatment studies using a sex and gender approach is needed. An important area of future study is the therapist characteristics and gender match that influence treatment for women with mood and anxiety disorders.

Traumatic experiences are almost considered universal in most women's lives and have featured in almost all chapters in this section. However, Karam and colleagues have discussed the issue in depth and have raised some important points for future research. The gendered experience of trauma including partner violence and sexual abuse has been widely recognised. However, the authors emphasise that most of the research in this area is from the western world and research from other cultures is minimal. Raising an interesting point, the authors mention how social taboos related to discussing intimate partner violence or sexual trauma may have resulted in this lack of data and research and stress the need for more research in this field from non western countries.

The chapter also focuses on how women are exposed to different forms of trauma compared to men. While men are exposed more to accidents, war and collective violence, women are exposed to more intimate forms of trauma such as those mentioned above. While men can report and discuss their traumatic experiences, women by virtue of the intimate and stigmatised nature of their traumatic experiences, are precluded from the process of disclosure. This has important implications for the higher prevalence of psychiatric disorders in relation to trauma among women compared to men. The authors also emphasise how in situations like war or disasters, women are exposed to trauma related to the war itself, such as loss of property and bereavement and in addition have to deal with trauma related to rape, abuse and childbirth, thus compounding the experience of trauma in these stressful situations.

The authors have also focused on women's responses to trauma and report the higher prevalence of posttraumatic stress disorder PTSD in women compared to men even if exposed to similar types of trauma. In addition, some symptoms of PTSD, specifically the anxiety and arousal symptoms are much higher in women than in men. In order to explain these gender variations, the authors have then discussed the biological aspects of trauma in women including relationship of glucocorticoid responses to peri-traumatic dissociation and the role of the hippocampus in mediating.

While biology offers some solutions to the riddle of higher PTSD and typical PTSD symptoms in women, temperament may also have a role to play both in the response to trauma and in its avoidance. The authors emphasise how a better understanding of the relationship between biology, temperament and availability of support during trauma may mediate the impact of trauma. This relationship needs to be studied in more detail in order to plan interventions for prevention in the aftermath of wars or disasters.

Finally, the authors have described how several psychiatric disorders in addition to PTSD including: depression, anxiety and substance use disorders may contribute to high levels of co morbidity in women exposed to trauma.

In the current state of the world where violence has become an increasing part of women's lives, be it interpersonal or collective, the authors stress the need for future research to address more interventions and study factors that contribute to vulnerability and protective factors.

Abbas and Palmer in their chapter on eating disorders have taken a no nonsense, practical and clinical approach which is useful to clinicians dealing with the condition. While dwelling at length on the reasons for the worldwide differences in rates of eating disorders, they discuss the relative role of socio cultural attitudes related to weight and eating with more individual factors such as self esteem and control that determine the path of an eating disordered adolescent. In a world that is preoccupied with issues related to obesity, eating disorders appear a paradoxical reaction to the public health messages stressing the problems of being overweight and the authors discuss this as a possible area of study. The authors mention that with globalisation, migration and change in lifestyles, eating disorders will probably emerge in many societies across the world and better reporting and research in non western cultures is required.

They also emphasise the nosological problems in eating disorders in the current classificatory systems, specially the AN/BN association and also make a case for giving the otherwise neglected category of eating disorder not otherwise specified (EDNOS), its right due both for diagnosis and research.

Finally, they discuss treatment models that show some promise, while acknowledging the role of mental health professionals in enhancing the sense of agency and responsibility among patients with eating disorders for any treatment to be successful. In countries where eating disorders are becoming an emerging problem, the lessons from this chapter on assessment and treatment including continuity of care issues are very relevant. Eating disorders can be disabling and frustrating experiences for the patient and the clinician and the authors give a few pointers on how to overcome them.

The chapter on suicide and self harm raises certain important issues related to self harm in women. Two important facets of understanding suicide rates between countries and between sexes have been discussed, which include the concepts of *ecological fallacy* and the *gender paradox*. Hadlaczky and Wasserman discuss the possible reasons for the marked gender differences in suicide rates, within and between countries and emphasise why this knowledge is important for prevention measures. Suicide intent appears to be equally strong in both sexes, however, the methods of suicide employed and substance use may explain the gender differences in completed suicide rates across the world, with a few exceptions. The authors also warn against generalising the gender related demographics of suicide to all societies and countries, especially in the context of countries in transition and those undergoing rapid urbanisation. Finally, they describe how suicide prevention programmes can address women specific issues including social isolation, help seeking patterns and the role of culture and reproductive events in suicide.

Women with severe mental illness (SMI) form one of the most vulnerable and weakest sections of society, the world over. The chapter on women with psychosis and bipolar illness discusses key gender differences in the clinical manifestations of SMI. Some important themes that emerge from this chapter include those related to problems that women with SMI face in marriage and parenting, especially in cultures where women's identities depend on their marital status.

An emerging research and service issue is the need for special services for rehabilitation among women. With advances in psychopharmacology, more and more women are getting better and becoming functional. However, their reintegration into society is far from easy, owing to the fact that most rehabilitation programmes do not emphasise issues such as parenting or socialisation – areas that women's roles require for them to gain acceptance. With new understanding about social cognition deficits in schizophrenia, it becomes important to address these issues as women are known to use more social networking and support and women with psychosis may have a disadvantage related to this.

Another area of research is related to the impact of psychopharmacology on women's health. It is now known that women are more vulnerable to side effects of psychotropic drugs than men and there are enormous implications related to fertility, reproduction, diabetes, cardiac effects and bone health [7]. However, a lot more needs to be studied in this area and more importantly, the knowledge needs to be incorporated into routine clinical guidelines.

Baingana has given a comprehensive description of the epidemiology and social issues among women with substance use. In many cultures, this is a hidden population. Conventionally, substance use is more among men and services cater predominantly to the male population. However, as the author illustrates, based on global data, not only is substance abuse in women, a significant problem in several parts of the world, the health and social implications are often enormous. HIV, sexual risk and violence are intertwined in a complex manner with substance use and have clearly emerged the world over as important areas for intervention.

Finally, the most important chapter in this section, or maybe even in the whole book, are the voices of consumers. A compilation of women's narratives from four different countries indicate the commonalities of stigma, myth and dogma that women with mental illness experience. Often, neglected and abandoned, these women, then have to strive 100 times harder than everyone else, to regain their foothold in society. Four women, describe their tryst with mental illness and their paths to recovery. The narratives have several lessons for health professionals, including the need to understand the lived experience for women with psychiatric disorders, to acknowledge the role of alternative medicines and different pathways to care in several cultures, to include the family in the recovery process as a valuable resource and finally, to develop services that handle the unique problems that women with mental illness face. Placed at the end of this section, mental health professionals, the world over, can learn a lot by reading this chapter.

Conclusions

Theodore Roszak [8] in his book, *The Gendered Atom* writes – 'The myths of gender work at so deep a level in us that it would take more than extraordinary personal awareness to bring them into the light of day. Will the sciences, still among the most gender biased institutions in our society, be courageous enough to restore the woman in us to her rightful place?'

As we enter an era where science is making new strides, with new drugs and advances in pharmacogenomics, psychosocial interventions and models of services should develop in parallel with equal speed and fervour. Unfortunately, this does not appear to be the case and there are major gaps between what we know and what we deliver to our patients, obviously linked to economics, lack of personnel and a dearth of research in the area of women specific interventions.

The next era of gender specific psychiatric research has to be faster and accommodate the rapid changes that are happening in society and biology. There are some examples of women themselves as consumers being participants in research in areas that are important to them. More research bodies need to bring consumers and scientists together and prioritise clinical and interventional research. Several models need to be developed simultaneously in different parts of the world, for different problems that have been highlighted in this section. There is a lot to be learned from cost effective models being evolved in the developing world, which are not very money intensive and are focused and useful in this era of uncertainty and change.

References

1. Kirmayer, L.J. and Young, A. (1998) Culture and somatization: clinical, epidemiological, and ethnographic perspectives. *Psychosomatic Medicine*, **60**, 420–30.
2. Halliburton, M. (2005) "Just some spirits": the erosion of spirit possession and the rise of "tension" in South India. *Medical Anthropology*, **24** (2), 111–44.
3. Pigott, T.A. (2003) Anxiety disorders in women. *Psychiatric Clinics of North America*, **26**, 621–72.
4. Bekker, M.H.J. and Mens-Verhulst, J. van (2007). Anxiety disorders: Sex differences in prevalence, degree, and background, but gender-neutral treatment. *Gender Medicine*, **4** (B), 178–93.
5. Moerman, C.J. and van Mens-Verhulst, J. (2004) Gender-sensitive epidemiological research: Suggestions for a gender-sensitive approach towards problem definition, data collection and analysis in epidemiological research. *Psychology Health Medicine*, **9**, 41–52.
6. Gillespie, B.L. and Eisler, R.M. (1992) Development of the feminine gender role stress scale: a cognitive/behavioral measure of stress, appraisal and coping for women. *Behaviour Modification*, **16**, 426–38.
7. Aichhorn, W., Whitworth, A.B., Weiss, E.M. and Marksteiner, J. (2006) Second-generation antipsychotics: is there evidence for sex differences in pharmacokinetic and adverse effect profiles? *Drug Safety*, **29** (7), 587–98.
8. Roszak, T. (1999) *The Gendered Atom-Reflections on the Sexual Psychology of Science*, Conary Press, Berkley, pp. 154–55.

1
Psychotic disorders and bipolar affective disorder

Rangaswamy Thara and Ramachandran Padmavati

Schizophrenia Research Foundation, Chennai, India

1.1 Psychotic disorders in women

If mental health is low in the priority of policy and programmes in many countries, women's mental health issues have been a subject of neglect and indifference for a long time. In women, severe mental illness, even if low in prevalence assumes importance largely on account of the social ramifications and human distress. Feminists often opine that they have not been involved in the complex process of understanding and dealing with the issues around women's mental health [1].

The 1998 World Health report states that 'Women's mental health is inextricably linked to their status in society'. It benefits from equality and suffers from discrimination [2]. Many women with severe mental illness stay outside treatment settings, especially in low income countries with poor and inadequate mental health facilities. Those who do enter treatment settings have varied experiences ranging from humane care to indifference and stigmatisation. This chapter outlines the clinical features of women with schizophrenia and bipolar disorder, BPD, but chooses to place greater emphasis on interpersonal and social ramifications of these disorders and the impact on their lives as a whole.

Contemporary Topics in Women's Mental Health   Edited by Chandra, Herrman, Fisher, Kastrup,
© 2009 John Wiley & Sons, Ltd   Niaz, Rondón and Okasha

1.2 Schizophrenia

Epidemiological indices

Incidence

Incidence of schizophrenia seems to be fairly stable in both genders across reported studies. The diagnostic definitions (broad vs restrictive) used have however determined differences as in the case of the Determinants of Outcome of Severe Mental Disorders DOSMED study [3].

The review of 55 core incidence studies by McGrath *et al.* [4], reported higher incidence rates in males; the male-female rate ratio median was 1.4 (0.9−2.4). Nine studies, which reported higher rates in women were examined in detail, but showed no features distinguishable from the other studies.

The Madras study on a population of 100 000 did not show any gender differences [5]. However, Dube and Kumar [6] in Agra reported a greater incidence in males (1.5 : 1). In the Chandigrah study, the incidence rates of broadly defined schizophrenia were the highest among rural women (0.47/1000) and lowest in urban males (0.37/1000).

Prevalence

Rates for genders have varied greatly across studies, and variations in methodology, sample sizes prevent any definitive conclusions to be drawn. A review of prevalence studies in schizophrenia by Saha *et al.* [7] did not find any striking sex differences.

Mortality

Morbidity risk for schizophrenia over the lifespans seems to be around 1% in both genders. In the 25-year follow-up of the Madras Longitudinal Study of 90 first episode schizophrenia patients, 25 patients have died, of whom males were 15. More males have had physical illnesses, while more women have committed suicide (unpublished data). The suicides in women were largely in response to symptoms as in the case of one woman who had the delusion that she appeared nude to others and resultant social embarrassment. Higher suicide risk in women with schizophrenia was also reported by Mortenesen and Juel [8].

A recent study in rural China by Ran *et al.* [9] found much more mortality and suicide in men than in women and ascribed the higher prevalence found in women to this.

A systematic review of mortality in schizophrenia revealed no sex differences [4]. Augier *et al.* [10] however, report more suicides in young males with schizophrenia.

Course and outcome

Women have a better outcome than men. It is unclear whether this is due to later age of onset, protective nature of hormones such as oestrogens or better drug response.

The Australian Study of Low Prevalence (Psychotic) Disorders looked at gender differences among 1090 cases of psychosis (schizophrenia, schizoaffective disorder, affective psychoses and other psychoses). Results within diagnostic groupings confirmed differences in how men and women experience and express their illness. Within each diagnostic group, women reported better premorbid functioning, a more benign illness course, lower levels of disability and better integration into the community than men. They were also less likely to have a chronic course of illness. There were no significant differences in age at onset. Differences between women across the diagnostic groups were more pronounced than differences between women and men within a diagnostic group. In particular, women with schizophrenia were severely disabled compared to women with other diagnoses [11].

The Madras Longitudinal study found better outcome in women after five years of follow-up, but this did not sustain through the rest of the 15 years of follow-up [12]. It is likely that several mechanisms are needed to explain the differences. Greater social integration and functioning in women across diagnostic groups may well reflect culturally and socially determined gender differences. In contrast, variability and attenuated findings with respect to symptom profiles beg the question of biological mechanisms with some degree of specificity [11, 13].

Psychopathology

It has been documented that women with schizophrenia tend to be more overtly hostile, physically active and dominating, have more sexual delusions and are more emotional than men.

A large sample of Chinese patients with schizophrenia had more paranoid subtype of schizophrenia in females. They also showed a different pattern of ongoing symptoms and severity with more severe positive and affective symptoms, and a greater number of suicide attempts whereas male patients were more likely to show severe deterioration over time [14].

Muller [15] studied gender specific differences in association of depression in persons with schizophrenia. In females, depression was independently associated with higher negative symptom scores ($P < 0.01$) and younger age ($P < 0.05$) whereas in males positive symptoms ($P < 0.05$) and short hospitalisation ($P < 0.05$) were the main factors associated with depression.

Age at onset

A higher mean age at onset of schizophrenia for women has been one of the very consistent findings in the last 20 years. Several independent reviews of many studies have shown that the disorder appeared later in women. Since the time between onset of symptoms and first hospitalisation were the same in both genders, it was evident that women did have a later onset. There have been however a few reports which have not replicated this finding. Some studies from India have not found a gender difference in the age of onset and have questioned the universality of the traditional view of earlier onset in men [16]. The Madras longitudinal study of almost equal numbers of men and women in a sample of 90 cases also did not find a gender difference in onset [12].

Alcohol and drug abuse

Women with chronic mental illness tend to use alcohol and drugs of addiction, especially if they have become victims of sexual abuse. This however may not be the case in some developing countries where almost all women live with families who keep a close watch on them. Besides, these women also do not have the financial independence to acquire these substances. Many studies from the developing world have reported very low rates of drug abuse in women with schizophrenia.

Response to treatment

There is an expanding literature on gender differences in psychopharmacology. It has long been observed that men and women seem to require different dosages of anti-psychotics and have different responses to them. The SOHO (Schizophrenia Outpatient Health Outcomes) study was a three-year, prospective, observational study of health outcomes associated with antipsychotic treatment in 10 European countries that included over 10 000 outpatients initiating or changing their antipsychotic medication in 4529 men (56.68%) and 3461 women (43.32%). Findings showed that gender was a significant predictor for response based on the Clinical Global Impression (CGI) scale and for improvement in quality of life. The highest gender differences were found in typical antipsychotics and clozapine. Olanzapine only showed differences in quality of life, and no differences were found for Risperidone [11].

In the Chinese study of Tang *et al.* [17], males received higher daily doses of antipsychotics and demonstrated a different pattern of antipsychotic usage, being less likely to be treated with second-generation antipsychotics. The clozapine blood level was 35% higher in women than in men.

In general, premenopausal women seem to require lower doses. The role of oestrogens in neuromodulation seems to account for this difference. It has to be kept in mind that the bulk of patients taking part in drug trials are men and much of the knowledge about dosing is therefore more applicable to men.

Side effects of medication

Neuroendocrine effects of antipsychotics, especially those secondary to hyper-prolactinaemia can cause a lot of distress to women patients. This is true with all First Generation Antipsychotics and to an extent risperidone and ziprasidone. Clozapine, olanzapine and quetiapine seem to spare prolactin. Amenorrhoea, galactorrhoea, decreased sexual interest and functioning and changes in bone density are the side effects of increased prolactin levels.

Obesity also seems to be more common among women and has its own psychological and medical effects.

Marriage and schizophrenia

While international research has largely dealt with marital rates in schizophrenia the outcome of the marriage itself has received sparse attention. Kreitman [18], Eaton [19], Odegaard [20], Saugstad [21] and Hafner [22] have all examined the relationship between marriage and schizophrenia and most of them have reported low marital rates. The issue of marital status vis àvis outcome of schizophrenia has been examined by few [23–26].

In countries like India, marriage is not just an indicator of social functioning, but is almost a mandatory event in life. Separation and divorce are still stigmatised and even unheard of in rural areas. In this context, we interviewed 75 women with schizophrenia/BPD who were separated/divorced. While 40 women (53%) had been rejected/abandoned by their spouses without going through any formal divorce/separation proceedings, only 16 had been legally divorced, 5 had their marriages annulled by local rural governing bodies (Panchayat), 7 had their cases pending in court. Three (4%) had been granted *talaq* by the Muslim court and four had not been granted divorce by the courts.

Only four of the women received any kind of financial support from their husbands. Thirty-three husbands (44%) had remarried after separation from the ill woman [27, 28]. The women experienced a gamut of emotions starting with denial and shock to deep depression and suicidal thoughts and attempts. Many of them retained their symbol of marriage since being separated was more stigmatising than being mentally ill. When asked about future plans, the characteristic reply was '. . . there is no future for me, so what's the point of thinking about it, this will only lead to more worries, I have enough as it is'.

Concerns of being a burden to their aged parents were widely expressed and many wanted to work to support themselves. Hostile criticisms from parents and siblings that openly ridiculed their uselessness further reinforced their sense of being a burden to their families and were also particularly painful to them. But faced with few options, they felt they had little choice but to carry on with their lives and leave it all to God and fate.

In contrast many of the women had extremely supportive and overly protective families on whom the patient was deeply dependent. These women were quite content to live under the protective umbrella of their parental homes. While some of them did express concerns about what was to become of them after the death of their loving parents, it was obvious that this was only a fleeting thought and not one which they liked to dwell on much. Avoiding, escaping and shifting the onus of care onto someone else seemed to be markedly present among these women.

This study brought into focus some issues that confront women with chronic mental illness in many developing countries. They are:

1. A lack of awareness of the illness and its disabilities resulting in a widespread belief that marriage is a panacea for all ills. This results in their families arranging their marriages, very often suppressing the fact of mental illness to the husband and his family.

2. Absence of legal protection including maintenance for such women.

3. Once they have a relapse after marriage, they are sent back to the parental home and the responsibility of caring for them falls on the ageing parents.

4. Lack of welfare programmes to offer physical, sexual and financial security for these women.

However, we see this as a priority area of intervention by governments, which should have some national policies and programmes to take of such women whose families are unable to continue caring for them. If not provided with a suitable shelter, these women can land on the streets and become prey to sexual abuse and other high-risk activities.

Homelessness

Homelessness is probably the most visible of all the social sequelae of psychotic disorders in women. It has been estimated that 20–40% of homeless women suffer from psychotic disorders. In many developing countries, family support notwithstanding, the numbers of mentally ill women who become homeless seems to be on the increase. This may well be due to breaking up of joint and extended families, and better transport facilities resulting in such women migrating from one part of the country to the other. In many countries, services for such women are either absent or totally fragmented and inadequate. Homeless mentally ill women have more pregnancy and childbirth related complications.

Though males who are ill are at grater risk of becoming homeless, homeless women seem to be sicker than their male counterparts [29], Goering *et al.* [30] spoke of demoralisation of the female homeless who wanted their rights respected and autonomy maintained.

A comparative study found substance abuse to be less in homeless women than in men. Symptom severity in homeless individuals with schizophrenia appears as an interaction of symptom profiles and risk behaviours that are gender specific [31].

There has been a dearth of systematic research in homelessness, especially in developing countries. As pointed out by Dinesh Bhugra in his book [32], the impact of risk factors such as poverty and poor environmental conditions and their association with ill health needs to be studied in various socio-cultural settings. In large countries like India, where the homeless travel long distances across the length and breadth of the country, the challenge is relocating them in their families. While some families are keen to receive them, others tend to be distinctly hostile or indifferent to them when they are sent back. Planning of care facilities for this group of persons with severe mental illness is hardly a priority in many countries.

Burden and stigma

Stigma faced by patients and families has also evinced a lot of international research interest and efforts are underway to plan major stigma reduction pro-grammes. The WHO's Dare to Care campaign and the WPA's global anti-stigma programmes are foremost among these. Knowledge of mental illness in the relative, the need to seek psychiatric treatment, which is still not looked upon very favourably in many traditional societies, the need for social restraints on account of behaviour problems and above all issues of employment and marriage contribute to the experience of stigma in families. Thara and Srinivasan [33] found that many caregivers felt depression and sorrow, which was more profound if the patient was a woman. Women caregivers reported more stigma than male carers. These feelings probably become even more severe when they have to deal with their daughters with uncertain futures and broken marriages and lack of social support.

Another Indian study [34] observed similar levels of burden among caregivers of patients of schizophrenia and BPD. They used similar types of coping methods to deal with it. Awad and Voruganti [35] in an article on burden of schizophrenia opine that 'there are no reliable estimates of the costs associated with care of persons with schizophrenia'. As there is a lack of reliable cost information about the family burden of care specific to schizophrenia, there is an urgent need to develop reliable approaches that can generate data that can inform in policy making and organisation of services.

Disabilities in women

The 1992 National Health Interview Survey NHIS data from the USA is a comprehensive published data set that contains domains of disabilities associ-ated with health conditions. The survey assessed three domains of disabilities: limitations in activities, work and self-care. A minimally greater proportion of women were more disabled than men in all three domains. However women who were mentally disabled were younger than their physically disabled counterparts. This was especially notable in limitations in personal care. It was pointed out by the authors that policy makers need to be aware of the special needs of service development and configuration for women disabled by mental disorders. Appropriate coverage for the care of disorders and disabilities would result in better short term and long term outcomes [36].

In the Madras Study, there were no differences in disabilities between genders at five-year follow-up. However, work in the case of men and daily activities in the case of women seemed critical to address and intervene [25].

Psychosocial rehabilitation in women

It has been observed that Psychosocial Rehabilitation programmes by and large have not paid much attention to the special needs of women. Carol Mowbray [37] points out that only 3% of the 127 articles published in the Psychiatric Rehabilitation Journal from 1999 to 2001, focused on women. For women, relationship and basic survival skills take precedence over substance abuse related skills. In many countries in Asia where women live in joint and extended families, there is a constant need to adjust to various emotions, critical comments and expectations of the family members. Married women in the west are often exposed to Psycosocial Rehabilition, PSR programmes with specific focus on motherhood and care of children. While the focus of PSR in the west is on independent living, it is on managing dependent relationships in large families in many Asian countries. Marriage and motherhood are also issues that need to be addressed during rehab.

Ageing women with schizophrenia

Like everybody, women with schizophrenia also age. And like the age, some of their problems can also increase. The gender differences seen in the younger years seem to plateau off as the age increases. Problems of ageing such as cognitive decline and chronic medical conditions may be exacerbated by schizophrenia and the disorder is associated with premature mortality. Older women with schizophrenia are at risk for neglect of psychiatric and other health needs that are further compounded by limited social support and low socioeconomic status.

In countries like India where families are the primary caregivers, older women, especially those widowed, meet with varying reactions from the younger members. As long as they are physically active and able to contribute to the household chores, they are quite welcome. However, a physical illness or relapse of schizophrenia upsets the balance and many women feel ignored and rejected. In the absence of any alternative boarding and care facilities, the families look upon them as a 'burden'.

1.3 Bipolar disorder

Introduction

Bipolar affective disorders are currently classified as illnesses separate from clinical depression. The spectrum of psychopathology under the rubric of 'bipolar disorder' is wide and includes bipolar I, bipolar II and mixed states, which is an admixture of both poles of the illness.

Epidemiology

The lifetime prevalence of bipolar disorders has been reported as 0.5–1.6% [38]. The differences in lifetime prevalence and current (12-month rates) are smaller than in major depression. In contrast to major depression, there are relatively few gender differences in bipolar disorder, a finding supported by large population studies across several countries and cultures, including studies in Asian countries like Hong Kong [39] or Taiwan [40]. There is preliminary evidence to suggest that women may be more likely to be diagnosed as bipolar disorder type II. In a chart review of 131 patients attending a Mood Disorder Clinic in Los Angeles, Hendrick *et al.* [41] found 48% of their clinic population to be women and 60% of the women were diagnosed as BPD II. Contrary to this, similar rates of BPD II in men and women was reported by Szadoczky *et al.* [42] in a Hungarian Epidemiological study.

Age of onset

There has been some suggestion that the onset of illness is later in women with BPD than men [43]. Several other studies have not demonstrated any difference in the age of onset between men and women [41, 44–47]. The findings need to be viewed cautiously, since they did not provide age at the time of first mania or first depression. Hendrick's study, which provided the data, did not show the effect of sex on age of onset. Taylor and Abrams subdivided patients into early and late onset based on a cutoff age of 30. Females accounted for 35% in early onset group versus 22% in late onset, a non-significant finding. More male patients were identified in case records of adolescents with a diagnosis of bipolar disorder over six years in India, indicating that males had an earlier age of onset in this group [48].

Pattern of course and outcome

Several longitudinal studies have shown that bipolar disorders are characterised by frequent recurrences. Only a few longitudinal evaluations have explored the course of illness in developing countries [40, 49–53]. Few have commented on gender differences. In the studies which have compared the course of illness in men and women [41, 45, 54] differences in the number of hospitalisations and the episodes of mental illness have been inconsistent. These results may be either due to different methodologies used or, it is more likely that sex probably does not impact the course of bipolar illnesses.

Mixed mania

The effect of gender on mixed mania is inconsistent through literature. There is some evidence that women with BPD may be more likely than men to experience mixed episodes. This finding is however not consistent across studies. Definitional and methodological limitations hinder comparisons. Arnold *et al.* [55] in a review of gender effects in mixed mania, suggested that as the definition of mixed mania involves an increasing number of depressive symptoms, the ratio of women to men increases This finding was supported by Akiskal [56]. In a comprehensive review of 17 mixed studies by McElroy *et al.* [57] female patients accounted for 58–90% of subjects with mixed mania in five studies. One study found that male patients accounted for 59% of the subjects with dysphoric mania. The remaining 11 studies did not report the sex of the subjects. Rob *et al.* [54] identified a trend towards females experiencing more mixed episodes in the previous one year.

Rapid cycling

Women are more likely than men to experience a rapid cycling phase in their bipolar illness. This finding has been consistent across several studies. Pooled data from 10 studies showed that women on an average accounted for 71.7% of the cases of rapid cycling, defined as at least four distinct mood episodes in a 12-month period [58]. Similar findings were reported by Wherr *et al.* [59] and Robb *et al.* [54]. In addition to finding more rapid cycling amongst women, Schneck *et al.* [60] also reported that rapid cyclers had a greater severity of illness than those without rapid cycling. Several explanations have been put forth to explain the effects of sex on rapid cycling. These have included higher rates of hypothyroidism in women, more frequent use of antidepressants and the effects of menstrual cycle on mood changes [43]. All these factors however remain speculative [61]. Hormonal fluctuations do not seem to influence rapid cycling in women. The possibility of greater use of antidepressants to explain the higher rates of rapid cycling in women remains untested.

Suicide

People with bipolar disorder are at great risk for suicide if they are not treated. The National Mental Health Association reports that 30–70% of suicide victims have suffered from a form of depression. Women had a significantly higher rate of suicidal attempt, but men a higher risk of suicide death [62]. The data from a study in an Italian tertiary care centre suggests that females were more likely to report a history of suicidal gestures and a comorbid panic disorder; males were more likely to present with a comorbid obsessive-compulsive disorder, and there was a trend for a more frequent history of alcohol or substance abuse [63].

Phenomenology and bipolar disorder

In a study on gender differences, Kawa *et al.* [64] reported that most gender comparisons showed no differences. Nonetheless, more men than women reported mania at the onset of bipolar I disorder. Men also had higher rates of comorbid alcohol abuse/dependence, cannabis abuse/dependence, pathological gambling and conduct disorder. Men were more likely to report 'behavioural problems' and 'being unable to hold a conversation' during mania. Women reported higher rates of comorbid eating disorders, weight and appetite change and little disorder during depression. Kessing [65] reported that significantly more women were treated as outpatients than as inpatients. Women were treated for longer periods as inpatients but not as outpatients. In both settings, the prevalence of depressive versus manic/mixed episodes was similar for men and women and the severity of manic (hypomanic/manic without psychosis/manic with psychosis) and depressive episodes (mild/moderate/severe without psychosis/severe with psychosis) did not differ between genders. The prevalence of psychotic symptoms at first contact was the same for both genders. Among patients treated in outpatient settings more men than women presented with comorbid substance abuse and among hospitalised patients, more women than men presented with mixed episodes.

The severity of the illness in the developing countries at onset is no less than in the west [66]. Although symptomatology appears not dissimilar to patients from developed countries, more pronounced distractibility and a persistent embarrassing behaviour are more common in the Indian Setting [67]. The same authors also reported a preponderance of mania in Indian patients in a more recent study, Shahul Ameen and Daya Ram [68] reported that there were no significant gender differences in the prevalence of negative symptoms in remitted bipolar disorder.

Cognitive dysfunction and bipolar disorder

Although several reviews of neuropsychological deficits in bipolar disorders have been reported [69, 70] few studies have commented on sex differences in cognitive deficits in bipolar disorders. Sex differences are not found in cognitive functioning of patients with bipolar disorder, both in acute phase as well as when in remission [71].

Substance abuse and bipolar disorder

Several studies have reported an association between alcoholism and mood disorders. Data from both developed and developing countries reveal high levels of comorbidity in bipolar illness [72]. Data collected on bipolar disorder show rates of substance abuse that are five to six times greater than those among general populations [73, 74]. Three studies found the rate of substance misuse in those with bipolar I disorder to be over 60%, and at least 35% of total bipolar disorder cases were complicated by alcohol abuse [75, 76]. A diagnosis of an underlying bipolar illness may be missed because of the high rate of comorbidity and the more conspicuous signs and symptoms of substance abuse [77]. Very little research has addressed the issue of substance abuse and bipolar comorbidity amongst women. Chandra et al. [78] reported that areca nut, commonly occurs amongst Indian psychiatric patients. Predictors of current areca nut use included less education, diagnosis of bipolar disorder and current tobacco use. Predictors of severe use were older age, female gender, less education and current tobacco use.

Bipolar disorder and pregnancy

Contrary results have been put forth on the impact of pregnancy on bipolar disorders. Some have suggested that pregnancy may be a time in which women may experience a relief from their mood symptoms. However, Blehar et al. [44] closely examined the timing of pregnancy and emotional problems in women with BPD Type 1 and found that 37% reported mood episodes during their pregnancy and 14 reported mood changes in pregnancy and postpartum periods.

Postpartum period and bipolar disorder

Nonacs and Covans [79] reported that women with BPD had a 20–50% risk of relapse during the postpartum period. The risk of postpartum relapse appears to be even higher in women with a past history of postpartum psychoses. Kendal et al. [80] provide the strongest evidence supporting these findings. Linking data from the Edinburgh Case Register to the Scottish maternity discharge database, they inferred that a psychiatric admission for psychoses during the first 90 days after childbirth was 14% more likely than before childbirth. Amongst women with a past history of bipolar disorder, 21.4% required admission during the first three months after childbirth. This risk was significantly greater than the risk of women diagnosed as schizophrenia (3.4% risk) or depressive neurosis (1.7% risk). In a study in Turkey, Kisa et al. [81] reported 32% patients were diagnosed as bipolar disorder in the postpartum period.

Menopause

The effects of menopause have not received much research attention and the reported findings have been contradictory. In a study of menopausal women, Blehar et al. [44] found 13% women with depression and 4% women with mania.

Management of bipolar disorders: Impact of sex on response rates

Possible sex differences in the responses to treatment with mood stabilisers has been an understudied area, although it has been well established that sex differences have been found in absorption, metabolism and excretion of medications. Endogenous hormone cycles have been known to influence the pharmacokinetics of the treatment agents, whatever the life cycle of the woman.

The sex differences in response to treatment with lithium have been extensively studied. Viguera *et al.* [82] reviewed 17 lithium studies comprising of 1548 patients. No significant differences were seen in the response rates. A recent large-scale efficacy study using divalproex [83] did not report efficacy on sex of the participant.

Decisions regarding treatment of bipolar disorder during pregnancy

Evidence base indicates that decision to treat must balance the risks associated with the untreated condition versus teratogenecity.

No treatment

Patients who discontinue mood-stabilising medication after conception increase their risk of relapse [84] either of which could lead to complications and untoward effects on the foetus. Untreated mania may be associated with perinatal risks, as a pregnant patient in a manic state may engage in impulsive, high-risk behaviours that endanger her and the foetus [85]. These effects may be mediated by the illness itself or by other factors that indirectly affect birth outcomes.

Antimanic (mood stabilising) agents

Patients vary in their response to antimanic agents. Therefore, there is no single preferred medication for bipolar disorder, regardless of reproductive status. The preferred medication is what has been effective for and has been tolerated by the individual patient.

Lithium

Lithium is a first line drug for acute and maintenance treatment of bipolar disorder. There is no evidence for an increased risk of miscarriage or intrauterine foetal death in women treated with lithium [86]. Recent controlled epidemiologic studies suggest a real, but modest, teratogenic risk of Ebstein's anomaly following first-trimester lithium exposure. Based on a pooled analysis of the data, Cohen *et al.* [87] estimated the risk of Ebstein's anomaly to between 1/1000 (0.1%) and 2/1000 (0.2%), which is 10–20 times higher than rates in the general population. Thus, while the relative risk for Ebstein's anomaly is increased, the absolute risk remains small. Pregnant women taking lithium should be evaluated with a high-resolution ultrasound and foetal echocardiography at 16–18 weeks gestation to screen for cardiac anomalies. Still birth was reported in a patient in whom lithium prophylaxis was considered essential for clinical and social reasons in India [88]. The authors suggested avoiding the use of lithium, at least in the first trimester.

Maternal lithium toxicity can occur due to various factors such as vomiting, febrile illness, alteration of sodium intake for treatment of pre-eclampsia or diuretic therapy. Toxicity is most likely to occur during the intrapartum period. Patients are encouraged to have their lithium level monitored every two to four weeks throughout pregnancy, weekly in the last month and every few days shortly before and after delivery [89]. Adverse neonatal outcomes are more extensive in the setting of higher lithium concentrations at delivery. Lithium delivery concentrations can be significantly reduced at delivery without compromising pharmacotherapeutic efficacy by withholding lithium therapy from the onset of labour [90]. While lithium is associated with significant risks in all stages of pregnancy, it arguably remains the safest medication for the pregnant woman with bipolar disorder.

There are no prospective studies to establish the incidence and risk factors for occurrence of lithium toxicity in the foetus and newborns, although this was reported in the mid 1970s [91]. This follow up study showed that attainment of major developmental milestones for 22 lithium-exposed subjects was comparable to controls. In a more recent study, serum lithium levels in nursing infants were reported to be low. No significant adverse clinical or behavioural effects were noted [92]. These findings encourage reassessment of recommendations against lithium during breast-feeding and underscore the importance of close clinical monitoring of nursing infants.

Anticonvulsants

Studies performed through the late 1990s suggest that the risk of morphologic malformations in infants exposed to valproate and carbamazepine is about two to three times higher than in the general population. The most common malformations in exposed offspring are similar to those seen in the general population (e.g. heart defects, hypospadias, club foot and cleft lip or palate). No single malformation has been associated with a specific antiepileptic drug, with the exception of spina bifida, which is more common with exposure to valproic acid (1–5% of exposed infants) and carbamazepine (0.5–1%). Malformations are also more common after exposure to polytherapy than after exposure to a single drug. Additional evidence for a higher teratogenic potential of valproate comes from the North American registry, in which malformations were four times more common among infants exposed to valproic acid than in those exposed to all other antiepileptic monotherapies combined.

The risk of birth defects after Lamitrogine exposure used in first trimester are similar to rates in general population. Intrauterine growth retardation is included in descriptions of the foetal valproate syndrome, but the incidence has not been established. Carbamazepine is associated with reductions in mean birth weight (about 250 g).

Other anticonvulsants, such as oxcarbazepine (Trileptal; Novartis), tiagabine (Gabitril; Cephalon, Inc., Frazer, PA) and topiramate (Topamax; Ortho-McNeil Neurologics, Inc., Titusville, NJ) are occasionally used in clinical practise as antimanic agents or to treat anxiety symptoms. Outcomes of 94 pregnancies in women exposed to oxcarbazepine found no anomalies related to its use; however, these are too few to rule out adverse effects with confidence. The safety of tiagabine and topiramate for use in pregnancy has not been investigated.

Neurobehavioural teratogenicity

A retrospective survey of British women between the ages of 16 and 40 who were exposed to antiepileptic drugs during pregnancy evaluated the subsequent need for special education for their exposed children. Those exposed to valproate monotherapy had a higher likelihood of needing special education (OR, 3.4; 95% CI 1.63–7.10). In contrast, carbamazepine had no statistically significant effect (OR, 0.26; 95% CI 0.06–1.15). Polytherapy including valproate had similarly high odds ratios for lower academic achievement (OR, 2.51; 95% CI 1.04–6.07) compared with those exposed to polytherapy excluding valproate (OR, 1.51; 95% CI 0.56–4.07). Although these findings should be treated with caution, they suggest that monotherapy or polytherapy with valproate during pregnancy carries particular risks for the neurodevelopment of children exposed in utero.

A prospective study of children's intelligence quotients (IQs; mean age seven years) compared IQs in children of epileptic mothers to the IQs of children in a control group. Again, children exposed to valproate prenatally had a mean IQ that was 11 points lower than those children who were not exposed. The same study found no association between carbamazepine and cognitive dysfunction. A single follow-up of 23 infants exposed to lamotrigine demonstrated no alterations or delays in development at 12 months of age. Data are still inadequate to determine the risks of developmental effects of foetal exposure to lamotrigine. No evidence of growth problems, post-birth discovery of occult malformations, neonatal seizures or deviations in psychomotor development to one year of age were observed in 62 infants exposed to lamotrigine in utero.

Neonatal toxicity

Manifestations of withdrawal, including irritability, jitteriness, abnormal tone, feeding difficulties and seizures have been described in infants whose mothers took valproic acid during pregnancy. The frequency of withdrawal symptoms was significantly related to the dose of valproate given to the mothers in the third trimester, and there was a tendency for both the frequency of the minor abnormalities and the major malformations to be related to the valproate dosage in the first trimester.

Maternal vitamin supplementation

Maternal folate supplementation reduces the risk of neural tube defects. However, risk reduction has not been confirmed in pregnant women treated with anticonvulsants. Some experts recommend a daily dose of 4–5 mg of folic acid before and during pregnancy, or at least through the first trimester, for all women who take antiepileptic drugs. Pernicious anaemia can be masked by folate supplementation; therefore, a B12 level obtained before beginning folate treatment is a prudent recommendation. Carbamazepine has been associated with vitamin K deficiency. Because adequate levels of vitamin K are necessary for clotting, in utero carbamazepine exposure could increase the risk of neonatal bleeding. Most experts recommend women on carbamazepine take an additional 20 mg of vitamin K supplement daily throughout pregnancy.

Other anticonvulsants

Other anticonvulsants, such as oxcarbazepine (Trileptal; Novartis), tiagabine (Gabitril; Cephalon, Inc., Frazer, PA) and topiramate (Topamax; Ortho-McNeil Neurologics, Inc., Titusville, NJ) are occasionally used in clinical practise as antimanic agents or to treat anxiety symptoms. Outcomes of 94 pregnancies in women exposed to oxcarbazepine found no anomalies related to its use; however, these are too few to rule out adverse effects with confidence. The safety of tiagabine and topiramate for use in pregnancy has not been investigated.

Antipsychotic agents

Antipsychotic drugs are often used as monotherapy or adjunctive medications for patients with bipolar disorder. Antipsychotics are commonly used in the management of acute mania. The largest body of evidence regarding safety for use in pregnancy exists for the older, first-generation antipsychotics.

The best-studied drug in this class is chlorpromazine, in a 1977 survey of more than 50 000 mother-child pairs that identified 142 first trimester exposures and 284 total exposures to chlorpromazine, there was no elevation in the rate of physical malformations. Several case reports have documented transient extrapyramidal symptoms, including motor restlessness, tremor, hypertonicity, dystonia and Parkinsonism in neonates exposed to antipsychotic agents during pregnancy. These problems have typically been of short duration and have been followed by apparently normal subsequent motor development.

In a 2004 review of the management of bipolar disorder in pregnancy, Yonkers [89] supports the role of first-generation antipsychotic agents both in the treatment of acute mania during pregnancy, and as an alternative to selected mood stabilisers. Psychiatric clinicians may elect to switch a patient's medication from lithium or an anticonvulsant to a first-generation antipsychotic either for the entire pregnancy or for the first trimester. This strategy is particularly recommended for patients who have benefited from mood stabilisation with antipsychotic medications in the past. First-generation antipsychotic medications may also be a choice for women with bipolar disorder who elect to discontinue medication during pregnancy but begin to experience a recurrence of symptoms while pregnant.

Atypical antipsychotic agents

McKenna *et al.* [93] examined 151 pregnancy outcomes from mothers enrolled in the Canadian Motherisk Programme to determine whether atypical antipsychotics increase the rate of major malformations. These included exposures to olanzapine (n = 60), risperidone (n = 49), quetiapine (n = 36) and clozapine (n = 6). The results suggest that atypical antipsychotics are not associated with an increased risk for major malformations; however, the limited numbers are inadequate to determine the risk of foetal exposure.

Olanzapine is associated with serious metabolic side effects that could potentially exacerbate maternal weight gain and gestational diabetes, which is associated with an increased risk for a large for gestational age newborn.

Antidepressants

Monotherapy with antidepressants – that is, use of an antidepressant without concomitant antimanic medication – is not appropriate in the management of bipolar disorder. Use of antidepressants in a patient with bipolar disorder may trigger a mood shift from depression to induction of a manic, hypomanic, mixed episode or rapid cycling.

Psychosocial management

A number of studies have addressed effectiveness of various psychosocial strategies [94–98]. There is limited literature on the role of gender in the effectiveness in these strategies. In an analysis of intensive family intervention, bipolar patients were reported to do better than depressive patients in terms of global ratings, symptoms social role functions and family attitudes. The beneficial effects seen were attributed to improvement in female patients [99].

1.4 Other psychoses

Schizoaffective psychoses

The definition of schizoaffective psychoses has undergone several changes through the years, making it difficult to get reliable epidemiological information. However, pooled data from various clinical studies have estimated that approximately

2–29% patients have been diagnosed as schizoaffective. Levinson *et al.* [100] estimated 19% patients were diagnosed as schizoaffective disorder. Women had a higher prevalence of the disorder. Relatives of women suffering from the disorder had a higher rate of schizophrenia and depression as compared to relatives of male schizophrenia patients [101].

Acute and transient psychoses

Acute and transient psychoses is a relatively new entrant into psychiatric nosology [102]. Female preponderance was noted in the occurrence of this category of psychoses [103–105].

Delusional disorder

Mixed results have been published on the gender differences in patients diagnosed as suffering from delusional disorder. A crude estimate of the condition has been reported to be between 0.7 and 3.0 per 100 000 population [106]. In a retrospective study from China, 0.83% of 10 418 outpatients met DSM IV criteria for delusional disorder, with equal gender distribution. Women were significantly older than men [107]. Yamada and associates [108] reported a 3 : 1 female to male ration in Japan. Hwu and colleagues [40] did not find any sex differences in their studies. In India, rates have varied: from 0.5 to 5% [109, 110]. In a study from North India, 55.7% of the patients diagnosed as delusional disorder were females [111].

Postpartum psychosis

Postpartum psychosis is a term used for all psychoses occurring during the postpartum period. All classic psychoses (i.e. the manic, the depressive or very often the schizoaffective type, but also schizophrenic or 'atypical' psychoses) can occur. In contrast to depressive disorders, risk for psychosis is excessively higher during the postpartum period than at other times of a woman's life – up to 20 times higher in the first month after parturition [80]. Recent evidence suggests that postpartum psychiatric illness is virtually indistinguishable from psychiatric disorders that occur at other times during a woman's life. Postpartum psychosis, a severe form of postpartum psychiatric illness, is a rare condition that typically has a dramatic onset and is characterised by psychotic symptoms including disorientation and disorganised behaviour. Epidemiological studies have reported rates of 1–2 cases per 1000 live births. Most studies have not distinguished postpartum psychosis from bipolar disorder or the proportion of the incidence attributable to pre pregnancy psychiatric morbidity [112]. The incidence of postpartum psychosis was reported as 0.07% from the USA. In a prevalence study of postpartum disorders, in Tamil Nadu, India, the estimate of psychoses was 0.63% [113]. Data from a psychiatric clinic in Hazara district in Pakistan reported 8.6% of the women attending the clinic over three years had a history of postpartum disorders. Of these, 60% had diagnoses of postpartum psychosis. This high rate was attributed to the selection of specialist clinics for the study, where only gravely ill subjects were brought [114].

1.5 Special issues in women with severe mental illness

Sexuality

Few studies describe sexual disturbance in schizophrenia and only a few of these describe sexual function or dysfunction in women [115]. Whereas men with schizophrenia frequently lose their sexual drive early in the course of illness and are not likely to be sexually active if their illness is severe, this is generally not true for women. They continue to be interested in relationships and to engage in sexual intercourse [116]. The relative passivity and isolation that accompany schizophrenia are fertile ground for sexual victimisation. For these reasons, women with schizophrenia are at special risk not only for unwanted pregnancy but also for sexually transmitted disease [117].

Two studies compared schizophrenia women to normal controls [118, 119]. Schizophrenia women are more likely than normal controls to have low sexual desire and difficulty becoming aroused or reaching orgasm. Several factors contribute to sexual dysfunction amongst women. Amongst women receiving conventional antipsychotic treatment, 50−90% experience menstrual irregularities [120]. Serum Prolactin irregularities are also hypothesised to contribute to sexual dysfunctions. Women may also experience dyspareunia due to vaginal dryness and atrophy.

Social skills deficits in schizophrenia is likely to make a woman vulnerable to sexual exploitation. Social consequences such as homelessness, vulnerability to sexual abuse and exposure to HIV and other infections contribute to the difficulties to rehabilitation of women [121].

Mothers with psychosis as parents

Many women with schizophrenia are mothers. This is particularly true in societies like India when women marry rather early and have children. The later age of onset of illness in women also seems to facilitate this. Research in this area has been sparse and has included some qualitative interviews with women who are mothers [122]. The problems faced by such women also differ across countries and cultures. Issues regarding day to day parenting, custody, foster care and dealing with welfare agencies are important in many western countries. In the east, where joint families provide substitute or supplementary mothering, the problems are lack of social welfare schemes and the additional burden and responsibility on the women's families. In a study on 75 women with schizophrenia who were separated or divorced, 29 women had children [27]. Twenty of these 29 who had children who continued to live with their ill mothers even after separation. When the mother was too ill or had multiple relapses, the ageing grandparents often had to take on the parental roles. Only six husbands of these 75 women came forward to take care of the children and only two provided financial support to the wife and children.

In a literature review of studies in the last five years [123], it has been pointed out that maternal mental illness can impact negatively on a child's life, especially where an insecure attachment is formed between mother and baby during the important early developmental years. Impaired cognitive development, behavioural difficulties and increased risk of psychiatric disorder seem to be some of the sequelae. Effective parenting skills are suggested to be a protective factor against these sequelae. It therefore becomes imperative to focus on providing parental skills as part of the general psychosocial programmes.

References

1. Davar, B.V. (1999) *Mental Health of Indian Women: A Feminist Agenda*, Sage Publications, New Delhi.
2. World Health Organization (1998) World Health Report, Geneva.
3. Sartorius, N., Jablensky, A., Korten, A. *et al.* (1986) Early manifestations and first: contact incidence of schizophrenia in different cultures: a preliminary report on the initial evaluation phase of the WHO Collaborative Study on determinants of outcome of severe mental disorders. *Psychological Medicine*, **16** (4), 909–28.
4. Saha, S., Chant, D. and McGrath, J. (2007) A systematic review of mortality in schizophrenia: is the differential mortality gap worsening over time? *Archives of General Psychiatry*, **64** (10), 1123–31.
5. Rajkumar, S., Padmavati, R., Thara, R. and Sarada Menon, M. (1993) Incidence of Schizophrenia in an urban community in Madras. *Indian Journal of Psychiatry*, **35** (1), 18–21.
6. Dube, K.C. and Kumar, N. (1972) Epidemiological study of schizophrenia. *Journal of Biosocial Science*, **4**, 187–95.
7. Saha, S., Chant, D., Welham, J. and McGrath, J. (2005) A systematic review of the prevalence of schizophrenia. *PloS Medicine*, **2** (5), e 141.
8. Mortensen, P.B. and Juel, K. (1993) Mortality and causes of death in first admitted schizophrenic patients. *The British Journal of Psychiatry*, **163**, 183–89.
9. Ran, M.S., Chen, E.Y., Conwell, Y. *et al.* (2007) Mortality in people with schizophrenia in rural China: 10-year cohort study. *The British Journal of Psychiatry*, **190**, 237–42.
10. Auquier, P., Lançon, C., Rouillon, F. *et al.* (2006) Mortality in schizophrenia. *Pharmacoepidemiology and Drug Safety*, **15** (12), 873–79.
11. Morgan, V.A., Castle, D.J. and Jablensky, A.V. (2008) Do women express and experience psychosis differently from men? Epidemiological evidence from the Australian National Study of Low Prevalence (Psychotic) Disorders. *The Australian and New Zealand Journal of Psychiatry*, **42** (1), 74–82.
12. Thara, R. (2004) Twenty-year course of schizophrenia: the Madras Longitudinal Study. *Canadian Journal of Psychiatry*, **49** (8), 564–69.
13. Canuso, C.M. and Pandina, G. (2007) Gender and schizophrenia. *Psychopharmacology Bulletin*, **40** (4), 178–90.

14. Usall, J., Suarez, D., Haro, J.M. SOHO Study Group (2007) Gender differences in response to antipsychotic treatment in outpatients with schizophrenia. *Psychiatry Research*, **153** (3), 225–31 [Epub 2007 Aug 2].

15. Müller, M.J. (2007) Gender-specific associations of depression with positive and negative symptoms in acute schizophrenia. *Progress in Neuro-Psychopharmacology and Biological Psychiatry*, **31** (5), 1095–100. [Epub 2007 Mar 30].

16. Murthy, G.V., Janakiramaiah, N., Gangadhar, B.N. and Subbakrishna, D.K. (1998) Sex difference in age at onset of schizophrenia: discrepant findings from India. *Acta Psychiatrica Scandinavica*, **97** (5), 321–25.

17. Tang, Y.L., Gillespie, C.F., Epstein, M.P. *et al.* (2007) Gender differences in 542 Chinese inpatients with schizophrenia. *Schizophrenia Research*, **97** (1–3), 88–96 [Epub 2007 Jul 12].

18. Kreitman, N. (1968) Married couples admitted to mental hospitals. *The British Journal of Psychiatry*, **114**, 679–718.

19. Eaton, W.W. (1975) Marital status and schizophrenia. *Acta Psychiatrica Scandinavica*, **52**, 320–29.

20. Odegaard, O. (1980) Fertility of psychiatric first admissions in Norway. *Acta Psychiatrica Scandinavica*, **62**, 212–20.

21. Saugstad, L.F. (1989) Social class, marriage and fertility in schizophrenia. *Schizophrenia Bulletin*, **15**, 9–43.

22. Hafner, H., Reicher-Rossier, A., Fatkenheuer, B. *et al.* (1991) Sex differences in schizophrenia. *Psychiatria Fennica*, **22**, 123–56.

23. Seeman, M.V. (1986) Current outcome in schizophrenia: women vs men. *Acta Psychiatrica Scandinavica*, **73**, 609–17.

24. Leon, C.A. (1989) Clinical course and outcome of schizophrenia in Cali, Columbia: a 10-year follow-up. *The Journal of Nervous and Mental Disease*, **177**, 593–605.

25. Thara, R. and Rajkumar, S. (1992) Gender differences in schizophrenia: results of a follow-up study from India. *Schizophrenia Research*, **7**, 65–70.

26. Thara, R. and Srinivasan, T.N. (1997) Outcome of marriage in schizophrenia. *Social Psychiatry and Psychiatric Epidemiology*, **32**, 416–20.

27. Thara, R., Kamath, S. and Kumar, S. (2003) Women with schizophrenia and broken marriages – doubly disadvantaged. Part I: patient perspective. *The International Journal of Social Psychiatry*, **49** (3), 225–32.

28. Thara, R., Kamath, S. and Kumar, S. (2003) Women with schizophrenia and broken marriages – doubly disadvantaged? Part II: family perspective. *The International Journal of Social Psychiatry*, **49** (3), 233–40.

29. Marshall, J.E. and Reed, J.L. (1992) Psychiatric morbidity in homeless women. *The British Journal of Psychiatry*, **160**, 761–68.

30. Goering, P., Paduchak, D. and Durbin, J. (1990) Gender and schizophrenia. Housing homeless women – a consumer preference study. *Hospital and Community Psychiatry*, **41**, 790–94.

31. Opler, L.A., White, L., Caton, C.L. *et al.* (2001) Gender differences in the relationship of homelessness to symptom severity, substance abuse, and neuroleptic noncompliance in schizophrenia. *The Journal of Nervous and Mental Disease*, **189** (7), 449–56.

32. Bhugra, D. (1996) *Homelessness and Mental Health*, Cambridge University Press.

33. Thara, R. and Srinivasan, T.N. (2000) How stigmatising is schizophrenia in India? *The International Journal of Social Psychiatry*, **46** (2), 135–41.

34. Chadda, R.K., Singh, T.B. and Ganguly, K.K. (2007) Caregiver burden and coping: a prospective study of relationship between burden and coping in caregivers of patients with schizophrenia and bipolar affective disorder. *Social Psychiatry and Psychiatric Epidemiology*, **42** (11), 923–30 [Epub 2007 Aug 13].

35. Awad, A.G. and Voruganti, L.N. (2008) The burden of schizophrenia on caregivers: a review. *PharmacoEconomics*, **26** (2), 149–62.

36. Kennedy, C., Carlson, D., Ustun, B. *et al.* (1997) Mental health, disabilities and women. *Journal of Disability and Policy Studies*, **8** (1 & 2).

37. Mowbray, C.T. (2003) Women and psychiatric rehabilitation practice. *Psychiatric Rehabilitation Journal*, **27** Fall (2), 101–3.

38. Goodwin, R.D., Jacobi, F., Bittner A. and Wittchen, H. (2006) Epidemiology of mood disorders, in *Textbook of mood disorders*, Chapter 3 (eds D.J. Stein, D. Kuppfer and A. Schatzberg), American Psychiatric Publishing Inc., Washington, pp. 33–54.

39. Chen, C.N., Wong, J., Lee, N. *et al.* (1993) The Shatin community mental health survey in Hong Kong, II: major findings. *Archives of General Psychiatry*, **50**, 125–33.

40. Hwu, H.G., Yeh, E.K. and Chang, L.Y. (1989) Prevalence of psychiatric disorders in Taiwan defined by the Chinese Diagnostic Interview Schedule. *Acta Psychiatrica Scandinavica*, **79**, 136–47.

41. Hendrick, V., Altshuler, L.L., Gitlin, M.J. *et al.* (2000) Gender and bipolar disorder. *The Journal of Clinical Psychiatry*, **61**, 393–96.

42. Szadoczky, E., Papp, Z., Vitrai, J. *et al.* (1998) The prevalence of major depressive disorders in Hungary: results from a national comorbidity survey. *Journal of Affective Disorders*, **50**, 153–62.

43. Leinbenluft, E. (1996) Women with bipolar illness: clinical and research issues. *The American Journal of Psychiatry*, **153**, 163–73.

44. Blehar, M.C., DePaulo, J.R., Gershon, E.S. *et al.* (1998) Women with bipolar disorder: findings from the NIMH genetics initiative sample. *Psychopharmacology Bulletin*, **34**, 239–43.

45. Roy-Byrne, P., Post, R.M., Uhde, T.W. *et al.* (1985) The longitudinal course of recurrent affective illnesses: life chart data from research patients at the NIMH. *Acta Psychiatrica Scandinavica*, **71** (317), 5–34.

46. Winokur, G., Coryell, W., Akiskal, H.S. *et al.* (1994) Manic depressive (bipolar disorder) course in light of a prospective ten-year follow up of 131 patients. *Acta Psychiatrica Scandinavica*, **89**, 102–10.

47. Taylor, M.A. and Abrahms, R. (1981) Gender differences in bipolar affective disorder. *Journal of Affective Disorders*, **3**, 261–77.

48. Jagadheesan, K. and Sinha, V.K. (2003) Course and outcome of adolescent onset bipolar affective disorder: a retrospective clinic-based study. *Hong Kong Journal of Psychiatry*, **13** (3), 2–6.

49. Lee, S. (1992) The first lithium clinic in Hong Kong: a Chinese profile. *The Australian and New Zealand Journal of Psychiatry*, **26**, 450–53.

50. Makanjoula, R.O.A. (1985) Recurrent unipolar manic disorder in Yoruba Nigerians: further evidence. *The British Journal of Psychiatry*, **147**, 434–42.

51. Khanna, R., Gupta, N. and Shankar, S. (1992) Course of bipolar disorders in eastern India. *Journal of Affective Disorders*, **24**, 35–41.

52. Khess, C.R.J., Das, J. and Akhtar, S. (1997) Four year follow up of first episode manic patients. *Indian Journal of Psychiatry*, **39**, 160–65.
53. Chopra, M.P., Kishore Kumar, K.V., Subbhakrishna, D.K. *et al.* (2006) The course of bipolar disorder in rural India. *Indian Journal of Psychiatry*, **48**, 254–57.
54. Rob, J.C., Young, L.T., Cooke, L.T. and Joffe, R.T. (1998) Gender differences in patients with bipolar disorders influence outcome in the medical outcomes survey (SF-20) subscale scores. *Journal of Affective Disorders*, **49**, 189–93.
55. Arnold, L.M., McElroy, S.L. and Keck, P.E. (2000) The role of gender in mixed mania. *Comprehensive Psychiatry*, **41**, 83–87.
56. Akiskal, H.S., Hantouche, E.G., Bourgeois, M.L. *et al.* (1998) Gender, temperament, and the clinical picture in dysphoric mixed mania: findings from a French national study (EPIMAN). *Journal of Affective Disorders*, **50**, 175–86.
57. McElroy, S.L., Keck, P.E., Pope, H.G. *et al.* (1992) Clinical and research implications of the diagnosis of dysphoric, or mixed mania or hypomania. *The American Journal of Psychiatry*, **49**, 1633–44.
58. Tando, L. and Baldessarini, R.J. (1998) Rapid cycling in women and men with bipolar manic-depressive disorders. *The American Journal of Psychiatry*, **155**, 1434–36.
59. Wher, T.A., Sack, D.A., Rosenthal, D.E. and Cowdry, R.W. (1998) Rapid cycling affective disorders: contributing factors and treatment responses in 51 patients. *The American Journal of Psychiatry*, **145**, 179–84.
60. Schneck, C.D., Miklowitz, D.J., Calabrese, J.R. *et al.* (2004) Phenomenology of rapid cycling bipolar disorder: data from the first 500 participants in the systematic treatment enhancement program. *The American Journal of Psychiatry*, **161** (10), 1902–8.
61. Shulman, K.I., Schaffer, A., Levitt, A. and Herrmann, N. (2002) Effects of gender and age on phenomenology and management of bipolar disorder: a review, in *Bipolar Disorder WPA Series. Evidence and Experience in Psychiatry*, Chapter 5 (eds M. Maj, H.S. Akiskal, J.J. Lopez Ibor and N. Sartorius), John Wiley & Sons, Ltd, UK.
62. Simon, G.E., Hunkeler, E., Fireman, B. *et al.* (2007) Risk of suicide attempt and suicide death in patients treated for bipolar disorders. *Bipolar Disorders*, **9** (5), 526–30.
63. Benedetti, A., Fagiolini, A., Casamassima, F. *et al.* (2007) Gender differences in bipolar disorder type 1: a 48-week prospective follow-up of 72 patients treated in an Italian tertiary care center. *The Journal of Nervous and Mental Disease*, **195** (1), 93–96.
64. Kawa, I., Carter, J.D., Joyce, P.R. *et al.* (2005) Gender differences in bipolar disorder: age of onset, course, comorbidity, and symptom presentation. *Bipolar Disorders*, **7** (2), 119–25.
65. Kessing, L.V. (2004) Gender differences in the phenomenology of bipolar disorder. *Bipolar Disorders*, **6**, 421–25.
66. Rao, V.A. (1996) Depression and bipolar affective disorder, in *Psychiatry in the Developing World*, Chapter 10 (eds D. Tantam, L. Appleby and A. Duncan), Gaskell.
67. Chatterjee, R.N. and Kulhara, P. (1989) Symptomatology, symptom resolution and short-term course in mania. *Indian Journal of Psychiatry*, **31**, 213–18.
68. Ameen, S. and Ram, D. (2007) Negative symptoms in the remission phase of bipolar disorder. *German Journal of Psychiatry*, **10**, 1–7.

69. Murphy, F.C. and Sahakian, B.J. (2001) Neuropsychology of bipolar disorders. *The British Journal of Psychiatry*, **178**, 120–27.

70. Trivedi, J.K. (2006) Cognitive deficits in psychiatric disorder: current status. *Indian Journal of Psychiatry*, **48**, 10–20.

71. Zalla, T., Joyce, C., Szöke, A. *et al.* (2004) Executive dysfunctions as potential markers of familial vulnerability to bipolar disorder and schizophrenia. *Psychiatry Research*, **121** (3), 207–17.

72. Khanna, R. (2001) Bipolar disorders, in *Neurological, Psychiatric, and Developmental Disorders: Meeting the Challenges of the Developing World*, Chapter 8. Committee on Nervous System Disorders in Developing Countries, Board on Global Health, institute of Medicine, National Academy Press, Washington, DC.

73. Tsai, S.Y., Lee, J.C. and Chen, C.C. (1999) Characteristics and psychosocial problems of patients with bipolar disorder at high risk for suicide attempt. *Journal of Affective Disorders*, **52** (1–3), 145–52.

74. Regier, D.A., Farmer, M.E., Rae, D.S. *et al.* (1990) Comorbidity of mental disorders with drug and alcohol abuse: results from the Epidemiologic Catchment Area (ECA) study. *The Journal of the American Medical Association*, **264**, 2511–18.

75. Kessler, R.C., McGognale, K.A., Zhoa, C. *et al.* (1994) Lifetime and 12 month prevalence of DSM-III-R, psychiatric disorders in the United States. *Archives of General Psychiatry*, **51**, 8–19.

76. Tohen, M. and Goodwin, F. (1995) Epidemiology of bipolar disorder, in *Textbook in Psychiatric Epidemiology* (eds M.T. Tsuang, M. Tohen and G.E.P. Zahner), Wiley-Liss, New York, pp. 301–17.

77. Helzer, J.E., Burnam, A. and McEvoy, L.T. (1991) Alcohol abuse and dependence, in *Psychiatric Disorders in America* (eds L.N. Robins and D.A. Regier), Free Press, New York, pp. 81–129.

78. Chandra, P.S., Care, M.P., Carey, K.B. and Jairam, K.R. (2003) Prevalence and correlates of areca nut use among psychiatric patients in India. *Drug and Alcohol Dependence*, **69** (3), 311–16.

79. Nonacs, R. and Cohen, L.S. (1998) Postpartum mood disorders: diagnosis and treatment guidelines. *The Journal of Clinical Psychiatry*, **59** (Suppl 2), 34–40.

80. Kendell, R.E., Chalmers, J.C. and Platz, C. (1987) Epidemiology of puerperal psychoses. *The British Journal of Psychiatry*, **150**, 662–73.

81. Kisa, C., Ayedemir, C., Kurt, A. *et al.* (2007) Long term follow up of patients with post partum psychosis. *Turk Psykiyatri Dergisi*, **18** (3), 223–30. PMID: 17853977 [PubMed – indexed for MEDLINE].

82. Viguera, A.C., Tondo, L. and Baldessarini, R.J. (2000) Sex differences in response to lithium treatment. *The American Journal of Psychiatry*, **157**, 1509–11.

83. Bowden, C.L., Calabrese, J.R., McElroy, S.L. *et al.* (2000) A randomized placebo controlled 12 month trial of Divalpoex and lithium in the treatment of outpatients with bipolar I disorder. *Archives of General Psychiatry*, **57**, 481–89.

84. Viguera, A.C., Nonacs, R., Cohen, L.S. *et al.* (2000) Risk of recurrence of bipolar disorder in pregnant and nonpregnant women after discontinuing lithium maintenance. *The American Journal of Psychiatry*, **157**, 179–84.

85. Curtis, V. (2005) Women are not the same as men: specific clinical issues in female patients with bipolar disorder. *Bipolar Disorders*, **7**, 16–24.

86. Jacobson, S.L., Jones, K., Johnson, K. *et al.* (1992) Prospective multicentre study of pregnancy outcome after lithium exposure during first trimester. *Lancet*, **339**, 530–33.

87. Cohen, L.S., Freidman, J.M., Jefferson, J.W. *et al.* (1994) A reevaluation of risk of in utero exposure to lithium. *The Journal of the American Medical Association*, **271**, 146–50.

88. Khandelwal, S.K., Sagar, R.S. and Saxena, S. (1989) Lithium in pregnancy and still birth: a case report. *The British Journal of Psychiatry*, **154**, 114–15.

89. Yonkers, K.A., Wisner, K.L., Stowe, Z. *et al.* (2004) Management of bipolar disorder during pregnancy and post partum period. *The American Journal of Psychiatry*, **161**, 608–20.

90. Newport, D., Viguera, A., Beach, B. *et al.* (2005) Lithium placental passage and obstetrical outcome: implications for clinical management during late pregnancy. *The American Journal of Psychiatry*, **162**, 2162–70.

91. Schou, M. (1976) What happened later to lithium babies? A follow up study of children born without malformations. *British Medical Journal*, **54**, 193–97.

92. Viguera, A.C., Newport, J., Rithchie, J. *et al.* (2007) Lithium in breast milk and nursing infants: clinical implications. *The American Journal of Psychiatry*, **164**, 342–45.

93. McKenna, K., Koren, G., Tetelbaum, M. *et al.* (2005) Pregnancy outcome of women using atypical antipsychotic drugs: a prospective comparative study. *The Journal of Clinical Psychiatry*, **66**, 444–49.

94. Simoneau, T.L., Milkowitz, D.J., Richards, J.A. and Saleem, R. (1998) Expressed emotions and interactional patterns in the families of bipolar patients. *Journal of Abnormal Psychology*, **107**, 497–507.

95. Milkowitz, D.J. and Goldstein, M.J. (1988) Family factors and the course of bipolar affective disorders. *Archives of General Psychiatry*, **45**, 225–31.

96. Scott, J. (1996) The role of cognitive behavior therapy in bipolar disorder. *Cognitive and Behavioral Practice*, **3**, 29–51.

97. Frank, E., Swartz, H. and Kupfer, D. (2000) Interpersonal and social rhythm therapy: managing the chaos of bipolar disorder. *Biological Psychiatry*, **48**, 593–604.

98. Lam, D.H., Bright, J., Jones, S. *et al.* (2000) Cognitive therapy for bipolar disorder-a pilot study for disorder prevention. *Cognitive Therapy and Research*, **24**, 503–20.

99. Clarkin, J.F., Glick, I., Haas, G. *et al.* (1990) A randomized clinical trial of inpatient family intervention. V. Results for affective disorders. *Journal of Affective Disorders*, **18**, 17–28.

100. Levinson, D.F., Umapathy, C. and Musthaq, M. (1999) Treatment of schizoaffective disorder and schizophrenia with mood symptoms. *The American Journal of Psychiatry*, **156**, 1138–48.

101. Keck, P.E. Jr., Reeves, K., Harrigan, E. *et al.* (1998) Ziprasidone in short term treatment of patients with schizoaffective disorder: results from two double blind placebo controlled, multicenter studies. *Journal of Clinical Psychopharmacology*, **21**, 27–35.

102. Malhotra, S. (2007) Acute and transient psychoses: a paradigmatic approach. *Indian Journal of Psychiatry*, **49**, 233–43.

103. Malhotra, S., Verma, V.K., Misra, A.K. *et al.* (1998) Onset of acute psychotic states in India: a study of sociodemographic, seasonal and biological factors. *Acta Psychiatrica Scandinavica*, **97**, 125–31.

104. Susser, E., Verma, V.K., Malhotra, S. *et al.* (1995) Delineation of acute and transient psychotic illnesses in a developing country setting. *The British Journal of Psychiatry*, **167**, 216–19.

105. Marneros, A., Pillmann, F., Rottig, S. *et al.* (2005) Acute and transient psychotic disorder: an atypical bipolar disorder, in *Bipolar Disorders: Mixed Sates, Rapid cycling and Atypical Forms* (eds A. Marneros and F. Goodwin), Cambridge University Press, pp. 207–51.

106. Patel, J.K., Pinals, D.A. and Breier, A. (2003) Schizophrenia and other psychoses, in *Psychiatry*, 2nd edn (eds A. Tasman, J. Kay and J.A. Lieberman), John Wiley & Sons, West Sussex, pp. 1131–206.

107. Hsiao, M.C., Liu, C.Y., Yang, Y.Y. *et al.* (1999) Delusional disorder: a retrospective analysis of 86 Chinese outpatients. *Psychiatry and Clinical Neurosciences*, **53**, 673–76.

108. Yamada, N., Nakajima, S. and Noguchi, T. (1998) Age at onset of delusional disorder is dependent on the delusional theme. *Acta Psychiatrica Scandinavica*, **97**, 122–24.

109. Srinivasan, T.N., Suresh, T.R., Vasantha, J. *et al.* (1993) Delusional parasitosis in an Indian setting. *Indian Journal of Psychiatry*, **35**, 218–20.

110. Hebbar, S., Ahuja, N. and Chandrasekhar, R. (1999) High prevalence of delusional parasitosis in an Indian setting. *Indian Journal of Psychiatry*, **41**, 136–39.

111. Grover, S., Biswas, P. and Avasthi, A. (2007) Delusional disorder: a study from North India. *Psychiatry and Clinical Neurosciences*, **61** (5), 462–70.

112. Harlow, B.L., Vitonis, A.F., Sparen, P. *et al.* (2007) Incidence of hospitalization for postpartum psychotic and bipolar episodes in women with and without prior prepregnancy or prenatal psychiatric hospitalizations. *Archives of General Psychiatry*, **64** (1), 42–48.

113. Prabhu, R.T., Asokan, T.V. and Rajeshwari, A. (2005) Postpartum psychiatric illness. *Journal of Obstetrics and Gynaecology of India*, **55** (4), 329–32.

114. Irfan, N. and Badar, A. (2008) Determinants and Pattern of Postpartum Psychological Disorders in Hazara Division of Pakistan, http://www.ayubmed.edu.pk/JAMC/PAST/15-3/naveedirfan.htm (accessed March 2008).

115. Kelly, D.L. and Conley, R.R. (2004) Sexuality and schizophrenia. *Schizophrenia Bulletin*, **30**, 4.

116. Seeman, M.V. (2000) Women and schizophrenia: Sexuality. *Medscape Women's Health* **5** (2). (Avaliable online http://www.medscape.com/viewarticle/408915_2)

117. Miller, L.J. (1997) Sexuality, reproduction, and family planning in women with schizophrenia. *Schizophrenia Bulletin*, **23**, 623–35.

118. Raboch, J. (1984) The sexual development and life of female schizophrenia patient. *Archives of Sexual Behavior*, **13** (4), 341–49.

119. Friedman, S. and Harrison, G. (1984) Sexual histories, attitudes and behaviour of schizophrenia and 'normal' women. *Archives of Sexual Behaviour*, **13**, 555–67.

120. Ghadirian, A.M., Chouinard, G. and Annable, L. (1982) Sexual dysfunction and plasma prolactin levels in neuroleptic treated schizophrenic outpatients. *Journal of Nervous and Mental Disease*, **170** (8), 463–67.

121. Thara, R. and Patel, V. (2001) Women's mental health: a public health concern. *Regional Health Forum WHO South-East Asia Region*, **5** (1), 24–33.

122. Nicholson, J., Sweeney, E.M. and Geller, J.L. (1998) Mothers with mental illness: I. The competing demands of parenting and living with mental illness. *Psychiatric Services*, **49** (5), 635–42.

123. Craig, E.A. (2004) Parenting programs for women with mental illness who have young children: a review. *The Australian and New Zealand Journal of Psychiatry*, **38** (11–12), 923–28.

2

Depression and anxiety among women

Nadia Kadri and Khadija Mchichi Alami

Ibn Rushd University Psychiatric Centre, Casablanca, Morocco

2.1 Introduction

Women are at least twice as likely as men to suffer from depression and anxiety disorders, including unipolar depression, dysthymia, panic disorder, post-traumatic stress disorder, generalised anxiety disorder (GAD), social anxiety disorder and phobias [1, 2]. These sex differences are seen in multiple, diverse countries and cultures, suggesting a biological basis.

On the other hand, several studies have indicated that this vulnerability is closely associated with marital status, work and roles in society. These findings have been replicated worldwide.

2.2 Epidemiology

Epidemiological studies have reported twice as high rates of depression in women compared to men [3]. Similarly, it has been shown that women, more often than men, suffer from anxiety disorders [4] and that the sexes differ in suicidal behaviour [5].

Data from the National Comorbidity Survey (NCS), a population-based epidemiological study, show that the prevalence of a major depressive disorder (MDD) is 21.3% in women and 12.7% in men [3]. This sex gap begins in

Contemporary Topics in Women's Mental Health Edited by Chandra, Herrman, Fisher, Kastrup,
© 2009 John Wiley & Sons, Ltd   Niaz, Rondón and Okasha

adolescence and continues to midlife, approximating the span of the childbearing years in women [3]. Similar female/male prevalence ratios have been documented across different countries and ethnic groups [6]. Data from a cross-national epidemiological study disclose a higher rate of MDD in women in the 10 countries surveyed (United States, Canada, Puerto Rico, France, West Germany, Italy, Lebanon, Taiwan, Korea and New Zealand) [6]. By contrast, lifetime rates of bipolar disorders are more consistent across countries (0.3/100 in Taiwan to 1.5/100 in New Zealand); the sex ratio is nearly equal; and the age at first onset was found earlier than the onset of major depression. In a recent Moroccan population based study which included 6000 subjects, Kadri et al. found that 40% of the sample had at least one mental disorder, according to the Mini International Neuropsychiatric Interview in its Moroccan validated version [7]. Prevalence of depressive disorder was the most important (26.5%) with predominance among women and in rural area while the prevalence of bipolar disorder was equal between the two genders.

Prevalence of anxiety disorders

Although the overall lifetime risk for psychiatric illness is equal in men and women, women have a greater propensity to develop both anxiety disorders and depressions. GAD and post-traumatic stress disorder occur twice as frequently in women as in men: 6.6% vs. 3.6% and 10.4% vs. 5.0%. Women develop panic disorder and simple phobia at rates far exceeding men: 5.0% vs. 2.0% and 15.7% vs. 6.7%, respectively. Although the gender gap for obsessive–compulsive disorder (3.1% in women vs. 2% in men) and social phobia (15.5% in women vs. 11.1% in men) is not as wide, these disorders are still more prevalent in women [8–12] (Figure 2.1).

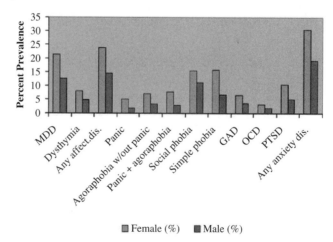

■ Female (%)   ■ Male (%)

Figure 2.1 Lifetime prevalence of depression and anxiety in men and women. Adapted from: Kessler et al. [9, 10]; Robins et al. [13]; Yonkers and Ellison [12]; Halbreich, U. and Kahn, L.S., *Journal of Affective Disorders* **102** (2007) 245–258

Weissman *et al.* [15] in the cross-national epidemiology study of panic disorder in 10 countries including over 40 000 subjects, found that lifetime prevalence rates for panic disorder ranged from 1.4 to 2.9%. Mean age at first onset was usually in early to middle adulthood. The rates were higher in female than male subjects in all countries. Panic disorder was associated with an increased risk of agoraphobia and major depression in all countries. On the other hand, Weissman *et al.* [16] also found a predominance of females in the one-month and six-month prevalence rates of panic disorder in most countries.

In Morocco, two studies were conducted in the general population showing that anxiety disorders are frequent and prevalent among females [17, 18].

Prevalence of depressive disorders

Women have a twofold greater risk for recurrent unipolar depressive disorder and MDD in general, as compared with men [19–22]. The sex difference is also supported by the NCS [16, 17] which found higher lifetime estimates for MDD (21% in women and 13% in men) with a preserved 2 : 1 women to men difference (Figure 2.1). Epidemiological studies from other countries including Switzerland [14, 23], Canada [24] and Germany [25], all report that women are at least twice as likely as men to suffer from MDD. In addition to MDD, dysthymic disorder occurs more often in women. Rates for dysthymic disorder in women and men were reported to be 4.1 and 2.2%, respectively [20]. In the NCS, the rates for dysthymic disorder were similarly skewed, with 8% women in 5% of men suffering from the illness [9, 10].

Comorbidity of depressions and anxiety disorders among women

Comorbidity between depressions and anxiety, particularly GAD and MDD is very common in both men and women [26–28]. In fact, some researchers argue that the majority of depression cases are not 'pure' [29] and that comorbid depression and anxiety may be the norm rather than the exception [30–32]. Several studies have reported that patients with comorbid anxiety and depression have poorer outcomes than those with either anxiety or depression alone [27–29]. Data derived from the Netherlands Mental Health Survey and Incidence Study (N = 7076) documented that in general population, comorbid anxiety disorders and mood disorders defined as depression, dysthymia, bipolar disorder were the most prevalent conditions [33]. Female gender, younger age, lower educational level and unemployment were associated with comorbid anxiety and mood disorders – but not with pure mood disorders. Women were more likely than men to have a pure anxiety disorder and anxiety – comorbid mood disorder, while men were more likely to have a substance use disorder either pure or comorbid. The prevalence of comorbid anxiety and mood disorders was 5.1% for females, and 1.9% for males while the prevalence for pure anxiety disorders was 10.7% for females, 4.7% for males. Compared to men, women have a documented higher frequency of comorbid depression and anxiety disorders, as well as coexisting anxiety disorders [12, 34–38]. The NCS reported that over half of all lifetime psychiatric disorders were concentrated among 14% of the population with a history of three or more comorbid disorders – and that the prevalence of both lifetime and 12 month comorbidity of three or more disorders was higher among women than men [9, 10]. The lifetime odds ratio of having ≥3 comorbid disorders was 1.24 for women vs. men; the 12 month odds ratio for ≥ comorbid disorders was 1.55 for women vs. men. The Zürich Cohort Study found that women had higher rates in nearly all categories of threshold and subthreshold level anxiety and depression – particularly those involving comorbidity of above threshold depression and anxiety [14, 39–41]. Female to male sex difference was far greater for comorbid anxiety and depression than for pure forms of these disorders [41]. The odds ratio (female to male) was 1.8 for threshold anxiety and threshold depression; and 2.4 for threshold depression and subthreshold anxiety while for pure depression and pure anxiety, there was almost no sex difference [41]. Another study, [14] confirms prior reports on the higher prevalence of comorbid depression and anxiety among women, as compared to men, in nearly all categories of threshold and sub-threshold depression and anxiety, females had higher rates – particularly those reflecting comorbidity (Figure 2.2).

Community studies have suggested that anxiety disorders often precede the onset of MDD [42, 43]. Breslau *et al.* [35] conducted a longitudinal epidemiological study to determine whether a relationship exists between sex, prior anxiety and MDD; and whether sex differences in rates of prior anxiety disorders might explain the observed sex differences in the prevalence rates for MDD. A significant part of the observed sex difference in the rate of MDD could be accounted for by

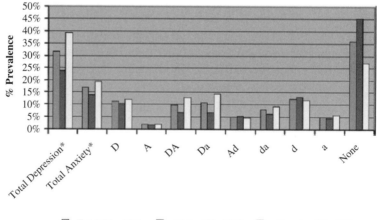

■ Total (N = 591) ■ Males (N = 292) □ Females (N = 299)

Figure 2.2 Depressions and anxieties in females and males. Classification code: D = DSM-III major depressive disorder. d = Subthreshold depressive syndrome. A = DSM-III panic disorder or GAD. a = Subthreshold anxiety syndrome. Adapted from: Preisig *et al.* [14]

prior anxiety disorder [35, 44]. Cumulative percentages begin to diverge at age 12, and by age 14 the proportions with a history of MDD were 1.3% in males and 3.1% in females. By age 10, 17% of females already had a history of any anxiety disorder, compared to 8% of males.

These results confirm that depression and some anxiety disorders are the most prevalent psychiatric conditions in non-clinical and clinical populations with a high female to male ratio. Several hypotheses were proposed to explain this phenomenon [45]:

1. Women may often seek help more than men for an equal prevalence of a given disorder.

2. Biological differences between men and women may account for some of the higher prevalence. The years of greatest risk of depression in women coincide roughly with the period between menarche and menopause. Moreover, reproductive events, particularly child birth, are robustly related to depressive symptoms and disorders [46, 47]. Careful prospective research has also confirmed that up to 10% of women meet criteria for premenstrual dysphoric disorder (PMDD). Women with PMDD are at higher risk for other mood disorders, suggesting a common factor in all of them [48–50]. Gender differences in depression hence could also be explained by hormonal factors. Oestrogen and progesterone may be the common factors contributing to women's vulnerability to depression, although the nature of this link is not clear. Disturbance of thyroid function, which is four to five times more common in women than men [51], may also contribute to the excess rate of depression in women. Another phase in which women experience great hormonal change occurs at menopause. However, there is no peak in the rate of MDD at the biological menopause.

3. Social effects of life stress, social vulnerability factors, absence of support and of women's role in society.

4. A difference in direction of distress depending on social factors such as family structure, social role and gender difference expectation [52, 53]. For example, Winokur [52] described a depressive spectrum disease, in which women tend to have depression, while male family members present with alcoholism and antisocial personality instead. Men may direct their distress in different directions.

2.3 Transcultural aspects of affective disturbances in sub-Saharan Africa

Depression may be defined in different languages by different cultures. In South Africa and many other contexts it may be referred to as 'the nerves', in East Timor as 'wind blowing through one's body' while in western countries it may be described as 'yuppie flu'. Acknowledging the fact that people throughout the world may have variable terminology for depression is not the same as the exoticising of Africa and other countries in the developing world. The danger is that when limitations are found in existing diagnostic and screening instruments that they are then discarded. There is no doubt that instruments need to be culturally sensitive, but there is also sufficient data from Africa that when people are sensitively and intensively questioned, even when people present with multiple somatic complaints, it is possible to assess mood. What is required is a clear understanding of the specific cultural terminology used, and sensitivity to the context within which presentation occurs.

Regardless of varying cultural manifestations of distress, the extent to which different idioms of distress are indicative of depression, anxiety, cultural meaning making or normative adaptation in adverse conditions are all ultimately empirical questions. Clearly, both qualitative and quantitative research skills are needed in order to develop a full understanding of the presentation and prevalence of affective disorders in women in sub-Saharan Africa, as well as risk factors for disorder, and models of the most appropriate care. Patel's [54] careful study of common mental disorders in Zimbabwe is something of a model in this regard, combining both epidemiological and anthropological approaches. More work using multiple methods is required, with a particular focus on risk and protective factors, about which we still know relatively little from a gender perspective. In particular, given indications that abuse of women is a major issue in sub-Saharan Africa [55], it would be helpful to know whether the relationship between abuse and affective disorder which has been found in women in USA [56], for example, is replicated in an African context.

2.4 Treatment effects

If gender roles deserve more attention in anxiety disorder therapies, it is not reflected in the research literature on treatment. In Europe, 26.1% of individuals with any anxiety disorder used formal health services, and among those, 30.8% received only drug treatment, 19.6% only psychological treatment and 26.5% a combination [8]. None of these percentages were specified for men and women separately. Empirical researches on the influence of sex/gender on treatment appear to be rare. Most of the 33 studies identified in the literature search that initially seemed relevant appeared to avoid sex/gender-specific analyses, although they provided data about sex distribution within the sample. Consequently, it remains unclear whether no sex-specific effects were found or whether the researchers omitted a comparison of the effects for both sexes. Table 2.1 shows the findings of the four studies examining the influence of gender on anxiety treatment. Two studies reported that sertraline was more effective than placebo in both women and men when used to treat panic disorder (PD) [57] or GAD [58]. According to Clayton *et al.*, this is in contrast with earlier findings that women may have a worse prognosis and a somewhat lower short-term treatment response than do men. In the PD study, women improved more than men did in panic frequency and time spent worrying about having a panic attack,

Table 2.1 Overview of studies on the influence of gender on anxiety treatment of adults

Author	Type of disorder	Type of treatment	Sample	Method	Instrument	Results
Clayton *et al.* [62]	PD with/without agoraphobia	Sertraline	F (n = 338); M (n = 335)	RCT, double-blind	HAM-A; CGH; PDSS; POMS; Q-LES-Q	Sertraline exceeded Placebo; women profited more than men
Steiner *et al.* [63]	GAD	Sertraline	Sertraline (n = 182) F:M = 59%:41% Placebo (n = 188) F:M = 51%:49%	RCT, double-blind RA	HAM-A; CGH	Sertraline exceeded placebo; no sex differences
Cottone *et al.* [64]	AD	CBT or psychodynamic gender therapy	Patients (N = 46) F:M = unknown therapists (N = 89)	RA	STAI	Men withdrew more often, showed more symptom reduction and profited more with woman therapist
Stewart *et al.* [65]	OCD	Intensive residential therapy	(N = 476) F:M = 58.7%:41.3% Age: M = 32.5 yr	MRA models (scatter plots); multiple RA	Y-BOCS; WSA; SOS-10; PGI	Female gender predicts decrease in complaints

PD = panic disorder; F = female; M = male; RCT = randomised, controlled trial; HAM-A = Hamilton Anxiety Scale; CGI = Clinical Global Impression-Improvement; PDSS = Panic Disorder Severity Scale; POMS = Profile of Mood States; Q-LES-Q = Quality of Life, Enjoyment and Satisfaction Scale; GAD = generalised anxiety disorder; AD = anxiety disorder; CBT = cognitive-behavioural therapy; RA = regression analysis; STAI = State-Trait Anxiety Inventory; OCD = obsessive-compulsive disorder; MRA = multiple regression analysis; Y-BOCS = Yale-Brown Obsessive-Compulsive Scale; WSA = Work and Social Adjustment Scale; SOS-10 = Schwarz Outcome Scale-10; PGI = Patient Global Impression Scale.

but this may be due partly to a lower placebo response in men. It should be noted that there were no sex differences in the other outcome measures. Cottone *et al.* [59] focused on the role of gender (for clients, therapists and psychotherapy dyads) in the reduction of symptoms and the duration of therapy in CBT or psychodynamic therapy. No sex differences occurred for the duration of therapy. However, male clients were more likely to withdraw from therapy after the initial intake assessment. If they participated, they showed a greater reduction of trait and state anxiety symptoms than did women. Additional searches performed for sex-specific studies of CBT in general (i.e. not specifically connected to anxiety disorders) did not yield new or relevant information. Subsequently, 36 meta-analyses encompassing treatment of anxiety disorders that were published after 1995 were manually reviewed for possible sex/gender information. Three relevant publications emerged reporting sex in relation to prevalence and demographics [60, 61]. These analyses of controlled trials examining anxiety disorders reported, at minimum, the sex distribution of the study participants: 60.2, 60 and 72.2% women, respectively.

Gould *et al.* [60] found that CBT and pharmacotherapy did not differ significantly in effect size for anxiety severity, but CBT was comparatively more effective for depression severity and maintenance of treatment gains. One study examined self-help interventions (e.g. books, audio/videotapes and computer/Internet-based programmes) [61]. According to the effect sizes, the effectiveness of self-help was higher than for control groups without treatment but lower than for therapist-directed interventions. Given the sex distribution of their sample (72.2% women), these findings relate mainly to women. Unfortunately, however, a check for sex differences was missing.

2.5 Sex differences in depression and anxiety disorders: Biological determinants

Sex differences in stress responses

Abnormalities in the regulation of the hypothalamic–pituitary adrenal axis and the sympathoadrenomedullary system have been identified in depression and anxiety disorders, and these disorders are clearly precipitated and exacerbated by stress [66]. Evidence from animal studies to date suggests that females are relatively resistant to the behavioural and neurobiological effects of acute and chronic stress.

For example, although chronic stress over 21 days produces reversible atrophy of apical dendrites of hippocampal pyramidal neurons in males [67], this effect is not seen in females [68]. Similarly, repeated swim stress over 30 days decreased CA3 and CA4 pyramidal cell number in gonadectomised male rats, but not in females [62].

Parallel results were found in a study of male and female vervet monkeys subjected to chronic social stress [63]. Males also had higher stress-induced c-fos gene expression in several brain areas compared to proestrus and diestrus females [64].

Consistent with these sex differences in structural responses to chronic stress, female rats do not show the impairment of spatial memory or object recognition memory after chronic restraint stress that is characteristic of males [65].

One way to reconcile relative resistance of females to neurobiological effects of stress with increased prevalence of affective illness in women is to consider the stress-induced neurobiological changes in males as adaptive, potentially preventing subsequent development of depression and anxiety symptoms.

Effects of reproductive hormones

Compared to men, women are subject to greater fluxes in reproductive hormones across the lifespan. Changes in reproductive hormones in utero, during puberty, the oestrus cycle, pregnancy and menopause clearly alter brain structure and function, and are likely to play a role in the increased prevalence of affective disorders in women. HPA (hypothalamic pituitary axis) responsiveness increases [69] and glucocorticoid feedback sensitivity [70] and brain GABA Gamma Amino Butyric Acid content decreases [71] in the luteal phase of the menstrual cycle, potentially destabilising these homeostatic systems in vulnerable women [70, 72]. In addition, both catecholamine and HPA axis stress response systems are suppressed during pregnancy [71, 73] and lactation [74, 75]. Several brain neurochemical systems known to modulate anxiety and fear, including oxytocin, prolactin, norepinephrine and GABA, appear to be altered in parallel during pregnancy and lactation [76]. Rapid weaning or lack of breastfeeding postpartum may precipitate more rapid decreases in these anxiolytic hormones, destabilising stress responses and exacerbating anxiety and depression symptoms.

Sex differences in the serotonin 1A receptor and serotonin transporter binding in the human brain measured by PET-SCAN

A growing body of evidence suggests major differences in brain structure, function and neurochemistry between healthy women and men [77]. Furthermore, women and men differ in serotonin associated psychiatric conditions, such as depression, anxiety and suicide [78, 79]. Of the biomarkers in the serotonin system, serotonin1A (5-HT1A) receptor is implicated in depression and anxiety and is a target for selective serotonin reuptake inhibitors, psychotropic drugs used in the treatment of these disorders.

A study conducted by Karolinska Institut, Department of Clinical Neuroscience, Psychiatry Section and the Department of Woman and Child Health, Stockholm, Sweden [80] found that compared to men, women had significantly higher 5-HT1A receptor and lower 5-HTT binding potentials in a wide array of cortical and subcortical brain regions. In women, there was a positive correlation between 5-HT1A receptor and 5-HTT binding potentials for the region of hippocampus. Sex differences in 5-HT1A receptor and 5-HTT binding potentials may reflect biological distinctions in the serotonin system contributing to sex differences in the prevalence of psychiatric disorders such as depression and anxiety.

2.6 Sex differences in depression and anxiety disorders: Social factors

The condition of women varies depending on the country, its policy and extent of opening towards universal human values. This variation can be found in the same country depending on whether it's a rural or urban area and it can change in the same city from one neighbourhood to another. But in general, women have an unequal social status with men, despite the major role they play in family and community tasks, in reproduction and in procreation.

Conditions of women's lives

Epidemiological studies conducted since the beginning of the twentieth century have shown an inverse relationship between socio-economic status and the occurrence of a variety of mental disorders [81–84].

These community population studies found that two-thirds of depressive patients are women, and that depression is the most prevalent disorder in women [85–87]. Factors linked to this finding are the lack of confidence, absence of child rearing assistance, employment, economic problems and chronic stressful conditions [88–92].

Multiple roles: Double shift

Since 1950, the number of women in western countries with paid employment increased significantly. In some Arab countries also, the number of employed women is steadily increasing year after year. In spite of this active contribution to the finances of the family income, there has been no significant change in the domestic division of labour. Women, at least 90% of them, still do the housework and childcare. In daily life, when a couple comes back home from work, the woman has to deal with the children and housework while the man has to rest from his fatiguing day.

Moreover, the reproductive life of women is a source of stress; to be pregnant, and having children to take care of contribute to her professional deterioration, and have, in general, a negative effect on her professional career. Moreover, women are sometimes paid less than men for the same work, and many of them suffer from sexual harassment at the workplace. From all these facts, we can see that a married woman who is professionally active has more sources of stress and discomfort than a man.

Marital status and number of children

The relationship between marital status and mental health has been well documented in western countries [93, 94]. Subjects with the best mental health would be employed married men, while those who have the worst mental health are the married unemployed women. Children are therefore a negative factor in this respect. These data were also confirmed in Arab countries. Weissman *et al.* [21] found that persons who were separated or divorced had significantly higher rates of major depression than married persons in most of the countries, and the risk was somewhat greater for divorced or separated men than women in most countries. For Mouchtaq [95] the typical profile of a depressive woman was a married one, a housewife, not educated, having a low socio-economical position, with several life stressors preceding the episode (marital conflict, repudiation, marriage of the partner, grief).

For housewives, other social factors can be found. Men have two sources of gratification, work and family while the wife has only the family. Childcare and housework can often be frustrating activities and the role of a housewife is invisible, not structured and not rewarded.

A study conducted by Plaisier *et al.* [96] examined the association of work and family roles with the prevalence of depression and anxiety disorders, and whether these social roles could explain the female preponderance in the prevalence of depression and anxiety disorders. Concerning their mental health, authors expected that men may profit more from certain social roles than women. This was particularly supported by the results regarding the work role. Both having a job and working full-time were associated with a lower prevalence of depression and anxiety disorders among men, but not among women, supported by significant gender interaction terms. The results showed that the associations of the partner role and the parent role with anxiety and depressive disorders were consistent for men and women. Thus, for both genders, the partner role was a strong protective factor for mental health, but the parent role did not have such a pronounced effect. On the other hand, they found two significant associations of role combinations with anxiety and depressive disorders among women. First, an increased prevalence of depression and anxiety was found among women with children but without a partner. Secondly, the effect of the work role was positive for women's mental health when they had no children, but not among those with children. Both men and women had a better mental health when they had more social roles.

Impact of physical and sexual violence

Ideally, the family provides an area of security and stability of mental health. In reality, it is 'the most frequent single locus of violence of all types' as Hillberman stated [97]. While the extra familial violence is recognised and publicly condemned, the one inside the family is hidden and considered by many as private and legitimate.

It's undeniable that women are the first victims of physical and sexual harassment. According to several authors [98, 99] the victims of sexual violence have significantly more psychiatric disturbances than non-victims. These disturbances are depression, anxiety and somatisation.

In the University Psychiatric Centre Ibn Rushd, Casablanca, Morocco, a study conducted on violence and depression has shown that 44% of depressive subjects suffered during their childhood from one form or another of violence (physical or sexual) vs 8% of control subjects [100]. In a Moroccan population based study on sexual abuse in a sample of 800 women Mchichi Alami and Kadri found that victims of sexual abuse during childhood and adolescence were at higher risk of depression, anxiety and sexual dysfunction [101].

In addition to these shared factors, others are specific to some conditions such as Muslim and Arab countries. In some of these societies, having a girl might be less desirable than a boy. For this phenomenon several reasons are evoked: the protective role played by the boy towards his mother and sisters when the father dies concerning inheritance; the non-possibility for the girl to perpetuate the name of the family across generations and finally a belief that by the nature of her gender, the girl is able to break social law and taboos, and bring the disgrace upon herself.

Zurayk *et al.* [102] reviewed key health problems of women in the Arab countries. She stressed the relevant context in which Arab women live: lingering illiteracy rates, lack of access to cash income and increasing poverty. Reproductive health is reviewed within this context pointing to trends of delayed marriage and declining fertility in some countries while other countries maintain high levels. The socio-cultural context is found to be particularly relevant regarding pregnancy and childbirth, menopause and violence against women, particularly female circumcision.

The right to education

Women are still the majority among victims of illiteracy. In many Arab countries, it affects more than 70% of them. In several studies this factor gives a risk of morbidity.

In our countries, especially in rural areas, girls are sent to school less than boys. The major reasons are economical or cultural.

Traditional marriage

Traditional marriage remains common in many Arab countries. It is defined as an arranged marriage often with cousins or with someone never met before consumption, or a forced marriage and rarely, a marriage preceded by a short period of courtship.

Chaleby [103] conducted a prospective study of 150 consecutive outpatients who were either married or divorced. Discord was found to be more likely to happen when the couple had never met before or when there had been a period of courtship. This was more likely to be associated with anxiety and dysthymic disorders and to affect females more. Polygamy was a definite stress. The consanguineous marriage had a higher rate of marital discord than the non-consanguineous, but this was found not to be statistically significant. In 40% of discordant, consanguineous marriages the discord was directly related to the degree of consanguinity.

Effects of polygamy

The practise of polygamy, although varying from culture to culture, is widespread in many areas of the world. In all Arab Muslim countries, except Tunisia, the Muslim man is allowed to have four spouses at the same time. Although sociologists and anthropologists, as well as common sense, have suggested that a polygamous marriage may have a negative effect on the wives involved, an extensive literature search failed to discover any research examining this situation.

Chaleby [104] found that the percentage of wives of polygamous marriages was significantly greater in the inpatient psychiatric population than in the general population of Kuwait. In addition, the results suggested a relationship between the nature of psychiatric disorder and the marital situation.

Sexuality

Sexuality has various aspects including biological, cultural, medical, forensic, ethical, social, psychological and psychiatric perspectives. It needs a multidisciplinary approach. It is well known that in the sexual field, disorders are of high frequency, leading to burden and handicap. As a matter of fact, sexuality has a large impact on women's mental health [105]. This aspect is amplified in societies in which the only authorised frame for sexuality is married housewife, not educated, having a low socio-economical condition, with several life stressors preceding the episode (marital conflict and where the single mothers have very stressful and hidden lives which interfere negatively with their mental health).

Effect of female circumcision

Female circumcision is a deeply rooted traditional practise that adversely affects the health of girls and women. At present, it is estimated that over 120 million girls and women have undergone some form of genital mutilation and that 2 million girls per year are at risk of being circumcised. Most of the girls and women affected live in African countries where the prevalence of genital mutilation is estimated to range from 5 to 98%.

Dirie *et al.* [106] conducted a study on female circumcision in Somalia. They investigated 200 Somalian women. One hundred per cent of these women were circumcised, despite their relatively high socio-economic status as shown by their educational level. Eighty-eight per cent of them had been circumcised, with excision and infibulation. The majority of these women justified the practise of female circumcision through religious reasons and all were willing to circumcise their daughters.

Lightfoot [107] interviewed over 400 Sudanese women and men in all walks of life on the physical, emotional and psychosexual effects of female genital circumcision and infibulation. He found that the adverse psychological effects of this practise on women were mitigated by a strong conviction that its performance purifies and ennobles them. Sudanese women said that they were able to experience orgasm in spite of their genital mutilation.

In Dorkenoo's opinion [108], the elimination of female genital mutilation will not only improve women's and children's health; it will also promote gender equity and women's empowerment in the communities where the practise persists.

2.7 Mood and anxiety disorders across lifespan in women

Menstrual cycle

This biological phenomenon has been the subject of myths and taboos within and among various cultures. These myths distort the reality surrounding menstruation and create ambivalent feelings about the value and usefulness of this function outside of its necessity as a means of reproduction. Thus, studies concerning menstruation need to take into account cultural and psychosocial factors that define the meaning, values and behaviour associated with this biological phenomenon.

Premenstrual syndrome (PMS) encompasses a variety of symptoms appearing during the luteal phase of the menstrual cycle. Although PMS is widely recognised, the aetiology remains unclear and it lacks definitive, universally accepted diagnostic criteria [109].

Prevalence of PMS/PMDD

The American College of Obstetricians and Gynaecologists states that as many as 20–40% of women of reproductive age experience difficulties during the period just preceding menstruation [110]. Such difficulties include depressed mood, irritability, anxiety and emotional lability [111]. Roughly 210% of women report a severe disruption of work or interpersonal relationships during the luteal phase of their menstrual cycle, thereby meeting the Diagnostic and Statistical Manual of Mental Disorders, Fourth Edition, criteria for PMDD – a condition more severe than PMS [110, 112].

Adewuya et al. [113] found the prevalence of PMDD amongst sub-Saharan Africans was 6.1%, comparable to that in western cultures. In this study, the correlates included older age, painful menstruation and high score on neuroticism scale. The presence of pain may cause distress and aggravate the emotional and behavioural response to such menstrual symptomatology. Compared with participants without PMDD, participants with PMDD have significantly higher rates for the following psychiatric diagnoses: dysthymia, MDD, panic disorder and GAD.

In a study conducted by Kh Mchichi Alami *et al.* in a Moroccan based population the same prevalence of symptoms of PMS and PMDD were found as in western countries [114].

Changes in the balance of sex hormones

PMS occurs during the luteal phase (progesterone) of a woman's cycle and disappears during the follicular phase (oestrogen). Hence, it has been theorised that hormonal fluctuations contribute to mood changes [115].

A strong similarity has been found among affects reported during the premenstrual period, during menopause, and as a side effect of oral contraceptives – a similarity that has been interpreted as providing support for the existence of a biological component of the depression that can occur at such times [116]. This idea is supported by the fact that the syndrome is absent during anovulatory cycles [117].

Role of serotonin

During the past decade, many reports have shown that the neurotransmitter serotonin may be involved in the pathophysiology of PMDD [118, 119]. Although there are as yet no clear findings suggesting that patients with PMDD differ from controls with respect to brain serotonergic activity, the indirect evidence supporting an involvement of serotonin is very strong [115]:

1. Animal experiments have established that brain serotonergic neurons mainly modulate aspects of behaviour that are also regulated by sex steroids [78]. Women with PMDD have been assumed to be under serotonergic control [119].

2. It is known that oestrogen, progesterone and testosterone influence brain serotonergic activity [120, 121].

3. Women with PMDD differ from controls with respect to a number of biological markers believed to reflect brain serotonergic transmission. These include platelet monoamine oxidase activity [122]; density of serotonin transporters in platelets [123]; ratios between the dopamine metabolite, homovanillic acid and the serotonin metabolite; 5-hydroxyindoleacetic acid in the cerebrospinal fluid [124] and serotonin-mediated release of prolactin [122].

4. The most cogent argument for involvement of serotonergic neurons in the pathophysiology of PMDD is the fact that pharmacologic agents facilitating brain serotonergic transmission effectively relieve PMDD symptoms in most patients [125].

2.8 Pregnancy

Although the idea of having a baby is an important and happy event in the life of a couple and family, pregnancy represents a critical moment in women's lives. For most of them, it is a stressor. Maladaptation leads to personal distress and threatens the integration in the family unit.

Depression and anxiety during pregnancy

It has been shown that the prevalence of depression during pregnancy is approximately 25–35%, with about 10% of women meeting the criteria for an MDD (equal to that in nonpregnant women) [126, 127]. Depressive symptoms most commonly occur during the first or third trimester.

Kh Mchichi Alami *et al.* conducted a follow up study among 100 women from the first trimester of pregnancy to nine months after delivery. They found that 19.2% of the pregnant women experienced a depression with positive association to psychosocial variables [128].

Bipolar disorders

The course of illness is not well determined during pregnancy. In our daily practise, patients might be stable throughout the whole pregnancy, have a recurrence of their depressive or manic state before or after delivery. In all cases very close monitoring is necessary. In the happiest cases all medications have to be withdrawn, or at least during the first trimester. But in the field patients need support: medical (antipsychotic, antidepressant, mood stabiliser) and psychotherapeutical. In our experience, group therapy with cognitive behavioural treatment is of great help. It allows patients to be seen as closely as need, to acquire the psychological means for monitoring their mood, and cognitions and to detect the smallest symptoms for a possible relapse. On the other hand psycho education is known to be very efficient in the field of bipolar disorder.

Anxiety disorders

Various courses of anxiety disorders are seen during pregnancy

Obsessive compulsive disorder might have its onset or worsen during pregnancy [129–131]. There is no case of post traumatic stress disorder observed regarding the period of labour or delivery even if these moments are painful and potentially dangerous. This fact begs a question: how are women protected against PTSD during these phases?

Regarding specific fears, the following were shown: a fear of delivery variable in intensity, a fear of death during delivery, fear of having a baby with various malformations. These fears have to be integrated in the whole story of the pregnant woman and need to be managed psychotherapeutically.

In all cases, the impact of stress in pregnancy on foetal outcome was widely explored:

- Prenatal life event stress might lead to a diminished birth weight of 55 g per event.

- 32% relative risk low birth weight (<2500 g).

- Prenatal maternal anxiety might lead to an incremental diminution in gestational age at delivery by three days/point.

- A positive association was shown between foetal growth and perceived social support [132–134].

For all these reasons, treating these patients is crucial to allow the mother and her baby to enjoy good mental and physical health. Regarding the treatment option, a question has to be discussed: What makes treating pregnant patients different from treating a non pregnant woman? Various aspects have to be considered in this case:

- Two individuals whose welfare must be considered.
- Any distress or illness affecting mother has the potential to affect the foetus.
- Treatment given to mother may have a direct impact on the foetus.
- It may have a conflict between the state of mother and foetus.

Thus, there is a considerable risk to the mother and the foetus of not treating depression during pregnancy. In mild-to-moderate cases, psychotherapy must be considered, and if an antidepressant must be used, it is advisable to wait until after the first trimester [135]. Clinicians have to take into account mother/foetus and be able to manage the treatment by balancing the advantages and inconvenience of each therapeutical decision.

2.9 Motherhood

Postpartum blues

A short-lived cluster of depressive symptoms often occurs in new mothers during the first two weeks after delivery [136]. It requires recognition, explanation, empathy and support. In our culture, women in childbirth are well supported by the other family members and the community (importance of neighbours).

Postpartum depression

Several studies were conducted in Arab countries to explore this disorder, and to compare it to the western data. Abou Saleh and Ghubash in the UAE [137, 138] found in the early postpartum a prevalence of psychiatric morbidity of 24% according to self report, of which 18% were of a depressive nature. In Morocco, Agoub *et al.* [139] in a prospective study of 120 women followed up during nine months after the childbirth in Casablanca, found that the prevalence of postpartum depression was 18.7%. A second study found a prevalence of 17% of depression during postpartum. In this group, 19.2% started their episode during pregnancy [140].

The two studies found a significant association with obstetrical and perinatal complications, life events, quality of relationship with the partner, psychiatric antecedents and primiparity. In all cases the impact of depression on the child might be severe including poor orienting skills, a decrease of motor tone, low activity levels, right EEG asymmetry (left hypofrontality), reflex, excitability, withdrawal clusters on the Brazelton scale [141–143].

Menopause

Menopause is a biologically induced event, which is specific to our species [144]. The menopause is defined literally as 'suspension of menstruation'. Naturally, women cease menstruation between the ages of 50 and 52 years on average. With the increase of life expectancy, women can expect to live more than a third of their lives beyond menopause. It should not be considered only from a physiological point of view as a hormonal imbalance without taking into account its psychological and social aspects.

Perimenopause is the period during which the transition from regular ovarian cycles to complete cessation of menstruation takes place. Absence of menses for 12 or more months denotes menopause. Demographic studies show that in 1990, there were 467 million postmenopausal women in the world. Population projections on the basis of these demographic studies predict that by the year 2030, the number of postmenopausal women will increase to 1.2 billion [145]. At this time, approximately 47 million women will be entering menopause each year. The median age of menopause in the Massachusetts Women's Health Study of 2570 women was 51.3 years [145]. Symptoms include, hot flushes, night sweats, headaches, vaginal dryness, sleep disturbances, fatigue, irritability and changes in appetite and libido. Factors that affect vulnerability to depression during menopause include: marital status, educational background, socioeconomic status, race, smoking, exposure to toxic substances, nutrition and history of previous depression [146].

The relationship between menopause and depressive and anxious symptoms is controversial. This relationship is mostly seen by gynaecologists. Women who often consult them have a higher prevalence of psychiatric morbidity [147, 148]. It was shown that the women who are the most disturbed during menopause had a higher prevalence of depression during pregnancy and menstruation phase [149]. However, this association was not confirmed in global population studies [150]. Most recent studies have demonstrated that the pre-menopause was more critical than menopause it self. The symptoms experienced are: insomnia, irritability, fatigue, lack of self esteem, anxiety, disturbance of memory and difficulties of concentration.

Kadri and Zarbib [151] explored the menopause in Moroccan and Tunisian samples, matched by age, level of education and socio-economical status. For the Moroccan sample, the highest prevalence score of depression and anxiety was found in pre-menopause (58.3% of anxiety and 48% of depression) while in the Tunisian group the highest prevalence happened during menopause (37.5% of anxiety and 37% of depression). The two groups reported a decline of their sexual activity. This study found, in accordance with literature that the complaints were significantly prevalent in women with low level of education and in women who were less informed about changes expected to happen in menopause [152].

In fact, biological reality is the same for all women around the globe. The real change is in the manner the woman perceives and lives her femininity, her fertility, her ageing, the kind of link she has with her environment, family, men and in general how she perceives and looks upon her body, her health and pain. For the anecdote, the translation of the term 'menopause' in Arabic language is 'the age of despair'!

2.10 Conclusion

Women are more prone than men to depression and anxiety and this increased vulnerability has been ascribed to events arising from changes in the endocrine control of the reproductive system. These changes occur during the menstrual cycle (PMS and PMDD), after parturition (postpartum depression) and during the menopause (perimenopausal and menopausal syndrome). Because the serious mood disorders that sometimes accompany these syndromes cannot be explained by changes in sex hormone balance alone, increasing attention has been given to the notion that women who develop these disorders are, for various reasons (psychosocial and/or metabolic), especially susceptible to changes in hormonal balance, which in turn are believed to affect the activity of certain neuronal systems (particularly the serotonin-specific ones). This interpretation is favoured by evidence indicating the existence of a powerful effect of the sex hormones on serotonin-specific neurotransmitter function, and on mood.

References

1. Regier, D., Narrow, W., Rae, D. *et al.* (1993) The de facto mental and addictive disorders service system. Epidemiologic catchment area prospective 1-year prevalence rates of disorders and services. *Archives of General Psychiatry*, **50**, 85–94.

2. Kessler, R., McGonagle, K., Zhao, S. *et al.* (1994) Life-time and 12-month prevalence of DSM-III-R psychiatric disorders in the United States. *Archives of General Psychiatry*, **51**, 8–19.

3. Kessler, R.C., McGonagle, K.A., Swartz, M. *et al.* (1993) Sex and depression in the National Comorbidity Survey. 1: lifetime prevalence, chronicity and recurrence. *Journal of Affective Disorders*, **29**, 85–96.

4. Pigott, T.A. (1999) Gender differences in the epidemiology and treatment of anxiety disorders. *Journal of Clinical Psychiatry*, **60** (Suppl 18), 4–15.

5. Lewinsohn, P.M., Rohde, P., Seeley, J.R. *et al.* (2001) Gender differences in suicide attempts from adolescence to young adulthood. *Journal of the American Academy of Child and Adolescent Psychiatry*, **40**, 427–34.

6. Weissman, M.M., Bland, R.C., Canino, G.J. *et al.* (1996) Cross-national epidemiology of major depression and bipolar disorder. *The Journal of the American Medical Association*, **276**, 293–99.

7. Kadri, N., Agoub, M., El Gnaoui, S. *et al.* (2005) Moroccan colloquial Arabic version of the Mini International Neuropsychiatric Interview (MINI): qualitative and quantitative validation. *European Psychiatry*, **20**, 193–95.

8. Kessler, R.C. (1995) Epidemiology of psychiatric comorbidity, in *Textbook in Psychiatric Epidemiology* (eds M.T. Tsuang, M. Tohan and G.E.P. Zahner), John Wiley & Sons, Inc., New York, pp. 179–97.

9. Kessler, R.C., McGonagle, K.A., Nelson, C.B. *et al.* (1994a) Sex and depression in the National Comorbidity Survey. II: cohort effects. *Journal of Affective Disorders*, **30**, 15–26.

10. Kessler, R.C., McGonagle, K.A., Zhao, S. *et al.* (1994b) Lifetime and 12-month prevalence of DSM-III-R psychiatric disorders in the United States. Results from the National Comorbidity Survey. *Archives of General Psychiatry*, **51**, 8–19.

11. Wittchen, H.U. and Hoyer, J. (2001) Generalized anxiety disorder: nature and course. *Journal of Clinical Psychiatry*, **62**, 15–19; discussion 20–21.

12. Yonkers, K.A. and Ellison, J.M. (1996) Anxiety disorders in women and their pharmacological treatment, in *Psychopharmacology and Women* (eds M.F. Jensvold, U. Halbreich and J.A. Hamilton), American Psychiatric Press, Washington, DC, pp. 261–85.

13. Robins, L.N., Helzer, J.E., Weissman, M.M., Orvaschel, H., Gruenberg, E., Burke, J.D., Jr, Regier, D.A. (1984) Lifetime prevalence of specific psychiatric disorders in three sites. *Arch Gen Psychiatry*. Oct, **41** (10), 949–58.

14. Preisig, M., Merikangas, K.R. and Angst, J. (2001) Clinical significance and comorbidity of subthreshold depression and anxiety in the community. *Acta Psychiatrica Scandinavica*, **104**, 96–103.

15. Weissman, M.M., Bland, R.C., Canino, G.J. *et al.* (1997) The cross-national epidemiology of panic disorder. *Archives of General Psychiatry*, **54** (4), 305–9.

16. Weissman, M.M., Canino, G.J., Greenwald, S. *et al.* (1995) Current rates and symptom profiles of panic disorder in six cross-national studies *Clinical Neuropharmacology*, **18** (Suppl 2), S1–S6.

17. Kadri, N., Agoub, M., El Gnaoui, S. *et al.* (2007) Prevalence of anxiety disorders: a population-based epidemiological study in metropolitan area of Casablanca, Morocco. *Annals of General Psychiatry*.. 6, 6 (Published online 2007 February 10).

18. Kadri, N., Agoub, M., Assouab, F. *et al*. Moroccan National Study on Prevalence on Mental Disorders: A Community-Based Epidemiological Study, http://www. Annals-general-psychiatry.com/content/6/1/6. (Submitted).

19. Weissman, M.M. and Klerman, G.L. (1977) Sex differences and the epidemiology of depression. *Archives of General Psychiatry*, **34**, 98–111.

20. Weissman, M.M., Livingston, B.M. and Leaf, P.J. (1991) Affective Disorders, in *Psychiatric Disorders in America* (eds L.N. Robins and D.A. Regier), Free Press, New York.

21. Weissman, M.M. and Olfson, M. (1995) Depression in women: Implications for health care research. *Science*, **269**, 799–801.

22. Wolk, S.I. and Weissman, M.M. (1995) Women and depression: an update, in *Review of Psychiatry*, Vol. 14 (eds J.M. Oldham and M.B. Riba), American Psychiatric Press, Washington, DC.

23. Ernst, C. and Angst, J. (1992) The Zurich Study XII. Sex differences in depression. Evidence from longitudinal epidemiological data. *European Archives of Psychiatry and Clinical Neuroscience*, **241**, 222–30.

24. Bland, R.C., Orn, H. and Newman, S.C. (1988) Lifetime prevalence of psychiatric disorders in Edmonton. *Acta Psychiatrica Scandinavica*, **77** (Suppl), 24–32.

25. Wittchen, H.U., Essau, C.A., Von Zerssen, D. *et al*. (1992) Lifetime and six-month prevalence of mental disorders in the Munich follow-up study. *European Archives of Psychiatry and Clinical Neuroscience*, **241**, 247–58.

26. de Graaf, R., Bijl, R.V., Smit, F. *et al*. (2002) Risk factors for 12-month comorbidity of mood, anxiety, and substance use disorders: findings from the Netherlands Mental Health Survey and Incidence Study. *The American Journal of Psychiatry*, **159**, 620–29.

27. Kessler, R.C., DuPont, R.L., Berglund, P. *et al*. (1999) Impairment in pure and comorbid generalized anxiety disorder and major depression at 12 months in two national surveys. *The American Journal of Psychiatry*, **156**, 1915–23.

28. Wittchen, H.U. and Essau, C.A. (1993) Comorbidity and mixed anxiety depressive disorders: Is there epidemiologic evidence? *Journal of Clinical Psychiatry*, **54** (Suppl), 9–15.

29. Wittchen, H.U., Lieb, R., Wunderlich, U. *et al*. (1999) Comorbidity in primary care: presentation and consequences. *Journal of Clinical Psychiatry*, **60**, 29–36; discussion 37–8.

30. Kessler, R.C., Sonnega, A., Bromet, E. *et al*. (1995) Posttraumatic stress disorder in the National Comorbidity Survey. *Archives of General Psychiatry*, **52**, 1048–60.

31. Sartorius, N., Ustun, T.B., Lecrubier, Y. *et al*. (1996) Depression comorbid with anxiety: results from the WHO study on psychological disorders in primary health care. *The British Journal of Psychiatry*, **168** (suppl. 30), 38–43.

32. Wittchen, H.U., Essau, C.A. and Krieg, J.C. (1991) Anxiety disorders: similarities and differences of comorbidity in treated and untreated groups. *The British Journal of Psychiatry*, Supplement 1991(12), 23–33.

33. de Jong, P.C. and Blijham, G.H. (1999) New aromatase inhibitors for the treatment of advanced breast cancer in postmenopausal women. *The Netherlands Journal of Medicine*, **55**, 50–58.

34. Angst, J. and Vollrath, M. (1991) The natural history of anxiety disorders. *Acta Psychiatrica Scandinavica*, **84**, 446–52.

35. Breslau, N., Schultz, L. and Peterson, E. (1995) Sex differences in depression: a role for preexisting anxiety. *Psychiatry Research*, **58**, 1–12.
36. Howell, H.B., Brawman-Mintzer, O., Monnier, J. *et al.* (2001) Generalized anxiety disorder in women. *The Psychiatric Clinics of North America*, **24**, 165–78.
37. Yonkers, K.A., Kando, J.C., Hamilton, J.A. *et al.* (2000) Gender differences in treatment of depression and anxiety, in *Pharmacotherapy for Mood, Anxiety, and Cognitive Disorders* (eds U. Halbreich and S.A. Montgomery), American Psychiatric Press, Washington, DC, pp. 59–74.
38. Yonkers, K.A. (1998) Assessing unipolar mood disorders in women. *Psychopharmacology Bulletin*, **34**, 261–66.
39. Angst, J. (1996) Comorbidity of mood disorders: a longitudinal prospective study. *The British Journal of Psychiatry*, (Suppl), 31–37.
40. Angst, J. and Merikangas, K.R. (2001) Multi-dimensional criteria for the diagnosis of depression. *Journal of Affective Disorders*, **62**, 7–15.
41. Angst, J., Merikangas, K.R. and Preisig, M. (1997) Subthreshold syndromes of depression and anxiety in the community. *Journal of Clinical Psychiatry*, **58**, 6–10.
42. Angst, J., Vollrath, M., Merikangas, K.R. *et al.* (1990) Comorbidity of anxiety and depression in the Zürich cohort study of young adults, in *Comorbidity of Mood and Anxiety Disorders* (eds J.D. Maser and C.R. Cloninger), American Psychiatric Press, Washington, DC, pp. 123–37.
43. Kessler, R.C., Nelson, C.B., McGonagle, K.A. *et al.* (1996) Comorbidity of DSM-III-R major depressive disorder in the general population: results from the US National Comorbidity Survey. *The British Journal of Psychiatry*, **168** (Suppl), 17–30.
44. Parker, G. and Hadzi-Pavlovic, D. (2001) Is any female preponderance in depression secondary to a primary female preponderance in anxiety disorders? *Acta Psychiatrica Scandinavica*, **103**, 252–56.
45. Kadri, N. and Moussaoui, D. (2001) Mental health in women in the Arab world, in *An Arab perspective* (eds A. Okasha and M. Maj), World Psychiatric Association, Scientific book House, Cairo.
46. Garvey, M.J., Tuason, V.B. and lumry, A.E. (1983) Occurrence of depression in the postpartum state. *Journal of Affective Disorders*, **5**, 97.
47. Hamilton, J.A. (1989) Postpartum psychiatric syndromes. *The Psychiatric Clinics of North America*, **12**, 89–103.
48. Arpels, J.C. (1996) The female brain hypoestrogenic continuum; from PMS to menopause. *The Journal of Reproductive Medicine*, **41**, 633–39.
49. Halbreich, U. and Endicott, J. (1985) The relationship of dysphoric premenstrual changes to depressive disorders. *Acta Psychiatrica Scandinavica*, **71**, 331–38.
50. Roca, C. and Schmidt, P.J. (1994) Models for the development and expression of symptoms in premenstrual syndrome. *Journal of General Internal Medicine*, **9**, 507–12.
51. Tunridge, W. (1993) prevalence of autoimmune endocrine disease, in *Autoimmune Endocrine Disease* (ed. T. Davies), John Wiley & Sons, Ltd, Chicester.
52. Winokur, G. (1979) Unipolar depression. Is it divisible into autonomous subtypes? *Archives of General Psychiatry*, **36**, 47–52.
53. Weissman, M.M. and Klerman, G.L. (1977) Sex differences and the epidemiology of depression. *Archives of General Psychiatry*, **34**, 98–111.

54. Patel, V., Todd, C.H., Winston, M. *et al.* (1998) The outcome of common mental disorders in Harare, Zimbabwe. *The British Journal of Psychiatry*, **172**, 53–57.

55. Jewkes, R., Penn-Kekana, L. and Rose-Junius, H. (2005) "If they rape me, I can't blame them": reflections on gender in the social context of child rape in South Africa and Namibia. *Social Science and Medicine*, **61**, 1809–20.

56. Kendler, K.S., Kuhn, J.W. and Prescott, C.A. (2004) Childhood sexual abuse, stressful life events and risk for major depression in women. *Psychological Medicine*, **34**, 1475–82.

57. Clayton, A.H., Steart, R.S., Fayyad, R. *et al.* (2006) Sex differences in clinical presentation and response in panic disorder: Pooled data from sertraline treatment studies. *Archives of Womens Mental Health*, **9**, 151–57.

58. Steiner, M., Allgulander, C., Ravindran, A. *et al.* (2005) Gender differences in clinical presentation and response to sertraline treatment of generalized anxiety disorder. *Human Psychopharmacology*, **20**, 3–13.

59. Cottone, J.G., Drucker, P. and Javier, R.A. (2002) Gender differences in psychotherapy dyads: changes in psychological symptoms and responsiveness to treatment during 3 months of therapy. *Psychotherapy: Theory, Research and Practice*, **39**, 297–308.

60. Gould, R.A., Otto, M.W., Pollack, M.H. and Yap, L. (1997) Cognitive behavioral and pharmacological treatment of generalised anxiety disorder: a preliminary metaanalysis. *Behaviour Research and Therapy*, **28**, 285–305.

61. Hirai, M. and Clum, G.A. (2006) A meta-analytic study of self help interventions for anxiety problems. *Behavior Therapy*, **37**, 99–111.

62. Mizoguchi, K., Kunishita, T., Chui, D.H. and Tabra, T. (1992) Stress induces neuronal death in the hippocampus of castrated rats. *Neuroscience Letters*, **138**, 157–60.

63. Uno, H., Else, J.G., Suleman, M.A. and Sapolsky, R.M. (1989) Hippocampal damage associated with prolonged and fatal stress in primates. *Journal of Neuroscience*, **9**, 1705–11.

64. Figueiredo, H., Dolga, C. and Herman, J. (2002) Stress activation of cortex and hippocampus is modulated by sex and stage of estrus. *Endocrinology*, **143**, 2534–40.

65. Luine, V. (2002) Sex differences in chronic stress effects on memory in rats. *Stress*, **5**, 205–16.

66. Gold, P.W. and Chrousos, G.P. (2002) Organization of the stress system and its dysregulation in melancholic and atypical depression: high vs. low CRH/NE states. *Molecular Psychiatry*, **7**, 254–75.

67. Conrad, C.R., Magarinos, A.M., LeDoux, J.E. and McEwen, B.S. (1999) Repeated restraint stress facilitates fear conditioning, independently of causing hippocampal CA3 dendritic atrophy. *Behavioral Neuroscience*, **113**, 902–13.

68. Galea, L.M., McEwen, B.S., Tanapat, P. *et al.* (1997) Sex differences in dendritic atrophy of CA3 pyramidal neurons in response to chronic restraint stress. *Neuroscience*, **81**, 689–97.

69. Altemus, M., Roca, C., Galliven, E. *et al.* (2001) Increased vasopressin and ACTH responses to stress in the mid-luteal phase of the menstrual cycle *The Journal of Clinical Endocrinology & Metabolism*, **86** (6), 2525–30.

70. Epperson, C.N., Haga, K., Mason, G.F. *et al.* (2002) Cortical gamma-aminobutyric acid levels across the menstrual cycle in healthy women and those with premenstrual

dysphoric disorder: a proton magnetic resonance spectroscopy study. *Archives of General Psychiatry*, **59**, 851–58.

71. Schulte, H.M., Weisner, D. and Allolio, B., 1990. The corticotropin releasing hormone test in late pregnancy: lack of adrenocorticotropin and cortisol response. *Clinical Endocrinology*, **33**, 99–106.

72. Roca, C.A., Schmidt, P.J., Altemus, M. *et al.* (2003) Differential menstrual cycle regulation of hypothalamic-pituitary-adrenal axis in women with premenstrual syndrome and controls. *The Journal of Clinical Endocrinology and Metabolism*, **88**, 3057–63.

73. Matthews, K.A. and Rodin, J. (1992) Pregnancy alters blood pressure responses to psychological and physical challenge. *Psychophysiology* **29**, 232–40.

74. Heinrichs, M., Meinlschmidt, G., Neumann, I. *et al.* (2001) Effects of suckling on hypothalamic-pituitary-adrenal axis responses to psychosocial stress in postpartum lactating women. *The Journal of Clinical Endocrinology and Metabolism*, **86**, 4798–804.

75. Mezzacappa, E.S., Yu, A.Y. and Myers, M.M. (2003) Lactation and weaning effects on physiological and behavioral responses to stressors. *Physiology and Behavior*, **78**, 1–9.

76. Altemus, M., Fong, J., Yang, R. *et al.* (2004) Changes in CSF neurochemistry during pregnancy. *Biological Psychiatry*, **56**, 386–92.

77. Cosgrove, K.P., Mazure, C.M. and Staley, J.K. (2007) Evolving knowledge of sex differences in brain structure, function, and chemistry. *Biological Psychiatry*, **62**, 847–55.

78. Gorman, J.M. (2006) Gender differences in depression and response to psychotropic medication. *Gender Medicine*, **3**, 93–109.

79. Weiss, L.A., Pan, L., Abney, M. *et al.* (2006) The sex-specific genetic architecture of quantitative traits in humans. *Nature Genetics*, **38**, 218–22.

80. Jovanovic, H. and Lundberg, J. (2007) Sex differences in the serotonin 1A receptor and serotonin transporter binding in the human brain measured by PET. *NeuroImage*, 2008 Feb 1: **39** (3), 1408–19. Epub 2007 Oct 25.

81. Dohrenwend, B.P. (1990) Socioeconomic status (SES) and psychiatric disorders. Are the issues still compelling? *Social Psychiatric Epidemiology*, **25**, 41–47.

82. Holzer, C.E. *et al.* (1986) The increased risk of specific psychiatric disorders among persons of low socioeconomic status: evidence from the epidemiological catchment area surveys. *The American Journal of Social Psychiatry*, **4**, 59–71.

83. Marmot, M.G., Kogenivas, M. and Elston, M.A. (1987) Social/economic status and disease. *Annual Review of Public Health*, **8**, 111–35.

84. Neugebauer, D.D., Dohrenwend, B.P. and Dohrenwend, B.S. (1980) The formulation of hypothesis about the true prevalence of functional disorder among adults in the United States, in *Mental Illness in the United States* (eds B.P. Dohrenwend, B.S. Dohrenwend, B. Link *et al.*), Preger, New York, pp. 45–94.

85. Benedek, E.P. (1981) Women's issues: a new beginning. *The American Journal of Psychiatry*, **138**, 1317–18.

86. Carmen, E., Russo, N.F. and Miller, J.B. (1981) Inequality and women's mental health: an overview. *The American Journal of Psychiatry*, **138**, 1319–29.

87. Lempert, L.B. (1986) Women's health from a woman's point of view: a review of the literature. *Health Care for Women International*, **7**, 255–75.

88. Belle, D. (1982) *Life's Stress: Women and Depression*, Sage, Beverley Hills.

89. Brown, G., Bhrolchain, M. and Harris, T. (1975) Social class and psychiatric disturbance among women in an urban population. *Sociology*, **9**, 225–54.

90. Makosky, V. (1982) Sources of stress: events or conditions? in *Lives in Stress* (ed. D. Belle), Sage Publications, Beverley Hills, pp. 35–53.

91. Pearlin, L.J. (1977) Marital status, life strains and depression. *American Sociological Review*, **42**, 704–15.

92. Radloff, L. (1975) Sex differences in depression: the effects of occupation and marital status. *Sex Roles*, **1**, 249–66.

93. Gove, W.R. and Tudoe, J.F. (1973) Adult sex roles and mental illness. *The American Journal of Economics and Sociology*, **78**, 50–73.

94. Guttentag, M., Salasin, S. and Belle, D. (eds) (1980) *The Mental Health of Women*, Academic Press, New York.

95. Mouchtaq, N. (1992) Enquête épidemiologique sur la dépression majeure en médecine générale. M.D. thesis number 21, Faculty of Medicine, Casablanca, Morocco.

96. Plaisier, I., De Bruijn, J.G.M., Smit, J.H. *et al.* (2008) Work and family roles and the association with depressive and anxiety disorders: differences between men and women. *Journal of Affective Disorders*, **105**, 63–72.

97. Hillbereman, E. (1980) Overview: the wife beater's wife reconsidered. *The American Journal of Psychiatry*, **137**, 1336–47.

98. Atkeson, B.M., Calhoun, K.S. and Resick, P.A. (1982) Victims of rape: repeated assessment of depressive symptoms. *Journal of Consulting and Clinical Psychology*, **50**, 96–102.

99. Winfield *et al.* (1990) Sexual assault and psychiatric disorders among a community sample of women. *The American Journal of Psychiatry*, **147**, 335–41.

100. Houssani-Skalli, H. and Kadri, N. (1999) Depression and violence. XI World Congress of Psychiatry, August 6–11, 1999, Hamburg. (Abstract).

101. Mchichi Alami, Kh. and Kadri, N. (2004) Moroccan women with a history of child sexual abuse and its long-term repercussion: population based epidemiological study. *Archives of Womens Mental Health*. 2004 Oct: **7** (4):237–42. Epub 2004 Sep 8.

102. Zurayk, H., Sholkamy, H., Younis, N. *et al.* (1997) Women's health problems in the Arab World: a holistic policy perspective. *International Journal of Gynecology and Obstetrics*, **58** (1), 13–21.

103. Chaleby, K. (1988) Traditional Arabian marriages and mental health in a group of outpatient Saudis. *Acta Psychiatrica Scandinavica*, **77** (2), 139–42.

104. Chaleby, K. (1985) Women of polygamous marriages in an inpatient psychiatric service in Kuwait. *The Journal of Nervous and Mental Disease*, **173** (1), 56–58.

105. Kadri, N. and Moussaoui, D. (2001) Mental health in women in the Arab World, in *An Arab Perspective* (eds A. Okasha and M. Maj), World Psychiatric Association, Scientific book House, Cairo.

106. Dirie, M.A. and Lindmark, G. (1991) Female circumcision in Somalia and women's motives. *Acta Obstetricia et Gynecologica scandinavica*, **70** (7–8), 581–85.

107. Lightfoot, K.H. (1989) Rites of purification and their effects: some psychological aspects of female genital circumcision and infibulation (Pharaonic circumcision) in

an Afro-Arab Islamic society (Sudan). *Journal of Psychology and Human Sexuality*, **2** (2), 79–91.

108. Dorkenoo, E. (1996) Combating female genital mutilation: an agenda for the next decade. *World Health Statistics Quarterly*, **49** (2), 142–47.

109. Halbreich, U., Backstrom, T., Eriksson, E. *et al.* (2007) Clinical diagnostic criteria for premenstrual syndrome and guidelines for their quantification for research studies. *Gynecological Endocrinology*, **23** (3), 123–30.

110. American College of Obstetricians and Gynecologists Committee on Gynecologic Practice. (1995) ACOG Committee Opinion: premenstrual syndrome. *International Journal of Gynaecology and Obstetrics*, **50**, 80–84.

111. Kornstein, S.G., Yonkers, K.A., Schatzberg, A.F. *et al.* (1996) Premenstrual exacerbation of depression. Presented at the 149th Annual Meeting of the American Psychiatric Association, New York.

112. American Psychiatric Association. (1994) *Diagnostic and Statistical Manual of Mental Disorders*, 4th edn, Vol. 4, American Psychiatric Association, Washington, DC.

113. Adewuya, A.O., Loto, O.M. and Adewumi, T.A. (2008) Premenstrual dysphoric disorder amongst Nigerian university students: prevalence, comorbid conditions, and correlates. *Archives of Women's Mental Health*, **11**, 13–18.

114. Mchichi Alami, Kh., Tahiri, S.M., Moussaoui, D. and Kadri, N. (2002) Evaluation des symptômes dysphoriques prémenstruels dans une population de femmes à Casablanca. *Encéphale*, **28**, 525–30, cahier 1.

115. Eriksson, E., Andersch, B., Ho, H.P. *et al.* (2002) Diagnosis and treatment of premenstrual dysphoria. *The Journal of Clinical Psychiatry*, **63** (Suppl 7), 16–23.

116. Bancroft, J. and Rennie, D. (1993) The impact of oral contraceptives on the experience of premenstrual mood, clumsiness, food craving, and other symptoms. *Journal of Psychosomatic Research*, **37**, 195–202.

117. Hammarback, S., Ekholm, U.B. and Backstrom, T. (1991) Spontaneous anovulation causing disappearance of cyclical symptoms in women with the premenstrual syndrome. *Acta Endocrinologica*, **125**, 132–37.

118. Eriksson, E., Sunblad, C., Yonkers, K.A. *et al.* (2000) Premenstrual dysphoria and related conditions: symptoms, pathophysiology, and treatment, in *Mood Disorders in Women*, Vol. 7 (eds M. Steiner, K.A. Yonkers and E. Eriksson), Martin Dunitz, London, pp. 269–329.

119. Eriksson, E. and Humble, M. (1990) Serotonin in psychiatric pathophysiology, a review of data from experimental and clinical research, in *The Biologic Basis of Psychiatric Treatment* (eds R. Pohl and S. Gershon), Basel,Karger, pp. 66–119.

120. Bethea, C.L., Pecins-Thompson, M., Schutzer, W.E. *et al.* (1998) Ovarian steroids and serotonin neural function. *Molecular Neurobiology*, **18**, 87–123.

121. Fink, G., Sumner, B., Rosie R. *et al.* (1999) Androgen actions on central serotonin neurotransmission: relevance for mood, mental state and memory. *Behavioural Brain Research*, **105**, 53–68.

122. Hallman, J., Oreland, L. and Edman, G. *et al.* (1987) Thrombocyte monoamine oxidase activity and personality traits in women with severe premenstrual syndrome. *Acta Psychiatrica Scandinavica*, **76**, 225–34.

123. Rapkin, A.J. (1992) The role of serotonin in premenstrual syndrome. *Clinical Obstetrics and Gynecology*, **35**, 629–36.

124. Eriksson, E., Alling, C., Andersch, B. *et al.* (1994) Cerebrospinal fluid levels of monoamine metabolites: a preliminary study of their relation to menstrual cycle phase, sex steroids, and pituitary hormones in healthy women and in women with premenstrual syndrome. *Neuropsychopharmacology*, **11**, 201–13.

125. Eriksson, E. (1999) Serotonin reuptake inhibitors for the treatment of premenstrual dysphoria. *International Clinical Psychopharmacology*, **14** (Suppl 2), S27–33.

126. Steiner, M. and Yonkers, K. (1998) *Depression in Women*, Martin Dunitz, London.

127. O'Hara, M.W., Schlechte, J.A., Lewis, D.A. and Varner, M.W. (1991) Controlled prospective study of postpartum mood disorders: psychological, environmental and hormonal factors. *Journal of Abnormal Psychology*, **100**, 63–73.

128. Mchichi Alami, K., Kadri, N. and Berrada, S. (2006) Prevalence and psychosocial correlates of depressed mood during pregnancy and after childbirth in a Moroccan sample. *Archives of Women's Mental Health*, **9** (6), 343–6.

129. Ingram, I.M. (1961) Obsessional illness in mental hospital patients. *Journal of Mental Science*. May, **107**, 382–402.

130. Neziroglu, F., Anemone, R., Yaryura-Tobias, J.A. (1992) Onset of obsessive-compulsive disorder in pregnancy. *American Journal of Psychiatry*. July, **149** (7), 947–50.

131. Hertzberg, T., Leo, R.J., Kim, K.Y. (1997) Recurrent obsessive-compulsive disorder associated with pregnancy and childbirth. *Psychosomatics*. Jul–Aug, **38** (4), 386–8.

132. Wadhwa, P.D., Sandman, C.A., Porto, M., Dunkel-Schetter, C., Garite, T.J. (1993) The association between prenatal stress and infant birth weight and gestational age at birth: a prospective investigation. *American Journal of Obstetric Gynecology*, Oct, **169** (4), 858–65.

133. Feldman, R. (2008) The intrauterine environment, temperament, and development: including the biological foundations of individual differences in the study of psychopathology and wellness. *Journal of American Academic Child Adolescent Psychiatry*. Mar **47** (3), 233–5.

134. McAnarney, E.R. and Stevens-Simon, C. (1990) Maternal psychological stress/depression and low birth weight - **Is there a relationship?** *American Journal of Diseases of the Child*, **144** (7), 789–92.

135. Cohen, L.S. and Rosenbaum, J.F. (1998) Psychotropic drug use during pregnancy; weighing the risks. *The Journal of Clinical Psychiatry*, **59** (Suppl 2), 18–28.

136. Gurel, S. and Gurel, H. (2000) The evaluation of determinants of early postpartum low mood: the importance of parity and inter-pregnancy interval. *European Journal of Obstetrics, Gynecology, and Reproductive Biology*, **91**, 21–24.

137. Abou Saleh, M.T. and Ghubash, R. (1997) The prevalence of early postpartum psychiatric morbidity in Dubai: a transcultural perspective. *Acta Psychiatrica Scandinavica*, **95**, 428–32.

138. Ghubash, R. and Abou Saleh, M.T. (1997) Postpartum illness in Arab culture: prevalence and psychosocial correlates. *The British Journal of Psychiatry*, **171**, 65–68.

139. Agoub, M., Moussaoui, D. and Battas, O. (2005) Prevalence of postpartum depression in a Moroccan sample. *Archives of Women's Mental Health*, **8** (1), 37–43. Epub 2005 May 4.

140. Mchichi Alami, K., Kadri, N. and Berrada, S. (2006) Prevalence and psychosocial correlates of depressed mood during pregnancy and after childbirth in a Moroccan sample. *Archives of Women's Mental Health*, **9** (6), 343–46. [Epub 2006 Oct 13].

141. Abrams, S.M., Field, T., Scafidi, F., Prodromidis, M. (1995) Newborns of depressed mothers, *Infant Mental Health Journal*, **16**(3), 233–9.

142. Jones, N.A., Field, T., Fox, N.A., Davalos, M., Lundy, B., & Hart, S. (1998) Newborns of mothers with depressive symptoms are physiologically less developed. *Infant Behavior and Development*, **21**, 537–41.

143. Lundy, B.L., Jones, N.A., Field, T., Nearing, G., Davalos, M., Pietro, P., Schanberg, S., & Kuhn, C. (1999) Prenatal depression effects on neonates. *Infant Behavior and Development*, **22**, 121–31.

144. Hardy, P., Feline, A. and Aminot, A. (1984) Psychologie et psychopathologie de la ménopause. *Revue Du Praticien*, **34** (5), 1339–46.

145. Hill, K. (1996) The demography of menopause. *Maturitas*, **23**, 113–27.

146. McKinlay, S.M., Brambilla, D.J. and Posner, J.G. (1992) The normal menopause transition. *American Journal of Human Biology*, **4**, 37–46.

147. Ballinger, C. (1990) Psychiatric aspects of the menopause. *The British Journal of Psychiatry*, **156**, 773–87.

148. Mc Kinlay, J., Mc Kinlay, S. and Brambilla, D. (1987) The relative contributions of endocrine changes and social circumstances to depression in mid-aged women. *Journal of Health and Social Behavior*, **28**, 345–63.

149. Stewart, D.E. and Boydell, K.M. (1993) Psychologic distress during menopause. Associations across the reproductive life cycle. *Journal of Psychiatry in Medicine*, **23**, 157–63.

150. Wolk, S.F. and Weissman, M.M. (1995) Women and depression. *Annual Review of Psychiatry*, **14**, 59–95.

151. Mc Kinlay, J., Mc Kinlay, S. and Brambilla, D. (1987) The relative contributions of endocrine changes and social circumstances to depression in mid-aged women. *Journal of Health and Social Behavior*, **28**, 345–63.

152. Kadri, N. and Zarbib, K. (2000) Ménopause et santé mentale. *Caducée*, **46**.

Further reading

Nielson, F.D., Videbech, P., Hedegaard, M. *et al.* (2000) Postpartum depression: identification of women at risk. *BJOG*, **107**, 1210–7.

3
Somatisation and dissociation

Santosh K. Chaturvedi and Ravi Philip Rajkumar

Department of Psychiatry, National Institute of Mental Health and Neurosciences, Bangalore, India

3.1 Introduction

The concepts of somatisation and dissociation have many similarities and differences. In diagnostic systems, disorders of somatisation and dissociation are identified as separate categories, but they show a substantial overlap. The understanding of the symptoms and syndromes of dissociation and somatisation, has continued to evolve over the years. Somatoform and dissociative disorders are distinct in terms of symptoms, however, they are highly comorbid with one another, as well as with depression, anxiety and post-traumatic stress disorder (PTSD) [1]. Moreover, they are both strongly associated with psychological stressors and trauma. Hence, they are often considered and studied together. Both somatoform and dissociative disorders range from acute and brief-lasting responses to stress to chronic and severe illnesses, whose disability and social outcome are comparable to or more severe than those of chronic physical illnesses. Patients with these conditions often present to primary care or general medical settings, rather than psychiatric services, due to the physical nature of their symptoms. Knowledge of somatisation and dissociation is essential when discussing the planning and implementation of general and mental health services for women, because they are much more frequently affected by these disorders.

This chapter presents the current concepts in the classification, diagnosis, clinical features, pathophysiology and management of women with these disorders.

Contemporary Topics in Women's Mental Health Edited by Chandra, Herrman, Fisher, Kastrup,
© 2009 John Wiley & Sons, Ltd   Niaz, Rondón and Okasha

3.2 Somatisation – definitions and concept

Somatisation, in its broadest sense, has been defined as the occurrence of physical symptoms for which no apparent medical cause can be found, and in which psychological factors are judged to play an important role. More simply, somatisation is the expression of psychological distress in physiological terms, and as such, is a nearly universal phenomenon in the general population [2]. The central concept remains the presentation of somatic complaints in the absence of an adequate 'physical' or 'general medical' explanation, and the presumption that psychological problems are thus being avoided, with an abnormal illness behaviour [3] or psychosocial distress is being communicated by somatic way.

For research purposes, somatisation has been operationalised in three main ways – (i) as medically unexplained physical symptoms (MUPS), (ii) as hypochondriacal worry or somatic preoccupation and (iii) as a somatic presentation of anxiety and other disorders [4]. Various terms have been used in literature that have a meaning similar to somatisation; these are hysteria (usually conversion; can also refer to dissociative disorders), medically unexplained symptoms, MUPS, somatic neurosis, psychophysiological disorders, psychosomatic disorders (a broad term; can also refer to medical conditions affected by psychosocial factors), psychogenic symptoms and idiopathic somatic complaints and syndromes (Table 3.1).

3.3 Dissociation – definitions and concept

Closely allied to somatisation, but distinct from it, is the concept of 'dissociation', in which a psychological stressor or conflict leads to loss of normal psychological integration. In dissociative disorders, symptoms reflect impairment of memory (*dissociative amnesia*), awareness of one's own actions (*dissociative fugue*) or the sense of self or identity (*dissociative identity disorder*) and cultural variants such as *trance and possession disorders*.

Table 3.1   List of terms equivalent to somatoform disorders

Hysteria (usually conversion; can also refer to dissociative disorders)

Medically unexplained symptoms

Medically unexplained physical symptoms (MUPS)

Somatic neurosis

Psychophysiological disorders

Psychosomatic disorders (a broad term; can also refer to medical conditions affected by psychosocial factors)

Psychogenic symptoms

Idiopathic somatic complaints and syndromes

Somatisation and dissociation are part of the complex array of responses to trauma and stress, though the individual mechanisms and pathways involved may differ, and are still being elucidated. Multiple factors, individual, social and biological play a role in shaping the nature and severity of individual symptoms in response to a given stressor. The chronic and disabling nature of somatisation and dissociation, poses a significant burden to affected women, leading to impaired quality of life [5], high social and occupational disability and increased health care utilisation and costs [6]. These disorders are often not recognised, and are difficult to treat, as a consequence many women suffering from these conditions receive sub-optimal care.

The role of cultural factors needs to be appreciated in the development, presentation and management of somatisation and dissociation disorders. Explanatory models employ the cultural formulation to get an understanding of the disorders (Table 3.2). The symptoms of somatisation and dissociation reflect

Table 3.2 Culture-related somatoform and dissociative syndromes

Syndrome	Cultural setting	Clinical features
Dhat	India, South-East Asia	Usually seen in men, with anxiety related to semen loss. An equivalent syndrome in women related to vaginal discharge has been described in India [113]
'The nerves'	Rural South Africa	Bodily disorders and pain, associated with emotional disturbances
Douleur de corps (pain in the body)	Haiti	Pain in the body, *faiblesse* (weakness), *gaz* (gastrointestinal disturbance), headaches
Ataque de nervios	Puerto Rico, Latin American countries	Headache, tremors, palpitations, shouting, crying, dissociative and conversion symptoms
Hwa-byung (fire illness)	Korea	Burning sensations in the head, epigastrium or other parts of the body
Trance and possession disorder	Various	Dissociative episodes in which the sufferer behaves as if possessed by a god, demon or the spirit of a deceased person
Multiple personality disorder	Chiefly in the United States	Presence of multiple 'personas' or identities in the same person, with shifts between 'personas' caused by stress

a cry for help, a failure of existing coping mechanisms and a need for support and understanding from family, friends and professionals. These need to be understood and addressed under the unique cultural framework of the individual. Idioms of distress have considerable conceptual overlap with the concepts of somatisation and dissociation, since the idioms of distress have a defensive purpose like in the erstwhile neurosis. Somatisation and dissociation may be construed as idioms of distress to communicate the distress or impact of trauma. The cognitions and idioms of distress are influenced by sociocultural factors [7].

3.4 The diagnosis and classification of somatoform and dissociative disorders

The current classificatory systems in use, ICD-10 and DSM-IV [8, 9], describe *somatisation disorder* as a condition with an onset before the age of 30, and a chronic course characterised by multiple unexplained physical complaints involving multiple systems.

The term *undifferentiated somatoform disorder* is used when symptoms are multiple and severe, but of insufficient number or duration to qualify for a diagnosis of somatisation disorder. A variant of this condition is the concept of *abbreviated somatisation*, described by Escobar *et al.* [10], which only requires a certain number (four for men and six for women) of somatic symptoms in the patient's lifetime. Kroenke [11] has proposed *multi somatoform disorder* as a similar, more easily applicable entity. When pain is the predominant or only symptom, a diagnosis of *somatoform pain disorder* (*pain disorder* in DSM-IV) is made.

Conversion disorder (DSM-IV) is diagnosed when the patient presents with symptoms referred to the central nervous system, for which no cause can be found despite adequate investigations, and which are presumably caused by psychological factors. In ICD-10, conversion disorder is grouped with the dissociative disorders (Table 3.3).

Dissociative disorders are classified according to the mental faculty or psychological function that is impaired. While DSM-IV provides a separate category for dissociative identity disorder and relegates trance and possession disorders to the 'not otherwise specified' category, the converse holds true in ICD-10. Finally, depersonalisation/derealisation syndrome, which is considered a separate disorder in ICD-10, is included as a dissociative disorder in DSM-IV.

The label 'somatisation' implying that the patient's symptoms are psychological, or 'all in the mind', is often stigmatising. As a result, the medical profession has, in parallel, devised diagnostic criteria for various 'functional somatic syndromes' that are, in essence, similar if not identical to somatoform disorders. These include, but are not restricted to:

1. Chronic fatigue syndrome (CFS), fibromyalgia and multiple chemical sensitivity in general medical practise.

2. Irritable bowel syndrome and functional dyspepsia in gastroenterology.

Table 3.3 Clinical subtypes of conversion disorders

Symptom and names	Clinical features
Non-epileptic seizures ('pseudoseizures', 'hystero-epilepsy', 'hysterical convulsions', 'non-epileptic attack disorder')	Triggered by stressors Duration >2 min Partial responsiveness Bizarre movements – such as sideways head movement or pelvic thrusts Resistance to eye opening Very brief or very prolonged episodes Flexor plantar reflexes Asynchronous motor movements 'Limp' muscles during the episode
Weakness ('functional weakness', 'hysterical paralysis', 'conversion hysteria')	Varying power of the limb Sudden collapsing weakness Hoover's sign Hemiparesis without facial weakness Normal tone and reflexes
Sensory loss	Distribution not conforming to anatomy Unilateral loss of all sensory modalities Sensory loss of a single limb
Gait disturbances ('astasia-abasia')	Fluctuation of gait disturbance Giving way without fall/injury Inconsistent Romberg's test Dragging an inverted/everted foot Normal cerebellar/sensory systems
Movement disorders ('dissociative motor disorder', 'psychogenic movement disorder')	Bizarre and flailing movements Inconsistent findings of tone, reflexes, and so on Relationship to stressors Varying site of movements

3. Chronic pelvic pain, urinary urgency and vulvar pain in gynaecology.

4. Temporomandibular joint dysfunction in dentistry.

5. Chronic pain syndromes.

Currently, there is still controversy about the nomenclature and classification of somatoform disorders [11]. Changes in diagnostic terms and criteria are expected in DSM-V and ICD-11 [12, 13]. However, regardless of any change in nomenclature, it is essential for psychiatrists to identify and treat these disorders appropriately, and not to consider them as being beyond their purview [14].

3.5 The neurobiology of somatisation and dissociation

Somatoform and dissociative disorders are often referred to as 'functional' disorders. Therefore, it is heuristically useful to consider somatisation, and dissociation as involving alterations in brain function (Table 3.4). It is possible that gender-related biological variations may underlie at least part of women's greater vulnerability to dissociation. These include:

Immunological mechanisms

Women are generally at higher risk for a variety of auto-immune disorders, and their hormonal milieu has important effects on immunological function (e.g. the exacerbation of systemic lupus erythematosus during pregnancy). Recent research in psychoneuroimmunology suggests that the symptoms of somatoform disorder may be explained by the central effects of inflammatory and immune mediators that are released in response to stress [15]. This model is attractive because: (i) it explains the association between stress and the genesis of somatoform

Table 3.4 Neurobiological factors related to somatisation in women

Aetiological factor	Description
Genetics	High-frequency somatisation in women may be a genetically distinct form of the illness, and is associated with type 2 alcoholism and criminality in male relatives.
Physiological awareness	Heightened sensitivity to pain and anxiety has been documented in women.
Neuroendocrine factors	A single study found increased cortisol levels in somatising patients, more than 60% of whom were women.
Gonadal hormones	Alterations in LHRH, and behavioural effects of ovarian hormones, may be associated with certain symptoms, especially those referred to the genital tract.
Neurocognition	Preliminary studies have found multiple cognitive deficits in women with somatisation; working memory deficits may lead to altered information processing
Neuroanatomy	Decreased cerebral glucose metabolism in bilateral caudate nuclei and left putamen; decrease in brain perfusion, possibly more in the non-dominant hemisphere.

symptoms and (ii) it may account for gender differences in somatisation, as women's hormonal and neurochemical milieu may make them more susceptible to develop abnormal immune activation in response to stress.

Sex hormonal influences

Changes in levels of oestrogen, progestogens and other gonadal hormones, as well as prolactin, could be associated with somatoform and mood symptoms. Some of the evidence cited to support this includes (Table 3.5):

1. The high occurrence of somatic symptoms during the premenstrual phase, pregnancy and the menopause [16].

Table 3.5 Aetiological factors related to conversion disorder in women

Aetiological factor	Description
Neuroanatomy	The anterior corpus callosum is larger in subjects with high hypnotisability, which shows some neurophysiological relationship with conversion
Emotional processing	Impairment of modulation between the limbic and sensory-motor networks has been postulated
Altered primary motor/sensory cortical function	Has been demonstrated in imaging studies. Electrophysiological studies have also found altered evoked potentials
Altered motor planning and volition	Imaging studies have shown activation of the anterior cingulate and orbitofrontal cortex in conversion paralysis, representing inhibition of movement.
Neurotrophic factors	A preliminary study has shown elevated serum brain-derived neurotrophic factor (BDNF) in patients with conversion disorder and depression, both disorders with a female preponderance
Self-monitoring	Increased self-monitoring has been shown in subjects with conversion disorder; this is known to be increased in women compared to men (see Somatisation, above)
Memory of traumatic events	An functional magnetic resonance imaging (fMRI) study in a woman with conversion disorder found activation of the amygdala and inferior frontal lobe in response to cues related to trauma, which was associated with the motor cortical anomalies described above.

2. Preliminary evidence that some hormonally-mediated conditions, such as primary dysmenorrhoea and secondary amenorrhoea, are associated with psychological variables and somatisation [17].

3. The documented physical and psychological effects of LHRH Luteinizing hormone-releasing hormone, oestrogen and progestogens, especially in response to stress [18].

4. The ability of gonadal hormones to affect the function of neurotransmitters such as dopamine, serotonin and gamma-amino butyric acid.

Neural circuitry

A few imaging studies have examined cerebral activation patterns in patients with somatoform disorders (Table 3.6). One such study, in which study subjects were exclusively women with somatisation, showed decreased metabolism in both caudate nuclei, as well as in the left putamen and right precentral gyrus [19]. Another study found hypoperfusion in a majority of subjects, with a preponderance in the right hemisphere; and right cerebellar hypoperfusion was more frequent in women than men [20]. Studies in conversion disorder have also demonstrated decreased activity of the primary motor or sensory cortex, and increased activation of the right orbitofrontal and cingulate cortices, as well as altered basal ganglia function [21]. As all these structures are involved in sensorimotor function and are interconnected with the limbic system, further investigations would help in understanding their role in the pathophysiology of somatisation, as well as the neural basis of gender differences. A role of the corpus callosum has been hypothesised, based on studies showing a larger anterior corpus callosum in subjects with high hypnotisability, a status linked to conversion [22], and activation of brain areas associated with traumatic recall has been reported in a woman experiencing motor conversion [23]. In dissociative disorders, smaller hippocampal and amygdalar volumes – perhaps related to childhood trauma [24] – and altered activity in cortical integrated areas in depersonalisation [25] have been described.

Neuropsychology

Neurocognitive deficits have been reported in women, primarily in the areas of verbal memory, semantic memory, visuospatial skills and speed of performance of attentional tasks. Such cognitive deficits are associated with a state of hyperarousal, and may lead to errors in monitoring of bodily phenomena and attribution, leading to the development of somatoform symptoms [26]. In dissociative disorders, impairments in memory, particularly autobiographical encoding, have been identified [27] and may play a role both in pathogenesis and the recovery process.

Table 3.6 Neurobiological factors involved in dissociation in women

Aetiological factor	Description
Neuroanatomy	Imaging studies have shown smaller volumes of the hippocampus and amygdala in dissociative identity disorder, and altered metabolism in integrative cortical areas in depersonalisation disorder
Cognitive deficits	Impairments in encoding of autobiographical memory have been proposed on theoretical and clinical grounds. A cognitive processing style known as the 'dissociative processing style', developed as a defence against trauma, has been described. Emotional cognitive deficits have been described in depersonalisation
Autonomic reactivity	Research has demonstrated heightened arousal responses to emotionally charged stimuli in dissociation
Neuroendocrine changes	High dissociators and depersonalisation show a greater cortisol response to stress. Hippocampus may be hyper reactive to cortisol in dissociation
Electrophysiology	Suppressed alpha activity and elevated theta band activity in electroencephalogram (EEG) of high dissociators
Neurotransmitter changes	Putative factors involved include noradrenaline and opioid peptides
Serum lipid levels	Associated with dissociation, impulsivity, aggression and suicidality
Neurodevelopment	Traumatic events may cause abnormalities of neurodevelopment that can produce dissociation through mechanisms involving the orbitofrontal cortex

Neuroendocrine dysregulation

Preliminary evidence suggests that patients with somatisation disorder, dissociative disorder and chronic unexplained pain [27, 28] have dysregulation of the hypothalamic-pituitary-adrenal (HPA) axis, specifically in the form of elevated cortisol levels. HPA axis dysregulation has for long been associated with stress, depression and psychological distress, and may affect hippocampal functioning [27].

Neurotransmitter dysfunction

Altered transmission involving the serotonergic system has been suggested in patients with hypochondriasis, but this is largely based on the response to serotonergic antidepressants [29]. Similarly, opioidergic and adrenergic dys-regulation have been proposed in dissociation and elevated brain-derived neurotrophic factor (BDNF) levels have been found in patients with conversion [30]. Though these theories are intriguing, much further work is needed to confirm their role in the pathophysiology of these disorders.

Autonomic dysfunction

In studies involving patients with hypochondriasis, differences in the response of heart rate to activity [31] and hyperarousal in response to illness-related imagery [32] have been documented, suggesting that these patients have heightened autonomic reactivity to various situations. Heightened autonomic reactivity has also been described in dissociation.

Complex integrative models

Models that attempt to explain conversion [33, 34] and dissociation [35, 36] have been proposed in recent years, using various perspectives. Certain common factors noted are:

1. The importance of the orbitofrontal and cingulate cortex, areas involved in the organisation of behaviour.

2. The role of stressful and traumatic events in early childhood.

3. The effect of these events on neurodevelopment, leading to deficits in emotional and behavioural regulation.

It seems that whatever the neural substrates of these disorders might be, early life experiences and adversities play a central role in their pathogenesis.

3.6 Psychosocial factors

Both somatisation and dissociation have been conceptualised as responses to traumatic or stressful life events and situations. However, a variety of factors determine the form and content of these responses, and these may operate at the individual or the larger social and cultural level.

The response to trauma in women

Somatisation and dissociation may reflect (Table 3.5) a 'cry for help' or 'idioms of distress' and a way of communication to the health care professionals that all is not well with their emotions and coping [37]. While trauma and the somatoform and dissociative disorders are inextricably linked, the differential response of men and women to the same traumatic situation is equally important. Women are more likely to respond to sexual trauma with 'internalising' symptoms such as anxiety, depression and somatisation. This response may be mediated by various mechanisms. Besides the biological variants described above, the following factors have also been found to play a significant role:

- *Alexithymia*: The term 'alexithymia' literally means 'no words for feelings'. Alexithymia is considered to play a central role in somatoform disorders [37]. High levels of alexithymia have been found in inpatients [38] as well as outpatients [39] with somatoform disorders. In studies examining the effects of gender, a recent study suggests that a component of alexithymia – 'difficulty identifying and expressing feelings' – was commoner in women [40]. Women with alexithymia seem to process emotion eliciting stimuli differently, and overactivate their 'bodily' brain regions in positron emission tomography (PET) scan studies: the motor and somatosensory areas are activated to a greater extent and anterior cingulate cortex to a lesser extent in women with alexithymia, and may be related to their tendency to somatisation [41].

- *Symptom perception in women*: For various reasons, women are more likely to report somatoform symptoms than men [42]. Various constructs have been invoked to explain this difference, such as anxiety sensitivity (fear and catastrophisation of the physical manifestations of anxiety), somatosensory amplification and sensitivity to pain. All these factors have been noted to be more common in women than men [43, 44] and have both been associated with somatisation disorder, though other factors are also involved [45].

- *Evolutionary explanations*: Some authors have sought to explain the preferential expression of somatoform symptoms in women on an evolutionary basis. Bracha *et al.* [46] have argued that certain 'medically unexplained symptoms', such as conversion and musculoskeletal pain, may be neurally mediated responses to stress and fear, which are sensitive to hormonal influences and conferred survival advantages on women – but not men – in primitive societies. Similarly, somatisation has been conceptualised as an appeasement display in response to real or perceived defeat [47]. Though such explanations must be regarded as speculative, they offer a novel perspective on the phenomenon of somatisation in women today.

- *Personality and coping styles*: Somatisation and dissociation can also be conceptualised as a maladaptive coping mechanism related to variations in temperament – specifically, traits such as harm avoidance [48] – and personality. A high degree of comorbidity with personality disorder (62.9%) was found in somatising patients in a recent study [49], and some authors have suggested that somatisation itself has the properties of a personality disorder [11] or a maladaptive trait [50]. Like somatisation, personality disorders – especially borderline disorders – are overrepresented in women, and are related to early childhood trauma and neglect, providing another potential pathway between trauma and somatoform or dissociative disorders.

The influence of culture

Somatisation reflects the dualism inherent in western biomedical practise, whereas in most traditional medicine (Chinese or Ayurvedic medicine) a sharp distinction between the 'mental' and the 'physical' does not occur [4]. People from traditional cultures may not distinguish between the emotions of anxiety, irritability and depression because they tend to express distress in somatic terms or they may organise their concepts of dysphoria in ways different from western ones. Gureje [51], reported that somatic distress varied across cultures in a complex way without any clear cultural explanation. Culture may influence the frequency of physical rather than psychological presentation, the form and content of somatic or dissociative symptoms and the specific effects of culture may place women at risk [52].

Culture and somatic presentations

It has been traditionally believed that somatisation is common in developing societies and among ethnic groups in the west. Early reports from Africa, India and China indicated that psychological disorders presented mainly with somatic symptoms [53]. This has sometimes been related to racial biases and lack of cultural understanding by western researchers. Recent and culturally sensitive studies [54] do confirm that syndromes of bodily distress are common in women across a variety of cultures, and are manifestations of underlying depression and anxiety. Women from developing countries are frequently less educated than men [55]. They may also have difficulty in communicating their feelings verbally, and therefore, somatise their emotional distress [56]. Culture may also provide explanatory models for symptoms, leading to specific patterns of presentation [52]. Certain cultures lack specific words for a variety of emotions. Expression of one's feelings overtly is regarded as an admission of weakness, and hence, socially undesirable in some Asian and African cultures [57, 58]. The deleterious social consequences of psychiatric labelling and stigmatisation may lead to the preferential expression of emotional distress in physical terms [57, 59]. In addition, the expression of physical distress may allow the patient to seek help that would otherwise not be available.

Culture and the form and content of symptoms

A significant number of culture bound syndromes can be construed as cultural variants of somatisation and dissociation. A list of some of these syndromes and their associated complaints is given in Table 3.2.

In addition, certain aspects of cultural practise may be more common in women, and may influence the form that symptoms take when distress is being expressed (Table 3.6). Dorahy *et al.* [60] found that religious ritual and dissociation were significantly correlated and that religious ritual scores were higher in Indian women than men, which was not the case for Australian women.

Culture as a risk factor for somatisation and dissociation in women

Certain cultural beliefs, values and practises may have an adverse impact on the physical and mental well-being of women, leading to traumatisation or chronic stress that is then expressed in somatic or dissociative symptoms. Each stage or transition of their life cycle is associated with its own adversities, for example:

1. *Puberty*: Ideas relating to the 'pollution' of menstruation, lack of knowledge, restrictions on the freedom of girls who have 'come of age'.

2. *Adolescence*: Taboos and conflicts related to contact with the opposite sex or sexual activity; a high premium placed on virginity; inability to pursue education or career goals; pressures to marry at a young age.

3. *Marriage*: Young age at marriage; societal restrictions on behaviour; demands for submissiveness and obedience; unsatisfactory personal and sexual relationships with spouses; domestic violence. In cultures where polygamy is common, fear of repudiation is also frequent. Indeed, a characteristic 'first wife syndrome', characterised by somatic symptoms resistant to treatment, has been described in Morocco [61] and probably exists elsewhere.

4. *Childbearing*: Early age at childbirth; malnutrition; poverty; unplanned pregnancy; lack of access to adequate pre- and postnatal care; religious beliefs against contraception; the stigma of bearing a daughter rather than a son.

5. *Infertility*: Loss of status; threat of divorce or rejection by the husband; stigmatisation.

6. *Widowhood*: Loss of status; loss of social support; economic deprivation.

These considerations are not of equal importance across cultures, but it is easy to see how treasured cultural values and beliefs can subject women to life events involving trauma, loss, humiliation, loss of support and, alone or in combination, significantly increase the risk of somatoform and dissociative disorders.

Epidemiology

The WHO cross-national study of mental disorders in primary care found a high prevalence of somatisation across all the 15 centres though rates varied markedly. Levels of somatic symptomatology and emotional distress were highly correlated at all the sites, thus suggesting a linear relationship between somatic symptoms and overt psychological expression of distress [62].

In a recent systematic review, a predominance of females in somatisation disorder was found in population or primary care based samples when DSM diagnostic criteria were used, but the female predominance was less clear on lowering the threshold of number of symptoms. A general tendency for females to report more somatic symptoms was noted. Hypochondriasis did not show a gender bias, suggesting that risk factors for multiple symptoms and illness worry may differ [14].

Dissociative symptoms appear to be relatively common in the population, while disorders may be less common. A 20 year follow-up study in West Bengal on changes in rate of hysteria showed declining rates, especially in women, perhaps due to improvement in their socioeconomic status [63].

Up to 60% of patients in general practise have at least one medically unexplained symptom, while a prevalence of 16.1–30.3% [64] of somato-form disorders was reported in general practise. If the 'unspecified' category is included, rates may be above 50% [64]. 'Pure' somatisation disorder is relatively infrequent, with a prevalence of 0.01–0.9% in the general population; however, abridged forms of somatisation were found to have a prevalence of 19.7% in a WHO cross-cultural study [4]. In general practise, partial syndrome presenta-tions are also frequent. They are generally more frequent in women, though ratios vary across populations and study settings. A high comorbidity with anxiety and depression has been consistently noted [1, 27].

Clinical features

The main clinical features are MUPS, which have usually been present for several years. Most patients have a long and complicated history of consulting several doctors. Common symptoms include aches and pains at different sites, headache, gastrointestinal sensations, cardiovascular symptoms, skin symptoms and sexual/menstrual complaints.

Somatoform disorders tend to run a chronic course, with fluctuations related to stressful situations. Diagnoses tend to remain stable over time, though there is some disagreement over this. While many studies suggest that the syndrome per-sists over several years [65], individual symptoms may show a high degree of varia-tion. The initiation of effective treatment may change this guarded prognosis [66].

Variations in presentation can take various forms. Those of significance in women are described below.

Cultural variations

Ataque de nervios reported in Puerto Rican and Caribbean subjects, are common in women, particularly those who are older, unmarried and with low levels of education. The common somatic manifestations of *ataque de nervios* are headache, trembling, palpitations, stomach disturbances, a sensation of heat rising to the head, numbness of extremities and at times pseudo seizures, fainting or unusual spells. *Douleur de corps*, described in Haitian immigrant women, is characterised by pain in the body, headache, fatigue and gastrointestinal symptoms. In Indian women, *genital complaints* associated with psychosocial factors are reported [67].

Similarly, in Muslim women in India, *somatic neurosis* characterised by multiple somatic symptoms, long-standing financial and family stressors and a lack of excessive concern over one's health, has been described [68].

Hwa byung is a Korean folk illness label commonly used by patients suffering from a multitude of somatic and psychological symptoms, including constricted, oppressed or pushing up sensations in the chest, palpitations, heat sensations, flushing, headache, epigastric mass, dysphoria, anxiety, irritability and difficulty in concentration. It is reported in the less educated, middle aged married women in times of stress.

Functional medical disorders

Fibromyalgia is the prototype of this group, characterised by pain and soft tissue tenderness in various parts of the body, in the absence of a known aetiology. Fibromyalgia shows a female preponderance, and many of the aetiological factors that have been suggested, such as neurotransmitter changes, immune dysregulation and abnormalities of self-monitoring [69], have also been implicated in somatisation.

Obstetric and gynaecological disorders

This topic has been extensively reviewed by Bitzer [16] and by Chandra and Ranjan [70]. There exists a group of conditions characterised by symptoms localised to the female genital tract, which mimic those of an organic disease, but for which no structural cause can be found [16], for example, chronic pelvic pain syndrome (CPPS). CPPS has shown some genetic relationship to somatic distress [71]. CPPS has also been associated with high rates of depression and anxiety and shares some vulnerability factors, such as sexual abuse and chronic life stress [47] with the somatoform disorders.

Syndromes with fatigue as a chief complaint

These include neurasthenia and CFS. Neurasthenia (*shenjing shuairuo*), is commonly diagnosed in China where other somatoform diagnoses are rare [72]. Similarly, CFS is a syndrome characterised by fatigue, weakness and associated physical complaints, which is frequently diagnosed in western settings. A major reason for the popularity of these diagnoses is that they are less stigmatising, and widely accepted by general practitioners in their respective cultures.

Treatment of somatoform disorders

General principles

Somatoform disorders are chronic and long-standing conditions, and the emphasis in management must be on care, not cure. A variety of treatment approaches has been tried in the management of somatisation, and there is little literature on gender variations in response to treatment, or on modalities that are especially effective for symptom variants such as CPPS. Considering the high prevalence of these complaints in primary care, certain principles should be universally applied by all medical professionals dealing with patients who are provisionally diagnosed with somatoform disorders [73, 74]:

1. Assessment for underlying medical disorders: this should be done only to the extent that is indicated by the patient's signs and symptoms. Clinicians should be careful to avoid either under- or over-investigation.

2. Explanation of the nature of the problem. It is useful to avoid stigmatising language ('there is nothing wrong', 'all in the mind'), to acknowledge the patient's symptoms as real, and to explain that the symptoms are not indicative of permanent structural damage or a life-threatening illness. Providing psychological explanations without appropriate preparation should be avoided. Education regarding the mind-body relationship, and the physical effects of stress and negative emotions, is also helpful.

3. Empathic listening to the patient's complaints and helping the patient to 'feel understood'.

4. Behavioural techniques to avoid abnormal illness behaviours. It is beneficial to make contract with the patient to follow-up consistently with one physician (to avoid 'doctor-shopping'), to have regular scheduled follow-ups, to agree on the extent of investigations and the duration of treatment trials, and to focus on specific targets – both with regard to symptom control and improving functioning; in other words, to 'change the agenda' [73].

5. Once the above steps have been completed, specific treatments as described below can be initiated. Central to the long-term management of somatisation is 'reattribution' – that is, modifying the attributions and meanings that patients attach to their symptoms, and providing them with the tools necessary to handle stressors and emotional conflicts.

6. Where simpler measures prove ineffective, or treatment becomes complicated by co-morbid psychiatric conditions, referral to a specialist should be considered.

Pharmacological interventions

Evidence to support the use of pharmacotherapy in somatisation is sparse, and most research has focused on antidepressants. Various classes of antidepressants have been used, with varying degrees of success; a review by O'Malley [75] concluded that both tricyclic and selective serotonergic (SSRI) antidepressants were beneficial in patients with medically unexplained symptoms, but the effect size was not large, and drop-outs were frequent. A meta-analysis by Fishbain et al. [76] concluded that antidepressants had analgesic properties in somatoform pain and related disorders. The evidence supporting the use of pharmacotherapy for somatisation is far less convincing than it is for depressive and anxiety disorders. However, if pharmacotherapy is contemplated, the use of tricyclic antidepressants or SSRIs appears reasonable; doses should be similar to those used in depressions, and trials of 6–12 weeks may be needed to assess efficacy. Medications should never be used as the sole treatment modality, as this may lead to iatrogenic reinforcement of somatisation-related behaviours; furthermore, drugs with an abuse potential, such as sedative-hypnotics and analgesics, should be avoided if possible. The primary indications for pharmacotherapy are the presence of comorbid depression and anxiety, and as an adjunct to well-established forms of psychotherapy.

Psychosocial interventions

A substantial body of evidence supports the use of cognitive-behavioural therapy (CBT) as a primary treatment for somatoform disorders. Two recent reviews [12, 77] both concluded that individual and group-based CBT are effective in the management of somatisation disorder as well as other medically unexplained symptoms and syndromes. CBT was found to improve both physical complaints and psychological distress, and resulted in better functioning. Escobar et al. [78] reported that a time-limited modification of CBT, which could be administered by primary care physicians, was highly efficacious. Other techniques include psychodynamic psychotherapy, reattribution therapy [73] and individual affective cognitive behavioural therapy (ACBT). The components of ACBT are relaxation training, behavioural management, cognitive restructuring, emotion identification, emotion regulation and interpersonal skills training [79]. CBT, where available, should be offered to all women with somatisation as a first choice, and can be implemented in individual or group settings. Where time or manpower constraints preclude this – as in primary care settings in developing countries – training of general practitioners in abbreviated CBT or reattribution techniques is a valuable and potentially cost-effective alternative.

3.7 Conversion disorder

Conversion disorder has always remained at the interface between neurology and psychiatry since the days of Charcot, Breuer and Freud. A recent study reported a significant overlap between conversion disorder and somatoform pain disorder; as both conditions can be referred to the nervous system, this may indicate shared aetiological or pathogenic mechanisms [80].

Epidemiology

It has been estimated that around 10–30% of patients presenting to neurology services will have symptoms that are 'medically unexplained' but appear to be referred to the nervous system [81]. A female preponderance has been noted, with a female-to-male ratio ranging from 1.5 to 15 : 1 [82].

A high degree of psychiatric comorbidity is seen, with the majority (75–90%) of patients having at least one other diagnosis [83]. Common comorbidities include depression, other somatoform disorders, anxiety disorders and personality disorders.

Clinical features

One of the commonest types of conversion disorder takes the form of non-epileptic seizures, which account for 20–40% of this group at all ages [84, 85]. Other common presentations include motor weakness, movement disorders, aphonia, sensory loss and disturbances in gait. Reuber *et al.* [86], have described various terms used in the literature to describe these disorders, along with clinical features to distinguish them from 'organic' neurological conditions.

While acute presentations may show a benign course conversion disorders presenting to specialist or tertiary services tend to run a chronic course, as has been shown by two long-term follow-up studies [87, 88] which showed that 40–80% of patients continue to be disabled and symptomatic even after a period of 10–12 years; In the study by Mace and Trimble, over 50% of patients were rated as improved, and about 30% were considered to be in remission; however, a sizeable number also developed the features of somatisation disorder. Certain symptom subtypes, such as non-epileptic seizures, may be associated with a worse prognosis [86]; factors predicting a poorer outcome include a longer duration of illness, the use of non-psychotropic medications and psychiatric co-morbidity.

Treatment

General principles

Current studies have shown that few patients with conversion disorder are eventually re-diagnosed with a neurological illness explaining their symptoms. Nevertheless, as in the case of patients with somatisation, appropriate investigations should be carried out. Once a diagnosis of conversion disorder is made, inappropriate treatments should be discontinued, as their continued use may itself contribute to morbidity and even mortality.

Steps involved in communicating a diagnosis of conversion have been summarised by Reuber *et al.* [86]. Briefly, the components are similar to those used in somatoform disorder, though specific reassurance regarding the absence of life-threatening or crippling illness needs to be given. Misconceptions regarding symptoms and diagnosis, which may originate with the patient, their family or social networks or previous contacts with doctors, should be corrected; it is sometimes important to tell the patient what s/he *does not* have, and not merely make the diagnosis. A biopsychosocial approach to complaints, in which the treating doctor examines the relative contributions of biological, individual psychological and social variables, and a stress-diathesis model are useful both in assessing patients and in communicating the diagnosis. Specific points that can be stressed initially include reversibility, emphasis on positive aspects, encouraging self-help and establishing an alliance with family members and other caregivers [74, 89].

Pharmacotherapy

The role of pharmacotherapy in conversion disorder is less well established. Drugs are probably best used as part of multi-modality treatment, and when a primary indication (such as depression or anxiety) exists for their use.

Specific psychotherapies

CBT has been widely advocated in the management of various forms of conversion symptoms, such as non-epileptic seizures and motor disorders. One of the advantages of CBT is that it can be used both for acute treatment and as part of rehabilitation; physiotherapy is often a part of the behavioural techniques used [90].

Other forms of therapy which have been used are psychodynamic psychotherapy, brief dynamic therapy, hypnosis and paradoxical intention. In women whose conversion symptoms are associated with family conflicts, family therapy may be a beneficial approach.

Physiotherapy and rehabilitation models

Physiotherapy and physical exercise are probably beneficial for a wide range of patients, though there are no controlled trials [74].

In conclusion, treating physicians can play a major role in the management of women with conversion disorders. The steps outlined above should be applied to all patients, and the exploration of specific stressors and traumatic situations should not occur prematurely.

3.8 Hypochondriasis

Hypochondriasis is characterised by 'a distressing preoccupation with the fear or thought, based on physical sensations, that one has a serious disease' (DSM-IV). Hypochondriasis has traditionally been classified along with the somatoform disorders, and has been thought to share pathogenic mechanisms with them. However, more recent work suggests that hypochondriasis may be even more closely related to anxiety disorders or obsessive-compulsive disorder [91]. Pilowsky [3] in the description of abnormal illness behaviour, suggested that there were three dimensions – disease phobia, disease conviction and somatic preoccupation.

Epidemiology

Prevalence rates of between 4 and 25% have been reported by earlier studies; however, an international study [62] conducted in 14 countries found a prevalence of 0.8%. Unlike somatoform and conversion disorders, no convincing evidence of a preponderance in women has been found. Comorbidity may be noted with anxiety, depressive and somatoform disorders.

Clinical features

Patients with hypochondriasis are preoccupied with the thought or fear of having a life-threatening illness. The illness is often named but sometimes is not specifically labelled. Patients are not so much preoccupied with symptoms as with the implications of their symptoms. Thus while a patient with somatisation may complain bitterly of a headache unresponsive to treatment, and describe her pain in great detail, a patient with hypochondriasis would report a fear or worry that her headache represents an underlying brain tumour.

Hypochondriasis tends to run a chronic course, though varying rates of persistence have been found depending on treatment setting. Barsky *et al.* [92] studied medical out-patients with hypochondriasis over four to five years and found that 63.5% of them still fulfilled the criteria for diagnosis at the end of the study. Noyes *et al.* [93] found similar results in a one-year follow-up of medical outpatients. The presence of concurrent somatisation, depression or anxiety may be associated with chronicity.

Treatment

1. *General principles*: Compared to somatoform symptoms, hypochondriasis is relatively rare in general practise. However, its clinical features are distinctive and easy to recognise by medical practitioners, once the boundaries between somatisation and hypochondriasis have been understood. Several interventions can be productively carried out in primary care. These include empathic validation of the patient's problems, regular visits and follow-ups, conservative use of investigations, emphasis on functioning, avoiding unnecessary treatments and education regarding the role of amplification in increasing symptoms.

2. *Pharmacotherapy*: Hypochondriacal symptoms are not exclusive to hypochondriasis, but occur in depressive, anxiety and psychotic disorders. This phenomenon, known as 'secondary hypochondriasis', has been known to respond to treatment of the underlying disorder. Primary hypochondriasis may also respond to pharmacotherapy, in particular serotonin reuptake inhibitors [29].

3. *Psychotherapies*: Cognitive and behavioural approaches – used either individually or together – show promise in the management of hypochondriasis.

The precursor of such therapy was Kellner's [94] explanatory therapy, which showed good results in the short-term.

3.9 Dissociative disorders

A normal person has a unitary sense of self and this unifying experience of self consists of an integration of a person's thoughts, feelings and actions into a unique personality and identity. The key dysfunction in the dissociative disorder is the loss of the unitary state of consciousness. This was first clearly stated by Pierre Janet, who considered dissociation to be 'an organised division of the personality' and a lack of integration between the 'systems of ideas and functions that constitute personality'.

Dissociative disorders were previously considered a subtype of hysteria, leading to a blurring of boundaries between dissociation and conversion [95]. Dissociation is best understood as a complex response to trauma, in the presence of certain predisposing factors. It shares many common aetiological factors with conversion and somatisation, especially trauma and early life adversity, as well as a high rate of comorbidity with anxiety, depression and PTSD. It differs from conversion in the exact nature of the psychological and pathophysiological processes involved, as well as in its clinical presentation.

Clinicians distinguish pathological from non-pathological forms of dissociation, and note that dissociation may be normative in some cultures, such as religious experiences. However, inclusion of normal phenomena like absorption, imagination and daydreaming, under the category of dissociation leads to a lack of clarity in the concept, and should be avoided [96].

Epidemiology

Large-scale cross-national epidemiological studies of dissociative disorders are lacking. In China up to 5% of psychiatric inpatients were reported to have a dissociative disorder, as opposed to around 1% of outpatients and less than 1% of a general population sample [97]. Similar rates were reported from Europe [98], suggesting that this may be an accurate estimate of the scope of the problem. A community-based study in New York found slightly higher rates of dissociation [99]. A study done in Turkey in women among the general population found that 18.3% met lifetime criteria for dissociation as per DSM-IV; [100]. About 35% of patients presenting to a psychiatric emergency ward in Turkey had a diagnosis of dissociative disorder, with dissociative identity disorder being the commonest. [101].

Dissociation has generally been considered to be commoner in females, but recent studies suggest it may be equally common across genders [99, 102] Dissociative disorder has been found to be a common comorbidity with borderline personality disorder, alcohol dependence, conversion disorder and obsessive-compulsive spectrum disorders.

Specific subtypes

Dissociative identity disorder

The important characteristic feature of multiple personality disorder is the presence of two or more distinct personalities within a single individual with only one of them being manifest at a time. A strong association with traumatic events in childhood, particularly physical or sexual abuse is reported. The change from one personality to another is often sudden and dramatic. Each personality is complete, with its own memories, characteristic personal preferences and behavioural patterns. The personalities may be of either sex and may be disparate and extremely opposite. Nothing unusual is found in the mental status of these patients except for amnesia for the events which occurred when the patient was in the previous personality state, or 'alter'. Often prolonged interviews and multiple contact with the patient may lead the clinician to arrive at a diagnosis of multiple personality disorder.

Trance and possession disorder

Dissociative trance disorder is characterised by temporary alteration in the state of consciousness or loss of customary sense of personal identity without replacement by an alternate identity. An associated narrowing of the awareness of surroundings and stereotyped behaviours may be present. Episodes occur in discrete attacks and there is amnesia for the trance state. In possession attacks, an episodic alteration in the state of consciousness is characterised by the replacement of customary sense of personal identity by a new identity. These could be stereotyped and culturally determined behaviours or movements that are experienced as being controlled by the possessing agent. Trance and possession states can occur in various religious and cultural contexts. It becomes a disorder only when it occurs involuntarily or is unwanted and also when it intrudes into ordinary activities by occurring outside religious or other culturally accepted situations. Possession states and trance are common in the Indian subcontinent.

Depersonalisation disorder

Depersonalisation has been defined as 'a type of dissociation involving a disrupted integration of self-perceptions with the sense of self . . . individuals experiencing depersonalisation are in a subjective state of feeling estranged, detached or disconnected from their own being' [103]. Patients with this syndrome are aware that their experience is abnormal, which has been referred to in literature as an 'as-if' feeling. Short-lived depersonalisation experiences are common in the general population, and transient depersonalisation in response to severe stressors is also well known. When such symptoms occur frequently, are persistent, and cause distress or disability, depersonalisation disorder is diagnosed. Unlike other dissociative disorders, depersonalisation is equally common in men and women, and tends to run a chronic course.

Somatoform dissociation

In somatoform dissociation, the individual fails to process somatic experiences adequately. Somatoform dissociation is linked to a number of psychiatric disorders that are relatively resistant to treatment. This needs to be differentiated from psychological dissociation – a failure to integrate cognitive, behavioural and emotional aspects of experience [102].

Somatoform dissociation can be understood as a set of adaptive psychophysiologic responses to trauma where there is a threat of inescapable physical injury. Clinicians may need to assess the nature and severity of childhood trauma and somatoform dissociation when there are high levels of somatic symptoms within psychiatric disorders that cannot be explained medically [104].

Cultural variations

While the mechanisms and functions of dissociation may be universal, the form that symptoms take may be shaped by culture. It has been argued, for example, that dissociative identity disorder is a culture bound syndrome [105], a view that is also echoed in ICD-10. Other examples include:

1. *ataque de nervios* in Puerto Ricans, which combines dissociative, conversion and somatoform symptoms (*vide supra*).

2. Group dissociation experiences, usually in response to cultural change.

3. Trance and possession in South Asian countries.

4. *amok* in Malaysia, which has been variously viewed as a psychotic disorder or a fugue state.

Changes in culture can also lead to changes in symptomatology – for example, Halliburton [106] found that, in India, spirit possession was being replaced by complaints of 'psychological tension', perhaps reflecting changing explanatory models and mental health-related beliefs.

Treatment of dissociative disorders

Treatment of dissociative disorders requires a multi-modal approach, involving assessment of the disorder, comorbid conditions and current and past stressors, as well as specific psychological interventions. The role of pharmacotherapy is limited, but studies supporting the use of specific medications have emerged in recent years. Gender-specific aspects of therapeutics have yet to be explored systematically.

1. *General principles*: Dissociative disorders generally present to psychiatrists, but they are not uncommon in primary care. Treatment has traditionally been thought to entail long-term psychotherapy. A multifaceted model for managing dissociative disorders in primary care has been described by Elmore [107] which includes psychoeducational, cognitive and behavioural techniques.

2. *Psychological therapies*: Psychodynamic, cognitive-behavioural and integrated therapies have all been advocated in the management of dissociative disorders. Much of this work comes from patients with complex dissociative disorders or dissociative identity disorder, and therapy is usually a long-term process, which needs to be individualised. Restoring a stable sense of self is a key aspect of therapy, and certain general principles are universal, regardless of theoretical orientation. Cognitive-analytic therapy, which combines techniques from CBT and dynamic therapy, may be effective. Techniques used in the management of PTSD, including eye movement desensitisation and reprocessing (EMDR), may also be used, given the central role of severe trauma in the genesis of these disorders. A rehabilitative approach, emphasising enhancement of functioning, communication and containment of the trauma, may be useful in patients with chronic symptoms.

3. *Pharmacological therapies*: The use of pharmacotherapy in dissociative disorder is still a growing area, without conclusive evidence. Medications that have been advocated include antidepressants for mood dysregulation, opioid antagonists for self-injurious behaviour, and neuroleptics for intrusive flashbacks, and hallucinatory voices [108]. Evidence from recent trials suggests efficacy for paroxetine, for dissociative symptoms in patients with comorbid PTSD and dissociation [109], clonidine for dissociative symptoms in women with borderline personality disorder [110] and the opioid antagonists naloxone and naltrexone for dissociation in women with borderline personality disorder [111, 112].

Conclusions

Somatoform and dissociative disorders in women represent, *par excellence*, the value of a biopsychosocial approach in understanding the aetiology, pathogenesis, clinical presentation and treatment of a disorder. Though traditionally viewed as difficult-to-treat and frustrating conditions, the use of various psychotherapeutic techniques, supplemented when necessary by pharmacotherapy, yields rewarding results. The influences of comorbidity, personality and cultural factors should always be taken into account when formulating a treatment plan. Given the female preponderance, chronicity and disability associated with these disorders, appropriate management can significantly improve women's quality of life, strengthen their coping skills and enable them to face the various stressors that are part of their lives.

References

1. Lieb, R., Meinlschmidt, G. and Araya, R. (2007) Epidemiology of the association between somatoform disorders and anxiety and depressive disorders: an update. *Psychosomatic Medicine*, **69**, 860–63.

2. Lipowski, Z.J. (1988) Somatization. The concept and its clinical application. *The American Journal of Psychiatry*, **145**, 1358–68.

3. Pilowsky, I. (1992) Somatic symptoms/somatization. *Current Opinion in Psychiatry*, **5**, 213–18.

4. Kirmayer, L.J. and Young, A. (1998) Culture and somatization: clinical, epidemiological, and ethnographic perspectives. *Psychosomatic Medicine*, **60**, 420–30.

5. Koch, H., van Bokhoven, M.A., ter Riet, G. *et al.* (2007) Demographic characteristics and quality of life of patients with unexplained complaints: a descriptive study in general practice. *Quality of Life Research*, **16**, 1483–89.

6. Barsky, A.J., Orav, E.J. and Bates, D.W. (2005) Somatization increases medical utilization and costs independent of psychiatric and medical comorbidity. *Archives of General Psychiatry*, **62**, 903–10.

7. Chaturvedi, S.K. and Bhugra, D. (2007) The concept of neurosis in a cross-cultural perspective. *Current Opinion in Psychiatry*, **20**, 37–45.

8. World Health Organization, WHO (1992). The ICD-10 Classification of Mental and Behavioural Disorders, Clinical Descriptions and Diagnostic Guidelines. World Health Organization, Geneva.

9. American Psychiatric Association, APA (1994). *Diagnostic and Statistical Manual of Mental Disorders*, 4th edn, American Psychiatric Association, Washington, DC.

10. Escobar, J.I., Burnam, M.A., Karno, M., Forsythe, A., Golding, J.M. (1987) Somatization in the community. *Archives of General Psychiatry*, **44**, 713–18.

11. Mayou, R., Kirmayer, L.J., Simon, G. *et al.* (2005) Somatoform disorders: time for a new approach in DSM-V. *The American Journal of Psychiatry*, **162**, 847–55.

12. Kroenke, K. (2007) Somatoform disorders and recent diagnostic controversies. *The Psychiatric Clinics of North America*, **30**, 593–619.

13. Dimsdale, J.E., Patel, V., Xin, Y. and Kleinman, A. (2007) Somatic presentations – a challenge for DSM-V. *Psychosomatic Medicine*, **69**, 829.

14. Creed, F. and Barsky, A. (2004) A systematic review of the epidemiology of somatisation disorder and hypochondriasis. *Journal of Psychosomatic Research*, **56**, 391–408.

15. Dimsdale, J.E. and Dantzer, R. (2007) A biological substrate for somatoform disorders: importance of pathophysiology. *Psychosomatic Medicine*, **69**, 850–54.

16. Bitzer, J. (2003) Somatization disorders in obstetrics and gynecology. *Archives of Women's Mental Health*, **6**, 99–107.

17. Goldstein-Ferber, S. and Granot, M. (2006) The association between somatization and perceived ability: roles in dysmenorrhea among Israeli Arab adolescents. *Psychosomatic Medicine*, **68**, 136–42.

18. Charney, D.S. (2004) Psychobiological mechanisms of resilience and vulnerability: implications for successful adaptation to extreme stress. *The American Journal of Psychiatry*, **161**, 195–216.

19. Hakala, M., Karlsson, H., Ruotsalainen, M. *et al.* (2002) Severe somatization in women is associated with altered cerebral glucose metabolism. *Psychological Medicine*, **32**, 1379–85.

20. Garcia-Campayo, J., Sanz-Carrillo, C., Baringo, T. and Ceballos, C. (2001) SPECT scan in somatization disorder patients: an exploratory study of eleven cases. *The Australian and New Zealand Journal of Psychiatry*, **35**, 359–63.

21. Vuilleumier, P., Chicherio, C., Assal, F. *et al.* (2001) Functional neuroanatomical correlates of hysterical sensorimotor loss. *Brain*, **124**, 1077–90.

22. Nash, M.R. (2005) Salient findings: a potentially groundbreaking study on the neuroscience of hypnotizability, a critical review of hypnosis' efficacy, and the neurophysiology of conversion disorder. *Journal of Clinical and Experimental Hypnosis*, **53**, 87–93.

23. Kanaan, R.A.A., Craig, T.K.J., Wessely, S.C. and David, A.S. (2007) Imaging repressed memories in motor conversion disorder. *Journal of Psychosomatic Medicine*, **69**, 202–5.

24. Vermetten, E., Schmahl, C., Lindner, S. *et al.* (2006) Hippocampal and amygdalar volumes in dissociative identity disorder. *The American Journal of Psychiatry*, **163**, 630–36.

25. Simeon, D., Guralnik, O., Hazlett, E.A. *et al.* (2000) Feeling unreal: a PET study of depersonalization disorder. *The American Journal of Psychiatry*, **157**, 1782–88.

26. Hammad, M.A., Barsky, A.J. and Regestein, Q.R. (2001) Correlation between somatic sensation inventory scores and hyperarousal scale scores. *Psychosomatics*, **42**, 29–34.

27. Allen, L.A., Gara, M.A., Escobar, J.I. *et al.* (2001) Somatization: a debilitating syndrome in primary care. *Psychosomatics*, **42**, 63–67.

28. McBeth, J., Chiu, Y.H., Silman, A.J. *et al.* (2005) Hypothalamic-pituitary-adrenal stress axis function and the relationship with chronic widespread pain and its antecedents. *Arthritis Research and Therapy*, **7**, 992–1000.

29. Magarinos, M., Zafar, U., Nissenson, K. and Blanco, C. (2002) Epidemiology and treatment of hypochondriasis. *CNS Drugs*, **16**, 9–22.

30. Deveci, A., Aydemir, O., Taskin, O. *et al.* (2007) Serum brain-derived neurotrophic factor levels in conversion disorder: comparative study with depression. *Psychiatry and Clinical Neurosciences*, **61**, 571–73.

31. Gramling, S.E., Clawson, E.P. and McDonal, L.K. (1996) Perceptual and cognitive abnormality model of hypochondriasis: amplification and physiological reactivity in women. *Psychosomatic Medicine*, **58**, 423–31.

32. Brownlee, S., Leventhal, H. and Balaban, M. (1992) Autonomic correlates of illness imagery. *Psychophysiology*, **29**, 142–53.

33. Kozlowska, K. (2005) Healing the disembodied mind: contemporary models of conversion disorder. *Harvard Review of Psychiatry*, **13**, 1–13.

34. Tallabs, F.P. (2005) Functional correlates of conversion and hypnotic paralysis: a neurophysiological hypothesis. *Contemporary Hypnosis*, **22**, 184–92.

35. Scaer, R.C. (2001) The neurophysiology of dissociation and chronic disease. *Applied Psychophysiology and Biofeedback*, **26**, 73–91.

36. Forrest, K.A. (2001) Towards an etiology of dissociative identity disorder: a neurodevelopmental approach. *Consciousness and Cognition*, **10**, 259–93.

37. Sifneos, P.E. (1996) Alexithymia: past and present. *The American Journal of Psychiatry*, **153** (Suppl 7), 137–42.
38. Subic-Wrana, C., Bruder, S., Thomas, W. *et al.* (2005) Emotional awareness deficits in inpatients of a psychosomatic ward: a comparison of two different measures of alexithymia. *Psychosomatic Medicine*, **67**, 483–89.
39. Burba, B., Oswald, R., Grigaliunien, V. *et al.* (2006) A controlled study of alexithymia in adolescent patients with persistent somatoform pain disorder. *Canadian Journal of Psychiatry*, **51**, 468–71.
40. Moriguchi, Y., Maeda, M., Igarashi, T. *et al.* (2007) Age and gender effect on alexithymia in large, Japanese community and clinical samples: a cross-validation study of the Toronto Alexithymia Scale (TAS-20). *BioPsychoSocial Medicine*, **1**, 1–15.
41. Karlsson, H., Naatanen, P. and Stenman, H. (2008). Cortical activation in alexithymia as a response to emotional stimuli. *The British Journal of Psychiatry*, **192**, 32–38.
42. Barsky, A.J., Peekna, H.M. and Borus, J.F. (2001) Somatic symptom reporting in women and men. *Journal of General Internal Medicine*, **16**, 266–75.
43. Bernstein, A., Zvolensky, M.J., Stewart, S.H. *et al.* (2006) Anxiety sensitivity taxonicity across gender among youth. *Behavior Research and Therapy*, **44**, 679–98.
44. Nakao, M., Tamiya, N. and Yano, E. (2005) Gender and somatosensory amplification in relation to perceived work stress and social support in Japanese workers. *Women and Health*, **42**, 41–54.
45. Mueller, J. and Alpers, G.W. (2006) Two facets of being bothered by bodily sensations: anxiety sensitivity and alexithymia in psychosomatic patients. *Comprehensive Psychiatry*, **47**, 489–95.
46. Bracha, H.S., Yoshioka, D.T., Masukawa, N.K., Stockman, D.J. (2005) Evolution of the human fear-circuitry and acute sociogenic pseudoneurological symptoms: the Neolithic balanced polymorphism hypothesis. *Journal of Affective Disorders*, **88**, 119–29.
47. Price, J.S., Gardner, R. Jr. and Erickson, M. (2004) Can depression, anxiety and somatization be understood as appeasement displays? *Journal of Affective Disorders*, **79**, 1–11.
48. Karvonen, J.T., Veijola, J., Kantojärvi, L. *et al.* (2006) Temperament profiles and somatization – an epidemiological study of young adult people. *Journal of Psychosomatic Research*, **61**, 841–46.
49. Garcia-Campayo, J., Alda, M., Sobradiel, N. *et al.* (2007) Personality disorders in somatization disorder patients: a controlled study in Spain. *Journal of Psychosomatic Research*, **62**, 675–80.
50. Chaturvedi, S.K., Desai, G., Shaligram, D. (2006) Somatoform disorders, somatization and abnormal illness behaviour. *International Review of Psychiatry*, **18**, 75–80.
51. Gureje, O. (2004) What can we learn from a cross-national study of somatic distress? *Journal of Psychosomatic Research* **56**, 409–12.
52. Kirmayer, L.J. and Sartorius, N. (2007) Cultural models and somatic syndromes. *Psychosomatic Medicine*, **69**, 832–40.

53. Tomlinson, M., Swartz, L., Kruger, L.M. and Gureje, O. (2007) Manifestations of affective disturbance in sub-Saharan Africa: key themes. *Journal of Affective Disorders*, **102**, 191–98.

54. Halbreich, U., Alarcon, R.D. and Calil, H. (2007) Culturally-sensitive complaints of depressions and anxieties in women. *Journal of Affective Disorders*, **102**, 159–76.

55. Douki, S., Zineb, S.B., Nacef, F. *et al.* (2007) Women's mental health in the Muslim world: cultural, religious, and social issues. *Journal of Affective Disorders*, **102**, 177–89.

56. Chaturvedi, S.K. (1993). Neurosis across Culture. *International Review of Psychiatry* **5**, 181–94.

57. Nicolas, G., Desilva, A.M., Subrebost, K.L. *et al.* (2007) Expression and treatment of depression among Haitian immigrant women in the United States: clinical observations. *American Journal of Psychotherapy*, **61**, 83–98.

58. Pereira, B., Andrew, G. and Pednekar, S., (2007) The explanatory models of depression in low income countries: listening to women in India. *Journal of Affective Disorders*, **102**, 209–18.

59. Raguram, R., Weiss, M.G., Channabasavanna, S.M. *et al.* (1996) Stigma, depression, and somatization in South India. *The American Journal of Psychiatry*, **153**, 1043–49.

60. Dorahy, M.J., Schumaker, J.F., Krishnamurthy, R., Kumar, P. (1997) Religious ritual and dissociation in India and Australia. *The Journal of Psychology*, **131**, 471–6.

61. El Sherbiny, L., El Nabulsi, M. and El Sendiouny, F. (2003) First Wife Syndrome. Paper Presented at the First Pan Mediterranean Conference on Psychiatry and Cultures, 9–13 November 2003.

62. Gureje, O., Ustün, T.B. and Simon, G.E. (1997) The syndrome of hypochondriasis: a cross-national study in primary care. *Psychological Medicine*, **27**, 1001–10.

63. Nandi, D.N., Banerjee, G., Mukherjee, S.P. *et al.* (2000) Psychiatric morbidity of a rural Indian community over 20 years. *The British Journal of Psychiatry*, **176**, 351–56.

64. Fink, P., Sørensen, L. and Engberg, M. (1999) Somatization in primary care. Prevalence, health care utilization, and general practitioner recognition. *Psychosomatics*, **40**, 330–38.

65. Rief, W. and Rojas, G. (2007) Stability of somatoform symptoms – implications for classification. *Psychosomatic Medicine*, **69**, 864–69.

66. Arnold, I.A., de Waal, M.W., Eekhof, J.A. and van Hemert, A.M. (2006) Somatoform disorder in primary care: course and the need for cognitive-behavioral treatment. *Psychosomatics*, **47**, 498–503.

67. Patel, V., Weiss, H.A., Kirkwood, B.R. *et al.* (2006) Common genital complaints in women: the contribution of psychosocial and infectious factors in a population-based cohort study in Goa, India. *International Journal of Epidemiology*, **35**, 1478–85.

68. Janakiramaiah, N. (1983) Somatic neurosis in middle-aged Hindu women. *International Journal of Social Psychiatry*, **29**, 113–16.

69. Karst, M., Rahe-Meyer, N., Gueduek, A. *et al.* (2005) Abnormality in the self-monitoring mechanism in patients with fibromyalgia and somatoform pain disorder. *Psychosomatic Medicine*, **67**, 111–15.

70. Chandra, P.S., Ranjan, S. (2006) Psychosomatic obstetrics and gynecology – a neglected field? *Current Opinion in Psychiatry*, **20**, 168–73.

71. Zondervan, K.T., Cardon, L.R. and Kennedy, S.H., (2005) Multivariate genetic analysis of chronic pelvic pain and associated phenotypes. *Behavior Genetics*, **35**, 177–88.

72. Lee, S. *et al.* (1998) Estranged bodies, simulated harmony, and misplaced culture: neurasthenia in contemporary Chinese society. *Psychosomatic Medicine*, **60**, 448–57.

73. Goldberg, D., Gask, L. and O'Dowd, T. (1989) The treatment of somatization: teaching techniques of reattribution. *Journal of Psychosomatic Research*, **33**, 689–95.

74. Stone, J., Carson, A. and Sharpe, M. (2005) Functional symptoms in neurology: management. *Journal of Neurology, Neurosurgery and Psychiatry*, **76**, 13–21.

75. O'Malley, P.G., Jackson, J.L., Santoro, J., Tomkins, G., Balden, E., Kroenke, K. (1999) Antidepressant therapy for unexplained symptoms and symptom syndromes. *Journal of Family Practice*, **48**, 980–90.

76. Fishbain, D.A., Cutler, R.B., Rosomoff, H.L., Rosomoff, R.S. (1998) Do antidepressants have an analgesic effect in psychogenic pain and somatoform pain disorder? A meta-analysis. *Psychosomatic Medicine*, **60**, 503–9.

77. Sumathipala, A. (2007) What is the evidence for the efficacy of treatments for somatoform disorders? A critical review of previous intervention studies. *Psychosomatic Medicine*, **69**, 889–900.

78. Escobar, J.I., Gara, M.A., Diaz-Martinez, A.M., Interian, A., Warman, M., Allen, L.A., Woolfolk, R.L., Jahn, E., Rodgers, D. (2007) Effectiveness of a time-limited cognitive behavior therapy type intervention among primary care patients with medically unexplained symptoms. *Annals of Family Medicine*, **5**, 328–35.

79. Woolfolk, R.L., Allen, L.A. and Tiu, J.E. (2007) New directions in treatment of somatization. *Psychiatric Clinics of North America*, **30**, 621–44.

80. Birket-Smith, M. and Mortensen, E.L. (2002) Pain in somatoform disorders: is somatoform pain disorder a valid diagnosis? *Acta Psychiatrica Scandinavica*, **106**, 103–8.

81. Carson, A.J., Ringbauer, B., Stone, J. *et al.* (2000) Do medically unexplained symptoms matter? A prospective cohort study of 300 new referrals to neurology outpatient clinics. *Journal of Neurology, Neurosurgery and Psychiatry*, **68**, 207–10.

82. Gigineïshvili, D.A. and Shakarishvili, R.R. (2006) Unexplained somatic symptoms and underlying psychologic disorders in the neurology clinic. *Georgian Medical News*, **132**, 50–53.

83. Sar, V., Akyuz, G., Kundacki, T. *et al.* (2004) Childhood trauma, dissociation, and psychiatric comorbidity in patients with conversion disorder. *The American Journal of Psychiatry*, **161**, 2271–76.

84. Kuloglu, M., Atmaca, M., Tezcan, E. *et al.* (2003) Sociodemographic and clinical characteristics of patients with conversion disorder in Eastern Turkey. *Social Psychiatry and Psychiatric Epidemiology*, **38**, 88–93.

85. Kozlowska, K., Nunn, K.P., Rose, D. *et al.* (2007) Conversion disorder in Australian pediatric practice. *Journal of the American Academy of Child and Adolescent Psychiatry*, **46**, 68–75.

86. Reuber, M., Mitchell, A.J., Howlett, S.J. *et al.* (2005) Functional symptoms in neurology: questions and answers. *Journal of Neurology, Neurosurgery and Psychiatry*, **76**, 307–14.

87. Stone, J., Sharpe, M., Rothwell, P.M. and Warlow, C.P. (2003) The 12 year prognosis of unilateral functional weakness and sensory disturbance. *Journal of Neurology, Neurosurgery and Psychiatry*, **74**, 591–96.

88. Mace, C.J. and Trimble, M.R. (1996) Ten-year prognosis of conversion disorder. *The British Journal of Psychiatry*, **169**, 282–88.

89. Stonnington, C.M., Barry, J.J. and Fischer, R.S. (2006) Conversion disorder. *The American Journal of Psychiatry*, **163**, 1510–17.

90. Shapiro, A.P. and Teasell, R.W. (2004) Behavioural interventions in the rehabilitation of acute v. chronic non-organic (conversion/factitious) motor disorders. *The British Journal of Psychiatry*, **185**, 140–46.

91. Castle, D.J. and Phillips, K.A. (2006) Obsessive-compulsive spectrum of disorders: a defensible construct? *The Australian and New Zealand Journal of Psychiatry*, **40**, 114–20.

92. Barsky, A.J., Fama, J.M., Bailey, E.D., Ahern, D.K. (1998) A prospective 4- to 5-year study of DSM-III-R hypochondriasis. *Archives of General Psychiatry*, **55**, 737–44.

93. Noyes, R. Jr., Kathol, R.G., Fisher, M.M., Phillips, B.M., Suelzer, M.T., Woodman, C.L. (1994) One-year follow-up of medical outpatients with hypochondriasis. *Psychosomatics*, **35**, 533–45.

94. Kellner, R. (1983) Prognosis of treated hypochondriasis. A clinical study. *Acta Psychiatr Scand.* Feb, **67** (2), 69–79.

95. Isaac, M. and Chand, P.K. (2006) Dissociative and conversion disorders: defining boundaries. *Current Opinion in Psychiatry*, **19**, 61–66.

96. Van der Hart, O., Nijenhuis, E., Steele, K. and Brown, D. (2004) Trauma-related dissociation: conceptual clarity lost and found. *The Australian and New Zealand Journal of Psychiatry*, **38**, 906–14.

97. Xiao, Z., Yan, H., Wang, Z. *et al.* (2006) Trauma and dissociation in China. *The American Journal of Psychiatry*, **163**, 1388–91.

98. Spitzer, C., Barnow, S., Grabe, H.J. *et al.* (2006) Frequency, clinical and demographic correlates of pathological dissociation in Europe. *Journal of Trauma and Dissociation*, **7**, 51–62.

99. Johnson, J.G., Cohen, P., Kasen, S. and Brook, J.S. (2006) Dissociative disorders among adults in the community, impaired functioning, and axis I and II comorbidity. *Journal of Psychiatric Research*, **40**, 131–40.

100. Sar, V., Akyüz, G. and Doğan, O. (2007) Prevalence of dissociative disorders among women in the general population. *Psychiatry Research*, **149**, 169–76.

101. Sar, V., Koyuncu, A., Ozturk, E. *et al.* (2007) Dissociative disorders in the psychiatric emergency ward. *General Hospital Psychiatry*, **29**, 45–50.

102. Maaranen, P., Tanskanen, A., Honkalampi, K. *et al.* (2005) Factors associated with pathological dissociation in the general population. *The Australian and New Zealand Journal of Psychiatry*, **39**, 387–94.

103. Simeon, D. (2004) Depersonalisation disorder: a contemporary overview. *CNS Drugs*, **18**, 343–54.

104. Waller, G., Hamilton, K., Elliott, P. *et al.* (2000) Somatoform dissociation, psychological dissociation, and specific forms of trauma. *Journal of Trauma and Dissociation*, **1** (4), 81–98.

105. Piper, A. and Merskey, H. (2004) The persistence of folly: a critical examination of dissociative identity disorder. Part I. The excesses of an improbable concept. *Canadian Journal of Psychiatry*, **49**, 592–600.

106. Halliburton, M. (2005) "Just some spirits": the erosion of spirit possession and the rise of "tension" in South India. *Medical Anthropology*, **24**, 111–44.

107. Elmore, J.L. (2000) Dissociative Spectrum Disorders in the Primary Care Setting. *Primary Care Companion to the Journal of Clinical Psychiatry*, **2**, 37–41.

108. Loewenstein, R.J. (2005) Psychopharmacologic treatments for dissociative identity disorder. *Psychiatric Annals*, **35**, 666–73.

109. Marshall, R.D., Lewis-Fernandez, R., Blanco, C. *et al.* (2007) A controlled trial of paroxetine for chronic PTSD, dissociation, and interpersonal problems in mostly minority adults. *Depression and Anxiety*, **24**, 77–84.

110. Philipsen, A., Richter, H., Schmahl, C. *et al.* (2004) Clonidine in acute aversive inner tension and self-injurious behavior in female patients with borderline personality disorder. *The Journal of Clinical Psychiatry*, **65**, 1414–19.

111. Philipsen, A., Schmahl, C. and Lieb, K. (2004) Naloxone in the treatment of acute dissociative states in female patients with borderline personality disorder. *Pharmacopsychiatry*, **37**, 196–99.

112. Bohus, M.J., Landwehrmeyer, G.B., Stiglmayr, C.E. *et al.* (1999) Naltrexone in the treatment of dissociative symptoms in patients with borderline personality disorder: an open-label trial. *The Journal of Clinical Psychiatry*, **60**, 598–603.

113. Chaturvedi, S.K., Chandra, P., Isaac, M.K. *et al.* (1993) Somatisation misattributed to non pathological vaginal discharge. *Journal of Psychosomatic Research*, **37**, 575–9.

Further reading

Chaturvedi, S.K. and Desai, G. (2007) Neurosis, in *Textbook of Cultural Psychiatry* (eds K. Bhui and D. Bhugra), Cambridge University Press, pp. 193–206.

4

Eating disorders

Sarvath Abbas[1] and Robert L. Palmer[1,2]

[1]*Leicestershire Eating Disorder Service, Leicestershire Partnership NHS Trust, Leicester, UK*
[2]*Department of Health Sciences, University of Leicester, Leicester, UK*

4.1 Introduction

The clinical eating disorders (EDs) – anorexia nervosa (AN), bulimia nervosa (BN) and similar states – have become much more prominent over the last two or three decades. Indeed it was as recently as 1979 that BN was first fully described and named [1, 2]. With remarkable speed, these disorders have moved from obscurity with at best brief mention in the small print of medical textbooks to a prominence where most people have some acquaintance with them and there is regular comment about them in the lay press. At least in Europe and North America, the public knows about the EDs and indeed holds opinions about them.

What has brought about this change? Are EDs now a worldwide problem? What causes them? What treatments are best? Do EDs represent a significant public health problem? These are some of the issues that will be addressed in this chapter.

But first it may be useful to mention briefly what seem to be the problematic preconceptions and prejudices that sometimes get in the way of the EDs being taken seriously at an individual or public health level. In the developed world these prejudices are of two broad types. The first is the view that sees EDs in general, and especially AN, as severe but puzzling and rare diseases that afflict and often kill their young victims; golden girls cut down before the prime of their lives. The second view is that EDs are widespread but are merely an exaggerated form of the common body preoccupations and slimming behaviours of adolescent girls. This latter view may sometimes be associated with an ambivalent link

Contemporary Topics in Women's Mental Health   Edited by Chandra, Herrman, Fisher, Kastrup,
© 2009 John Wiley & Sons, Ltd   Niaz, Rondón and Okasha

between EDs and glamour; the press often featuring famous 'victims' and their 'battles' with EDs. Both views have some small basis in truth but both lead to a trivialisation of the disorders; the first by suggesting that they are rare and the second through minimising the degree of morbidity and indeed excess mortality arising from them. An additional complication is that now the EDs must be viewed against the background of what has been called a worldwide epidemic of obesity [3]. Obesity is conventionally excluded from classification amongst the EDs and this chapter will follow that convention. Nevertheless the two areas of concern are not entirely separate and the rhetoric of public health messages about the dangers of being overweight have a distorted echo in the beliefs and preoccupations of many of those with EDs.

The EDs are complex and may be fascinating to the detached observer. However, to those who suffer them they are sources of unhappiness and misery. Indeed, they are commonly life blighting and may even be life destroying [4, 5]. They are important causes of ill health and are not uncommon. In severe form they place a burden upon carers similar to that of psychosis [6] and hence deserve to be taken seriously.

4.2 Risk factors and pathogenesis

The causes and pathogenesis of the EDs are difficult to specify in detail with any degree of confidence. Nevertheless many people, including members of the public and the lay press, hold firm views on the topic. Indeed some would claim to know how these disorders arise. They have strong intuitions that social factors are crucial, most notably the idealising of a thin body and the pressure upon adolescent girls and young women to attain and maintain it. Indeed, there is evidence that eating restraint is a risk factor for the development of EDs [7–9]. However, widespread social influences cannot be the whole story because only a small minority of any relevant population develop EDs. Most encounter the potentially noxious pressures, many are influenced but few fall ill. There must be other factors that make particular individuals susceptible. What might these factors be?

Genetic factors are almost certainly involved. There is evidence that EDs run in families in ways that suggest that susceptibility is inherited with coaggregation between the two main EDs [10, 11]. Indeed there is some evidence of shared risk of anxiety, mood disorders and alcohol abuse [10, 11]. Some studies have produced figures for heritability of over 50%. However, this should not be taken to mean that environmental issues are not important. Heritability may vary with circumstance. Thus, estimates of heritability will be high when noxious environmental factors are uniformly high since genetic factors would then determine who would fall into EDs and who would remain well. So genetypic variation may underlie much of the variation in individual risk but, the nature of the corresponding phenotype is uncertain. Might it be manifest as a behavioural trait, as a variation of mechanisms of the regulation of appetite or satiety or as an endophenotype difficult to define in other than biochemical terms? As with other disorders, genetics seem to offer the prospect of both greater understanding and therapeutic potency in the future, but for the present such benefits have yet to be delivered. Indeed, more generally the active field of research into the biology of EDs has produced findings in neuro-chemistry, neuro-psychology and neuro-imaging, but there has been thus far little that has directly influenced clinical practise [12, 13].

Research suggests that there are risk factors that are clearly related to weight, shape and eating and others that are more general risk factors for mental disorder [14]. Fairburn and colleagues from Oxford conducted a series of case control studies seeking risk factors for AN, BN and binge eating disorder (BED) [15–17]. The study revealed broadly two sets of risk factors, those reflecting factors to do with weight and eating (family dieting, special pressure to be slim, critical comments about shape, etc.) and those of a more general kind (childhood adversity, abuse, low self-esteem, perfectionism).

Two further risk factors are well established. These are gender – being female – and age – being in the teens and 20s. Most reports, both of clinical or population samples, find that for every male with an EDs there are at least 10 females. But which of the many differences between males and females are relevant to this differential risk? The different social meanings of body size and shape are clear candidates. Age and developmental issues are relevant here also. Thus for the female, the marked change of shape with puberty and the associated increase of body fat are harbingers of adulthood, of sexual attraction and of potential fertility. The equivalent changes in the male are less dramatic. However, there are also hidden gender differences of a biochemical nature. For instance, serotonin mechanisms, which have important roles in the regulation of both satiety and mood, differ between the genders when the individual restrains their intake of food [18]. Furthermore, genes may play a part in determining the age of risk since it has been shown that relevant genes 'switch on' during an individual's passage through puberty [19]. Especially for girls, puberty and adolescence involve changes which are not only profound in their implications but also evident with each glance in the mirror. These changes come unbidden and cannot be switched off except perhaps imperfectly by self-starvation. The young female with ED and especially with AN can be thought of as battling with her own body and indeed with her biological destiny [20].

In brief, the evidence to date suggests that when adolescent girls and young women find themselves within a culture or a sub-culture that values a slender body ideal and they are themselves troubled and have low self-esteem, they are at a raised risk of developing EDs. However, our ability to predict who will and who will not fall ill remains poor. There may well be important risk factors that are currently overlooked or neglected.

4.3 Distribution

There are troubled people everywhere. It is an open question whether people with EDs are to be found everywhere. It is plausible that EDs are mainly confined to countries and populations that might be described as 'western' or that are becoming 'westernised'. However, little is known with confidence about the prevalence of EDs in most countries of the world because there are no adequate studies. Nevertheless, some cases have been reported from many countries and EDs are increasingly thought of as being worldwide in their distribution [21]. It remains plausible that EDs are endemic throughout the world and would become evident were appropriate studies to be done; as the saying goes 'lack of evidence is not evidence of lack'. Alternatively, EDs may be spread throughout the world but only – or at least mainly – in westernised elites.

4.4 Presentation, assessment, diagnosis and engagement

Presentation

The detection and diagnosis of EDs is straightforward when there is evident physical abnormality such as emaciation and/or evident behaviour. Thus many people may suspect AN when they encounter a young woman who weighs say 30 kg – giving her a body mass index of 12 – and who behaves in a manner apparently motivated by a desire to sustain that position. However, strictly speaking the diagnosis cannot be clinched unless the psychopathology is made manifest which nearly always involves the individual being willing to talk about what she is thinking and feeling. Many are so willing but some are not.

It is characteristic of people with EDs in general, and especially AN, that they have some reticence in talking about themselves and their disorder. Indeed, people with AN are often reluctant patients, presenting to the clinic only when persuaded or cajoled by others. This stance is sometimes described as 'part of the illness' and may be discussed with the patient as such. However, a somewhat more complex but arguably better way of construing the patient's reluctance is as a result of truly mixed feelings within an interpersonal context.

The person who is stuck within AN is likely to find much of the experience at the least irksome or uncomfortable and not uncommonly as destructive and terrifying. There may be some positives – such as a strange sense of achievement or control – but in the main the experience is negative. However, she – or occasionally he – is reluctant to strive straightforwardly for change because the prospect of such change and in particular weight gain feels as if it will bring consequences that could be even more negative. The patient may find it difficult to put such feelings into words even to herself. But the sense of change as threatening some sort of loss of control is powerful and scary. This may be discussed in terms of weight, shape and eating but somehow such issues are experienced as resonating in a wordless way with issues that are both wider and deeper. At worst the patient can feel that the very existence of her self is in danger. Thus the person with AN will be experiencing painful internal conflict and is likely to employ any available mechanism from plain denial through to plain courage in managing her internal struggle.

And what of the interpersonal context? The patient experiencing truly mixed feelings about both changing and not changing is likely to find herself surrounded by others who are unequivocally pushing for weight gain and other positive change. They may include family, friends and crucially clinicians. The temptation for any or all of these people is to push the patient towards what seems to be positive change. However, if the mixed feelings have not been explored and expressed, their well meaning efforts may have unintended negative consequences. Thus, in simplified terms the patient with her inner dialogue of conflicting fears ('I need to eat' v 'I can't eat') when confronted by the simple message of those who would help her ('You must eat') finds that the positive half of her dilemma is now spoken by others. She becomes more likely to express the other more negative side and finds herself saying and indeed perhaps experiencing only one side of the conflict – 'I can't eat'. Thus the interpersonal context may amplify and distort the way in which the patient and the clinician experience the problem. As Charles Lasegue, the nineteenth century French psychiatrist, wrote well over a 100 years ago, 'an excess of persistence begets an excess of resistance'. What had been an internal tussle within the patient comes to be an external battle with others. Tragically, it can sometimes it be a battle to the death.

Such issues may come into play from the very beginning of the first meeting with the patient. The clinician is wise to spend as much time as is required on exploring the patient's feelings even if this involves proceeding more slowly than might otherwise be the case. The simple initial question, 'What do you feel about coming along here today?' may open up a whole seam of invaluable conversation. Assessment and engagement should go hand in hand. And of course, it is important to remember that the patient is assessing you, the clinician, every bit as much as you are assessing her. Do you listen? Do you seem to know what is what? To what degree might it be possible to trust you?

If the stereotypical person with AN has mixed feelings around issues of control, the equivalent stance of the person with BN is one of wariness mixed with shame and self-criticism. But as with any stereotypes, the actual individual thoughts, feelings and attitudes are what matter and these will need to be explored; a process that starts in assessment and should continue within psychological treatment.

Assessment

The assessment of a patient with an ED includes several elements. These include categorical diagnosis of the ED, examination of the mental state and diagnosis of any psychiatric co-morbidity and assessment of the physical state. A detailed account of the many physical complications of the EDs and how they may be detected and managed is beyond the scope of this chapter. However whatever the profession of the clinician involved with a person with severe ED some arrangement needs to be made to assess physical risk. There are a number of useful accounts of what issues are involved [22–24]. Assessment of risk should include risk of suicide and self-harm in all cases. The clinician should also develop some provisional understanding of the patient's 'story' including how she views her present position. The inclusion of family members or important others at some stage in the assessment can be valuable and is almost universal when the patient is a child or early adolescent. Adult patients should usually have a veto as to what third parties are involved if any.

Diagnosis

Unfortunately, the available diagnostic classifications of the EDs are importantly flawed. The better of the two international systems is probably the American DSM-IV (Diagnostic and Statistical Manual of Mental Disorders of the American Psychiatric Association 1994) although the ICD-10 (World Health Organization) is widely used for clinical coding [25, 26]. Essentially, DSM-IV has three diagnoses. The two dominant categories are AN and BN which, respectively, have low weight and binge eating as their central features. Each of these main categories has subdivisions (The DSM-IV criteria are set out in Box 4.1)

The DSM-IV classification has at least two major flaws. The first and lesser problem concerns the way in which the system deals with the issue of overlap between AN and BN or rather to avoid begging the question, with people who are at low weight but who also binge in a way that would qualify for a diagnosis of BN all other things being equal. An earlier version of the DSM allowed the dual diagnoses of both AN and BN to be made in such circumstances but DSM-IV makes AN 'trump' BN using the sub-category of AN, binge/purge sub-type.

The second and more important problem concerns the third major diagnosis available in DSM-IV namely Eating Disorder not Otherwise Specified (EDNOS); a term that is increasingly being referred to as 'EDNOS' in both speech and writing. As the name implies EDNOS is essentially a residual category included to sweep up what is left of EDs once AN and BN have been excluded. However, this residual category, EDNOS has been repeatedly shown to be common in clinical samples and indeed is often the biggest diagnostic group [27, 28]. This is probably the case in non-clinical community samples also [29]. This is somewhat embarrassing. Furthermore since the sole positive criterion for EDNOS is that it should be used only for EDs of clinical severity, the argument that EDNOS can be excluded because it is not serious or of no clinical relevance cannot prevail. Indeed, a recent study has shown that in the clinic EDNOS and BN do not differ in overall symptom severity, functional impairment, length of history or response to treatment [30]. Some EDNOS patients fall into the provisional DSM-IV sub-type, BED which approximates to BN without compensatory behaviours such as vomiting and with diagnostic criteria that do not specify specific weight and shape related psychopathology [31, 32]. However, in most EDs clinics only a minority of EDNOS cases may be classified as having BED although it is more common in obesity clinics. Nevertheless, BED has been

Box 4.1 DSM IV Diagnostic Criteria for the Eating Disorders – Slightly Simplified

Anorexia Nervosa (AN)

- Refusal to maintain body weight at or above a minimally normal weight for age and height.

- Intense fear of gaining weight or becoming fat even though underweight.

- Disturbance in the way in which one's body weight or shape is experienced, undue influence of body weight or shape on self-evaluation, or denial of the seriousness of the current low body weight.

- Amenorrhoea in postmenarcheal females.

Types: Restricting Type – no regular binge-eating or purging behaviour; Binge-Eating/Purging Type.

Bulimia Nervosa (BN)

- Recurrent episodes of binge-eating characterised by eating in a discrete period of time an amount of food that is definitely lager than most people would eat under similar circumstances. During the episode there is a sense of lack of control over eating.

- Recurrent inappropriate compensatory behaviour in order to prevent weight gain, such as self-induced vomiting, misuse of laxatives, diuretics, enemas or other medications; fasting excessive exercise.

- Binge-eating and compensatory behaviours occur on average at least twice a week for three months.

- Self-evaluation is unduly influenced by body shape or weight.

- The disturbance does not occur exclusively during episodes of anorexia nervosa.

Types: Purging type – regular use of self-induced vomiting or the misuse of laxatives, diuretics or enemas; Non-purging type – use of non-purging methods of inappropriate compensation such has fasting or excessive exercise.

Eating Disorder Not Otherwise Specified (EDNOS)

Disorder of eating that does not meet the criteria for any specific eating disorder. The disorder must be of clinical significance and severity.

widely studied. In the community, the commonest form of EDNOS is probably a syndrome characterised by the use of purging – induced vomiting and/or laxative abuse – for weight control but without either low weight or binging for which the term 'purging disorder' has been proposed [29, 33].

One response to the flawed classification of the EDs and the EDNOS problem has been to emphasise the many things that the different EDs have in common and the way in which an individual may pass through states which fulfil different diagnostic criteria at different times in their eating disordered 'career'; the pathway from AN to BN or EDNOS being especially well travelled. This has led Fairburn and others to champion what they call the 'transdiagnostic' position in which the basic diagnosis is of ED and different features such as low weight or binge eating are included as mere qualifiers to that diagnosis [34]. However, the transdiagnostic position does not eliminate classificatory problems. Practically, severe AN does seem often to demand a different management and a different way of thinking. Theoretically, the approach raises in an especially stark form the question of how ED itself should be defined [35, 36]. This is a surprisingly tricky matter but lengthy discussion would be out of place in a chapter such as this. The next version of the DSM is due to appear early in the next decade and it will be of interest to see what changes are made. In the meantime, services, funding bodies and clinicians should not exclude EDNOS cases from their treatment programmes. In the light of what is known about their typical severity, and so on it would be unethical to do so.

Engagement

The issue of engagement was discussed above somewhat in relation to the early presentation of the patient. This was appropriate because without an adequate relationship with the patient the whole process of assessment and moving on to treatment may well be derailed. The nurturing of the relationship and the establishment of some degree of common understanding of her situation and that of the clinician in relation to it is crucial. Even if one has doubts about its causal potency it is useful to develop some sort of 'story' as too why the patient has fallen ill when she has and perhaps in the manner that she has. Such a story should be tailor made to the person although it may include elements derived from the clinician's theoretical position or previous experience with others. Any account should be constructed provisionally and held tentatively. Imposing a rigid model is likely to provoke resistance. Above all the clinician should keep an open mind.

4.5 Treatment and management

The treatment of mental disorders in general and of EDs in particular should aim to combine evidence-based interventions with enough knowledge, empathy, good communication and clinical nous to sustain the therapeutic relationship and find a way forward when the map of good evidence is inadequate or runs out. When good evidence is in short supply, it is tempting to place more reliance than is sensible upon the few nuggets that are available. The clinician needs to combine enthusiasm and confidence in proposing interventions with a critical stance with regard to both evidence and what might be called received wisdom or clinical tradition.

The person stuck within an ED is confronting what may be usefully thought of as one or more vicious circles. And vicious circles are vicious because the easiest thing to do is to keep going around them. Escape requires that the patient does things that may feel 'wrong' such as eating regular substantial meals even though she construes her problem as one of eating too much. The well informed confidence of the clinician is crucial. The patient needs to be able to trust the clinician and the situation just enough to feel sufficiently safe to try changing. Whatever the details of the treatment the clinician needs to be able to gain and sustain such trust.

It may sometimes be useful to make a distinction between 'treatment' – interventions designed to change the disorder itself – and 'management' which covers the attempts to ameliorate the consequences and complications of the disorder or to contain and hold the patient's state whilst treatment occurs [37]. In practise what is offered to a particular patient may also be determined by a third issue namely that of 'service organization'. Thus for instance, although it may seem better in general for there to be continuity of contact with a particular treating clinician or therapist before, during and after a hospital admission, this may not be feasible for reasons to do with service organization. Sometimes the reasons for discontinuity are clear. For instance, if a patient with severe AN comes from a distant region with no availability of the special treatment and management that she is judged to need, then she may need to be admitted to a hospital hundreds of kilometres away and treated and managed by different clinicians whilst she is there. However, sometimes discontinuity is less rationally based in the quirks of local service organization or even by a legal framework that artificially divides hospital from 'office' practise.

In the United Kingdom, where the bulk of healthcare is provided within the state run and taxation funded National Health Service (NHS), a government sponsored organisation the National Institute for Clinical Excellence (NICE) has produced a guideline document on the treatment and management of EDs [25, 38]. It does not discuss service organisation and concentrates upon what should usually be offered to people with EDs but not how. NICE guidelines are based wherever possible on careful and systematic review of the evidence. The following discussion will draw upon the NICE guideline. However, guidelines are neither cookbooks nor sacred texts. In at least a significant minority of cases it may be appropriate that treatment and/or management differs from what is suggested.

Psychological treatment

Few would disagree with the idea that EDs are psychological and behavioural disorders even though they may have important, even lethal physical consequences. Furthermore, most would think of them as potentially open to empathetic understanding as in the traditional view of 'neurosis' rather than showing the 'non-understandability' of psychosis. However, the old split between the understandable and not is less compelling in the age of neuroscience.

Most psychological treatment for EDs is delivered on an outpatient basis. This is cheaper and less disruptive of the person's life. Nevertheless, some countries notably Germany, make much greater use of residential treatment even for BN.

There is a contrast between the substantial available evidence supporting different treatments for BN and the meagre evidence concerning treatments for AN or for EDNOS other than for the minority who have BED.

Two kinds of time limited psychological treatment for BN, namely a specific version of Cognitive Behaviour Therapy (CBT-BN) and Interpersonal Psychotherapy (IPT) have substantial evidence supporting their efficacy [39–43] (see Boxes 4.2 and 4.3). Interestingly, CBT-BN seems to be associated with greater improvement at end of treatment but IPT catches up in the following months. These treatments are effective but are not universally so with at best only about half of patients escaping from their disorder in relation to the treatment. There is little evidence to illuminate what to offer next when patients do not do well. People with co-morbid borderline personality disorder associated with behavioural problems such as recurrent self-harm and drug misuse may be helped by special inpatient programmes and/or by Dialectical Behaviour Therapy (DBT) [44, 45]. In contrast, some people with BN and EDNOS including BED may improve with lesser treatments, notably various forms of self-help from books or CDs offered with or without professional help and guidance [46–49]. The idea of stepped care whereby simpler and cheaper interventions are offered first and before more substantial treatments has some merit although there is a danger that more severely affected patients may drop out rather than persist after the initial steps [50].

CBT and IPT have come to be viewed as the standard treatments for BN and BED against which other treatments should be compared. Furthermore, CBT is currently the dominant theoretical framework and several centres are developing

---

Box 4.2 Cognitive Behavioural Therapy for Bulimia Nervosa

Cognitive Behaviour Therapy (CBT) is outpatient based and involves 15–20 one-to-one treatment sessions. The treatment has three stages

- *Stage 1*: The first aim is to engage the patient. The second is educating the patient. The third is to help the patient regain control of their eating.

- *Stage 2*: Here there is continued emphasis on their eating and regularising it. Overevaluation of shape and weight is addressed.

- *Stage 3*: Here the aim is to maintain progress.

Box 4.3 Interpersonal Psychotherapy for Bulimia Nervosa

Interpersonal Psychotherapy (IPT) is a short term psychological treatment. IPT was developed for the treatment of depression. There has been strong indication for its use in Bulimia Nervosa. There is some evidence for its use in Anorexia Nervosa.

- *Stage 1 (Sessions 1–4)*: In the first phase interpersonal problem areas are identified. Problem areas are divided into four broad groups: grief (abnormal grief reaction); role disputes; difficulty with role transitions and interpersonal deficits. Among patients with eating disorders role disputes and role transitions are common. The first phase ends in the therapist and patient agreeing on the problem area that will become the focus of treatment.

- *Stage 2 (Sessions 5–15)*: In the second phase the patient identifies solutions for the problem areas with the help of the therapist. The therapist is active but not directive.

- *Stage 3 (Sessions 16–20)*: In the final phase of treatment the work is often at two weekly intervals. It becomes more future oriented. Future times of difficulty are thought of and the problem areas are reviewed.

---

treatments that build upon it by adding different elements in order to improve its efficacy or widen its scope. Therapists working outside the framework of CBT sometimes take heart at the efficacy of IPT. However, evidence for other therapies is limited although they are doubtless widely used. Unfortunately, there has been little relevant research [51].

It seems likely that CBT-BN and IPT promote change differently. CBT-BN focuses largely upon the weight, shape and eating issues and IPT, at least how it was delivered in the relevant trials, does not [40]. Christopher Fairburn and the Oxford group who pioneered much of the work on both CBT-BN and IPT have recently evaluated two 'enhanced' versions of CBT, called CBT-Ef and CBT-Eb. The 'f' stands for focused on weight, shape and eating and the 'b' for broad because that treatment includes flexibility to include modules on perfectionism, low self-esteem, emotional regulation and interpersonal issues. In a trial, both CBT-Ef and CBT-Eb did well with the latter seeming to be better only for people with more complex general psychopathology [52]. The trial was unusual in recruiting people with EDNOS other than BED and showing that they too responded well to CBT-E.

Offering some sort of psychological treatment to people with AN is almost universally thought of as a good thing. Trying to escape from this disorder is personally demanding and having a therapeutic relationship with an understanding and trusted person is likely to be helpful. However, at least for adults, there is little evidence that any one therapy is better than any other. There are of course, plenty of opinions and some consensus that a therapist for a person with AN needs to find the right combination of being more active than would be typical of psychodynamic approaches whilst being more reflective and less pushy than might be typical of some cognitive-behavioural treatments. Interestingly a recent trial in New Zealand found that a general supportive approach – named 'non-specific supportive clinical management' – was superior to versions of CBT and IPT adapted for this diagnostic group [53].

The single psychological treatment for AN deemed to be evidence based within the NICE guideline is the family approach for adolescent patients. There is more than one style of treatment although what has come to be known as the Maudsley Method is widely used [54–57] (see Box 4.4). However, comparisons between such conjoint family therapy where the family meet together and family

---

Box 4.4 The Maudsley Model of Family Therapy

The Maudsley Model of Family Based Treatment for Anorexia Nervosa was first developed by Christopher Dare and his colleagues at the Maudsley Hospital in London in the mid-1980s [62]. In this model parents were given a primary role in treatment working together as a team. The main features were:

1. Refeeding their child and confronting anorectic behaviour.

2. Blaming the anorexia rather than the child.

3. Reducing expressed emotion.

4. Once safe eating and weight were achieved through parental intervention, responsibility was handed back to the adolescent.

While the Maudsley model has been found to be effective it does not necessarily work for all patients. This has led to two proponents of the Maudsley model. In the United States there has been commitment to the original model by manualising the treatment and subjecting this to further randomised controlled trials [63]. In the United Kingdom and Germany there has been an adaptation of the Maudsley approach into a multiple therapy format [59–61].

The benefits of multiple family therapy have not been experimentally demonstrated. However its potential lies in the solidarity that can be promoted between families in their fight against anorexia nervosa.

counselling where patient and parents are seen separately failed to detect a difference in efficacy [58]. Over the last few years there has been considerable enthusiasm for bringing several families together for a few lengthy meetings in so-called multi-family therapy however, it has yet to be adequately evaluated [59–61].

Pharmacological treatment

Once again, there is a useful evidence base for BN but not for AN. Many clinical trials of various antidepressant medication show efficacy in reducing binge frequency in BN or BED. Mood disturbance and preoccupation with shape also show improvement although the presence or absence of depression does not affect this response [64]. Antidepressants may be used as an adjunct to psychological treatment and as 'first aid' in BN. Drugs alone are rarely if ever an adequate response. Fluoxetine in high dosage (40–80 mg daily) has been most widely used and studied and is probably the drug of choice [65].

There are no drugs of proven worth in the treatment of AN. Anti-depressants may be less effective at low weight even in the treatment of co-morbid depression. There were claims that fluoxetine reduced the risk of relapse in people with AN who had restored weight in hospital but subsequent work has not supported this claim [66]. Likewise, there is only minimal evidence to support the use of 'new' neuroleptics such as Olanzepine or Quetiapine but they are widely used in attempts to relieve the mental anguish experienced by many people with AN [67].

Management

In general, outpatient treatment is cheaper, more straightforward and less disruptive than inpatient treatment. People with BN or EDNOS at normal weight can – and arguably should – almost always be treated as outpatients unless risks and issues associated with co-morbidity require otherwise.

People with AN can pose such risks too but in addition may be at risk because of their low weight and associated physical ill health. These complications may be many and various. Sometimes they may require urgent inpatient management often under a physician. Such admissions aim to regain some physical safety and stability and are usually quite short.

Admissions for treatment involving greater weight restoration together with psychological treatment are usually arranged in psychiatric units and preferably in units in which the staff of all disciplines have experience in dealing with such patients. Physical monitoring is essential. Typically such admissions are longer and they may last for months. In many such units the aim is that the patient achieves an average weekly weight gain of 0.5–1 kg. Thus even on the optimistic estimate of the higher figure restoration of a weight deficit of 20 kg would take perhaps six months allowing some time for stabilisation.

The length and cost of long admissions to hospital has been one spur to the creation of alternatives. These include intensive home treatment and various forms of partial hospitalisation of which day treatment is most widespread. The former are rare and have yet to be evaluated. Day treatment programmes are more numerous and vary from being intensive but relatively separate from other aspects of the service to being an integral part of a unified response to AN which includes both outpatient and inpatient facilities [68–71].

There is little formal evidence concerning the merits or otherwise of inpatient treatment for AN. Attempts to examine the issue in randomised trials have been flawed and the results have been equivocal [72–74]. However few clinicians confronted with the full range of severity in people with AN would want to be without the option of offering admission. But the point at which they seek to invoke this possibility varies. The American Psychiatric Association guidelines recommend that patients with weight loss to below 85% of healthy body weight should be admitted [75]. Elsewhere admission is usually reserved for more severe cases. Some clinicians advocate admission at a Body Mass Index (BMI) of 13.5 or below whilst others, including the present authors, have no such limit but include body weight in an overall appraisal of the risks and benefits of both the option of admitting and the option of not admitting the patient [76].

A similar decision arises in relation to the use of legal compulsion. The law varies from country to country but there is usually some relevant power. In the United Kingdom, it is clear that AN is a 'mental disorder' and 'feeding' a treatment within the meaning of the act [77]. Nevertheless some clinicians seek to avoid using whatever legal powers are available and prefer to persist in attempting to achieve collaboration even when the patient is severely ill. The aim is to push the dilemma about what to do back into the patient who is helped to experience anxiety about her condition so that weight restoration can occur as a venture in which she has some sense of agency and responsibility. Other clinicians are more active in using compulsion and feel that not to do so is to take unnecessary risks. There is little empirical data to support either view and this important topic is unlikely ever to be the subject of a randomised controlled trial. One follow up study compared detained and non-detained patients and showed that the former did less well in the long run [78]. However, severity was an inevitably confounding issue. Whichever broad approach is taken the treatment of people with very severe AN is a specialised business and this applies even more if compulsion is used. It is likely to go better if the team is experienced and the circumstances suitable. Just as with other specialised procedures, for instance transplantation surgery, the compulsory treatment of AN is difficult if attempted on a one off basis.

In the main, treatment of AN under legal compulsion does not involve anything that could be called 'forced feeding'. However, occasionally clinicians may decide that feeding through a naso-gastric tube is the only way forward. Even more uncommon is the situation where such feeding is carried out against resistance. The perceived need to resort to such intervention should always lead to a complete review of the case and the options for treatment and management.

Another extreme measure that is occasionally considered is the terminal care of people with very chronic and very severe AN who have come to think of themselves as cases entirely without hope. Some clinicians advocate hospice care or something similar to give the person a well managed and dignified death [79]. To others – including the present authors – this seems to be to miss the point about the nature of AN which is not a 'psychic cancer' as it were. Improvement or even recovery is thought of as always possible and therefore to arrange hospice care seems to be collude with the patient's hopelessness and to go along with what is essentially her suicide. However, there is major room for improvement in the definition and delivery of what would be good care for people with truly chronic AN.

4.6 Conclusion

EDs are a common problem in many parts of the world. In the Netherlands the annual incidence of new cases of AN in primary care is about 8 per 100 000 and 12 per 100 000 for BN [80]. The rates for EDNOS are probably higher. Many cases continue for several years constraining the person's life at a crucial time in personal development. In perhaps 1 in 10, the disorder will be truly chronic and last for decades. And some will die prematurely because of their disorder either through its physical consequences or through despair and suicide [4, 5]. For the present we cannot be sure how widespread and prevalent the EDs are outside of 'western' countries. The disorders may already be present but hidden in less affluent countries. However, even if this is not the case it is at least plausible that they will emerge in due course, as a largely unforeseen side effect of globalisation and increasing wealth. If they do arrive apparently associated with affluence and modernity they may provoke, perhaps even in heightened form, the distorted and ambivalent attitudes that have complicated both the public and professional response to them elsewhere. As stated above they deserve to be taken seriously. They need to be thought of as ordinary mental disorders.

References

1. Russell, G.F.M. (1979) Bulimia nervosa: an ominous variant of anorexia nervosa. *Psychological Medicine*, **9**, 429–48.
2. Vandererycken, W. (1994) Emergence of bulimia nervosa as a separate diagnostic entity: review of the literature from 1960 to 1979. *International Journal of Eating Disorders*, **16**, 105–16.
3. World Health Organization (1998) Obesity: Preventing and Managing the Global Epidemic: Report of a WHO Consultation on Obesity, WHO/NUT/NCD/98, WHO, Geneva.
4. Sullivan, P.E. (1995) Mortality in anorexia nervosa. *American Journal of Psychiatry*, **152**, 1073–74.
5. Neilsen, S., Moller-Madsen, S., Isager, T. *et al.* (1998) Standardised mortality in eating disorders – a quantitative summary of previously published and new evidence. *Journal of Psychosomatic Research*, **44**, 413–34.

6. Treasure, J., Murphy, T., Szmuckler, G. *et al.* (2001) The experience of care giving for severe mental illness: a comparison between anorexia nervosa and psychosis. *Social Psychiatry and Psychiatric Epidemiology*, **36**, 343–47.

7. Palmer, R.L. (2005) Concepts of eating disorders, in *The Essential Handbook of Eating Disorders* (eds J. Treasure, U. Schmidt and E. van Furth), John Wiley & Sons, Ltd, Chichester.

8. Polivy, J. and Herman, C.P. (1993) Etiology of binge eating: psychological mechanisms, in *Binge Eating: Nature, Assessment and Treatment* (eds C.G. Fairburn and G.T. Wilson), Guilford Press, New York.

9. Wilson, G.T. (1995) The controversy over dieting, in *Eating Disorders and Obesity: A Comprehensive Handbook* (eds K.D. Brownell and C.G. Fairburn), Guilford Press, New York and London.

10. Strober, M. and Bulik, C.M. (2005) Genetic epidemiology of eating disorders, in *Eating Disorders and Obesity: A Comprehensive Handbook*, 2nd edn (eds C.G. Fairburn and K.D. Brownell), Guilford Press, New York and London.

11. Strober, M., Freeman, R., Lampert, C. *et al.* (2000) A controlled family study of anorexia nervosa and bulimia nervosa: evidence of shared liability and transmission of partial syndromes. *American Journal of Psychiatry*, **157**, 393–401.

12. Kaye, W. (2002) Central Nervous system neurotransmitted activity in anorexia nervosa and bulimia nervosa, in *Eating Disorders and Obesity: A Comprehensive Handbook*, 2nd edn (eds C.G. Fairburn and K.D. Brownell), Guilford Press, New York and London.

13. Treasure, J. and Campbell, I. (1994) The case for biology in anorexia nervosa. *Psychological Medicine*, **24**, 3–8.

14. Schmidt, U., Humphress, H. and Treasure, J. (1997) The role of general family environment and sexual and physical abuse in the origins of eating disorders. *European Eating Disorders Review*, **5**, 184–207.

15. Fairburn, C.G., Welch, S.L., Doll, H.A. and Davies, B.A. (1997) Risk factors for bulimia nervosa: a community based case-control study. *Archives of General Psychiatry*, **54**, 509–17.

16. Fairburn, C.G., Doll, H., Welch, S. *et al.* (1998) Risk factors for binge eating disorder: a community-based case-control study. *Archives of General Psychiatry*, **55**, 425–32.

17. Fairburn, C.G., Cooper, Z., Doll, H. and Welch, S.L. (1999) Risk factors for anorexia nervosa: three integrated case comparisons. *Archives of General Psychiatry*, **56**, 468–76.

18. Goodwin, G.M., Fairburn, C.G. and Cowen, P.J. (1987) Dieting changes serotonergic function in women, not men: Implications for the aetiology of anorexia nervosa. *Psychological Medicine*, **17**, 839.

19. Klump, K.L., Burt, A., McGue, M. and Iacono, W.G. (2007) Changes in genetic and environmental influences on disordered eating across adolescence. *Archives of General Psychiatry*, **64**, 1409–15.

20. Crisp, A.H. (1980) *Anorexia Nervosa: Let Me Be*, Academic Press, London.

21. Nasser, M. (1997) *Culture and Weight Consciousness*, Routledge, London.

22. Crow, S. (2005) Medical complications of eating disorders, in *Eating Disorders Review Part 1* (eds S. Wonderlich, J. Mitchell, M. de Zwaan and H. Steiger), Radcliffe Publishing, Oxford and Seattle.

23. Pomeroy, C. and Mitchell, J. (2005) Medical complications of anorexia nervosa and bulimia nervosa, in *Eating Disorders and Obesity*, 2nd edn (eds C.G. Fairburn and K.D. Brownell), Guilford Press, New York and London.

24. National Collaborating Centre for Mental Health (2004) Eating Disorders: Core Interventions in the Treatment and Management of Anorexia Nervosa, Bulimia Nervosa and Related Eating Disorders, National Clinical Practice Guideline no. CG9, British Psychological Society & Gaskell, London.

25. American Psychiatric Association (1994) *Diagnostic and Statistical Manual of Mental Disorders*, 4th edn, American Psychiatric Association, Washington, DC.

26. World Health Organization (1992) The ICD-10 Classification of Mental and Behavioural Disorders: Clinical Descriptions and Diagnostic Guidelines, WHO, Geneva.

27. Fairburn, C.G. and Harrison, P.J. (2003) Eating disorders. *Lancet*, **361**, 407–16.

28. Button, E.J., Benson, E., Nollett, C. and Palmer, R.L. (2007) Don't forget EDNOS (eating disorder not otherwise specified): patterns of service in an eating disorders service. *Psychiatric Bulletin*, **29**, 134–36.

29. Wade, T.D., Bergin, J.L., Tiggerman, M. *et al.* (2006) Prevalence and long-term course of lifetime eating disorders in an adult Australian twin cohort. *Australian and New Zealand Journal of Psychiatry*, **40**, 121–28.

30. Fairburn, C.G., Cooper, Z., Bohn, K. *et al.* (2007) The severity and status of eating disorder NOS: implications for DSM V. *Behavior Research and Therapy*, **45**, 1705–25.

31. Murphy, R., Perkins, S. and Schmidt, U. (2005) The empirical status of binge eating disorder, in *EDNOS: Eating Disorder Not Otherwise Specified; Scientific and Clinical Perspectives on the Other Eating Disorders* (eds C. Norring and B. Palmer), Routledge, London and New York.

32. de Zwaan, M. (2005) Binge eating, EDNOS & obesity, in *EDNOS: Eating Disorder Not Otherwise Specified; Scientific and Clinical Perspectives on the Other Eating Disorders* (eds C. Norring and B. Palmer), Routledge, London and New York.

33. Keel, P. (2007) Purging disorder: Sub-threshold variant or full-threshold eating disorder? *International Journal of Eating Disorders*, **40**, S89–94.

34. Fairburn, C.G., Cooper, Z. and Shafran, R. (2003) Cognitive behaviour therapy for eating disorders: a "transdiagnostic" theory and treatment. *Behavior Research and Therapy*, **41**, 509–28.

35. Fairburn, C.G. and Walsh, B.T. (2002) Atypical eating disorders (Eating Disorder not Otherwise Specified), in *Eating Disorders and Obesity*, 2nd edn (eds C.G. Fairburn, and K.D. Brownell), Guilford Press, New York and London.

36. Fairburn, C.G. and Cooper, Z. (2007) Thinking afresh about the classification of eating disorders. *International Journal of Eating Disorders*, **40**, S107–10.

37. Palmer, R.L. and Treasure, J. (1999) Providing specialised services for anorexia nervosa. *British Journal of Psychiatry*, **175**, 306–9.

38. Wilson, G.T. and Shafran, R. (2005) Eating disorders guideline from NICE. *Lancet*, **365**, 79–81.

39. Fairburn, C.G., Marcus, M.D. and Wilson, G.T. (1993) Cognitive-behavioral therapy for binge eating and bulimia nervosa; A comprehensive treatment manual, in *Binge Eating: Nature, Assessment and Treatment* (eds C.G. Fairburn and G.T. Wilson), Guilford Press, New York.

40. Fairburn, C.G. (1997) Interpersonal psychotherapy for bulimia nervosa, in *Handbook of Treatment for Eating Disorders* (eds D.M. Garner and P.E. Garfinkel), Guilford Press, New York.

41. Fairburn, C.G., Jones, R., Peveler, R.C. *et al.* (1991) Three psychological treatments for bulimia nervosa. *Archives of General Psychiatry*, **48**, 463–69.

42. Agras, W.S., Walsh, T., Fairburn, C.G. *et al.* (2000) A multicenter comparison of cognitive-behavioral therapy and interpersonal psychotherapy for bulimia nervosa. *Archives of General Psychiatry*, **57**, 459–66.

43. Fairburn, C.G., Jones, R., Hope, R.A. and O'Connor, M. (1993) Psychotherapy and bulimia nervosa: the longer term effects of interpersonal psychotherapy, behaviour therapy and cognitive behaviour therapy. *Archives of General Psychiatry*, **50**, 419–28.

44. Lacey, J.H. (1995) Inpatient treatment of multi-impulsive bulimia nervosa, in *Eating Disorders and Obesity: A Comprehensive Handbook* (eds K.D. Brownell and C.G. Fairburn), Guilford Press, New York and London.

45. Palmer, R.L., Birchall, H., Damani, S. *et al.* (2003) A Dialectical behavior therapy program for people with eating disorder and borderline personality disorder – description & outcome. *International Journal of Eating Disorders*, **33**, 281–86.

46. Fairburn, C.G. (1995) *Overcoming Binge Eating*, Guilford Press, New York.

47. Schmidt, U. and Treasure, J. (1993) *Getting Better Bit(e) by Bit(e)*, Lawrence Erlbaum Associates, London.

48. Sysko, R. and Walsh, B.T. (2008) A critical evaluation of the efficacy of self-help interventions for the treatment of bulimia nervosa and binge eating disorder. *International Journal of Eating Disorders*, **41**, 97–112.

49. Palmer, R.L., Birchall, H., McGrain, L. and Sullivan, V. (2002) Self-help for bulimic disorders: a randomised controlled trial comparing minimal guidance with face-to-face or telephone guidance. *British Journal of Psychiatry*, **181**, 230–35.

50. Fairburn, C.G. and Peveler, R.C. (1990) Bulimia nervosa and the stepped care approach to management. *Gut*, **31**, 1220–22.

51. Murphy, S., Russell, L. and Waller, G. (2005) Integrated psychodynamic therapy for bulimia nervosa and binge eating disorder: theory, practice and preliminary findings. *European Eating Disorders Review*, **13**, 383–91.

52. Fairburn, C.G., Cooper, Z., Doll, H.A., O'Connor, M.E., Bohn, K., Hawker, D.M., Wales, J.A., Palmer, R.L. (2009) Transdiagnostic cognitive-behavioral therapy for patients with eating disorders: a two-site trial with 60-week follow-up. *American Journal of Psychiatry*. Mar, **166** (3), 311–19. Epub 2008 Dec 15.

53. McIntosh, V., Jordan, J., Carter, F. *et al.* (2005) Three psychotherapies for anorexia nervosa: a randomized controlled trial. *American Journal of Psychiatry*, **162**, 741–47.

54. Eisler, I., le Grange, D. and Asen, E. (2005) Family interventions, in *The Essential Handbook of Eating Disorders* (eds J. Treasure, U. Schmidt and E. van Furth), John Wiley & Sons, Ltd, Chichester.

55. Russell, G.F.M., Szmuckler, G.I., Dare, C. and Eisler, I. (1987) An evaluation of family therapy in anorexia nervosa and bulimia nervosa. *Archives of General Psychiatry*, **44**, 1047–56.

56. Lock, J., le Grange, D., Agras, W.S. and Dare, C. (2001) *Treatment Manual for Anorexia Nervosa: A Family – Based Approach*, Guilford Press, New York.

57. Lock, J., Agras, W.S., Bryson, S. and Kraemer, H.C. (2005) A comparison of short-and long-term family therapy for adolescent anorexia nervosa. *Journal of the American Academy of Child and Adolescent Psychiatry*, **44**, 632–39.

58. Eisler, I., Dare, C., Hodes, M. *et al.* (2000) Family therapy for adolescent anorexia nervosa: the results of a controlled comparison of two family interventions. *Journal of Child Psychology and Psychiatry*, **41**, 727–36.

59. Asen, E. (2002) Multiple family therapy: an overview. *Journal of Family Therapy*, **24**, 3–16.

60. Colahan, M. and Robinson, P. (2002) Multi-family groups in the treatment of young adults with eating disorders. *Journal of Family Therapy*, **24**, 17–30.

61. Dare, C. and Eisler, I. (2000) A multi-family group day treatment programme for adolescent eating disorder. *European Eating Disorder Review*, **8**, 4–18.

62. Dare, C., Eisler, I., Colahan, M. *et al.* (1995) The listening heart and the chi square: clinical and empirical perceptions in the family therapy of anorexia nervosa. *Journal of Family Therapy*, **17**, 31–57.

63. Lock, J. and Le Grange, D. (2001) Can family-based treatment of anorexia nervosa be manualised? *Journal of Psychotherapy Practice and Research*, **10**, 253–61.

64. Bacaltchuk, J. and Hay, P.J. (2003) Anti-depressants versus placebo for bulimia nervosa. *Cochrane Database of Systematic Reviews*, 4 (Art. No.: CD003391v).

65. Goldstein, D., Wilson, M., Thompson, V. *et al.* The Fluoxetine Bulimia Nervosa Collaborative Study Group (1995) Long-term fluoxetine treatment of bulimia nervosa. *British Journal of Psychiatry*, **166**, 660–66.

66. Walsh, B.T., Kaplan, A.S., Attia, E. *et al.* (2006) Fluoxetine after weight restoration in anorexia nervosa: a randomised controlled trial. *Journal of the American Medical Association*, **295**, 2605–12.

67. Mehler-Wex, C., Romanos, M., Kirchheiner, J. and Schulze, U.M.E. (2008) Atypical antipsychotics in severe anorexia nervosa in children and adolescents – review and case reports. *European Eating Disorders Review*, **16**, 100–8.

68. Olmsted, M.P. (2002) Day hospital treatment of anorexia nervosa and bulimia nervosa, in *Eating Disorders and Obesity: A Comprehensive Handbook*, 2nd edn (eds C.G. Fairburn and K.D. Brownell), Guilford Press, New York and London.

69. Robinson, P. (2003) Day treatments, in *The Essential Handbook of Eating Disorders* (eds J. Treasure, U. Schmidt and E. van Furth), John Wiley & Sons, Ltd, Chichester.

70. Gerlinghoff, H., Backmund, H. and Franzen, U. (1998) Evaluation of a day treatment programme for eating disorders. *European Eating Disorders Review*, **6**, 96–1006.

71. Birchall, H., Palmer, R.L., Waine, J. *et al.* (2002) Intensive day programme treatment for severe anorexia nervosa – the Leicester experience. *Psychiatric Bulletin*, **26**, 334–36.

72. Crisp, A.H., Norton, K., Gowers, S. *et al.* (1991) A controlled study of the effect of therapies aimed at adolescent and family psychopathology in anorexia nervosa. *British Journal of Psychiatry*, **159**, 325–33.

73. Gowers, S., Clark, A., Roberts, C. *et al.* (2007) Clinical effectiveness of treatments for anorexia nervosa in adolescents: randomised controlled trial. *British Journal of Psychiatry*, **191**, 427–35.

74. Meads, C., Gold, I. and Burls, A. (2003) How effective is outpatient care compared to inpatient care for the treatment of anorexia nervosa? A systematic review. *European Eating Disorders Review*, **9**, 229–41.

75. American Psychiatric Association (2006) *Practice Guideline for the Treatment of Patients With Eating Disorders*, 3rd edn, American Psychiatric Association, Washington, DC.

76. Palmer, R.L. (2000) *Helping People with Eating Disorders: A Clinical Guide to Assessment and Treatment*, John Wiley & Sons, Ltd, London.

77. Radcliffes Mental Health Law Briefing No. 34 (2000). Radcliffes Solicitors, London.

78. Ramsay, R., Ward, A., Treasure, J. and Russell, G.F.M. (1999) Compulsory treatment in anorexia nervosa: short term benefits and long term mortality. *British Journal of Psychiatry*, **175**, 147–53.

79. O'Neill, J. Crowther, T. and Sampson, G. (1994) Anorexia nervosa: palliative care of terminal psychiatric disease. *American Journal of Hospice and Palliative Care*, **11**, 36–38.

80. van Hoeken, D., Seidell, J. and Hoek, H.W. (2002) Epidemiology, in *The Essential Handbook of Eating Disorders* (eds J. Treasure, U. Schmidt and E. van Furth), John Wiley & Sons, Ltd, Chichester.

5
Suicidality in women

Gergö Hadlaczky and Danuta Wasserman

National Prevention of Suicide and Mental Ill-Health at Karolinska Institutet, Stockholm, Sweden

Suicide and attempted suicide is a significant global problem for both males and females. Most research in this field has been targeted at men, as their mortality exceeds that of women. Whilst presenting selected research findings regarding epidemiology, risk factors and prevention, we argue for the importance of better knowledge regarding female suicidal behaviour and for understanding and preventing suicidal behaviour as a whole. Another important aspect, namely the role of culture and transition is discussed, as well as some methodological issues regarding research in this field.

5.1 Definitions

Terms like suicide, attempted suicide and self-harm can have broader or narrower definitions and consequentially incorporate more or fewer behaviours. Much of the validity and reliability of the findings generated in research depends on the precision of definitions and how consequently they are used among researchers. If the terms are defined imprecisely, a large amount of variation in the collected data will be due to factors which are irrelevant to the study objectives. If they are too precise, valuable information might be excluded. Therefore, giving operational definitions to those terms which are the object of suicidology is of great importance.

The word 'suicide' is fairly unproblematic in terms of operational definition, however gathering data can sometimes be difficult due to legal and practical

Contemporary Topics in Women's Mental Health Edited by Chandra, Herrman, Fisher, Kastrup,
© 2009 John Wiley & Sons, Ltd   Niaz, Rondón and Okasha

issues surrounding recording procedures [1]. The World Health Organizations (WHO) proposal for an operational definition of suicide is:

> For the act of killing oneself to be classed as suicide, it must be deliberately initiated and performed by the person concerned in the full knowledge, or expectation, of its fatal outcome [2].

This definition requires knowledge that the death of a person was caused by a conscious intent and the act was caused by the person themselves. It should be mentioned that assisted suicide, which is not performed by the person committing suicide, falls outside this definition. In this chapter, the term suicide will be used according to this WHO definition.

Terms related to non-fatal suicidal behaviour such as attempted suicide, parasuicide, self-harm, deliberate self-harm, self-mutilation and self-poisoning, and so on vary between researchers and in different parts of the world [3]. In this chapter, the term attempted suicide will be used synonymously to the word 'parasuicide' as defined in the WHO/EURO Multicentre Study on Parasuicide:

> An act with nonfatal outcome, in which an individual deliberately initiates a non-habitual behavior that, without intervention from others, will cause self-harm, or deliberately ingests a substance in excess of the prescribed or generally recognize therapeutic dosage and which is aimed at realizing changes which the subject desired via the actual or expected physical consequences [4].

5.2 Epidemiology

Suicide rates

According to WHO suicide represents approximately 1.5% of the global burden of disease in the world, and is the cause of approximately 1 million deaths per year [5, 6]. Table 5.1 shows the suicide rates (the number of suicides per 100 000 people) for all ages [7] in increasing order of male/female ratios. The ratio was calculated as the male suicide rates divided by the female suicide rates. It is important to note that these figures would be considerably higher if young people (those under 15 years old) were excluded. Children under the age of 15 decrease the statistic considerably, as suicide is very low in this age group (0.7 per 100 000 worldwide). The global suicide rate is 7.4 per 100 000 for young people aged 15–19, and increased for boys between 1965 and 1999 in Europe and worldwide [8, 9]. These young suicides add up to almost 10% of the deaths amongst 15–19 years olds, being the third leading cause of death worldwide, after accidents and homicide [9, 10].

More suicides are committed by young boys (10.5 per 100 000) than girls (4.1 per 100 000) [9]. This gender difference is also found in adult suicides. Although gender ratios vary between countries and across all ages (Table 5.1), every country has lower suicide rates in women compared to men, with the exception of China.

Table 5.1 Suicide rates and male/female ratios in order from lowest to highest ratio
[7] (the suicide ratios have been calculated by the authors)

	Year	Males	Females	M/F
China (selected rural and urban areas)	99	13	14.8	0.88
Tajikistan	1	2.9	2.3	1.26
India	98	12.2	9.1	1.34
Albania	3	4.7	3.3	1.42
Malta	4	7	4.9	1.43
Philippines	93	2.5	1.7	1.47
Singapore	3	12.5	7.6	1.64
Kuwait	2	2.5	1.4	1.79
Peru	0	1.1	0.6	1.83
China (Hong Kong SAR)	4	25.2	12.4	2.03
Zimbabwe	90	10.6	5.2	2.04
Saint Lucia	2	10.4	5	2.08
Switzerland	4	23.7	11.3	2.10
Netherlands	4	12.7	6	2.12
Norway	4	15.8	7.3	2.16
Republic of Korea	4	32.5	15	2.17
Ecuador	4	8.6	3.7	2.32
Denmark	1	19.2	8.1	2.37
TFYR Macedonia	3	9.5	4	2.38
Sri Lanka	91	44.6	16.8	2.65
Uzbekistan	3	8.1	3	2.70
Slovenia	4	37.9	13.9	2.73
Belgium	97	31.2	11.4	2.74
Sweden	2	19.5	7.1	2.75
Serbia and Montenegro	2	28.8	10.4	2.77
Japan	4	35.6	12.8	2.78
Suriname	0	17.8	6.4	2.78
Paraguay	3	4.5	1.6	2.81
Iceland	4	17.7	6.2	2.85
El Salvador	3	12.2	4.2	2.90
Bulgaria	4	19.7	6.7	2.94
Luxembourg	4	21.9	7.4	2.96
Nicaragua	3	11	3.7	2.97
Germany	4	19.7	6.6	2.98
Iran	91	0.3	0.1	3.00
France	3	27.5	9.1	3.02
Cuba	4	20.3	6.6	3.08
Croatia	4	30.2	9.8	3.08
Georgia	1	3.4	1.1	3.09
Thailand	2	12	3.8	3.16
Austria	5	26.1	8.2	3.18

continued overleaf

Table 5.1   (*continued*)

	Year	Males	Females	M/F
Spain	4	12.6	3.9	3.23
United Kingdom	4	10.8	3.3	3.27
Finland	4	31.7	9.4	3.37
Colombia	99	8.2	2.4	3.42
Guyana	3	42.5	12.1	3.51
Mauritius	4	12.7	3.6	3.53
Portugal	3	17.5	4.9	3.57
Brazil	2	6.8	1.9	3.58
Azerbaijan	2	1.8	0.5	3.60
Australia	3	17.1	4.7	3.64
Canada	2	18.3	5	3.66
Italy	2	11.4	3.1	3.68
Hungary	3	44.9	12	3.74
Guatemala	3	3.4	0.9	3.78
Uruguay	1	24.5	6.4	3.83
Turkmenistan	98	13.8	3.5	3.94
Argentina	3	14.1	3.5	4.03
United States of America	2	17.9	4.2	4.26
Trinidad and Tobago	0	20.9	4.9	4.27
Greece	4	5.2	1.2	4.33
Czech Republic	4	25.9	5.7	4.54
Bahamas	0	6	1.3	4.62
Venezuela	2	8.4	1.8	4.67
New Zealand	0	19.8	4.2	4.71
Dominican Republic	1	2.9	0.6	4.83
Estonia	5	35.5	7.3	4.86
Israel	3	10.4	2.1	4.95
Kyrgyzstan	4	15	3	5.00
Lithuania	4	70.1	14	5.01
Latvia	4	42.9	8.5	5.05
Ireland	5	16.3	3.2	5.09
Mexico	3	6.7	1.3	5.15
Romania	4	21.5	4	5.38
Republic of Moldova	4	29.3	5.2	5.63
Kazakhstan	3	51	8.9	5.73
Chile	3	17.8	3.1	5.74
Russian Federation	4	61.6	10.7	5.76
Ukraine	4	43	7.3	5.89
Puerto Rico	2	10.9	1.8	6.06
Poland	4	27.9	4.6	6.07
Belarus	3	63.3	10.3	6.15
Bosnia and Herzegovina	91	20.3	3.3	6.15
Armenia	3	3.2	0.5	6.40

Table 5.1 (*continued*)

	Year	Males	Females	M/F
Slovakia	2	23.6	3.6	6.56
Costa Rica	4	12.1	1.6	7.56
Panama	3	11.1	1.4	7.93
Belize	1	13.4	1.6	8.38
Bahrain	88	4.9	0.5	9.80
Antigua and Barbuda	95	0	0	
Barbados	1	1.4	0	
Egypt	87	0.1	0	
Haiti	3	0	0	
Honduras	78	0	0	
Jamaica	90	0.3	0	
Jordan	79	0	0	
Saint Kitts and Nevis	95	0	0	
Saint Vincent and The Grenadines	3	6.8	0	
Seychelles	87	9.1	0	
Syrian Arab Republic	85	0.2	0	
Sao Tome and Principe	87	0	1.8	0.00

Countries with the highest male suicide rates are in Eastern Europe and those with highest female rates are found in Asia as well as in Eastern Europe, as shown in Table 5.2.

Gender paradox

One of the most consistent findings in suicidology is that more men die as a result of suicide than women (with the exception of China). Another, equally consistent finding is that females attempt suicide more often than males (with the exception of Finland [11]). This discrepancy between the sexes is known as

Table 5.2 Highest rates of suicide worldwide for males and females

Countries with the highest suicide rates					
Males			**Females**		
	Year	Males		Year	Females
Lithuania	2004	70.1	Sri Lanka	1991	16.8
Belarus	2003	63.3	Republic of Korea	2004	15
Russian Federation	2004	61.6	China (selected rural and urban areas)	1999	14.8
Kazakhstan	2003	51	Lithuania	2004	14
Hungary	2003	44.9	Slovenia	2004	13.9

'the gender paradox', due to the contradiction that the group which displays more self-destructive acts is the group where fewer number of deaths occur.

Relatively few studies have investigated completed suicides in women [12] despite this puzzling phenomenon and the large number of attempted suicides. This is in part due to a focus on mortality by suicide, and since the mortality is highest amongst men, that is where most research is focused. Suicide attempts however, are approximately 10–20 times as common as completed suicides, and the gender difference, in many countries, is much greater than for completed suicide [13]. It can be said that suicidal morbidity is much higher in women, but also for the whole disease burden for suicidality, if morbidity and mortality are combined. While suicide is a predominantly male phenomenon, suicidality as a whole is predominantly a female phenomenon [12, 14]. Regardless of which of the sexes carries the greater burden, the paramount reason for a deeper understanding of the gender paradox is to increase our arsenal in the battle to prevent attempted and completed suicide.

The importance of understanding female suicidal behaviour

Female suicidal behaviour is often viewed as characterised by low intent [15] and as a call for help. However a number of studies have shown that suicidal intent does not differ between the genders [16–19]. Lester [20] suggested that poor physical strength in women compared to men, makes them less able to shoot, stab or hang themselves, reflected in lower suicide rates. This theory can be considered somewhat absurd, considering the relatively minute difference in physical strength between men and women and how little strength is necessary to shoot a gun or kick a chair away.

A more potent attempt at explaining the gender paradox is based on the different methods used by females and males. A number of studies have shown that females use less lethal methods such as poisoning resulting in fewer completed suicides, while males often prefer methods of hanging and shooting which increase the likelihood of death [16, 21]. However, this finding is not entirely consistent. For example, a study by Kposowa and McElvain [22] showed that although the use of firearms was more common amongst men, it was the second preferred choice for women in California and both sexes were equally likely to choose hanging. Another issue is that the frequency of suicidal acts are not equally distributed between the genders, women perform suicidal acts more often than men.

The gender differences in depression and alcohol abuse could also be, in part, responsible for the gender paradox. There is a strong association between clinical depression, and attempted and/or completed suicide. Women have a higher prevalence of clinical depression than men [23–26] which could go some way to explain elevated suicide attempts in women. On the other hand it is inconsistent with the higher ratio of completed suicides found in men. Alcohol abuse, which is more common in males, could be responsible for transforming what might be attempted suicide into completed suicide. Intoxication at the time of suicide is common in depressed men [24, 27, 28]. It has also been shown that some men may have a biological predisposition for suicide when they are depressed [25].

The gender paradox relates to two important methodological questions in suicide research: Is it possible to make generalisations about completed suicides from data about attempted suicides? Is it possible to make generalisations about men using data from women and vice versa?

The explanations above rest on the implicit assumption, that the population of attempters and completers are the same, or at least very similar with the obvious difference in outcome. However, another possibility is that there are two different populations, as shown in Figure 5.1, with two different aetiologies. If the latter view is correct, it is difficult to justify a generalisation from studies of attempted suicide to completed suicide. The debate regarding populations is ongoing. It appears, however, that there is at least one group which has the same, or almost identical clinical and psychosocial profiles as completers: those who survived extremely lethal suicide attempts [1, 29].

Even if the assumption about the two populations being the same is true, there seems to be another obstacle in generalising from attempted to completed suicide. Studies on attempted suicide yield predominantly information on female suicidal behaviour as more females attempt suicide, while studies on completed suicide tell us about male suicidal behaviour, as more males complete suicide. Therefore, even if we accept that we can generalise from attempters to completers within the sexes, it is not for sure that we have the right to generalise between the sexes. In short, without knowing the relationship between female and male suicidal behaviour, it is difficult to fully understand the relationship between suicide and attempted suicide. These aspects appear to go hand in hand.

Focusing on suicidal behaviour in women, and the similarities and differences with male suicidality, is an important step in coming closer to the ultimate goal of suicidology: preventing both male and female suicides and attempted suicides.

Ecological fallacy and male/female ratios

One source of variation in the suicide rates between countries is the composition of the population [30]. If one country has an elevated at-risk subpopulation, its

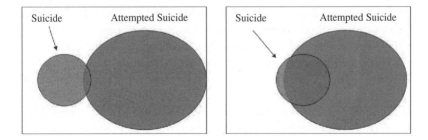

Figure 5.1 Suicide and attempted suicide as the same or as different populations

national suicide rate is likely to be elevated too. When such a unique composition remains unrecognised, it may incorrectly appear as though the country's suicide rate is uniformly high, that is, that a randomly chosen individual in that country is more likely to die due to suicide than in another country with a lower national suicide rate. Extrapolating incorrect conclusions from national to individual levels is called an ecological fallacy.

Yip and Liu [31] examined whether any specific subpopulation could be responsible for the uniquely low male/female ratio in China, the only country in the world with a ratio less than 1. In most age groups in rural and urban areas, suicide-rates for women were either the same or lower compared to men. In China, the only subpopulation where women had significantly higher suicide rates than their male counterparts were those who were living in rural areas and were between the ages 20 and 34. This is a quite substantial group, considering that 60% of the Chinese population lives in rural areas and that 68% of the men and women are below the age of 40 [32]. This interesting finding is a good reminder of how it can be difficult to draw valid conclusions when comparing countries, especially countries as large and heterogeneous as China, a country with double the population of Europe, without having a relatively good idea of the composition of their population. In addition, it can be said that it is not uncommon that male/female suicide ratios are below one in young people as suggested by Wasserman *et al.* [9]. In 14 out of 90 countries studied by Wasserman, young people aged 15–19, had higher suicide rates in females than in males. However due to the relatively small size of these groups, these population subgroups have an insignificant impact on their national suicide ratios.

Countries with low ratios

Despite the observation that it is a specific group of women aged 20–34 from rural areas in China, who may account for the low national male/female ratio in China, it is still important to ask why this specific group differs from the usual pattern. Women, in general, are more likely to poison themselves, both as a self-harming and as a suicide strategy as mentioned previously [16, 33]. Due to the high availability and lethality of pesticides in rural areas of China, these attempts are probably more likely to occur and more likely to result in death, compared to other countries. This is supported by the observation that pesticides or raticides are used in 62% of the suicides in China [34]. This is also common in Indian women, where the male/female ratio is also relatively low; and is true especially for the same subpopulation, which is responsible for the low suicide ratio in China: young adult females in rural areas [35].

There are a number of cultural differences between some developing countries and the so-called developed countries, which is the source of most suicide research. Some cultures and traditions may be responsible for the increased suicide rates in females. Some traditions may have a direct effect on female suicide, such as Sati in India which is still practised occasionally. This tradition involves a wife burning herself to death on her husband's funeral pyre [36]. In

China too, it was common in the past that the wife killed herself out of loyalty to the husband following his death. While these traditions probably explain a very small part of the variance in the suicide rates, women in some Asian and developing countries are under considerable psychosocial pressure. It is not uncommon, especially among rural women to face social and religious discouragement regarding employment, interest in education and/or independence. In many cases the women move to their husband's family and home and due to the geographical distance they may lose important supportive social networks such as family and friends to whom they would usually turn for help in stressful situations. Leaving an unhappy marriage is often seen as socially unacceptable, even in the case of domestic violence [12, 37, 38]. In many cultures women are also under the pressure to deliver male children often turning pregnancy, a protective factor against suicide, into abortion and a serious risk factor (see below) [12].

Phillips *et al.* found a number of unique characteristics in suicide completers in China. Besides the high frequency of women in rural areas, more than half of the victims had friends, associates or relatives who displayed suicidal behaviour, much higher numbers than in studies from elsewhere and more than a third had never attended school. Even though only 7% had ever seen a mental health professional, mental illness was found to be slightly lower amongst the completers in the west (63% compared to the 90–98%) [34, 39]. This finding could be explained by stigma and taboo surrounding mental ill-health, resulting in less people seeking help and victims' families are less likely to divulge information that may lead to a diagnosis. Interestingly, despite these differences in characteristics, the risk factors for suicide such as high levels of depression, previous attempts, acute stress at time of death were found to be very similar, in western countries.

Suicide in countries in transition

Many countries are currently going through rapid and significant modernisation. There are a number of theories regarding the effects of modernisation on male/female suicide ratios. Durkheim's [40] view was that due to processes that occur during modernisation, such as urbanisation and increased education, the traditional family ties and religious devotion would fade away. As these are important protective factors, their disappearance would lead to increased likelihood of suicide. However these protective factors would be more likely to disappear in men, because women, due to their nature and position in society, were more resilient to the forces attempting to destroy these protective factors. As a result modernisation would cause divergent suicide rates: an increase in males and little or no change in females.

Stack and Diangelis [41] studied the change in suicide in 17 industrialised countries between 1919 and 1972 and concluded that, contrary to Durkheim's prediction, suicide rates increased more in females than males, suggesting a convergent trend in suicides. However suicide rates in Australia from 1901 to 1985, in a study by Hassan and Tan [42], propose that an increase in female suicides is only true for the beginning of the modernisation period. After 1960, suicide rates decreased so much that it resulted in a divergent trend. Another empirical theory advocated by Stack [43] and Pampel [44], is a 'curvilinear relationship' where suicides in women increase initially, due to the hardships of urbanisation, but as they become adjusted to urban life, the rates plateau and finally decline. This theory predicts a convergent trend followed by a divergent trend. Finally, a study by Steen and Mayer [45], using time-series analysis on suicide rates in India from 1967 to 1997, showed that there was no significant relationship between modernisation and male/female suicide ratios. No change was observed. A significant decrease in suicide mortality for both males and females was observed in all 15 republics of the Soviet Union during the period of 'Perestroika' (1985–1990) [46, 47]. This period was characterised by a number of social changes, one of which was the considerable increase in alcohol prices. The result of lowering alcohol consumption had a large effect on suicide, for both sexes, although the effect was somewhat larger for males, suggesting a downward, divergent trend at first, but this was later followed by increased male suicide and stable female suicide [28, 48].

While the results of the above mentioned studies may appear confusing, they are actually a crystal clear demonstration of how futile it can be to generate rules of thumb regarding modernisation and suicide. It appears that each country is transformed in its own way during this process. Furthermore, the transformation may have different effects on suicide rates depending to some extent on the part of the population (different age-groups, gender, social classes, etc.). They may be affected by the changes, the way risk factors are altered or whether the composition of the population is modified in a way relevant for suicide. In the example of China, Yip and Liu [31] argue that due to the decrease in the number of women who live in rural areas (responsible for the low national male/female ratio) during the urbanisation in China a convergence of male/female suicides will occur until the ratio reaches 1, which will be followed by a divergence as the female suicide rates continue to decrease.

5.3 Suicidality and mental disorders and risk

Familial and biological factors

Most current models of the suicidal process incorporate biological, psychological and societal factors. According to the stress-diathesis model, genetic factors and psychosocial stressors are together responsible for suicidal behaviour. People with a greater predisposition for suicide require fewer psychosocial stressors, such as conflicts with life partners, loss of a loved one, abuse, stress, psychological disorders, and so on in order to induce a suicidal act and are therefore at greater risk of suicide [49, 50].

Several studies involving twins, adopted people and families have shown support for familial transmission of suicidal behaviour [51–54]. Interestingly it appears to occur independently of psychiatric disorders [55, 56], which supports a possible distinction between an hereditary susceptibility to mental illness and hereditary susceptibility to suicide. The latter is likely to manifest itself in personality traits or states such as aggression, impulsivity and hopelessness as well as in mental illnesses which all have been associated with suicidal behaviour [57].

There are several theories regarding the different neurotransmitter and neuroendocrine systems that may be involved in suicidal behaviour. The dopaminergic and noradrenergic systems have both been associated with depression, anxiety and stress but with somewhat inconsistent results to suicide [24]. There is however a consistent relationship between abnormalities in the serotonin system and with attempted and completed suicides [58, 59].

The angry/hostility personality trait, which is of special interest in impulsive suicides, appears to be more common in people with a genetic variant of a regulatory factor T-box 19 in the hypothalamic-pituitary–adrenal axis [60]. Furthermore, the novel finding of a polymorphism in the corticotrophin releasing hormone receptor 1 (CHRH1) gene suggests the involvement of a genetic susceptibility for suicidality, which was linked with depression among the males, but not among females [50].

Mental illnesses

Psychiatric illnesses are very common in both completed suicides and suicide attempts. Most studies use psychological autopsies to identify the presence of mental illnesses in suicide victims. During this method, the deceased is diagnosed by assessment of available medical records and interviews with family and friends. Such studies have shown that in more than 90–98% of the cases there is at least one of diagnosable mental disorder [61–63]. Around two thirds of suicide victims are in psychiatric populations and one third of the general population suffer from a mood disorder [64]. Other psychiatric conditions are common, such as substance-related disorders (especially alcohol), personality disorders, schizophrenia and anxiety disorders [61, 64]. It is important to mention that the vast majority of the studies regarding psychopathology and suicide come from countries in Europe, North America, Australia and New Zealand and their results may be difficult to generalise to countries outside this sphere.

Major depression is a serious risk factor for suicide found in 30–80% of the victims [65] and present in 59–91% of women who commit suicide [66]. While depression is considered to be a severe risk factor, especially in males, it is nonetheless frequent amongst female victims of attempted and completed suicide [67–69]. However despite this, the lifetime mortality of depression is approximated to be no more than 6–8% [24], which means that only a handful of those with depression complete suicide. Paradoxically, major depressive disorder is twice as common in young and middle aged women as in males of the same age, but frequency of suicide is more common [66]. The risk varies with the type of mood disorder, and of course with the likelihood of getting treatment. For instance the probability of completed and attempted suicide is greater if the severity of bipolar disorder symptoms is stronger. This is particularly the case when another disorder is also present [70]. Comorbidity (having several disorders) of any constellation is likely to increase suicidality, partly due to poor treatment of co-morbid disorders and partly because of the burden caused by the diseases. A substantial proportion (44–72%) of the suicide victims have more than one diagnosable mental disorder [68, 71–73].

The most common type of constellation of comorbidity found in suicide victims is a mood disorder and substance abuse/dependence [65, 73]. Substance abuse and dependence, especially alcohol, is more common in males but it is also a significant factor in female suicides. This is supported by a study where Wasserman *et al.* [48] observed the effect of the perestroika on suicide in the USSR. Although the decrease of suicide in men was more substantial, approximately 27% of the variation in women's suicides could be attributed to alcohol consumption.

Eating disorders, such as bulimia and anorexia nervosa are a type of mental illness found almost exclusively in women. Around 90–95% of the victims of this disorder are young females, living in developed countries between the ages of 17 and 30 [74]. One to five per cent of the women develop at least one of these disorders in their lifetime. Attempted suicide is equally common in both bulimia and anorexia [75]. However whilst the mortality rate is low in bulimia, it is the highest of all psychiatric disorders in anorexia. Contrary to expectations, the cause of death by anorexia is less often related to starvation, however, starvation is more likely in bulimia than in anorexia [76]. Pompili *et al.* [77] found that suicide is eight times more common in anorexia compared to the general population and it appears to be the most common cause for death amongst people with this disorder (2% die of suicide).

A simple explanation for the increased lethality of suicide attempts when they are carried out by anorexics compared to bulimics and persons with other mental illnesses, is that anorexia victims have often a low state of health due to inanition (lack of nourishment), an attack which might otherwise not be lethal, is more likely to end up in death on such a damaged system. Also, some behaviours that are common in both anorexia and bulimia, such as purging (removal of food from the body by artificial means) have also been associated with elevated rates of suicide in both eating disorders [76, 77]. Further, comorbidity, an important risk factor for suicide, is common in people with eating disorders: more than 65% also have at least one type of anxiety disorder [78], 30% a mood disorder [79] and 20% a personality disorder [80].

Suicidality and self harm in pregnancy

There appears to be a reduced risk of suicide for women during pregnancy compared to non-pregnant women in the same age group [81, 82]. In England and Wales, pregnant women had suicide rates that were 20 times lower than non-pregnant women. At greatest risk within this group were teenagers and non-married pregnant women. Those who did commit suicide showed a high frequency of violent suicide methods, such as jumping and self-incineration, which is supposedly uncharacteristic to female suicides.

In New York, suicide rates were found to be lower for pregnant women. The rates were only one third of the expected number [82]. This difference may be due to the inclusion of pregnancies in the study which ended in abortion. But not in the one England and Wales study. In Finland it was shown that suicide rates were elevated amongst women with uncompleted pregnancies. This was most pronounced amongst those with abortions. This group had suicide rates three times as high as non-pregnant women [83]. Despite these observations, it is dangerous to draw the conclusion that uncompleted pregnancy itself is responsible to suicide. It is possible that uncompleted pregnancy is associated with factors that are themselves linked with elevated suicide risk, such as depression, poor financial situation, drug abuse, lack of social support, loneliness, and so on. In other words, the cause of the uncompleted pregnancy might also be the cause of the suicide.

Even attempted suicide and self harm seems to be less frequent amongst those pregnant women who complete their pregnancy. According to a study by Greenblatt, the amount of pregnant women hospitalised for attempted suicide in Maryland, was half that of their non-pregnant counterparts of the same age group [84, 85]. Similar results were found in Pennsylvania [86].

Despite approximately 10–15% of the mothers getting at least one episode of depression during the first year following childbirth [85], lowered rates of suicide and attempted suicide have been observed even during this so-called postpartum period [81]. However, teenagers as well as women hospitalised with psychiatric disorders, are at a greater risk than women in the general population during the postpartum period. According to a Danish study [87], hospitalised women with psychiatric disorders are at an extreme (approximately 70 times greater) risk of suicide than the general population. The suicide risk appears to be highest in the first two months of the postpartum period.

5.4 Suicide prevention

Suicide prevention can be divided into the healthcare approach and public health approaches. The healthcare approach in suicide prevention is aimed at identifying the at-risk individuals and providing treatment and rehabilitation for them. The public health approaches target the whole population with the intention of reducing suicide, by identifying and eliminating risk factors associated with suicide. Ideally both public health and healthcare approaches ought to be exercised together to achieve the best possible effect.

In most cases, mental illness is a precursor to suicide, leading to the inevitable conclusion that the early diagnosis and adequate treatment of mental illnesses should be among the first priorities in suicide prevention. Improving the skills of general practitioners and other healthcare professionals to make early diagnosis of mental disorders in the general population and providing adequate treatment of mental illnesses, has been shown to be an effective way to prevent suicide

[88, 89]. This method is especially useful for preventing suicides in females, as in a number of cultures, females have a greater tendency than males to seek help from healthcare professionals, as well as from family and friends. It is important to take advantage of this help-seeking behaviour by increasing the availability of healthcare personnel and making sure their response is effective.

It is also important to destigmatise mental health problems and suicidal behaviour, in order to encourage help seeking behaviours, as well as to spread information about the availability of treatment amongst the general public [90]. As help is often sought from friends and family, it is essential that both the person seeking help and those near to them are aware of what options are available and how to make use of them.

Treatment interventions such as pharmacotherapy and/or psychotherapy focus on reducing suicide through the treatment of at risk individuals. Studies regarding antidepressants have shown little success in suicide prevention in young people [91]. In fact, some have been shown to increase suicidal behaviour in the early stages of administration [92]. For persons aged over 30, antidepressants appear to have a protective effect against suicidal behaviour [93]. However regardless of age, a close monitoring of the patient is recommended, in the beginning and termination of the treatments [94]. Psychotherapy treatment interventions, such as cognitive therapy, problem-solving therapy and interpersonal psychotherapy, have shown promising results in preventing suicide [88], but there are insufficient numbers of qualified personnel to support this.

Another example of an effective public health strategy is the restriction of the means of suicide, such as detoxification of domestic gases, restrictions in the use of fire-arms and pesticides [88]. Restriction of pesticides seems specifically potent in reducing female suicides in certain areas of the world, such as rural China and India, as mentioned earlier. It should be remembered that by removing the object used for the suicide one does not remove the desire to die, as life circumstances leading to suicide remain [95]. However it can be an effective way to buy time during which the desire can be targeted and eliminated, by for instance developing psychological support networks for women in rural areas living with their husbands' families. One action that may support networks is the education of key persons, for instance school teachers, who are often in contact with such at risk individuals about suicide prevention.

While it may be too costly and time consuming to give extensive education to all key persons, the teaching of the basic principles of suicide prevention can be done quickly and cost-efficiently by using short booklets and information leaflets. One example is the WHO suicide prevention resource for teachers and school staff, a 22 page, pocket-sized booklet [96]. Several key concepts for suicide prevention in schools are discussed, such as how to identify and give support to students with psychiatric disorders, when to refer students to treatment for drug or alcohol abuse, how to identify means of suicide and limit students' access to them, and so on. A series of resource guides has been published including resources for physicians, media professionals, primary healthcare workers as well as prison officers. (To download the material for free visit http://www.who.int/mental_health/resources/suicide/en/ it is available in several languages.)

Lowering alcohol consumption, for instance by increasing the price of alcoholic drinks or increasing the age at which alcohol may be purchased, can be an effective way to reduce suicide [48]. While it is true that these effects are more profound in males, they are also considerable in females both directly and indirectly. There are, especially in western countries, an increasing number of young females who have lifestyles similar to males who are at an increased suicide risk, characterised by increased alcohol consumption, violence and high prevalence of mental illness. Lowering the alcohol consumption of these young women will probably have a high effect in decreasing suicide similarly to their male counterparts. Other 'male-oriented' suicide prevention strategies may also be effective for women with destructive lifestyles. The reduction of alcohol in males can also have an indirect effect on females by, for instance, diminishing stressors that arise from having an alcohol dependent/abusing life partner. This is just one example of the importance of culture and gender in suicide prevention. Just like in suicide research, one-size-fits-all strategies and rules of thumbs are best avoided [36, 63].

Finally, it is of great importance that regardless what type of suicide prevention strategy is employed, critical evaluation of its efficacy should be facilitated and encouraged. Funds for suicide prevention are limited and it can be difficult to decide which strategy to invest in, without scientific evidence of its effect on reducing suicide. With critical evaluation one would be able to exclude less effective strategies from the list of available options and encourage the use of better ones.

It is important for the prevention of both female and male suicide to eradicate the incorrect views that suicidality is not a serious possibility when displayed by a certain gender [97]. It has been shown that in the cities of Bern, Wurzburg and Guipuzcoa young girls were less likely to receive recommended care after suicide attempts compared to boys, while in Odense, Oxford and Stockholm the opposite was true [98]. The moulding of the attitudes due to the education of caretakers can lead to increased confidence and knowledge regarding suicidal behaviour and is helpful in eliminating the erroneous beliefs and stigma which are associated with the gender biases that lead to certain suicide attempters receiving less care [99]. Furthermore, education of caretakers may also encourage gender oriented treatment, which takes into consideration the differences in risk factors and treatment options between females and males.

For further reading regarding specific strategies see, Suicide – An Unnecessary Death [63], the proposal for the Swedish national suicide prevention programme [100] a review by Mann *et al.* [88] and by Nordentoft [101].

References

1. Linehan, M.M. (1986) Suicidal people. One population or two? *Annals of the New York Academy of Sciences*, **487**, 16–33.

2. WHO (1998) Primary Prevention of Mental, Neurological and Psychosocial Disorders, World Health Organisation, Geneva.

3. Skegg, K. (2005) Self-harm. *Lancet*, **366** (9495), 1471–83.

4. Bille-Brahe, U., Schmidtke, A., Kerkhof, A.J. *et al.* (1995) Background and introduction to the WHO/EURO Multicentre Study on Parasuicide. *Crisis*, **16** (2), 72–78, 84.

5. World Health Organization (2001) World Health Report: Mental Illness: New Understanding, New Hope, WHO, Geneva.

6. World Health Organization (2003) World Health Report 2003: Shaping the Future, WHO, Geneva.

7. World Health Organization (2005) Suicide Rates Per 100,000 by Country, Year and Sex (Table), WHO.

8. Rutz, E.M. and Wasserman, D. (2004) Trends in adolescent suicide mortality in the WHO European Region. *European Child and Adolescent Psychiatry*, **13** (5), 321–31.

9. Wasserman, D., Cheng, Q. and Jiang, G.X. (2005) Global suicide rates among young people aged 15–19. *World Psychiatry Journal*, **4** (2), 114–20.

10. Pelkonen, M. and Marttunen, M. (2003) Child and adolescent suicide: epidemiology, risk factors, and approaches to prevention. *Paediatric Drugs*, **5** (4), 243–65.

11. Schmidtke, A., Bille-Brahe, U., DeLeo, D. *et al.* (1996) Attempted suicide in Europe: rates, trends and sociodemographic characteristics of suicide attempters during the period 1989–1992. Results of the WHO/EURO Multicentre Study on Parasuicide. *Acta Psychiatrica Scandinavica*, **93** (5), 327–38.

12. Beautrais, A.L. (2006) Women and suicidal behavior. *Crisis*, **27** (4), 153–56.

13. Bertolote J.M. (2001) Suicide in the world: an epidemiological overview, 1959–2000, in *Suicide: An Unnecessary Death* (ed. D. Wasserman), Martin Dunitz, London, pp. 1–11.

14. Canetto, S. and Lester D. (1995) The epidemiology of women's suicidal behavior, in *Women and Suicidal Behavior* (eds S. Canetto and D. Lester), Springer, New York, pp. 35–57.

15. Canetto, S.S. (1997) Gender and suicidal behavior: theories and evidence, in *Review of Suicidology* (eds R.W. Maris, M.M. Silverman and S.S. Canetto), Guilford, New York, pp. 138–67.

16. Denning, D.G., Conwell, Y., King, D. and Cox, C. (2000) Method choice, intent, and gender in completed suicide. *Suicide and Life-Threatening Behavior*, Fall **30** (3), 282–88.

17. Caldera, T., Herrera, A., Kullgren, G. and Renberg, E.S. (2007) Suicide intent among parasuicide patients in Nicaragua: a surveillance and follow-up study. *Archives of Suicide Research*, **11** (4), 351–60.

18. Hjelmeland, H., Knizek, B.L. and Nordvik, H. (2002) The communicative aspect of nonfatal suicidal behavior – are there gender differences? *Crisis*, **23** (4), 144–55.

19. Hjelmeland, H., Nordvik, H., Bille-Brahe, U. *et al.* (2000) A cross-cultural study of suicide intent in parasuicide patients. *Suicide and Life-Threatening Behavior*, Winter **30** (4), 295–303.

20. Lester, D. (1972) *Why Do People Kill Themselves*, Charles C. Thomas Publisher, Springfield.

21. Moscicki, E.K. (1994) Gender differences in completed and attempted suicides. *Annals of Epidemiology*, **4** (2), 152–58.

22. Kposowa, A.J. and McElvain, J.P. (2006) Gender, place, and method of suicide. *Social Psychiatry and Psychiatric Epidemiology*, **41** (6), 435–43.

23. Kessler, R.C., McGonagle, K.A., Swartz, M. *et al.* (1993) Sex and depression in the National Comorbidity Survey. I: lifetime prevalence, chronicity and recurrence. *Journal of Affective Disorders*, **29** (2–3), 85–96.

24. Wasserman, D. (2006) *Depression: The Facts*, Oxford University Press, Oxford.

25. Wasserman, D., Geijer, T., Sokolowski, M. *et al.* (2007) Genetic variation in the hypothalamic-pituitary-adrenocortical axis regulatory factor, T-box 19, and the angry/hostility personality trait. *Genes, Brain, and Behavior*, **6** (4), 321–28.

26. Weissman, M.M., Bland, R.C., Canino, G.J. *et al.* (1996) Cross-national epidemiology of major depression and bipolar disorder. *The Journal of the American Medical Association*, **276** (4), 293–99.

27. Suokas, J., Suominen, K. and Lonnqvist, J. (2005) Chronic alcohol problems among suicide attempters – post-mortem findings of a 14-year follow-up. *Nordic Journal of Psychiatry*, **59** (1), 45–50.

28. Varnik, A., Kolves, K., Vali, M. *et al.* (2007) Do alcohol restrictions reduce suicide mortality? *Addiction (Abingdon, England)*, **102** (2), 251–56.

29. Stengel, E. (1964) *Suicide and Attempted Suicide*, Penguin Books, Baltimore.

30. Moksony, F. (1990) Ecological analysis of suicide, in *Current Concepts of Suicide* (ed. D. Lester), Philadelphia,Charles Press, pp. 121–38.

31. Yip, P.S. and Liu, K.Y. (2006) The ecological fallacy and the gender ratio of suicide in China. *The British Journal of Psychiatry*, **189**, 465–66.

32. Zhou, Y. and Ma, L.J.C. (2003) China's urbanization levels: reconstructing a baseline from the Fifth Population Census. *The China Quarterly*, **173**, 176–96.

33. Moscicki, E. (1994) Gender differences in completed and attempted suicides. *Annals of Epidemiology*, **4** (2), 152–58.

34. Phillips, M.R., Yang, G., Zhang, Y. *et al.* (2002) Risk factors for suicide in China: a national case-control psychological autopsy study. *Lancet*, **360** (9347), 1728–36.

35. Kanchan, T. and Menezes, R.G. (2008) Suicidal poisoning in Southern India: gender differences. *The Journal of Forensic and Legal Medicine*, **15** (1), 7–14.

36. Canetto, S.S. (2009) Prevention of suicidal behavior in females: opportunities and obstacles, in *Oxford Textbook of Suicidology* (eds D. Wasserman and C. Wasserman), Oxford University Press, New York, in press, chapter 29, Part V, April, 2009.

37. Khan, M.M. (2005) Suicide prevention and developing countries. *Journal of the Royal Society of Medicine*, **98** (10), 459–63.

38. Vijayakumar, L., John, S., Pirkis, J. and Whiteford, H. (2005) Suicide in developing countries (2): risk factors. *Crisis*, **26** (3), 112–19.

39. Li, X.Y., Phillips, M.R., Zhang, Y.P. *et al.* (2008) Risk factors for suicide in China's youth: a case-control study. *Psychological Medicine*, **38** (3), 397–406.

40. Durkheim, E. (1951) *Suicide: A Study in Sociology*, Free Press, New York.

41. Stack, S. and Danigelis, N. (1985) Modernization and the sex differential in suicide, 1919–1972. *Comparative Social Research*, **8**, 203–16.

42. Hassan, R. and Tan, G. (1989) Suicide trends in Australia, 1901–1985: an analysis of sex differentials. *Suicide and Life-Threatening Behavior*, Winter **19** (4), 362–80.

43. Stack, S. (2000) Suicide: a 15-year review of the sociological literature. Part II: modernization and social integration perspectives. *Suicide and Life-Threatening Behavior*, Summer **30** (2), 163–76.

44. Pampel, F.C. (1998) National context, social change, and sex differences in suicide rates. *American Sociological Review*, **63**, 744–58.

45. Steen, D.M. and Mayer, P. (2004) Modernization and the male-female suicide ratio in India 1967–1997: divergence or convergence? *Suicide and Life-Threatening Behavior*, **34** (2), 147–59.

46. Wasserman, D., Varnik, A. and Dankowicz, M. (1998) Regional differences in the distribution of suicide in the former Soviet Union during perestroika, 1984–1990. *Acta Psychiatrica Scandinavica Supplementum*, **394**, 5–12.

47. Wasserman, D., Varnik, A. and Eklund, G. (1994) Male suicides and alcohol consumption in the former USSR. *Acta Psychiatrica Scandinavica*, **89** (5), 306–13.

48. Wasserman, D., Varnik, A. and Eklund, G. (1998) Female suicides and alcohol consumption during perestroika in the former USSR. *Acta Psychiatrica Scandinavica Supplementum*, **394**, 26–33.

49. Wasserman, D. (2001) A stress-vulnerability model and the development of the suicidal process, in *Suicide an Unnecessary Death* (ed. D. Wasserman), Martin Dunitz Publishers, Taylor and Francis Group, London, pp. 13–26.

50. Wasserman, D., Sokolowski, M., Rozanov, V. and Wasserman, J. (2007) The CRHR1 gene: a marker for suicidality in depressed males exposed to low stress. *Genes, Brain, and Behavior*, **7** (1), 14–19. Epub 2007 March 21.

51. Fu, Q., Heath, A.C., Bucholz, K.K. *et al.* (2002) A twin study of genetic and environmental influences on suicidality in men. *Psychological Medicine*, **32** (1), 11–24.

52. Qin, P., Agerbo, E. and Mortensen, P.B. (2003) Suicide risk in relation to socioeconomic, demographic, psychiatric, and familial factors: a national register-based study of all suicides in Denmark, 1981–1997. *American Journal of Medical Psychiatry*, **160** (4), 765–72.

53. Roy, A. and Segal, N.L. (2001) Suicidal behavior in twins: a replication. *Journal of Affective Disorders*, **66** (1), 71–74.

54. Wender, P.H., Kety, S.S., Rosenthal, D. *et al.* (1986) Psychiatric disorders in the biological and adoptive families of adopted individuals with affective disorders. *Archives of General Psychiatry*, **43** (10), 923–29.

55. Brent, D.A. and Mann, J.J. (2005) Family genetic studies, suicide, and suicidal behavior. *American Journal of Medical Genetics. Part C; Seminars in Medical Genetics*, **133** (1), 13–24.

56. Mittendorfer-Rutz, E. (2005) Perinatal and Familial Risk Factors of Youth Suicidal Behaviour. Doctoral Thesis, Karolinska Institutet, Stockholm.

57. Joiner, T.E. Jr., Brown, J.S. and Wingate, L.R. (2005) The psychology and neurobiology of suicidal behavior. *Annual Review of Psychology*, **56**, 287–314.

58. Mann, J.J. and Currier, D. (2007) A review of prospective studies of biologic predictors of suicidal behavior in mood disorders. *Archives of Suicide Research*, **11** (1), 3–16.

59. Samuelsson, M., Jokinen, J., Nordstrom, A.L. and Nordstrom, P. (2006) CSF 5-HIAA, suicide intent and hopelessness in the prediction of early suicide in male high-risk suicide attempters. *Acta Psychiatrica Scandinavica*, **113** (1), 44–47.

60. Wasserman, D., Geijer, T., Sokolowski, M. *et al.* (2006) Genetic variation in the hypothalamic-pituitary-adrenocortical axis regulatory factor, T-box 19, and the

angry/hostility personality trait. *Genes, Brain, and Behavior*, **6** (4), 321–8. Epub 2006, Aug. 7.

61. Bertolote, J.M. and Fleischmann, A. (2002) Suicide and psychiatric diagnosis: a worldwide perspective. *World Psychiatry Journal*, **1** (3), 181–85.

62. Mann, J.J. (2002) A current perspective of suicide and attempted suicide. *Annals of Internal Medicine*, **136** (4), 302–11.

63. Wasserman, D. (ed.) (2001) *Suicide, An Unnecessary Death*, Martin Dunitz, London.

64. Bertolote, J.M., Fleischmann, A., De Leo, D. and Wasserman, D. (2004) Psychiatric diagnoses and suicide: revisiting the evidence. *Crisis*, **25** (4), 147–55.

65. Bertolote, J.M., Fleischmann, A., De Leo D. and Wasserman, D. (2003) Suicide and mental disorders: do we know enough? *The British Journal of Psychiatry*, **183**, 382–83.

66. Chaudron, L.H. and Caine, E.D. (2004) Suicide among women: a critical review. *Journal of the American Medical Womens Association*, Spring **59** (2), 125–34.

67. Asgard, U. (1990) A psychiatric study of suicide among urban Swedish women. *Acta Psychiatrica Scandinavica*, **82** (2), 115–24.

68. Beautrais, A.L., Joyce, P.R., Mulder, R.T. *et al.* (1996) Prevalence and comorbidity of mental disorders in persons making serious suicide attempts: a case-control study. *The American Journal of Psychiatry*, **153** (8), 1009–14.

69. Shaffer, D., Gould, M.S., Fisher P. *et al.* (1996) Psychiatric diagnosis in child and adolescent suicide. *Archives of General Psychiatry*, **53** (4), 339–48.

70. Goldstein, T.R., Birmaher, B., Axelson D. *et al.* History of suicide attempts in pediatric bipolar disorder: factors associated with increased risk. *Bipolar Disorders*, **7** (6), 525–35.

71. Henriksson, M.M., Aro H.M., Marttunen M.J. *et al.* (1993) Mental disorders and comorbidity in suicide. *The American Journal of Psychiatry*, **150** (6), 935–40.

72. Lonnqvist, J.K., Henriksson, M.M., Isometsa, E.T. *et al.* (1995) Mental disorders and suicide prevention. *Psychiatry and Clinical Neurosciences*, **49** (Suppl 1), S111–16.

73. Seguin, M., Lesage, A., Chawky, N. *et al.* (2006) Suicide cases in New Brunswick from April 2002 to May 2003: the importance of better recognizing substance and mood disorder comorbidity. *Canadian Journal of Psychiatry*, **51** (9), 581–86.

74. Gelder, A., Gath, D., Mayou, R. and Cowen, P. (1996) *Oxford Textbook of Psychiatry*, 3rd edn, Oxford University Press, Oxford.

75. Corcos, M., Taieb, O., Benoit-Lamy, S. *et al.* (2002) Suicide attempts in women with bulimia nervosa: frequency and characteristics. *Acta Psychiatrica Scandinavica*, **106** (5), 381–86.

76. Franko, D.L. and Keel, P.K. (2006) Suicidality in eating disorders: occurrence, correlates, and clinical implications. *Clinical Psychology Review*, **26** (6), 769–82.

77. Pompili, M., Mancinelli, I., Girardi, P. *et al.* (2004) Suicide in anorexia nervosa: a meta-analysis. *The International Journal of Eating Disorders*, **36** (1), 99–103.

78. Kaye, W.H., Bulik, C.M., Thornton, L. *et al.* (2004) Comorbidity of anxiety disorders with anorexia and bulimia nervosa. *The American Journal of Psychiatry*, **161** (12), 2215–21.

79. Garcia-Alba, C. (2004) Anorexia and depression: depressive comorbidity in anorexic adolescents. *The Spanish Journal of Psychology*, **7** (1), 40–52.

80. Muller, B., Wewetzer, C., Jans, T. *et al.* (2001) Personality disorders and psychiatric comorbidity in obsessive-compulsive disorder and anorexia nervosa. *Fortschritte der Neurologie-Psychiatrie*, **69** (8), 379–87.

81. Appleby, L. (1991) Suicide during pregnancy and in the first postnatal year. *The British Medical Journal*, **302** (6769), 137–40.

82. Marzuk, P.M., Tardiff, K., Leon, A.C. *et al.* (1997) Lower risk of suicide during pregnancy. *The American Journal of Psychiatry*, **154** (1), 122–23.

83. Gissler, M., Hemminki, E., Lonnqvist J. (1996) Suicides after pregnancy in Finland, 1987–94: register linkage study. *The British Medical Journal*, **313** (7070), 1431–34.

84. Greenblatt, J.F., Dannenberg, A.L. and Johnson, C.J. (1997) Incidence of hospitalized injuries among pregnant women in Maryland, 1979–1990. *American Journal of Preventive Medicine*, **13** (5), 374–79.

85. Lindahl, V., Pearson, J.L., Colpe L. (2005) Prevalence of suicidality during pregnancy and the postpartum. *Archives of Womens Mental Health*, **8** (2), 77–87.

86. Weiss, H.B. (1999) Pregnancy-associated injury hospitalizations in Pennsylvania, 1995. *Annals of Emergency Medicine*, **34** (5), 626–36.

87. Appleby, L., Mortensen, P.B. and Faragher, E.B. (1998) Suicide and other causes of mortality after post-partum psychiatric admission. *The British Journal of Psychiatry*, **173**, 209–11.

88. Mann, J.J., Apter, A., Bertolote, J. *et al.* (2005) Suicide prevention strategies: a systematic review. *The Journal of the American Medical Association*, **294** (16), 2064–74.

89. Szanto, K., Kalmar, S., Hendin, H. *et al.* (2007) A suicide prevention program in a region with a very high suicide rate. *Archives of General Psychiatry*, **64** (8), 914–20.

90. Hegerl, U., Wittmann, M., Arensman, E. *et al.* (2007) The 'European Alliance Against Depression (EAAD)': a multifaceted, community-based action programme against depression and suicidality. *The World Journal of Biological Psychiatry*, **9** (1), 51–8.

91. Bridge, J.A., Iyengar, S., Salary, C.B. *et al.* (2007) Clinical response and risk for reported suicidal ideation and suicide attempts in pediatric antidepressant treatment: a meta-analysis of randomized controlled trials. *The Journal of the American Medical Association*, **297** (15), 1683–96.

92. Apter, A., Lipschitz, A., Fong R. *et al.* (2006) Evaluation of suicidal thoughts and behaviors in children and adolescents taking paroxetine. *Journal of Child and Adolescent Psychopharmacology*, **16** (1–2), 77–90.

93. Leon, A.C. (2007) The revised warning for antidepressants and suicidality: unveiling the black box of statistical analyses. *The American Journal of Psychiatry*, **164** (12), 1786–89.

94. Sihvo, S., Isometsa, E., Kiviruusu, O. *et al.* (2008) Antidepressant utilisation patterns and determinants of short-term and non-psychiatric use in the Finnish general adult population. *Journal of Affective Disorders*.

95. Wasserman, D., Thanh, H.T.T., Minh, D.P.T. *et al.* (2008) A case study of suicidal behaviour among young suicide attempters in a rural Vietnamese community: when there is no one to talk to. *World Psychiatry Journal*. 2008, Feb **7** (1), 47–53.

96. WHO (2000) Preventing Suicide: A Resource for Teachers and Other School Staff, World Health Organization, Geneva.

97. Canetto, S. and Lester, D. (1995) Suicidal women: intervention and prevention strategies, in *Women and Suicidal Behavior* (eds S. Canetto and D. Lester), Springer, New York, pp. 237–55.

98. Hulten, A., Wasserman, D., Hawton, K. *et al.* (2000) Recommended care for young people (15–19 years) after suicide attempts in certain European countries. *European Child and Adolescent Psychiatry*, **9** (2), 100–8.

99. Ramberg, I.L. and Wasserman, D. (2004) Benefits of implementing an academic training of trainers program to promote knowledge and clarity in work with psychiatric suicidal patients. *Archives of Suicide Research*, **8** (4), 331–43.

100. NASP (2006) Proposal for a National Program for Suicide Prevention (Förslag till nationellt program för suicide prevention), National Centre for Suicide Research and Prevention of Mental Ill-Health, Stockholm.

101. Nordentoft, M. (2007) Prevention of suicide and attempted suicide in Denmark. Epidemiological studies of suicide and intervention studies in selected risk groups. *Danish Medical Bulletin*, **54** (4), 306–69.

6
Alcohol and substance abuse

Florence Baingana

Makerere University School of Public Health, Kampala, Uganda

6.1 Introduction

This chapter focuses on alcohol and substance abuse in relation to women. The orientation is that of a socio-ecological model, so the discussion will not be so much on the signs and symptoms and the treatment methods; information about which is widely available. The discussion will focus more on how women are differently impacted by alcohol and substance abuse, either as the persons with the problem, or as wives, sisters, daughters or mothers of a person with an alcohol or substance abuse problem. Very often the challenge for women is not that the signs and symptoms are not recognisable, but that women are impacted differently, and thus solutions will not only be devising methods for greater access to treatment programmes for women, but also addressing issues of differential risks and vulnerabilities and this may have to be not just in the health/mental health field but addressing the broader social factors.

Terminologies

The term 'substance abuse' encompasses 'a maladaptive pattern of use indicated by . . . continued use despite knowledge of having a persistent or recurrent social, occupational, psychological or physical problem that is caused or exacerbated by the use (or by) recurrent use in situations in which it is physically hazardous' [1]. Within the term is included alcohol use disorder or AUD, alcohol dependence, as well as the use/abuse of tobacco, heroin, cocaine, pharmaceutical drugs and others. Another commonly used term is injection drug use (IDU); injections may

Contemporary Topics in Women's Mental Health   Edited by Chandra, Herrman, Fisher, Kastrup,
© 2009 John Wiley & Sons, Ltd   Niaz, Rondón and Okasha

be intra-muscular, subcutaneous or intravenous [1]. An illicit drug is one where the 'production, sale or use of which is prohibited. Strictly speaking, it is not the drug that is illicit, but its production, sale or use in particular circumstances in a given jurisdiction' [1].

There is an hierarchy of drug abuse according to 'hardest illicit drug used', with six levels beginning with none, marijuana, non injected cocaine other than crack, non injected heroin, crack or IDU [2] AUDs are on a continuum from abstinence, initiation, when the first full alcoholic drink is consumed, to 'alcohol related problem', when first alcohol abuse or dependence symptom occurs, and 'alcohol dependence', when full Diagnostic and Statistical Manual (DSM) IV criteria for alcohol dependence are first met [1].

The drugs being abused have increased in complexity, with newer drugs such as ecstasy, crystal methamphetamine, Phencyclidine (PCP) among others, having been introduced. These newer drugs are manufactured, some even in the bathroom amongst common household items or drugs available over the counter from pharmacies. Addiction to these newer drugs happens very quickly.

6.2 Genetics of alcohol and drug abuse

Genetics of alcohol and drug abuse disorders have until recently only focused on men. Alcohol dependence heritability is estimated at about 50–60% in both men and women [3, 4]. Studies do not just look at heritability of disorders, but also at stages of transition from initiation to problem development to alcohol dependence, how fast the transition takes as well as whether or not one progresses to the next level. Sartor *et al.*, studying genetic and environmental factors in the rate of progression to alcohol dependence in young women, found that the first transition from nonuse to initiation of alcohol use is greatly influenced by shared environment [3]. In the same study, variance in the speed of transition from one stage to another is explained 30–47% by heredity [3]. Women who transitioned quickly from one stage to the next were also at increased risk for transition to the next stage. Early initiators tended to transition much more slowly [3].

Items in the alcohol dependence symptomatology have been grouped into either genetic or environmental. Those that are considered genetic are 'job trouble because of drinking or lost job; alcohol-related health problems and/or continued drinking despite health problems, drinking binges lasting at least a couple of days and needing a drink in the morning just after waking' [4]. A study on sex differences in hereditability of alcohol problems found that three symptoms had significant hereditability in females, and these were 'increased risk of injury or harm', 'emotional problem related to drinking' and the 'desire to drink' [4].

6.3 Burden of the problem and patterns of drinking

In relation to alcohol, in general, abstention is greater in the developing world [5, 6] and women abstain at a greater rate than men in almost all countries [7]. In almost all countries of the world, drinking rates fall off in women over 50 years, except for Uganda and Nigeria, where rates are lower in the younger age groups [5]. Rates of 'heavy episodic drinking' or 'binge drinking' are also at a lower rate for women then for men; however, trends in binge drinking are higher in women where the rates for men are also high, as in Australia (15% in males and 12% in females), Canada (28% in males and 11% in females), Finland (49% in males and 14% in females), Germany (42% in males and 13% in females) and Iceland (43% in males and 20% in females). Rates for heavy episodic drinking were 40% in females in Nigeria (with 52% in males), the highest globally [7].

Women have lower rates of heavy drinkers than men in general, except for Burkina Faso (10% males and 13% females), Dominican Republic (1% males, 3% females), Ethiopia (8% males and 11% females), Nigeria (28% males and 36% females), Norway (3% males and 5% females), Slovakia (5% males and 8% females), South Africa (7% males and 9% females) and United Kingdom (39% males and 42% females) [7]. In general, women in Africa seem to drink more than in other parts of the world, and to drink almost as much as the men drink, and with similar drinking patterns [5–7].

Data on drug abuse and especially on women as drug abusers is much more difficult to find [8]. Since treatment facilities, the sources of most drug abuse data, may not admit women, the extent of the problem among women is under reported [8, 9]. What data is available seems to indicate almost similar rates between males and females for drug abuse in the developed countries [2, 9], although there is evidence to suggest that more men than women report using stigmatised drugs [2]. A National Household Survey carried out in the US in 1997 found 34% of white women, 19% of Latinas and 25% of African American women reported lifetime prevalence of illegal drug use [9]. The increase in drug abuse seen, especially in the developed countries, is linked to the transition of women from traditional roles in the home to economic provider as well as linked to emancipation and greater economic independence [9].

Post traumatic stress disorder is associated with higher levels of alcohol and substance abuse, as well as other co-morbid mental disorders in both males and females [10]. Women with acute post traumatic stress disorder (PTSD) have higher levels of mental health problems, substance use disorders as well as more risky sexual behaviours.

6.4 Alcohol and drug abuse, risky sexual behaviour and HIV vulnerability

More young people are initiating alcohol use and sexual activity earlier than in previous years [6]. In young people, alcohol is taken to facilitate the first sexual encounter [6], and in girls, the alcohol and the first sexual encounter may both be coerced. Even in adult women, rates of forced sex are higher among women who drink alcohol or abuse drugs than among those who do not [11]. Alcohol may not be the instigating factor, but is viewed as a 'pretext or cueing mechanism for socially scripted behaviour' [12, 13]. In some cultures, the link between alcohol and sex is such that drinking alcohol is part of a conscious strategy that leads to sexual encounters.

Male dominance makes it difficult for women to initiate condom use, especially when they are under the influence of alcohol or drugs [6]. Studies have also found that among young people, unsupervised time after school is a risk factor for alcohol and drug use as well as engaging in sexual activity. Cohen *et al.* found that tobacco and alcohol use are associated with unsupervised time for boys, but not for girls [14], and this risk increased for boys with the length of unsupervised time.

Alcohol and drugs are also associated with more instances of sex with strangers, casual sex, group sex and transactional sex [2, 6, 13]. This risk is higher for women on crack and injection drug users [11, 15], and they were more likely to have had 'concurrent partners, multiple partners, a history of commercial sex work, partners shared with a network member and unprotected sex' [2, 13, 15]. A study in Tijuana found that women IDU had a threefold higher HIV rate than male IDU [11]. In Botswana, women who were problem or heavy drinkers had over eight times the odds of providing sex for money or other items, compared to non drinkers [13]. There is a dose-response relationship between amount of alcohol consumed and unprotected sex. In a study carried out in Botswana, those who did not drink were at lowest risk for unprotected sex, while heavy drinkers had higher odds of unprotected sex than moderate drinkers [13].

There is increased prevalence of alcohol and drug use among commercial sex workers [2, 6, 11, 16], and this alcohol and drug abuse is linked to increased sexual risk behaviour, such as penetrative sex without condoms, anal sex and oral sex [2, 6, 13, 15]. Among commercial sex workers, alcohol is taken to deal with the difficult work and clients [6]. Women who engage in transactional sex often do so to support other family members [16].

Some women believe that having sex under the influence of alcohol will lead to greater satisfaction [6]. In the process of socialisation, purchasing of alcohol for a woman is often taken to be a first step to a sexual encounter with that woman [6, 12, 13]; it is agreed that the woman will have to 'pay back'. Even if this is not overtly prostitution, it may lead to risky sexual behaviour, without the use of a condom, or involving violence and anal and or oral sex. In many cultures, women who drink outside the home are perceived to be violating the socially accepted norms of behaviour for women and so put themselves at risk for sexual abuse, and or easy sexual liaisons [12]. In sub Saharan Africa, women who are involved in intergenerational relationships have higher rates of alcohol abuse and are also at an increased risk for HIV infection [13].

Women who have sex with women are especially vulnerable as they have been found to begin sexual activities earlier, engage in sex and unprotected sex more frequently and more often trade sex for money or drugs, all activities putting them at increased risk for HIV transmission [17]. Women who have sex with women use tobacco, alcohol, amphetamines, heroin and cocaine at higher rates than women who have never had sex with women [18].

Women and girls who abuse alcohol and drugs have higher HIV and AIDS rates, and those who are IDU are even more at risk. Women who drink alcohol are more likely to be infected with HIV than those who do not drink [12, 13]. In China, provinces bordering the Golden Triangle, where drug trafficking is common, have the highest HIV prevalence, and rates can be as high as 80% among IDU in the prefectures where drug abuse rates are highest [19]. There is a fear that the high rates of HIV in IDU who are also commercial sex worker (CSW) may lead to spread of HIV to the general population, such CSW are termed 'bridge populations' [11, 19]. Many IDU are CSW who engage in sex without use of condoms.

6.5 Stigma, women and alcohol and drug abuse

Women who abuse alcohol or drugs are stigmatised, it is often viewed as a weakness on the part of the women [6, 8, 9, 20]. Shelters for abused women will often not admit women who abuse alcohol or drugs, and drug treatment facilities are also not designed to admit women with alcohol or drug abuse problems. This arises from the stigma and discrimination of the health and social service providers, who believe that it is a weakness for women to abuse alcohol or drugs.

6.6 Health consequences

Women who abuse alcohol and drugs are at increased risk for HIV, and hepatitis C and or B infection, through sharing of needles, prostitution as well as increased incidence of casual sex with strangers [2, 8, 11, 12, 15, 19, 20]. There is an increase of co-morbidity with other mental disorders among people who abuse alcohol and drugs, including women [10, 20].

Excessive consumption of alcohol and its consequences can impact on the mental well-being of family members, including anxiety, fear, depression and physical or verbal aggression by the drinking person towards other family members [7]. Risks include infection with HIV. Women who abuse alcohol or drugs often have a partner who drinks or uses drugs even more than the woman. Some women who do not abuse drugs may provide sexual favours for drugs for their drug-abusing partner, thus putting themselves at risk for HIV [8].

6.7 Social and economic consequences

Gender, Alcohol, and Culture: an international Study (GENACIS), a study of gender, alcohol and drinking problems in eight countries around the world found that self-reported alcohol problems are low among women in all societies except in the two African countries studied, Uganda and Nigeria [5]. Social consequences include family disintegration, issues to do with money, children dropping out of school; child neglect is another consequence, especially if the woman is the one abusing alcohol [7, 8]. In some parts of sub Saharan Africa, a vicious cycle is created, with women as the brewers of alcohol, then sellers, they then become excessive consumers [7].

Impacts on children include giving children alcohol to keep them quiet or to stave off hunger, compounded with child abuse; these children may then drop out of school, resort to begging and stealing of food and other delinquent behaviours [7]. Daughters of drug abusing fathers or mothers may be pushed into prostitution in order to provide funds for the purchase of drugs [8].

GENACIS, found that Uganda, one of the countries with the highest rates of per capita alcohol consumption as well as a relatively high hazardous drinking score, also had the biggest impacts of drinking on their social lives, both in men and in women [5]. Problems included harmed marriage/intimate relations, harmed family relations, harmed friendships, fights while drinking, drink driving, harmed work, harmed chores, harmed finances, harmed physical health and guilt and remorse. Problem scores are highest for women in Uganda followed by Nigeria; problem scores for Nigerian women are the same as those for Nigerian men [5].

Alcohol, drug abuse and domestic violence

Very often, women who abuse alcohol and drugs also have a partner who abuses alcohol and drugs, sometimes at a rate higher than that of the woman [20]. Alcohol is commonly associated with domestic violence, with both the perpetuator and the victim abusing alcohol [6, 7]. Studies have also found that excessive consumption of alcohol by the victim is more associated with violence than if the victim is abstinent, as well as the instances where the perpetrator is the one abusing alcohol or drugs [7].

Women, mothers, wives, sisters and daughters, who live in a household where there is a man abusing alcohol or drugs are also affected by the abuse; they may experience social, health and economic disadvantages as well as domestic violence [8]. Women who abuse drugs may have had abusive fathers, or may have been sexually abused as children [8, 20].

6.8 Interventions

There are not too many reports of specific interventions for women substance users. A model of a successful intervention is a special child welfare clinic in Norway that provides support to pregnant substance abusing women. The intervention, a low threshold initiative, is to provide support to drug dependent women throughout the pregnancy. The women receive counselling as well as help with housing, economy and necessary health services. Normal pregnancy checks are held, the pregnant woman is encouraged to attend clinics regularly, if she does not, she is followed up in the home. It was found that there was a reduction of alcohol and substance use among the pregnant women in this programme [20]. This is an example of how a low cost intervention can be integrated into primary health units without an exorbitant increase in the funds required.

Since women tend to have a combination of PTSD as well as substance abuse disorders, programmes have been developed that provide an integrated approach [10]. Such programmes include routine screening for trauma and other health problems, and an approach that builds on safety and empowerment. Studies have found that such programmes lead to better outcomes in abstinence from drug use as well as in mental health and PTSD symptomatology [10].

6.9 Challenges

In many parts of the world, drug abuse treatment centres are not designed to have women as in-patients, those that do often do not admit those who may be pregnant or HIV positive [8]. Also, shelters for women who are homeless or abused may not be willing to take in women who abuse alcohol or drugs [8]. A barrier to services is that the women themselves may not seek care for fear that their children will be taken away and put into care [8]. The stigma attached to women who abuse alcohol or drugs also prevents them from seeking care [9]. In Pakistan, male to female rates of people in care are 99 : 1 [9].

Women are rarely questioned about their sexual behaviours or even about drug use during routine medical examinations [18].

6.10 Research

1. There is need to do further research to understand the sexual and drug behaviours of women who have sex with women, especially in the developing world where these communities may be highly stigmatised and thus marginalised. This would be important to provide targeted interventions for the drug problems but also as way to provide preventive interventions for HIV.

2. Further research is needed, into the social and ideological contexts of drinking behaviour of women and girls that are context specific. Some of the research questions could be what are the practises and attitudes towards women who drink outside the home? What is the understanding of society towards women who drink outside the home? How does this put these women at risk for HIV and AIDS, as well as sexual violence? How do we make socialisation outside of the home safer for women and girls?

6.11 Recommendations

1. Taking into account what we know about hereditability and environment in the initiation of alcohol use, targeted programmes could be developed for young women and girls with a history of alcohol abuse in the family to encourage them to delay initiation of the use of alcohol.

2. There needs to be stronger linkages between alcohol and drug abuse programmes with HIV/AIDS prevention and care especially in relation to
   prevention of HIV transmission among alcohol and drug abusing women.
   Interventions designed for commercial sex workers should target crack users
   and injection drug users for specific programmes to decrease risky sex
   behaviour. Interventions should also target women who are problem or heavy
   drinkers of alcohol for HIV prevention programmes.

3. There is a need to strengthen the linkage between violence against women
   intervention programmes and alcohol and drug abuse programmes, especially
   during the acute state following the traumatic event. This could be through
   training of Trauma Unit health personnel so they are able to recognise and
   refer women who have been abused to counselling programmes, but to also
   inquire about faulty coping mechanisms like alcohol and or drug abuse, and
   promiscuous sexual behaviour.

4. Programmes that promote the economic independence of women are likely
   to contribute to decreasing their risks for HIV infection. Higher levels of
   economic independence among women are associated with higher negotiating
   power over condom use.

5. Drug and alcohol treatment programmes for couples could be developed,
   since many women who abuse alcohol and or drugs often have a partner who
   also abuses alcohol and or drugs.

6.12 Conclusions

This chapter briefly discussed the socio-ecological factors related to alcohol and
drug abuse among women. Although hereditability of alcohol and drug abuse
are similar in men and women, social factors determine when the disorder will
manifest as well as how the problem is perceived and the response to the disorder
in women. Women also have different risks as well as differing consequences;
women become much more vulnerable to sexual and gender based violence as
well as to HIV infection. Drug and alcohol treatment programmes are presently
not very gender sensitive, many programmes do not admit women, those that
could, due to the stigma attached to women who abuse alcohol and or drugs, are
not welcoming to women.

Recommendations for the way forward include further research to better
understand the different social factors that play a role in increased risks to
women to sexual and gender based violence and HIV when they drink alcohol.
Interventions should be integrated so that alcohol and drug abuse can be
managed with trauma, especially that related to sexual and gender based violence.
Interventions should also be developed that target women who are heavy drinkers
of alcohol and as well as those who abuse hard drugs, since they are at increased
risk for HIV infection. Such interventions should also focus on how to prevent
the spread of HIV from CSW who are heavy drinkers or who abuse hard drugs,

since they are likely to be HIV positive and to prevent the spread of the HIV in the general population.

References

1. WHO (2008) Lexicon of Alcohol and Drug Terms Published by the World Health Organization, http://www.who.int/substance_abuse/terminology/who_lexicon/en/index.html (cited 13 October 2008).
2. Flom, P.L., Friedman, S.R., Kottiri, B.J. *et al.* (2001) Stigmatized drug use, sexual partner concurrency, and other sex risk network and behaviour characteristics of 18 to 24-year-old youth in a high-risk neighbourhood. *Sexually Transmitted Diseases*, **28** (10), 598–607.
3. Sartor, C.E., Agrawal, A., Lynskey, M.T. *et al.* (2008) Genetic and environmental influences on the rate of progression to alcohol dependence in young women. *Alcoholism, Clinical and Experimental Research*, **32** (4), 632–38.
4. Hardie, T.L., Moss, H.B. and Lynch, K.G. (2008) Sex differences in the heritability of alcohol problems. *The American Journal on Addictions*, **17** (4), 319–27.
5. Obot, I.S. and Room, R. (eds) (2005) Alcohol, Gender and Drinking Problems: Perspectives from Low and Middle Income Countries, World Health Organization, Geneva.
6. WHO (2005) Alcohol Use and Sexual Risk Behaviour: a Cross-cultural Study in Eight Countries, World Health Organization, Geneva.
7. WHO (2005) WHO Global Status Report on Alcohol 2004, World Health Organization, Geneva.
8. UNIFEM (2008) Women and Drugs: from Hard Realities to Hard Solutions, UNIFEM.
9. UNDCP (2002) Drug Abuse among Women: Emerging Global Trends. Women and Drug Abuse: The Problem in India, New York.
10. Amaro, H., Dai, J., Arevalo, S. *et al.* (2007) Effects of integrated trauma treatment on outcomes in a racially/ethnically diverse sample of women in urban community-based substance abuse treatment. *Journal of Urban Health*, **84** (4), 508–22.
11. Strathdee, S.A., Lozada, R., Ojeda, V.D. *et al.* (2008) Differential effects of migration and deportation on HIV infection among male and female injection drug users in Tijuana, Mexico. *PLoS ONE*, **3** (7), e2690.
12. Wolff, B., Busza, J., Bufumbo, L. and Whitworth, J. (2006) Women who fall by the roadside: gender, sexual risk and alcohol in rural Uganda. *Addiction*, **101**, 1277–84.
13. Weiser, S.D., Leiter, K., Heisler, M. *et al.* (2006) A population-based study on alcohol and high-risk sexual behaviours in Botswana. *PLoS Medicine*, **3** (10), 1940–48.
14. Cohen, D.A., Farley, T.A., Taylor, S.N. *et al.* (2002) When and where do youths have sex? The potential role of adult supervision. *Pediatrics*, **110** (6), e66 (DOI:10.1542/peds.110.6.e66)
15. Wang, M.Q., Collins, C.B., Kohler, C.L. *et al.* (2000) Drug use and HIV risk-related sex behaviours: a street outreach study of black adults. *Southern Medical Journal*, **93** (2), 186–90.

16. Wechsberg, W.M., Luseno, W.K. and Lam, W.K. (2005) Violence against substance-abusing South African sex workers: intersection with culture and HIV risk. *AIDS Care*, **17** (4), 55–64.

17. Gonzales, V., Washienko, K.M. and Kroner, M.R. (1999) Sexual and drug use risk factors for HIV and STDs: a comparison of women with and without bisexual experiences. *American Journal of Public Health*, **89** (12), 1841–46.

18. Bell, A.V., Ompad, D. and Sherman, S.G. (2006) Sexual and drug risk behaviours among women who have sex with women. *American Journal of Public Health*, **96** (6), 1066–72.

19. Kretzschmar, M., Zhang, W., Mikolajczyk, R.T. *et al.* (2008) Regional differences in HIV prevalence among drug users in China: potential for future spread of HIV? *BMC Infectious Diseases*, **8**, 108 (available at http://www.biomedcentral.com/1471-2334-8-108)

20. Hjerkinn, B., Lindbaek, M. and Rosvold, E.O. (2007) Substance abuse in pregnant women. Experiences from a special child welfare clinic in Norway. *BMC Public Health*, **7**, 322 (http://www.biomedcentral.com/1471-2458/7/322)

7

Psychiatric consequences of trauma in women

Elie G. Karam,[1,2,3] **Mariana M. Salamoun**[3] **and Salim El-Sabbagh**[1]

[1] *Department of Psychiatry and Clinical Psychology, Faculty of Medicine, Balamand University, Beirut, Lebanon*
[2] *Department of Psychiatry and Clinical Psychology, St. Georges Hospital University Medical Center, Beirut, Lebanon*
[3] *Institute for Development Research Advocacy and Applied Care (IDRAAC), Beirut, Lebanon*

7.1 Introduction

Epidemiologic research in mental health is now growing to be more global in comparing different cultures across the world with an emergent call for application of its findings in the public health and community services [1]. For most of the history of science, most research on human behaviour was with an assumption that (in the best scenarios) what applies to males does so largely to females. With the major advances in biological studies, it has become evident that women are living entities independent of men, with a different biological framework and environmental risk factors. This in turn has initiated a move towards conducting research on women to induce change, better services and treatment in all fields including psychopathology [2, 3].

From another point of view, it is clear that the role of women has changed over the past century as they have become more independent economically and socially. Women can live and travel alone; and such change, in no doubt, affects the type of experiences that women are subjected to. Thus, while females remain a target for many traumata, they are increasingly being exposed to other

Contemporary Topics in Women's Mental Health   Edited by Chandra, Herrman, Fisher, Kastrup,
© 2009 John Wiley & Sons, Ltd   Niaz, Rondón and Okasha

traumata, and to cite a few (that shadow their changing role): industrial and traffic accidents, mugging, combat exposure, and so on. However, the disadvantaged role of women is accentuated in less industrialised countries and consequently in many women in the Arab world where, for example, reports suggest that women receive less nutrition and healthcare from birth, which leads to poorer development on many levels including mental health [4]. In some Arab countries, a score of females are forbidden to travel or live alone, are bound by a duty to virginity, are forced to have abortions, accept arranged marriages, are more passive in divorce, are more subject to domestic violence (assault, beating, . . .), as well as being victims of honour killing [4].

The relation of trauma to mental health has been the subject of voluminous work since the 1900s with the works of S. Freud and the psychoanalytical school [5] where it is considered related to many mental conditions. This relation was revived in the 1970s especially with the concept of post traumatic stress disorder (PTSD) where for the first time a specific diagnostic mental entity was linked to trauma, in the newer diagnostic classification system (diagnostic and statistical manual, DSM) that had avoided until then precipitating factors all together. More recently, genetic work has shed clearer light on negative life events and trauma and their relation to the genetic make up of individuals [6]. It is however, beyond the scope of this chapter to review the extensive research on the relation of trauma to mental health.

We will rather, try in this chapter to focus more on traumata that are more common to women (compared to men) and their possible differential effect on well-being. In this chapter, we have attempted to summarise data spanning mostly the years 2004–2007 that dealt with these issues, unless otherwise warranted. In an effort to be global, we have limited our search to review articles.

First, we will begin with defining what constitutes a trauma, and discussing what types of traumatic events are more common among women.

7.2 What types of traumata are more common among women?

What constitutes a trauma is still a debate. From a cross-cultural perspective, different societies are exposed to different types of traumata. The World Health Organization-World Mental Health (WHO-WMH) consortium had conducted in 2001–2003 a global assessment of mental health that allows for cross-national comparisons across more than 27 developed and developing countries who have participated so far. The WMH group had come up with a list of possible traumatic events that an individual may experience across the lifespan (Table 7.1). This comprehensive list is part of the PTSD section of the Composite International Diagnostic Interview (CIDI) used in the survey [7]. The WMH surveys are instrumental in showing cross-national differences in exposure to traumata by gender; however, results are not available yet at the time of writing this chapter.

Table 7.1 List of possible traumatic events that an individual may be exposed to [7]

Group 1: Traumatic personal experiences

- Combat experience
- Relief worker in war/terror zone
- Civilian in war zone, for example, military war, revolution, invasion
- Civilian in region of terror, for example, political, religious or ethnic conflicts
- Refugee
- Kidnapped
- Toxic chemical exposure
- Automobile accident
- Other life-threatening accident
- Natural disaster, for example, flood, hurricane, earthquake
- Man made disaster, for example, fire. Bomb explosion
- Life-threatening illness

Group 2: Personal violence

- Beaten up as a child by caregiver
- Beaten up by a spouse or romantic partner
- Beaten up by someone else
- Mugged or threatened with a weapon
- Raped
- Sexually assaulted or molested
- Stalked
- Witnessed physical fights at home

Group 3: Events affecting others

- Unexpected death of a loved one
- Child's life-threatening/serious illness
- Traumatic event to loved one
- Witnessed death or dead body or saw someone seriously hurt
- Accidentally caused serious injury or death
- Purposely injured, tortured or killed someone
- Saw atrocities

Most existing research on trauma comes from the industrialised western world. In more traditional and conservative cultures, this issue remains a taboo, especially when it comes to reporting traumata in sensitive areas such as sexual abuse and domestic violence. A review on epidemiological studies has shown that the prevalence of lifetime exposure to traumata among women ranges from 15 to 88% in countries such as USA, Canada, Germany and Australia [3]. In general, women in western-based studies are more likely to experience some types of traumatic events than men do, for example, in the line of abuse and harassment [8]. A pooled analysis of 64 articles concluded that women are subjected more often than men to adult sexual assault, child sexual abuse, nonsexual abuse/neglect, while men are more likely to be exposed to accidents, nonsexual assault, combat, war, terrorism, fire, witnessing death or injury and illness [8]. There is an increasing demand to address actively the issue of violent acts against women and girls, including rape, domestic violence, stalking and sexual harassment. Calls for intervention and policymaking strategies are being initiated secondary to a more recent finding that violence increased injuries and deaths among women [9, 10]. Three types of violence against women have been identified across several cultures: self-directed, interpersonal and collective [11–13].

Self-directed violence

Women report more self-harm and self-mutilation behaviour than men [14]. Suicide attempts are widely known to be more frequent among females, and in some parts of the world, women use more often painful methods of suicide such as self-immolation (burning themselves) than men [15]. While self-mutilation and suicide are frequently consequences of mental disorders, they undoubtedly cause an enormous burden to women in terms of life scripts and social roles [14, 15].

Interpersonal violence

A second type of violence is the interpersonal type, which can be inflicted by a family member or by a stranger in the community and can be sexual, physical or psychological. Several studies have shown that about 15% of women suffer sexual abuse before age 18 [16]. A survey on women's health in 1998 showed that about 40% of American women experienced 'any type' of violence, 34.6% had experienced intimate partner violence and 8% were physically abused by their partners within the past year ([17] as cited in [18]). In reviewing intimate partner violence among US duty servicemen and veterans, Marshall et al. [19] found that 13.3–47% of active US duty servicemen and 13.5–42% of veterans reported intimate partner violence in the past year (the victim being mainly the wife).

A review on intrafamilial childhood sexual abuse in Australia [20] reported that more than 50% of women who had mental health problems were sexually abused in childhood. Kinz and Biebl ([21]; as cited in [20]) studying the mental health of 165 Australian women patients, found that among the 20% who were sexually abused, 72% were abused by their fathers, 15% by brothers/stepbrothers and 13% by uncles or grandfather. Other studies have shown that fathers were the most frequent, violent, threatening, penetrative and prolonged sexual abusers [20]. In some settings, such as the workplace, women are more likely to be sexually harassed than men are. This type of abuse has been noticeably reported among nurses [22].

Collective violence

Collective violence, common to both genders, is another type of violence: this could be nature made (hurricanes, flooding, earthquakes) or man made such as armed conflict (war) or in specific cultures, women might be the victims of cultural traditions and convictions (blood vengeance, arranged marriages, etc.).

The global life expectancy of women at birth is 68 years vs. 64 for men [23]. Women are more likely to outlive their husbands, and consequently be exposed to bereavement related trauma. This gets worse in countries exposed to military conflicts. More men participate in combat and get killed leaving behind widows who have to deal not only with the trauma of losing a husband, but also the burden of being the sole breadwinners and caregivers to children and families. Nevertheless, women are more prone to be sexually abused and raped during times of war. As an illustration, our group (Institute for Development Research Advocacy and Applied Care (IDRAAC)/St. George Hospital University Medical Center/Balamand University), following the July 2006 war in Lebanon, assessed the psychosocial situation of women in target regions [24]. During wartime, Lebanese women reported having to face more responsibilities, the death or injury of a loved or close person, separation from family due to displacement, witnessing atrocities and taking care of the dead bodies. Women also reported other additional lifetime non-war related stressors such as neglect or discrimination related to religion or political belonging, sexual harassment mostly among adolescents and hostility at home.

In the national Lebanese WMH survey (Lebanese Evaluation of the Burden of Ailments and Needs Of the Nation, L.E.B.A.N.O.N), Karam *et al.* [25] reported on the relationship between the past Lebanese internal wars (1975–1990) and lifetime mental disorders. Women reported being more exposed to specific types of war-related traumatic events than men. Compared to men, women were more likely to be civilians in a war zone and refugees, yet both genders were equally exposed to war-related events such as death of someone or trauma to a loved one.

One peculiar and, happily a fading tradition, which persists especially among tribes, is blood vengeance. Although blood vengeance is not perceived as violent per se and seems to be declining, its negative effects on women have been highlighted in a study on adolescent females [11]. Another issue that is not infrequent in many cultures and seen in clinical practise is 'arranged marriages', which is traumatic especially when enforced on women [4].

Other types of traumata

Other types of traumata that women might experience are related to specific conditions such as miscarriage and still birth [26, 27], having a life threatening illness or being a mother of a childhood cancer survivor [28, 29].

We have shown so far that some specific types of traumatic events are more common among women across different cultures; the next question is how do women respond to trauma?

7.3 How do women respond to trauma?

Most individuals are likely to experience at least one traumatic event in their lifetime, yet only a subgroup of individuals develops impairment and dysfunction secondary to trauma. The US National Comorbidity Study reported that 50–70% of the US population aged between 15 and 45 years had lifetime exposure to trauma, but only 5–12% developed PTSD [30]. For a more complete picture, some have shown that there might be a potentially positive side to trauma, whereby exposure to a traumatic event might induce in some individuals personal growth, better rearrangement of priorities and more goal-oriented activities [31].

Several studies have shown that although men were more likely to report exposure to traumatic experiences than women, mental disorders such as PTSD were more common among women [8, 18]. For example, Tolin and Foa [8] have conducted a meta-analysis on 290 articles comparing trauma and PTSD differences between genders. Pooled analyses showed that adult males were more likely to report experiencing a traumatic event than females, while the latter were 1.98 times more likely to meet criteria for PTSD. It has been suggested that the higher rates of PTSD might be attributed to the fact that women have higher rates of sexual abuse. However, when comparing both genders exposed to the same traumatic events, women still had more lifetime PTSD. This remained true even after controlling for specific types of events that were more commonly reported by men [32]. Additionally, emotional traumata are major risk factors that might shape neurobiological processes for, not only PTSD, but major depressive disorder (MDD) as well [16, 33].

Several attempts have been made to explain the mechanisms of response to trauma and possible gender differences. It seems that the higher rates of psychopathology among women in response to trauma may be attributed to risk factors other than the trauma itself (A1 criterion of DSM-IV PTSD). In a comprehensive review on gender differences in PTSD, Olff *et al.* [3] presented a schema of how women respond to trauma as compared to men. Several factors have been proposed to interact in response to trauma and these include immediate emotional responses, genetics and neurobiological processes.

Immediate emotional responses

The immediate emotional responses to trauma include trauma-related factors, cognitive evaluation and coping strategies. The type of trauma, rate of exposure, history of exposure to traumata and age at exposure are some of the many trauma related factors. As noted above, several studies showed that although men have higher rates of exposure to trauma than women, yet women are exposed more to certain types of events such as sexual abuse and neglect. Women report being exposed to traumatic events at a younger age and are more likely to report more often a history of exposure to trauma too [3]. One of the markers in the immediate response to trauma according to DSM-IV is the A2 criterion, and research is active in looking at the differential immediate responses and significance of the A2 criterion [34], and of peri-traumatic numbing. Are these markers of future pathology? Answers will be clearer hopefully with ongoing research such as the upcoming international and transcultural studies such as the ones conducted by the WMH consortium [1]. For example, the A2 criterion of the DSM-IV PTSD diagnosis (intense fear, helplessness and horror) is more common among women and this remains true even after adjusting for race, education and event type [34].

It is hypothesised that right after a trauma, women experience gender-specific acute physiological and psychological reactions that put them at greater risk for PTSD. Emotional responses and acute peri-traumatic dissociation (distorted awareness) are more common among women than men. In addition, these are thought of being important in increasing the risk for PTSD and alcohol use in response to trauma [3]. Many have addressed gender differences in the reactions and perceptions of traumatic experiences [32], especially in the light of empirical evidence about the important role of the subjective cognitive evaluation and interpretation in response to trauma. Cognitive factors have been linked to resilience and vulnerability [35]. Women are more likely to perceive events as threatening and stressful than men, they are more aroused by threat, and more resistant to extinction after danger has passed. They report more distress, loss of control and blame. Looking at the issue from another angle, women seem to have the tendency for maladaptive interpretations of acute traumatic symptoms that, in turn, could increase the likelihood for PTSD and persistence. Furthermore, women tend to use less effective coping strategies, such as avoidance, dissociation, passivity and emotionality, which are associated with posttraumatic morbidity [3].

Genetics and neurobiological responses

There is no doubt that neurobiological responses to trauma, whether adaptive or maladaptive, depend on many variables such as the context, timeframe, previous experiences, and so on. Genetic studies are additional variables that are increasingly coming to the forefront. It is suggested, for example, that two heritable factors might explain differences among individuals in response to trauma, namely their likelihood of being exposed to traumatic experiences, and their vulnerability of developing a mental disorder (or comorbid disorders) as a consequence of having experienced a traumatic event (DSM-IV PTSD criterion A) [35].

Animal neurobiological models tried to recreate traumatic paradigms in order to understand better not only immediate responses but also the lasting ones. They suggest that lower cortisol levels, reduced hypothalamic-pituitary-adrenocortical

(HPA) axis responses and serotonin transporter gene promoter polymorphism are related to women's response to stress [3]. In fact, peri-traumatic dissociation has been linked to lower cortisol levels and reduced HPA axis activity. It is suggested that females' brains pick up threat more readily than males and process more traumatic and emotional memories. Evidence from clinical work point to a relationship between peri-traumatic dissociation and stress-induced release of glucocorticoids. It is suggested that women have higher levels of nonsulfated dehydroepiandrosterone (DHEA) while men have higher levels of sulfated DHEA. It could be that the non-sulfated DHEA plays a role in inhibiting the release of glucocorticoids and thus affecting the HPA axis in PTSD. Others added that there might be a role of receptor signalling pathways in the brain mediating the function of the HPA axis. Yet all this needs to be examined further [3]. Another neurobiological model suggests an interplay between dissociation and hyperarousal in response to trauma. It is thought that women have sensitised dissociative systems that more likely show anxiety and somatoform symptoms, while men have hyperarousal systems that show conduct problems, impulsivity and hyper-vigilance [3].

Numerous studies have found that exposure to early adverse events is linked to the pathophysiology of depression and anxiety. The association between early life stress (abuse, neglect or maternal loss) and adult onset of depression and anxiety is thought to be mediated by an increased activity of corticotrophin releasing factor (CRF) [36]. Furthermore, some have shown that there is an increase in stress reactivity and a specific shaping of brain regions, which leads to a change in the neural circuits. If this change occurs in genetically vulnerable individuals, such as females, it may progress into psychiatric disorders [33]; in brains during early developmental phases (children) it would possibly lead to changes in hippocampal volume [37].

A recent biological model hypothesised that females possess hormones such as oxytocin and oestrogen which mediate a 'tend-be-friend' response in women versus a 'fight or flight' response in men. Oxytocin is thought to have an evolutionary role in mediating nurturing behaviours in women to reduce risk and preserve oneself and offspring. In addition, Oxytocin is involved in emotional regulation, and has a calming effect that suppresses arousal and HPA axis responses to stress. Lack of social support, sadness and exposure to childhood trauma reduce the effect of oxytocin, consequently making women more vulnerable for PTSD [3].

Women seem to have more negative responses to trauma that could cause drastic consequences such as mental health disorders [3, 18]. Next, we will review other risk factors that might have a role in response to trauma.

7.4 What are the trauma related risk factors?

In addition to acute emotional responses, genetics, cognitive and coping strategies and neurobiological responses (discussed above), several risk factors (which are related directly to or mediate neurobiological responses) are found to increase the likelihood of having a mental disorder because of experiencing a traumatic event. These factors could be physiologically, psychologically or socio-culturally determined.

Physiological factors

Some physiological responses seem to affect how women respond to a trauma such as forgetting the traumatic event, fainting and auditory startle in response to trauma. A remarkable concept is the capacity or inborn differences for 'forgetting' the trauma [31]. Women endorse more emotional and traumatic memories, and it could be that the *inability to forget* that increases the likelihood of having psychopathology. In addition and quite interestingly, there might be some evolutionary traits that seem more common in females such as 'faintness' [38]. It has been hypothesised, in the context of an evolutionary perspective that females upon exposure to violence would faint as a protective factor to avoid being killed by attacking tribes. However, what was protective (fainting at sight of blood, for example) has become 'less desirable' nowadays. Another predisposing trait (although not proven yet to be gender specific) is the elevated auditory startle response as measured by the orbicularis oculi (eye blink) in studies on Australian firefighters which found that it could be a risk factor for posttraumatic stress symptoms [35, 39, 40].

Psychological factors

Recently, there has been a global interest in understanding the role of the individual's emotional reactivity traits, otherwise known as temperament, in predicting psychological well-being. Temperament is a genetically determined trait, which is rather stable across the individual's lifetime [41], and is thought to affect individuals' lives through the choices they make (career, partner, etc.), experiences they get exposed to, paths they follow, education they achieve, and so on. It is believed by leading researchers in this field that temperament and psychopathology fall on the same spectrum and that there is continuity between temperament at one side and mental disorders at the other extreme [42]. Cloninger, the developer of the temperament and character inventory (TCI), outlines four types of temperament: reward dependence, novelty seeking, harm avoidance and persistence [43]. The TCI has been widely used to assess the relationship among temperament, character and mental disorders. Some studies found that there is an association between temperament and the HPA axis activity, whereby novelty seeking temperament, as opposed to harm avoidance and reward dependence, is inversely related to HPA hyperactivity [44]. Conceivably individuals would be more predisposed not only to suffer from mental disorders but also expose themselves (e.g. among low harm avoidance and high novelty seeking individuals) to risky and violence laden situations.

More recently, HS Akiskal [42] has developed the Temperament Evaluation of Memphis Pisa Paris and San Diego-Auto questionnaire (TEMPS-A) to assess five types of affective temperaments: dysthymic, cyclothymic, hyperthymic, irritable and anxious [45]. It is hypothesised that individuals with anxious temperament are by nature less exposed to traumatic events because they carry an evolutionary survival trait of 'worry' that plays a protective role against harm, as opposed to hyperthymics who are by nature risk taking and adventurous which increases their chances of being exposed to specific traumatic experiences [46].

On the other extreme of the spectrum, individuals with pre-existing mental disorders seem to expose themselves more to trauma [47]. For example, bipolarity in its classical or softer form (cyclothymia) could be an early risk to exposure to specific types of traumata such as sexual abuse. Children with bipolar symptoms might be overly friendly and giggling in the presence of a stranger (Akiskal personal communication, 2007 [48]). This could be theoretically misperceived by the potential predator thus leading to catastrophic consequences of sexual intimacy (this is yet to be proven). However, this is only a theoretically possible idea that needs to be proven by research. Substance abuse is another disorder that by mere fact might drive abusers to more violent or impaired capacity of judgement in evaluating the risks of exposure. In fact, substance use is known to alter basic judgement, besides inducing inattention and bringing about an inevitable chain of reactions. More so, alcohol abuse was shown to be a risk factor not only for being a perpetrator but also to be the victim [49]. It is beyond the scope of this chapter to review the evidence of the risk taken, by not only subjects with bipolar affective disorder, but also substance use disorder, impulse control disorders and other disorders common to both genders, yet it is worth noting here that, for example, sexual abuse is a common trauma to females with such disorders.

Other mental disorders that have been linked to trauma include mass psychogenic illness (epidemic sociogenic attacks), which is found to be more common in women. Living under extreme stress, without memories of immediate and clear traumatic perception, could induce what was referred to as 'mass hysteria' [50].

Sociocultural factors

Social support, whether structural (number of resources, frequency of interactions, etc.) or functional (quality of resources and victim's perceptions to resources, etc.), seems to be a mediating factor in alleviating the burden of trauma. Lack of social support seems to affect the psychological health of women more than men. Women receive and benefit from social support more than men, in addition to being more affected by the emotional burden of the support process [51]. In sexual abuse, clearly a taboo, particularly in conservative groups, women are less likely to come forward and report such incidents. Even a husband, a parent or mother is unlikely to report that incident too. An abused woman has to live not only the trauma but also the surrounding shame, and at times the guilt of what has happened to her. This may not occur in other traumatic experiences such as being mugged where the victim or family are more likely to report on it. Several studies confirmed the relationship between poor social support and higher rates of mental disorders such as PTSD and depression [3, 51]. In this context, Arab women have a disadvantage since quite frequently they still receive very minimal, if any, social support [4]. A study on Iranian refugees settling in Sweden, have shown that psychopathological manifestations of exposure to traumata can be resisted by coping strategies and social support [52]. However, more research is needed to clarify the issue further. In the following section, we will look at psychiatric consequences of traumatic events.

7.5 Which mental disorders are related to trauma?

Exposure to stress has been shown to be linked, not only to psychopathology, but to high comorbidity among mental disorders too. This high comorbidity in response to trauma may be explained in terms of the overlap of symptoms of many DSM-IV Axis I disorders such as PTSD, MDD, generalised anxiety disorder (GAD), panic, and so on, in addition to the setting and nature of the trauma, as well as individual vulnerability [35].

Anxiety disorders

Among the various anxiety disorders, PTSD is the most commonly reported psychiatric consequence of trauma. According to the DSM-IV, PTSD is a full blown mental disorder defined by criteria related directly to being exposed to a traumatic event and having intense reactions to it (criterion A). A meta-analysis by Tolin and Foa [8] concluded that although men were more likely to report traumatic experiences than women, PTSD was more common among women. The US National Comorbidity Survey (NCS) has shown that following the exposure to at least one traumatic event, 5% of women developed PTSD [30].

PTSD has been reported among women who were exposed to any of a variety of traumatic events such as sexual and physical abuse [18], nature made disasters [53], war [12, 54, 55], still birth and miscarriage [27, 56], cancer [29], and so on.

In the aftermath of disasters, women are considered to be among the most vulnerable groups to mental health problems. Acute stress disorder and PTSD were the most reported mental disorders associated with environmental disasters (such as earthquakes, hurricanes, flooding, etc.) [53]. Other common anxiety disorders were GAD and panic disorder [31]. On another level, several studies have pointed to the fact that traumatic events are a significant risk factor for developing psychogenic non-epileptic seizures (PNES), and high levels of trauma and PTSD have been recorded in patients with PNES. Women are more prone to trauma and abuse, resulting in a higher chance of developing trauma-related disorders. Compared to control women, women with PNES had higher rates of PTSD, trauma and childhood sexual abuse; however, no statistical difference was found between the two groups [57].

There is growing alertness towards the effect of mass violence on the mental health of exposed populations. Several mental disorders were identified in the aftermath of war including PTSD [12, 55]. Studies highlighting the psychiatric consequences of mass violence vary by the sample studied and methodology used. Most western studies were conducted on military samples with PTSD being the main psychopathological consequence [35]. However, studies from the Middle East were more community based. The Middle East has been a region of armed conflict for a long time. Arab countries such as Palestine, Iraq, Lebanon are still bearing the consequences of war to-date; war remains one of the most devastating causes of mental health deterioration in this region.

In Lebanon, the internal wars started since 1975 and ended in 1990. However, sporadic episodes of war have occurred since the early 1990s up until July 2006 when Lebanon was the target of foreign military attacks. Karam *et al.* [12, 25, 55, 58], in order to delineate the psychiatric consequences of war on the Lebanese community, have conducted a series of studies since the 1980s.

The first community study conducted in four regions in Lebanon with differential exposure to war by Karam *et al.* included three phases. Phase I was a retrospective phase covering the prewar years up to the Lebanon wars in 1989 and Phase II corresponded to the internal military Lebanon wars in 1990 [59]. The prevalence of lifetime PTSD among women up to 1989 was 7.5 and 8.9% in year 1990. Recently, and more than 10 years after the end of the internal Lebanese wars, Karam *et al.* [12, 25] conducted a national study that assessed the differential effect of war on 12-month and lifetime mental disorders among the Lebanese adult population. The authors found that differential exposure to war was significantly related to having any 12-month anxiety disorder. Additionally, exposure to three or more war events was significantly related to having a more serious DSM-IV disorder [12]. In another publication, Karam *et al.* [25] reported on the relationship between the Lebanese internal wars (1975–1990) and lifetime mental disorders. Women exposed to cumulative war events were not only at a higher risk for developing anxiety, but also to have it for the first time in their lives.

De Jong *et al.* [54] assessed the effect of war in four post conflict low-income countries. The prevalence rates of DSM-IV PTSD among women were 43.8% in Algeria, 34.2% in Cambodia, 15.2% in Ethiopia and 13.5% in Gaza. In Afghanistan, a national study assessing mental health post war showed that 83.5% of women had anxiety symptoms and 48.3% had PTSD symptoms [60].

A quarter to one third of women see labour and giving birth as a traumatic experience, and around 2–6% of these women develop full blown PTSD, however this has not been shown to be linked to the event of labour or giving birth [56]. Miscarriage has been shown to cause severe emotional reactions such as anxiety [27]. A review on PTSD and childbirth reported that the lifetime rate of PTSD after stillbirth is 29%, 25% at one month of pregnancy loss, miscarriage and 7% at four months [26]. However, after premature birth between 26 and 41% of mothers experienced posttraumatic stress symptoms. Still regular childbirth could cause full-blown PTSD or PTSD syndrome. The highest prevalence of PTSD (5.6%) was found at four to six weeks after delivery, with a minority possibly developing chronic PTSD.

Anxiety disorders are common not only among cancer patients, but also among mothers of childhood cancer survivors [29]. A review of 24 studies on PTSD in mothers of childhood cancer survivors has shown a range of 20–44% showing symptoms indicative of cancer related PTSD [28].

Mood disorders

Whereas most research has focused primarily on PTSD, we now know that trauma is a potential risk factor for the development of a variety of mental health disorders and the rule rather than the exception is to develop more than one disorder. Women having a history of early life trauma and MDD are at higher risk for concurrent PTSD than women who had early life trauma but no MDD [61]. Sensitisation in the context of stress is thought to increase the risk of developing depression or to cause relapse in individuals already having MDD [61].

Hegadoren *et al.* [62] reviewed the consequences of interpersonal violence on women and showed that there is a direct association between the number of childhood adversities and future adult psychopathology. If the person suffered from both physical and sexual abuse there is a higher occurrence of ill health, and women with histories of childhood adversity had much higher risk for depression. In another study, childhood sexual abuse caused a 35% increase in MDD rates among women. MDD rates among physically abused women ranged from 66 to 80% ([63, 64]; as cited in [62]). Women who were sexually abused by fathers had the most disabling psychiatric consequences [20]. Kinz and Biebl ([21]; as cited in [20]) found that 75% of sexually abused Australian women had repeated penetrative sexual abuse and had a high lifetime prevalence of psychiatric morbidity. Depression has been reported as a major consequence of intimate partner violence [18].

In response to disasters, whether natural or man made, depression has been recognised more recently as being at least as common if not more common than PTSD [31, 47, 55]. In order to determine the relationship between war events and depression, a sample of Lebanese adults who resided in regions differentially exposed to war in 1988–1989 were assessed; 23.1% of women in this sample had MDD [65]. The prevalence of depression differed across the different regions. Out of women in Ain Remaneh (where the war started and remained for 15 years) 19.4% had MDD; 13.3% in Ashrafieh (which was heavily bombarded), 13.6% in Bijjeh (which had one hour of bombing since the onset of war for 14 years) and 6.7% in Kornet Chehwan (which had sporadic shelling) [58]. Additionally, Karam *et al.* [47] reported on the comobidity between depression and PTSD in a sample of Lebanese women exposed to war and followed up a year later. Just over 34% of women had lifetime depression and 46.7% had one year depression caused by any precipitant, while 28.9% met criteria for lifetime and 34.1% for one year DSM III-R MDD and 11.1% had one year PTSD. When looking at the relation of comorbidity to war, the authors found that higher levels of exposure to war were strongly related to concurrent development of depression and PTSD. Moreover, prior exposure to war not only predisposed individuals to depression and PTSD, but more so increased comorbidity. Now and more than 10 years after the end of the Lebanon wars, Karam *et al.* [12, 25] found that differential exposure to war was significantly related to having mood disorders in the past 12 months and that being exposed to cumulative war events increased the likelihood of having first onset of mood disorders among women. As mentioned above, for women, death of a loved one is another precipitant for bereavement related depression especially at times of war where it becomes a more common traumatising event [66].

In Palestine, Khamis [67] investigated the psychological well-being of 253 traumatised women during the 'Intifada' as compared to 52 non-traumatised women. The traumatised group had higher scores on distress than the non-traumatised group as measured by anxiety and depression subscales symptom checklist (SCL) SCL-90R. Differences were not noted by type of trauma, however, women who belonged to families of those imprisoned reported higher scores of distress than non-traumatised. Punamaki *et al.* [68] reported that exposure to lifetime traumata was associated with mood disorders and peri-traumatic dissociation was linked to depression. In Afghanistan, it was found that 73.4% of a national sample had depression post war [60].

As mentioned above, other events such as miscarriage, cancer and other physical morbidities can be traumatising and thus cause not only anxiety disorders, but mood disorders as well. Depression and anxiety are generally considered to be the most important psychopathological comorbidities in cancer patients [29].

Substance use disorders

Many studies have shown a relation between trauma and substance use disorders. In a review of trauma and addictions, Hien *et al.* [69] reported that around 80% of women who sought treatment for substance use disorders had lifetime sexual or physical abuse. One of the cited articles in this review [70] showed that among 113 African American women those with a history of sexual/physical abuse had higher rates of alcohol consumption (22%) as compared to 'other' women populations (15%). However, another study by Widom *et al.* [71] found in a sample of 676 adults (50% of which were females) that whether one was abused or neglected as a child did not affect one's lifetime drug abuse in comparison with control groups; but both abuse and neglect were related to higher *current* drug abuse. From another angle, comorbidity of PTSD and substance use disorders is frequently reported [72]. Patients with PTSD not only reported abuse of substances but also have poor treatment outcomes and retention [69].

Substance use disorders were not only common in sexual/physical abuse related trauma, but also in nature made disasters [31], and war-related events as well. In a study assessing the prevalence of alcohol abuse or dependence, [73], found that 2.9% women had alcohol abuse or dependence during the war but no comparative group was available. A possibly indirect comparison (although the sample selection and interview techniques are totally different) but from the same population more than 10 years after war has ended found that abuse with or without dependence among females is only 0.4% [25].

Self-harm and suicidality

Adverse childhood experiences like emotional, physical and sexual abuse have been reported to increase the risk of self-harm among women. The greater the number of adverse events the greater the risk for suicide attempts among females having a history of childhood physical abuse [18]. Some authors believe that women with a history of sexual abuse may suffer from what is referred to as 'trauma re-enactment syndrome' where they do to themselves what was done to them in childhood; they would develop not only eating disorders and substance abuse but also self-mutilation [14]. As mentioned above, self-harm among women could be traumatic per se leading to psychiatric disorders such as depression, anxiety and substance use disorders [14, 15]. Some studies have linked suicide to war; for example, in Lebanon, rates of suicide ideation in times of war in year 1989 and one year after war (1991) were 6.7 and 3.8% respectively, and for suicide attempt 2.7 and 0.4% respectively [59]. Currently, Karam *et al.* are in the process of analysing the national rates of suicide ideation, plan and attempt in Lebanon, more than 10 years after war.

Other mental problems

In addition to the above, a variety of consequences have been described to follow violence in women, including, for example, somatic symptoms in those exposed to intimate partner violence [18]. Exposure to childhood maltreatment and adulthood military violence were also associated with somatoform disorders [68, 74].

From another perspective, traumatic exposure, whether early childhood or adult abuse, are factors that influence sexual decision making [75]. Physical and sexual trauma can influence decisions made by women in relation to their sexual relationships, choice of partner and use of protection; also, women who have a history of such trauma are at higher risk for sexually transmitted infections and Human Immunodeficiency Virus (HIV). In a vicious cycle, women's immigration status, socio-economic status, legal factors related to work and the nature of employment, are all factors that are directly correlated to constant exposure to physical and verbal abuse, and consequently HIV risk behaviours.

From another perspective, Karam *et al.* [12] revealed in their recent national study that being exposed to two or more war events increased the likelihood of having impulse control disorders by nine times in the past year among Lebanese adults more than 10 years after war has ended.

7.6 Future directions

Women are in many ways different from men in exposure and reaction to trauma. Prevention of exposure is the obvious ideal goal, but this is difficult to implement in many areas. History of Homo sapiens has been alas fraught and punctuated by violence. Women have been victims of gender specific violence, in addition to the other traumata that males have been exposed to. A new exciting area of research is the realm of factors predisposing women to trauma and thus possibly platforms for intervention. These factors are cultural, social, inherited and would call for more targeted research. Modes and timing of interventions on social and individual levels are other areas that need rigorous scientific studies not only to build solid prevention schemas but also to construct effective alleviating strategies.

References

1. WHO World Mental Health (2004) Prevalence, severity, and unmet need for treatment of mental disorders in the World Health Organization World Mental Health Surveys. *The Journal of the American Medical Association*, **291** (21), 2581–90.
2. Bentley, K.J. (2005) Women, mental health, and the psychiatric enterprise: a review. *National Association of Social Workers*, **30** (1), 56–63.
3. Olff, M., Langeland, W., Draijer, N. and Gersons, P.R.B. (2007) Gender differences in posttraumatic stress disorder. *Psychological Bulletin*, **133** (2), 183–204.
4. Douki, S., Zineb, S.B., Nacef, F. and Halbreich, U. (2007) Women's mental health in the Muslim world: cultural, religious, and social issues. *Journal of Affective Disorders*, **102**, 177–89.
5. Fine, R. (1973) *The Development of Freud's Thought: from the Beginnings (1886–1900) through Id Psychology (1900–1914) to Ego Psychology (1914–1939)*, Jason Aronson, Inc., New York.
6. Hariri, A.R. and Holmes, A. (2006) Genetics of emotional regulation: the role of the serotonin transporter in neural function. *Trends in Cognitive Science*, **10**, 182–91.
7. Kessler, R.C., Haro, J.M., Heeringa, S.G. *et al.* (2006) The World Health Organization World Mental Health Survey Initiative. *Epidemiologia e Psichiatria Sociale*, **15**, 161–66.
8. Tolin, D. and Foa, E. (2006) Sex differences in trauma and posttraumatic stress disorder: a quantitative review of 25 years of research. *Psychological Bulletin*, **132** (6), 959–92.
9. Chrisler, J.C. and Fergusan, S. (2006) Violence against women as a public health issue. *Annals of the New York Academy of Sciences*, **1087**, 235–49.
10. Humphreys, C. (2007) A health inequalities perspective on violence against women. *Health and Social Care in the Community*, **15** (2), 120–27.
11. Al-Krenawi, A., Slonim-Nevo, V., Maymon, Y. and Al-Krenawi, S. (2001) Psychological responses to blood vengeance among Arab adolescents. *Child Abuse and Neglect*, **25**, 457–72.

12. Karam, E.G., Mneimneh, Z.N., Karam, A.N. *et al.* (2006) Prevalence and treatment of mental disorders in Lebanon: a national epidemiological survey. *Lancet*, **367**, 1000–6.

13. Krantz, G. and Garcia-Moreno, C. (2005) Violence against women. *Journal of Epidemiology and Community Health*, **59**, 818–21.

14. Skegg, K. (2005) Self-harm. *Lancet*, **366**, 1471–83.

15. Karam, E.G., Hajjar, R. and Salamoun, M. (2007) Suicidality in the Arab world part I: community studies. *Arab Journal of Psychiatry*, **18** (2), 99–107.

16. Craighead, W.E. and Nemeroff, C.B. (2005) The impact of early trauma on response to psychotherapy. *Clinical Neuroscience Research*, **4**, 405–11.

17. Plichta, S.B. and Falik, M. (2001) Prevalence of violence and its implications for women's health. *Womens Health Issues*, **11**, 244–58.

18. Nemeroff, C.B., Bremner, J.D., Foa, E.B. *et al.* (2006) Posttraumatic stress disorder: a state-of-the-science review. *Journal of Psychiatric Research*, **40**, 1–21.

19. Marshall, A.D., Panuzio, J. and Taft, C.T. (2005) Intimate partner violence among military veterans and active duty servicemen. *Clinical Psychology Review*, **25**, 862–76.

20. Geanellos, R. (2003) Understanding the need for personal space boundary restoration in women-client survivors of intrafamilial childhood sexual abuse. *International Journal of Mental Health Nursing*, **12**, 186–93.

21. Kinz, J. and Biebl, W. (1991) Sexual abuse of girls: aspects of the genesis of mental disorders and therapeutic implications. *Acta Psychiatrica Scandinavica*, **83**, 427–31.

22. Kane-Urabazzo, C. (2007) Sexual harassment in the workplace: it is your problem. *Journal of Nursing Management*, **15** (6), 608–13.

23. WHO (2007) WHO Report 2005. World Health Statistics.

24. Karam, A.N., Fayyad, J.F., Cordahi, C. *et al.* (2007) Assessment of Psychosocial and Mental Health Needs of Women in War-Affected Region, IDRRAC, UNFPA Report, Beirut, Lebanon.

25. Karam, E.G., Mneimneh, Z.N., Fayyad, J.A. *et al.* (2008) Lifetime prevalent of mental health disorders: first onset, treatment and exposure to war- the LEBANON study. *PLOS Medicine*, **5** (4), e61.

26. Olde, E., Van der Hart, O., Kleber, R. *et al.* (2006) Posttraumatic stress following childbirth: a review. *Clinical Psychology Review*, **26**, 1–16.

27. Rai, R. and Regan, L. (2006) Recurrent miscarriage. *Lancet*, **368**, 601–11.

28. Bruce, M. (2006) A systematic and conceptual review of posttraumatic stress in childhood cancer survivors and their parents. *Clinical Psychology Review*, **26**, 233–56.

29. Frick, E., Tyroller, M. and Panzer, M. (2007) Anxiety, depression and quality of life of cancer patients undergoing radiation therapy: a cross-sectional study in a community hospital outpatient centre. *European Journal of Cancer Care*, **16**, 130–36.

30. Kessler, R.C., Sonnega, A., Bromet, E. *et al.* (1995) Posttraumatic stress disorder in the National Comorbidity Survey. *Archives of General Psychiatry*, **52** (12), 1048–60.

31. Ursano, R.J., Li, H., Zhang, L. *et al.* (2008) Models of PTSD and traumatic stress: the importance of research "from bedside to bench to bedside", in *Progress in Brain Research*, Vol. **167** (eds E.R. de Kloet, M.S. Oitzl and E. Vermetten), pp. 203–15.

32. Seedat, S., Stein, D.J. and Carey, P.D. (2005) Post-traumatic stress disorder in women epidemiological and treatment issues. *CNS Drugs*, **19** (5), 411–27.

33. Heim, C., Plotsky, P.M. and Nemeroff, C.B. (2004) Importance of studying the contributions of early adverse experience to neurobiological findings in depression. *Neuropsychopharmacology*, **29**, 641–48.

34. Breslau, N. and Kessler, R.C. (2001) The stressor criterion in DSM-IV posttraumatic stress disorder: an empirical investigation. *Biological Psychiatry*, **50**, 699–704.

35. Friedman, M.J. and Karam, E.G. (2009) Posttraumatic stress disorder: looking toward DSM-V and ICD-11, in *Stress-Induced and Fear Circuitry Disorders: Refining the Research Agenda for DSM-V* (eds G. Andrews, D.S. Charney, P. Sirovatka and D.A. Regier), American Psychiatric Association Press, pp. 3–29.

36. Heim, C., Newport, D.J., Heit, S. *et al.* (2000) Pituitary-adrenal and autonomic responses to stress in women after sexual and physical abuse in childhood. *The Journal of the American Medical Association*, **284**, 592–97.

37. Vythilingam, M., Heim, C., Newport, J. *et al.* (2002) Childhood trauma associated with smaller hippocampal volume in women with major depression. *American Journal of Psychiatry*, **159**, 2072–80.

38. Bracha, H.S., Yoshioka, D.T., Masukawa, N.K. *et al.* (2005) Evolution of the human fear-circuitry and acute sociogenic pseudoneurological symptoms: the Neolithic balanced polymorphism hypothesis. *Journal of Affective Disorders*, **88**, 119–29.

39. Guthrie, R. and Bryant, R. (2005) Auditory startle response in firefighters before and after trauma exposure. *American Journal of Psychiatry*, **162**, 283–90.

40. Morgan, C.A. (1997) Startle response in individuals with PTSD. *Clinical Quarterly*, **7**, 65–69.

41. Karam, E.G., Mneimneh, Z., Salamoun, M.M. and Akiskal, H.S. (2007) Suitability of the TEMPS-A for population-based studies: ease of administration and stability of affective temperaments in its Lebanese version. *Journal of Affective Disorders*, **98**, 45–53.

42. Akiskal, H.S. (1989) Validating affective personality types, in *The Validity of Psychiatric Diagnosis* (eds L.N. Robins and J.E. Barrett), Raven Press, New York.

43. Cloninger, C.R., Svrakic, D.M. and Przybeck, T.R. (1993) A psychobiological model of temperament and character. *Archives of General Psychiatry*, **50**, 975–90.

44. Tyrka, A.R., Mello, A.F., Gagne, G.G. *et al.* (2006) Temperament and hypothalamic-pituitary-adrenal axis function in healthy adults. *Psychoneuroendocrinology*, **31**, 1036–45.

45. Akiskal, H.S., Akiskal, K.K., Haykal, R.F. *et al.* (2005) TEMPS-A: progress towards validation of a self-rated clinical version of the temperament evaluation of the Memphis, Pisa, Paris and San Diego Auto questionnaire. *Journal of Affective Disorders*, **85**, 3–16.

46. Akiskal, K.K. and Akiskal, H.S. (2005) The theoretical underpinnings of affective temperaments: implications for evolutionary foundations of bipolar disorder and human nature. *Journal of Affective Disorders*, **85**, 231–39.

47. Karam, E.G. (1997) Comorbidity of posttraumatic stress disorder and depression, in *Posttraumatic Stress Disorder. Acute and Long-Term Responses to Trauma and Disaster* (eds R.J. Ursano and C.S. Fullerton), American Psychiatric Association Press, pp. 77–90.

48. Karam, E.G., Salamoun, M.M. and Yeretzian, J. (2007) Temperaments and Psychiatric Disorders. 3rd ICBB, Nov 28–Dec 1, Thessaloniki, Greece.

49. Brismar, B. and Bergman, B. (1998) The significance of alcohol for violence and accidents. *Alcoholism: Clinical and Experimental Research*, **22** (Suppl 7), 299S–306S.

50. Karam, E.G. and Khattar, L.H. (2007) Mass psychogenic illness (epidemic sociogenic attacks) in a village in Lebanon. *Lebanese Medical Journal*, **55** (2), 112–15.

51. Guay, S., Bilette, V. and Marchand, A. (2006) Exploring the links between posttraumatic stress disorder and social support: processes and potential research avenues. *Journal of Traumatic Stress*, **19** (3), 327–38.

52. Ghazinour, M., Richter, J. and Eisemann, M. (2004) Quality of life among Iranian refugees resettled in Sweden. *Journal of Immigrant Health*, **6** (2), 71–81.

53. Shalev, A.Y., Tuval-Mashiach, R. and Hadar, H. (2004) Posttraumatic stress disorder as a result of mass trauma. *Journal of Clinical Psychiatry*, **65** (1), 4–10.

54. de Jong, J.T.V.M., Komproe, I.H., Ommeren, M.V. *et al.* (2001) Lifetime events and posttraumatic stress disorder in 4 post conflict settings. *The Journal of the American Medical Association*, **286** (5), 555–62.

55. Karam, E. and Bou Ghosn, M. (2003) Psychosocial consequences of war among civilian populations. *Current Opinion in Psychiatry*, **16**, 413–19.

56. Slade, P. (2006) Towards a conceptual framework for understanding post-traumatic stress symptoms following childbirth and implications for further research. *Journal of Psychosomatic Obstetrics and Gynecology*, **27** (2), 99–105.

57. Fiszman, A., Alves-Leon, S.V., Nunes, R.G. *et al.* (2004) Traumatic events and posttraumatic stress disorder in patients with psychogenic nonepileptic seizures: a critical review. *Epilepsy and Behavior*, **5**, 818–25.

58. Karam, E.G., Howard, D.B., Karam, A.N. *et al.* (1998) Major depression and external stressors: the Lebanon wars. *European Archives of Psychiatry and Clinical Neuroscience*, **248**, 225–30.

59. Karam, E.G. (1999) Women and the Lebanon wars: depression and post-traumatic stress disorder, in *Women and War in Lebanon* (ed. L. Shehadeh), University Press of Florida, Gainesville, pp. 272–81.

60. Cardozo, B.L., Bilukha, O.O., Gotwat Crawford, C.A. *et al.* (2004) Mental health, social functioning, and disability in postwar Afghanistan. *The Journal of the American Medical Association*, **292** (5), 575–84.

61. Gillespie, C.F. and Nemeroff, C.B. (2007) Corticotropin-releasing factor and the psychobiology of early-life stress. *Current Directions in Psychological Science*, **16** (2), 85–89.

62. Hegadoren, K.M., Lasiuk, G.C. and Coupland, N.J. (2006) Posttraumatic stress disorder part III: health effects of interpersonal violence among women. *Perspectives in Psychiatric Care*, **42**, 163–73.

63. Follingstad, D.R., Wright, S., Lloyd, S. *et al.* (1991) Sex differences in motivations and effects in dating violence. *Family Relations: Interdisciplinary Journal of Applied Family Studies*, **40** (1), 51–57.

64. Goodman, L.A., Koss, M.P. and Fitzgerald, L.F. (1993) Male violence against women. Current research and future directions. *American Psychology*, **48** (10), 1054–58.

65. Weissman, M.M., Bland, R.C., Canino, G.J. *et al.* (1996) Cross-national epidemiology of major depression and bipolar disorder. *The Journal of the American Medical Association*, **276** (4), 293–99.

66. Karam, E.G. (1994) The nosological status of bereavement-related depressions. *British Journal of Psychiatry*, **165**, 48–52.

67. Khamis, V. (1998) Psychological distress and well-being among traumatized Palestinian women during the Intifada. *Social Science and Medicine*, **46** (8), 1033–41.

68. Punamaki, R., Komproe, I., Qouta, S. *et al.* (2005) The role of peritraumatic dissociation and gender in the association between trauma and mental health in a Palestinian community sample. *American Journal of Psychiatry*, **162**, 545–51.

69. Hien, D., Cohen, L. and Campbell, A. (2005) Is traumatic stress a vulnerability factor for women with substance use disorders? *Clinical Psychology Review*, **25**, 813–23.

70. Jasinki, J.L., Williams, L.M. and Siegel, J. (2000) Childhood physical and sexual abuse as risk factors for heavy drinking among African-American women: a prospective study. *Child Abuse and Neglect*, **24**, 1061–71.

71. Widom, C.S., Weiler, B.L. and Cottler, L.B. (1999) Childhood victimization and drug abuse: a comparison of prospective and retrospective findings. *Journal of Consulting and Clinical Psychology*, **67**, 867–80.

72. Morrissey, J.P., Jackson, E.W., Ellis, A.R. *et al.* (2005) Twelve-month outcomes of trauma-informed interventions for women with co-occurring disorders. *Psychiatric Services*, **56**, 1213–22.

73. Yabroudi, P., Karam, E., Chami, A. *et al.* (1999) Substance use and abuse: the Lebanese female and the Lebanon wars, in *Women and War in Lebanon* (ed. L. Shehadeh), University Press of Florida, Gainesville, pp. 282–320.

74. Punamaki, R., Komproe, I., Qouta, S. *et al.* (2005) The deterioration and mobilization effects of trauma on social support: childhood maltreatment and adulthood military violence in a Palestinian community sample. *Child Abuse and Neglect*, **29**, 351–73.

75. Wyatt, G.E., Myers, H.F. and Loeb, T.B. (2004) Women, trauma, and HIV: an overview. *AIDS and Behavior*, **8**, 401–3.

Further reading

Littleton, H.L., Breitkopf, C.R. and Berenson, A.B. (2007) Correlates of anxiety symptoms during pregnancy and association with perinatal outcomes: a meta-analysis. *American Journal of Obstetrics and Gynecology*, 424–32.

8

Voices of consumers – women with mental illness share their experiences

Shoba Raja

BasicNeeds, Bangalore, India

The 2001 WHO report estimates that 450 million people are affected by mental disorders worldwide. Hidden within these statistics are human lives, human stories of suffering, neglect, abuse and for those that are lucky . . . hope.

The four stories here are of four women told in their own voices. They talk about their lives, their experience and their feelings. They come from different countries, different cultures but have two things in common – they are women and they have all suffered from mental illness (MI).

8.1 'Ni Tagibebu' – 'I will change my lifestyle'

Nineteen-year-old Ibrahim Zulfawu lives in Tamale. She used to be a headstrong young girl. It was a sign of rebellion when she dropped out of school in defiance of her father's wishes and headed for Accra to savour life on her own independent terms. Soon, Ibrahim Zulfawu was in bad company, and a lethal cocktail of alcohol, marijuana, cocaine and other drugs led her to MI. She recovered quickly through traditional healing practises, and BasicNeeds forged her reconciliation with her angry, estranged father. He supported her apprenticeship as a hairdresser, a vocation for which she has innate flair. Ibrahim Zulfawu is now fully focused on life, and looks forward to establishing her own business.

Ibrahim Zulfawu's Life Story

As told to: Interviewer and Writer: Sayibu Montia, Assistant Development Officer, BasicNeeds Northern Ghana

From shackles to freedom

I am 19 years old. I live with my mother and my brother in house number K 413 at Ward K, a suburb of Tamale. I am my mother's firstborn. My brother, Adam, is seven years old. I am currently learning hairdressing.

Sayibu Montia of BasicNeeds met me at Alhaji Hussein's house during one of his routine visits to traditional healers. Alhaji Hussein is a traditional healer. I was then under his treatment and my condition was severe. I was very aggressive and insulted people. I was shouting and accusing people of raping me. I had been put in iron shackles by the traditional healer.

Sayibu Montia had empathy for me, so he decided to monitor my progress. He asked about me every time he visited Alhaji Hussein. My condition improved steadily. I was treated and discharged a month after I was admitted at Alhaji's house. My shackles were removed. I was well. I was free.

A message, an appeal

Sayibu Montia visited me one day when traditional healers were about to observe World Drug Abuse Day. He invited me to talk on the radio and share my experience with drugs with the youth of my city. This radio discussion was part of the activities held to mark World Drug Abuse Day. Traditional healers, partnering with BasicNeeds and the Ghana Health Service (a government institution responsible for healthcare delivery in the country), organised this programme to sensitise the public about the effects of drug abuse. It also served to highlight the contribution of traditional healers to treating people suffering from drug abuse-related MI.

To help lend credence to the message of traditional healers, two mentally ill people who received treatment from them for drug abuse were included in the panel discussion. I was one of them. I admitted that my illness was a result of taking alcohol, marijuana, cocaine and other drugs with my friends, especially at night clubs. I used the opportunity to appeal to the youth, and to young women in particular, to pursue their goals in life and stay away from drugs since that might hinder them from realising them.

Drug abuse is not a common habit among the youth in the cities of Ghana although it is steadily becoming a social problem.

After the programme Sayibu discussed with me the possibility of documenting my story and sharing it with others who might find themselves in similar situations. I readily agreed and we fixed a date for it.

'My family'

My parents are Ibrahim Adam and Zuweira Musah. They live in Tamale. They are divorced. Both my parents are Dagombas by tribe and Moslems by religion. My father is a commercial truck driver while my mother is a petty trader. She sells consumables around the Central Police Station in Tamale.

Paying the price for drugs

I refused to go to school after Junior Secondary School One (JSS1). I left home to live an independent life in Accra. I started taking drugs with a group of friends. I got this sickness through alcohol and drug abuse. I cannot remember what happened to me after that. I cannot recall my situation, or what it was that brought me to the traditional healer's place.

After some time my mother got a message from one of my colleagues that I was not well. This friend of mine described my condition as MI. My mother sent my brother to look for me. It was several days before my brother spotted me one day at Osu, a suburb of Accra. He also confirmed, after seeing me that I was suffering from MI.

My brother called my mother on the phone and told her that he found me with several cuts all over my body, probably as a result of being beaten. He said he suspected that people had beaten me because I had perhaps misbehaved with them due to my illness. I was finally brought back to Tamale. In fact, when my mother saw me she immediately knew I was suffering from MI.

Healing, in three weeks

When I came back from Accra, my father took me to Shekhinah Clinic (Basic-Needs' partner organisation in Tamale). I was on psychotropic drugs for about a month and my symptoms reduced. After a month, however, my condition worsened, to the extent that I stripped naked. My parents were advised by a friend to take me to the traditional healer, Alhaji Hussein.

Before that, my parents had already spent a great deal of money on buying rams and fowls for sacrifices to aid my recovery. They were forced to abandon their business and run helter-skelter to get treatment for my illness. The healer, Alhaji Hussein, asked my parents to buy a pot in which he boiled some herbal concoction for me. I drank this concoction and bathed with it for two weeks and then my condition began to improve. By the third week, I was completely well.

I did not get a diagnosis from Alhaji Hussein. I learnt that traditional healers do not classify MIs into categories such as mania, schizophrenia or depression. Their diagnosis is simply that the person is mentally ill. They do, however, explain the causes of illness. In my case, Alhaji Hussein's impression was that

I had developed MI because of substance abuse. I was not surprised. It was a destabilising cocktail I used to have – alcohol, marijuana, cocaine. It made me see images; it made me aggressive and violent. The healer diagnosed me with a brain disorder, which he felt was the result of drug abuse.

Building anew – BasicNeeds takes the initiative

Sayibu Montia spoke to me on several occasions when I was under treatment, and all the statements I made indicated my regrets about my past life. I told him I wished so much to change my situation for the better. However, I did mention to him that I needed support from my parents, especially my father, to rebuild my life. For me, then, this was far from reach because my father was furious with me about the life I had led, the life that had brought on my illness.

Sayibu Montia told me later that after this discussion with me, he felt the urge to seek my parents and interact with them because it seemed that everybody in my family was fed up with me. He took directions from me and located my mother at our residence. He briefed her on the activities of BasicNeeds and advised her that my effective recovery depended largely on how well I am accepted and reintegrated into the family. My mother promised to inform my father about their discussion. Sayibu Montia also encouraged her to invite my father to the cleansing ceremony, a ritual that Alhaji Hussein would conduct before discharging me, as BasicNeeds would be taking part in it.

A tearful reconciliation

Alhaji Hussein invited BasicNeeds to witness my cleansing ceremony. Cleansing ceremonies are held by traditional healers to discharge patients they have successfully treated. Peter, Programme Manager, BasicNeeds Northern Ghana and Sayibu participated in this ceremony. They used the opportunity to counsel me to avoid bad friends, live a life free of drugs and seek a better life than I had previously lived.

At the ceremony my father recounted how he had striven to make sure I succeeded in life. He said, 'I did my best to educate Zulfawu and she refused to be in school. When she dropped out of school, I opened a grocery shop for her to enable her to earn a living. She abandoned the shop and ran to Accra. She joined a group of bad friends and started smoking marijuana, only to bring shame and disgrace upon me. I think I have been responsible enough, as a father'.

At this point, I couldn't take it any more. I knelt down in tears and pleaded that my father should give me another chance. I requested him to forgive me and support me to learn hairdressing. Peter added his voice to my pleas and encouraged my father not to turn a deaf ear to my request. After a long discussion, he agreed to support me to learn a new vocation.

Zulfawu's new life

I have successfully undergone a two-year apprenticeship at a hairdressing salon called Mariam Shop, located close to the Tamale market. I remember Sayibu Montia visiting me at my workplace on the 16th of October 2007. I felt proud to be nicely clad in my uniform and busy working with my colleagues. I told him my trainer would see that I graduated by the end of the year. I told him I needed support to start work on my own.

My trainer, Mariam, remarked that it usually takes about three years for an apprentice to learn hairdressing, but I had been able to make it in two years. It was a great moment for me when Mariam said that she had added me to her group that was graduating that year. It proved to me that I was good at my work, that I was being acknowledged for it.

'I am so happy . . . '

It feels good to say I have recovered. I am not ashamed to call myself a stabilised mentally ill person. What shames me is that episode with drugs, straying away and embarking on that thoughtless course in life.

I have not been on any treatment after I achieved stability and was discharged by Alhaji Hussein. I, however, visit the traditional healer from time to time for a review.

It is amazing, this transformation I see in myself – how an iron-shackled and aggressive person has turned into a hairdresser now. I am so happy, Sayibu Montia is happy for me, just as my parents are. I am determined to mend the broken pieces of my life. I think my determination is amply demonstrated by the way I took my lessons seriously and completed my course within two years. I feel my progress should not be interrupted, it should continue. I would like to have financial support to open a hairdressing shop and start my own business.

8.2 Determined to go against the odds

Mary Monari has bipolar affective disorder. A gutsy lady in her early forties, she is undeterred by MI. Her narrations have striking clarity and her insight into her condition is strong and illuminating. MI is a challenge she is learning to overcome, every new day. She pleads lucidly for understanding and sensitivity in dealing with mentally ill people. Mary Monari lives in Nairobi, Kenya.

Mary Monari's Life Story

As told to: Interviewer and Writer, Faith Wanjiru, Project Officer, Schizophrenia Foundation of Kenya

> Don't turn your back on me just because I don't fit into your world. My torment is real, and I would change it if I could. If you take the time to understand me you will make my world a less painful place.
>
> Mary Monari

A positive person

My name is Mary Monari. When Mrs. Lillian Kanaiya, the Director of Schizophrenia Foundation of Kenya, and Faith Wanjiru, its Project Officer, called me for the interview, I requested them to meet me at a shop where I was delivering juice.

'I have just found a market for my home made juice', I told them when they arrived. 'This is my first customer', I told them happily, pointing to someone who had come in to buy my drink.

I am a middle aged woman in my early forties. Faith told me I am worthy of admiration, right from the time people start engaging with me. It felt good. I am cheerful, I have a ready smile and a very positive attitude despite my illness. I am determined to go against the odds caused by MI and am more than willing to help other mentally ill people.

Looking back

I graduated in Agriculture from Baraton University in the Rift Valley Province in Kenya. Before this disease – bipolar affective disorder – stopped me, I was working for the agricultural sector of the Magarini Integrated Rural Development programme in Malindi, 30 km north of Mombasa. It was a project funded by the Austrian government. I was attending a course on Women in Management in the south coast of Mombasa on the shores of the Indian Ocean. This was in 1995. I fell sick during this workshop. At the time I was nursing my first and only child, Solomon.

We had just come from Kilindini harbour, a tourist attraction in Mombasa, and had bought a lot of gifts for my family. On coming back I locked myself in my hotel room and did not want to associate with anyone. This went on for a while and the hotel management had to use the master key to open the door. The next day during the discussions at the workshop, I did not want to talk to anyone and was really scared.

I remember when I returned home to Malindi, I experienced breathing problems and could only see a mirage. I remember telling my now-deceased niece, 'Nikikufa, when I die please do not torture my baby'.

I was taken to Galana Hospital and my husband had to be called from Nairobi. I do not recall what happened at the hospital. I later gathered what had happened to me from friends and relatives. According to them I wanted to beat people at the hospital and at times I pulled at the hospital beds. Also when arrangements were being made for my return flight to Nairobi, at one point I seem to have said that I was going to jump off the plane. In fact I had to miss the flight since the airline staff insisted that without an immediate letter from a doctor assuring them that it was safe for me to travel, they would not allow me on the plane.

I was transferred to Masaba Hospital on arrival in Nairobi and later to the Nairobi Hospital. In Nairobi, I was mostly cheerful and even spoke well to members of my family and friends. However, I could not remember the exact nature of the conversations. Two weeks after my arrival from Mombasa, I was discharged from the Nairobi Hospital under heavy medication that made me drowsy and increased my appetite. This led to weight gain. I recovered and later went back to work with the same employer in Malindi in 1996, resuming my duties as the Agricultural Officer, but I was doing light duty. However, in June 1997, due to my need to be close to my family, I resigned, in the hope of getting a new job in Nairobi.

Never giving up

However, finding a job as a mentally ill person is not easy.

I was not about to give up, though, and I kept searching for a job. I eventually found a light job at Hundreds of Original Projects for Employment (HOPE), an Austrian non-governmental organisation, where I worked for the Hope projects in western Kenya.

It was during this period, in 1998, that I got an assignment from Gallinde Darnhoffer, who was then in charge of Hope '87 projects. I completed the assignment and handed in the report, which I believe can be found in the Hope '87 files. Gallinde asked me to take up another assignment but I was unable to do so because I had to be on medication for some time.

Since then I have been knitting chunky woollen cardigans and pullovers. However, this is not giving me job satisfaction. I love community work because it gives me an opportunity to interact with people and serve humanity. It gives me contentment to know that I have made a difference to someone's life.

Reaching out to a network

MI for me is usually accompanied by cold feet and breathing problems. I vividly remember seeing the streets of gold in heaven. At times I see images on television making faces at me.

I felt that most people did not understand my situation and therefore I needed to meet people with the same condition as I, particularly mothers and wives like myself. During one of my hospital visits to Menelik Hospital in Nairobi I came across a brochure from the Schizophrenia Foundation of Kenya. I contacted its Director, Lillian Kanaiya, and attended her first meeting at the Muteero PCEA Church in Karen (located in the outskirts of Nairobi). I was warmly welcomed and I enjoyed the sharing that took place, listening to the experiences of other people with schizophrenia and allied disorders. Nyawira, also a mentally ill patient, sang a nice welcome song for me, and since then, I have learnt a lot from her and other members. My family members occasionally attend the organisation's monthly group meetings.

I realise now in hindsight that, had I joined a self-help family support group in 1995, my life would have been different. Support groups provide emotional support, information about MI, allow people to share their experiences and give us a ray of hope.

Daring to dream

I like to be vibrant and independent. I have to be doing something. Later at home, I decided to take more interest in my hobby of knitting. I spend a lot of my time taking care of my 10 year old son. I also take care of my 13 year old nephew. I also spend some of my time reading, and the most inspiring book I have read is, 'How To Stop Worrying and Start Living' by Dale Carnegie.

I sew and sell sweaters, rear chickens and my newest project is making and selling fruit juices. I also wish to acquire more skills in decorating cakes, achieve computer literacy and master driving.

I visit mentally ill people at Mathari Hospital, the national mental health referral hospital in Nairobi, at least once a week and take presents for them. I wish to start a patient delivery service at this hospital where people who have recovered and stabilised can drop presents and share their experiences with mentally ill people in hospitals. I wish to identify the skills of mentally ill people and help them develop them.

I have a dream. I visualise a rehabilitation home or garden where mentally ill patients can get solace and revitalise themselves after leaving a mental hospital. I dream of land on which to put up income generating facilities and other facilities that will enhance the recovery of patients. I would like water to irrigate my garden where I would grow organic vegetables. I dream of an orchard of fruit trees. I hope for a Ray of Hope Nature Trail and Resurrection Hope Garden with beautiful flowers and messages on positive thinking, inscribed on stone and on paper for patients to read as they enjoy their walk. A music and video system can play hope-inspiring messages, a showroom can display the talents of patients. There will be counselling services, a cyber café, a poultry unit, possibly a bakery too, and promotional material like t-shirts and caps with anti-stigma messages.

I dream of funds. Funds to make my dream possible.

The lesson I have learnt is that mentally ill people should be assisted to start projects that will keep them busy, but with little stress. They would then spend less time on hospital beds. This will also enable them to acquire their basic needs.

The challenges of mental illness

MI is a cruel illness. Due to the strong stigma about it in Kenya, patients feel they are the hopeless and the useless of the earth. Mentally ill people are ridiculed, laughed at and treated as non-persons. Stigma is like a wall between those suffering from MI and the rest of the world.

I often asked God why it had to happen to me. I wanted to know the cause of my illness so that I could do something about it. I would read any disease-related material I could lay my hands on. I had the urge to share my troubles with someone who has suffered from MI, so that I could make better sense of my own.

People do not understand you and when you recover they don't trust you. Some of them want to manage your life and think you can't do a thing for yourself. Many of them are not even involved in decision-making that revolves around your life. Mentally ill people feel they are a burden to their families and carers. At times, your priorities do not seem their priorities, and you get tired of asking for money for everything.

I often complain about the high cost of medicine. Marketing goods made by mentally ill people has also not been easy. The sweaters I make face a lot of competition from second-hand clothes. There was a time when my machine broke down and I was idle for quite a while.

I have lost contact with many of my close friends since I fell sick. Some of my relatives too no longer visit me. I am however lucky to have a supportive family. Some people have advised me to visit a 'mganga', a witch doctor. Such people believe I am bewitched. For a long time I did not know what I was suffering from. At one point I was diagnosed with cerebral malaria. It is only very recently that I insisted on finding out my condition and went in for a proper diagnosis. I now know my condition: bipolar affective disorder or mood swings.

Don't turn your back on me just because I don't fit into your world. My torment is real, and I would change it if I could. If you take the time to understand me you will make my world a less painful place. This is a cry from the heart. I believe the cry of all those who suffer from MI would go something like this.

8.3 Brilliant madness – a narrative by a young woman from India who is recovering from mental illness

The 'mind' is the most complex yet simple tool the human race is conferred with and any extreme of its functioning good or bad is an out-of-this-world experience. The first prime minister of India, Jawahar Lal Nehru had coined the term 'scientific temper'. This term if related to the mind makes for an obvious correlation of the present technology-driven society's mental, physical, financial, spiritual and emotional state of being.

Now, what does all this have to do with MI one wonders? The problem is the pace at which the current human lifestyle is heading towards an over-emphasis on technology rather than the basic human spirit. The fallout has been a rise in MI among the young, middle-aged and the old. I was diagnosed with 'Schizo-affective Disorder' in 1999. The crescendo to my obsession to succeed in the world of cut-throat competitiveness was my illness.

However, over the last nine years as a mentally ill patient I have evolved as a functional person. From being a 12–14 hours (sometimes even more) sleeping person, unfit and vulnerable to relapses every six months – today I am a normal person with a part-time job and filling the rest of my day with music, exercises, reading, writing and socialising.

I have had my challenges as a woman from a traditional Hindu, Indian family with MI. The Indian society shuns a person with MI more overtly than the western world. An average Indian girl is made to play second fiddle to the male-dominated-world right from birth. However, the urban Indian woman is way ahead in this aspect (they make for only a small fraction!). Just like any other middle-class Indian family, my parents coaxed me into marriage. Ironically, it was a marriage that took place when I was beginning to become psychotic.

I don't blame my folks. Indian women are always made to feel that marriage, husband and children make up her reality – no matter what you do or where you come from.

Challenges I faced as a woman with mental illness in India

Schizophrenia usually occurs in youngsters in their twenties and I was 25 when I was diagnosed. It is that phase of a woman's life when she is seeking success in her career and preparing herself for the married life which is yet to come. I was bent on going abroad for my further studies, however, my illness struck at my self esteem very badly. I suddenly felt useless, lonely and outcast. My family could not handle this as they had always seen me as an independent woman. I became a burden to them and they wanted me to move away from home as people were finding me at home throughout the day. Another major component was that they were not able to accept my illness and denied the psychotic state I was in. They said I was responsible for this condition. They urged me to be positive and fight it – positive mental attitude could do it all they claimed. They also took me to various faith healers and I had my share of amulets and magico religious healers. A result of going through all this non medical treatment was a relapse because I stopped medication.

The heartening thing, however, was that I was brave and fought the illness in my own way. I knew a lot about the illness before it struck me because I had read about it. I set myself to gain my former physical fit form. I knew most MIs make people physically unfit and lethargic. I used to read up the information on the Internet about MI and also tried making online efriends to fight my loneliness.

After all this, I did get married and move to the United States. The marriage failed because of a relapse which my then husband was unable to fathom. He felt that my family had cheated him (even though I had told him everything about my illness). I was alone again and sick. To cut a long story short – I moved to a shelter for the homeless and struggled in a strange country, with no friends or support, but I survived. After a while I got a job and moved to my own apartment. But alas! This was temporary too and I ultimately moved back to India. I am a lot better now but I still stay with my family. Hopefully I will find a partner and move out and become completely functional one day. Till then, I will try and continue to work, exercise, write and most importantly survive in Indian society with self esteem.

To sum up, I have a couple of pointers for mental health professionals:

For women, no matter what their geographical, educational, economic and professional background – MI is a devastating condition. The initial years of battling the illness or accepting it is very burdensome and debilitating. My personal view after meeting patients like mine, in India and abroad, has been that.

- Mentally ill patients need to be given time and space to become functional members of society (something I found in plenty with a widowed mother and an understanding younger brother).

- Pressure and criticism from your circle of family and friends only excruciates the condition.

- The mentally ill are intelligent and proactive people and need to be given due recognition and a sense of agency.

- A nurturing environment goes a long way in uplifting these latent potential citizens.

- Co-ordination between mental health professionals and employers to offer gainful employment makes them nearer to normal.

- Constant feedback and co-ordination of the mental health professionals with family and employers make the ill feel more supported.

- My personal view is that not just educational qualifications, but the SKILL SET of the mentally ill makes them very confident.

- Skills like cooking, house-keeping, driving, writing, tutoring are fun activities and enumerative too.

- To end, I found that being proactive makes one foresee the symptomatic conditions that occur at very short intervals during the initial years of the illness.

A decade on the banks of MI, I have deeply connected to certain beautiful truths and otherwise:

1. MI is just another complicated state of being – but needs constant support from oneself, family, society and also the medical fraternity.

2. Mentally ill patients are deeply connected to the truths of the Cosmos *aka* 'Brahmanda'.

3. Women from traditional societies such as India (urban and rural) face challenges right from childhood. These are often overt and deeply traumatic such as, preference for boys and for light skinned girls. These are issues that start impacting on the self esteem of young girls and makes them fragile from very early on.

4. Indian women though strong in many ways, are often emotionally naïve compared to their western counterparts because of the nature of socialisation.

5. The Indian society, progressive as it is on the economic front – needs to pay attention to social and psychological issues of women.

Even as the Indian society's cultural values date to eons of suppression and domination of women, Indian psychiatrists need to note the above pointers to create a balanced person who is able to survive despite MI.

To sum up my experience as a survivor of mental trauma, I propagate an Indian society which should:

- Nurture women in a jovial, supportive, disciplined environment.

- Networking among people outside your cultural background.

- Support groups, discussions, writing and campaigning for the rights of Indian women in bad marriages and with mental health problems.

- Teenage is among the most trying time in the life of youngsters and depression usually sets in here. Educational institutions need to wake up to the need of employing mental health professionals and counsellors.

- Indian women need to be exposed to varied activities right from childhood to have a more balanced outlook to life.

PS: I thank my mental health professionals, family, friends and fellow beings for my turn around.

8.4 From illness to purpose and recovery . . .

> Imagine a butterfly caught in a spider's web frantically trying to escape. The more the brightly coloured creature flutters and panics, the more enmeshed it becomes. Terror and paralysis sets in. The butterfly is unable to move or fly, awaiting impending doom. Being caught helplessly in a sticky web is an apt metaphor to describe an episode of clinical depression.
>
> (mh@work®, beyondblue 2004)

Since I commenced my journey into mental health advocacy some seven years ago, not a day has gone past where I haven't had the conversation turned to depression and some form of mental health. Whenever I share my passion and activities it is like setting a grass fire. People's reactions have been varied, at times emotional and moving, and other times, controversial and divided. Mostly though, people would acknowledge and nod their head. They knew of someone who had been touched by some form of mental illness, but did not really understand what it meant. It was as if by the very mention of my vulnerability a green light was switched on and allowed people to talk about previously unspoken and personal issues. Others, however, believe the whole depression concept is a self-inflicted modern day malady that doesn't deserve time or attention and that in so doing it would talk people into being depressed.

Seven years on, the climate is slowly changing in Australia; depression and anxiety disorders are being talked about more widely than ever.

I remember at the beginning of my advocacy training those painful pioneering days, when the struggle to prick our society's conscience and build awareness began in earnest.

Depression and anxiety disorders have surrounded me in many different guises all my life, personally and professionally. As a workforce member I witnessed MI being poorly dealt with in the workplace repeatedly in many of the organisations and positions where I was employed. I felt out of my league when faced with these situations. Not ever having been trained in this area of people management, nor was there anyone else around me who was qualified or trained appropriately. Through lack of understanding and knowledge, I noticed many of my employers demonstrate discriminating and stigmatising attitudes and practises.

It was in my presence that a young woman had been asked by her manager if she could write 'a report outlining how many sick days she would be requiring in the next six months for this depression thing...' that was the catalyst for what would prove to be a life changing move. Something needed doing and I wanted to be a part of it.

This led me to dipping my toe into the small world of mental health advocacy and it was here where I met a group of inspiring people who courageously shared their experiences with a range of mental health issues. I could feel their pain acutely, it felt too familiar. We had so many things in common, not just the condition, but the stigma, the fear of rejection, isolation and frustration of being misunderstood by family and the community at large.

This would prove to be the beginning of many new experiences and where I would find myself regularly out of my comfort zone.

My first foray into media – was excruciatingly painful. I was invited to share my story of illness to wellness on national television, ABC's 7.30 Report. My anxiety levels went into overdrive. I was riding the porcelain bus before the filming, after the filming and after I knew the programme had aired. During the taping I was fighting my dry throat, fearing my voice would close up and nothing would come out. I felt like someone was choking me. Drinking fluids didn't make any difference. My brain felt scrambled, my body didn't feel like it belonged to me. I felt so vulnerable, so exposed. I may as well have been naked.

I could not bring myself to watch those few minutes of footage of that interview or any other. The pain and distress in doing them was overwhelming and stressful enough. The self-stigma and paranoia was constantly testing me. What would people say? How would my family and friends respond? I was imagining the '...she just wants attention...five minutes of fame...what has she got to be depressed about? She is so ungrateful'. I couldn't answer these questions myself and thought maybe I had made all this up. Why wasn't I more appreciative of my blessings? I have a wonderful life. So why did I choose to come out with my vulnerability to 400 000 Australians when I knew that reactions would be mixed? People wouldn't understand.

I had no idea what was driving me to do this on this occasion and those following after, but I did feel something powerful surging deep within me. This unwavering belief that depression needed championing and that I had the skills to do it, but only if I could just walk through the pain and fight the overpowering fear and anxiety. This wasn't a sexy topic with lots of high profile people and celebrities clamouring to tell their stories, like other health conditions, at that time there weren't many others coming out with this health condition. That would take a little time. Depression and anxiety disorders were not widely talked about or written about well. The very word depression was misunderstood and carried great stigma.

Growing up in a family where MI was too common, I knew no differently. It was something that wasn't talked about but accepted. This is the way things are; this is our lot in life. We kept so many secrets. In my late mother's case her psychiatric diagnosis and treatment was shrouded in secrecy. All we knew was that mum was going into hospital for a 'rest'. When she came out she was so medicated that all she could do was sleep for days and weeks. Later in life I would learn that it was during these times she was having Electro Convulsive Therapy (ECT) treatment. Through our lack of support, understanding and knowledge we didn't know how to recognise the signs and symptoms, or how to support each other within the family. We thought, hoped, we were helping but we may well have been hindering recovery in our loved one. In hindsight, we were exasperated carers who at times harshly judged each other.

I know first hand the havoc and devastating damage depression and anxiety disorders causes. There have been occasions I have wanted to die and I have tried to do just that. Not being able to rid my very being of undescribable grief and sorrow, my body, my heart, a cushion full of invisible machetes and knives. My very being was being held captive, leaving my body and mind tortured and aching, living in its private psychological prison everyday, every night, for what seemed like an eternity. How do I get through this pain? Especially when I couldn't function, couldn't love or live or work. Death seemed a way to end the pain.

Where my mother and other close family members and friends had experienced poor or frightening experiences of care from service providers, I was one of the fortunate few who had experienced positive mental healthcare. With loving non-judgemental support from my partner and daughter I have been able to experience wellness and contribute productively to our community and life.

Too many people's very lives and being have been and are threatened and relationships destroyed through this health condition. Over time I developed sensitivity and antennae for others with similar experiences. I was getting tired of the secrets that I was seeing in families and the community more broadly.

During the early days of beyondblue and the establishment of blueVoices of which I became Chair, invitations increased for me to share my journey of illness to wellness through various forums; print media, radio, television, in the development of educational films and DVDs. The more I received, the more I kept saying yes, even though each time was an enormous challenge and took all the strength I could find within me. Many people commented that I made it look so easy. If they only knew what was going on inside. At those times I was still physically ill, somehow carrying on with crippling anxiety and nausea, pretending I could do this. In essence I was undressing myself emotionally in public time after time. Somehow I believed that what I was doing was the right thing; this was one way to move people to action. In my thinking, if we didn't move people or get them by the heart we won't get attitude change. I needed to be brutally honest with myself and my journey, the good, the bad and all within a safe context. I was still terrified it would backfire and sometimes it did backfire.

I did have to face what I feared: negativity, criticism, misunderstanding and even rejection. It was difficult at times to read another person's interpretation of my words and reality in print. Would they portray what I shared fairly, honestly or would they change it? My meetings with the journalists who wrote or filmed my story were mostly positive. They were empathic and sensitive; some even disclosed their own emotional connections to depression.

There was, however, a heavy price to pay for voicing my experiences. Some family members didn't cope well with my honesty. Years on and some no longer ask me how my work is going or what activities I am doing in my life, preferring to ignore that part of me. Some relationships have even ended whilst others have been very supportive and have grown even stronger.

These instances forced me to ask myself if I was really doing the right thing, should I step back? My honesty and my illness were causing discomfort and pain to others. We all have differing realities. I was sharing my life's reality without pointing fingers or blaming anyone as no one was or is to blame. It was these reactions that tell me we still have a bit of work ahead of us to change old and harmful paradigms about MIs.

The beyondblue team and blueVoices executive provided back up support and debriefing to each other every step of the way, especially in the early days. I know that those of us voicing our stories couldn't have continued without it.

After having appeared on Channel 9's Kerri-Anne Kennerly's Morning programme, I cried when their producer invited me to come back the following week. It was as if it was ok, I was ok in going 'there'. He floored me when he said that the Channel 9 switch board had been jammed with calls from our segment. We had been a ratings winner . . . '*It was ok to talk about depression* . . .' I knew in my heart it was, but I needed the numbers to tell me to keep me doing this work.

When we did give a little of ourselves, we found we received so much more back. Our audience shared their painful secrets and tears with us.

Most overwhelming were the many letters, emails, cards, phone calls, hugs, hand holding and emotional appreciation I received from strangers each time my story appeared or I presented. It was their 'Thank yous . . .' and comments like ' . . . You're telling my story, thank you for bringing it out into the open, I didn't know, I didn't understand . . . . I will go and visit a doctor . . . You have helped me so much . . .'. These all became my keep going meter.

There was a chapter of my life in which I became involved in advocacy and soon after established my own business mentalhealth@Work (mh@work). Together, they have proven to be the most therapeutic and empowering experiences, an unexpected yet very enriching part of my recovery.

To be able to use my vulnerability to help others in a small way has been deeply gratifying and life changing. To participate in this way has now become a powerful personal crusade from what started as very painful beginnings. The journey has bestowed many surprises, lessons and powerful life gifts – all playing an important part in helping me to stay safe and well and becoming who I am today.

Surprisingly, I am now in a position where I wake up every day looking forward to what I love doing. There have been many occasions when I have pinched myself and thought . . . wow I am doing this because of my MI! So there is an upside to depression.

Through the exposing exercise of retelling my story on numerous occasions I discovered a new confidence and strength I never knew I had. By facing what I most feared and forcing myself to be honest, I found their power and hold has lessened. Somewhere along the line the terror and severe anxiety passed, a new peace settling in its place as I gained a new sense of self and new understandings of my past.

The power of education and knowledge has been a key for me to better manage my own mental health and to educate my immediate family to help support each other and myself appropriately without passing judgement. The lessons have helped me with managing my health and wellbeing which at times have called for difficult decisions.

In turn these lessons have also helped in teaching me to judge others and myself less harshly, the power of social connectedness and reaching out – it can and does save lives. The greatest gift we can give to another human is showing them they are valued.

So many opportunities have emerged during my journey to recovery. Acquiring new knowledge and skills about Australia's mental health sector and system(s) was a necessary responsibility that came with participating in the many advocacy, lobbying and advisory group activities.

It was through these memberships that submissions to various enquiries including the Senate Select Enquiry into Mental Health, the Human Rights and Equal Opportunity Commissioner's and Mental Health Council of Australia's 'Not for Service Report' were made.

National board membership with the Mental Health Council of Australia enabled my participation in the COAG process that was headed by the Prime Minister of Australia in 2006 and saw the Commonwealth place this health issue highly on the agenda with more than $1.8 billion towards the improvement of services and treatments for the mental health sector.

A desire to broaden knowledge about mental health and how to support the vulnerable in the community was the motivator for me to pursue a postgraduate qualification in Community Mental Health.

I have felt a special emotional affinity to the butterfly. It has become a part of me, and symbolises so much about freedom and hope. In the early days the butterfly helped me explain what depression was like. I could so easily imagine being that creature . . . flying freely and hopefully enjoying the bright blue sky and green grass until caught in a spider's web. Then trying to fight the entrapment until worn out and exhausted. I would be paralysed with fear, feeling helpless and hopeless, unable to fly, move or escape.

This metaphor also proved helpful in understanding how I manage my recovery.

Education and knowledge has proven to be significantly important in my recovery. The more I learnt about depression and my health condition the more empowered I have become. In so doing I am better able to take responsibility for my own well-being, becoming an informed participant rather than a submissive recipient of treatment. I am learning how to befriend the spider and the spider's web, to recognise, negotiate and manage my health.

Mounting evidence of workplaces being unable to manage mental health issues, my own personal and professional experiences, the earlier mentioned catalyst that prompted me to commence this leap into a totally new working space and the realisation that one didn't need be medically qualified to save a life or make a difference to someone with MI was what instigated the establishment of my business, mentalhealth@work (mh@work) ...

School, university and professional associations offer and offered nothing in the way of preparing or educating the workforce for dealing with these commonly occurring and treatable health problems.

As one of those ill-equipped workforce members, I decided to use my story, my advocacy skills and experiences and my passion to change this situation.

I am a happily married mother, educated, self-employed and rich with friendships, with a bubbly façade that belies a chameleon who manages life with a health condition: Depression.

Today, through mh@work® we are able to share the lived perspective in many boardrooms, demonstrating that these are real health conditions that deserve respect and that with basic understanding and skills they can be managed and supported more appropriately with better outcomes for employers, employees and ultimately the community.

mh@work® has been working successfully with Telstra and other Australia's blue chip organisations over many years developing their mental health strategies. A variety of communication elements have been developed and designed: intranet package, an interactive elearning tool mh@work®, a booklet 'Creating Supportive Workplaces', national awareness forums and workshops for employers, employees and their families, HR advisors and line managers.

mh@work's philosophy has revolved around sharing the lived experience, role modelling recovery, resilience and what it means to be touched directly and or indirectly by these illnesses, to show that MI does not mean mental incompetence. Through boldness and courage, mh@work® is open in its effort to build awareness and destigmatise this health issue. For a health and wellbeing strategy to be successful and long-lasting, an organisation needs to undergo a culture change – this takes time, so the investment and commitment to such a process is a long term one and needs leadership and passion to come from the top. mh@work® guides businesses through the obstacle course.

Now other major organisations are following Telstra's pioneering footsteps placing the issue of mental health high on the corporate agenda, bringing heart and wellbeing back into business using our model and approach.

My partner and daughter have been by my side throughout the seasons of my life and staunch supporters in all my activities, having taken more than a passing interest in what I do. During a personal crisis where I was experiencing a severe depressive episode, they continued lovingly to support me.

'We will help you through this, we can do it together'. Were the pearls of wisdom from my young daughter. She could read my mood and asked me directly if I was depressed and unwell. When I said yes, she took me by the hand and escorted me to bed. After tucking me in, she raced away for a little time and came back with a pile of books. She crawled into bed next to me and started reading aloud, looking at me between the lines, smiling and touching my face. Every so often she would say 'I love you mummy, we will get through this together'. She was only seven years old but with her childlike magic she pushed the wall I had built around myself. This was the best dose of Prozac I could have asked for.

Through my activities today, I go beyond educating the community and workplaces about depression and anxiety disorders and even beyond MIs It is about teaching us, reminding us about the importance to reach out to one another not just in well meaning words but in actions.

Knowledgeable workplaces and communities need to learn how to befriend the enemy, and navigate through the web.

By nurturing and celebrating uniqueness and vulnerability, we, as a society will be better able to take responsibility for ourselves and each other by supporting those not able to care for themselves. People can't recover from MIs on their own. They need to be supported and valued.

With support and compassion, workplaces are ideally placed to help enormously with empowering its people to lead healthier, fulfilling and productive lives. This goes to the core, the heart of our very humanity so that all the butterflys in our community can soar highly and live life more productively and fully.

> My wings haven't been clipped because of my episodes of depression. If anything they are as bright and healthy as they have ever been, scars and all.
>
> (beyondblue 2004).

8.5 Conclusions

Research suggests that there are major gender differences in the impact of MI. Women face greater and more varied forms of vulnerability to abuse, denial, neglect and overall human rights violations. While MI affects both men and women it's every day consequences within families and even communities could be gender determined to a large extent [1]. Stigma can operate differently for men and women, and women with MI appear to be more vulnerable to its impact. In several societies, which place a premium on male children and an emphasis on familial responsibilities for women, gender can influence family response to MI. For example, family resources invested for treatment, care giving or for social-familial opportunities such as marriage, childcare can be denied to women. Economic contribution to family often plays a significant role in determining a family member's role and position within families especially when it comes to involvement in decision making, use of family resources for treatment and care. In this context the combined influence of gender and MI considerably diminishes women's capacities and opportunities for earning income or contributing towards the family's livelihoods and financial stability.

At the policy level too, much like poverty, mental health and related polices remain deeply gendered leading again to comparatively greater treatment inadequacies and consequent poor mental health outcomes for women.

Arguments for positive mental health often quote the global burden of disease study to emphasise the magnitude and urgency of the problem. Listening to the women in the four stories here it seems that it is this very notion of being a burden that really hurts. It makes them vulnerable because they are made to feel dependent and useless, this coming on top of the havoc and devastation that MI – schizophrenia, depression, bipolar affective disorder, substance abuse – has caused in their lives. Their families, struggling along with them to cope with the severe practical and emotional disruptions that follow onset of the illness, are in need of help and support themselves. The support that affected persons seek goes beyond treatment and therapy. It is acceptance, opportunity and dignity which can enable them to regain control over their lives.

If you look at their lives as they themselves have been able to see it – it is not all despair. For they have dared to hope. The women also talk of their return to normal living, engaging with family and community, beginning to work and the revival of confidence and self esteem. By withstanding societal pressure and loneliness of a marriage failed or making a determined effort to work and earn, finding the courage to share their story on a public platform or forging an emotional reconciliation with estranged family – none of it has been easy. The tough decisions each of them have had to make and the even more difficult actions that followed illustrate the courage and fortitude with which they have dealt with their MI.

Each of them speak of two very important things that have helped – the understanding and support they have needed to recover and the support that their families have needed in order to help them. After their own recovery they have all reached out – to support and help others come out of the effects of MI. They have found this to be deeply gratifying and even therapeutic in sustaining their own recovery.

> Don't turn your back on me . . . . If you take the time to understand me you will make my world a less painful place . . .

References

1. Miranda, J. and Green, L. (1999) The need for mental health services research for poor young women. *Journal of Mental Health Policy and Economics*, **2**, 73–80.

SECTION 2

The interface between reproductive health and psychiatry

Prabha S. Chandra

Department of Psychiatry, National Institute of Mental Health and Neurosciences, Bangalore, India

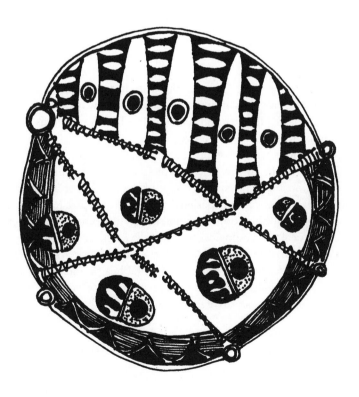

Contemporary Topics in Women's Mental Health   Edited by Chandra, Herrman, Fisher, Kastrup,
© 2009 John Wiley & Sons, Ltd   Niaz, Rondón and Okasha

Commentary

Introduction

The three chapters in this section deal with transitional points in women's lives which include pregnancy, childbirth, menopause and certain gynaecological conditions that have a major psychosocial impact. One paragraph quoted below from the chapter on menopause in this section probably sums up in many ways the truth about women's mental health in most contexts including that related to reproductive health:

> The classical social and contextual determinants of depression, such as unemployment, socioeconomic adversity, negative life events, lack of social support, loss of partner through bereavement or separation, or lack of a confiding relationship with a partner, continue to exercise a powerful influence [1].

The above statement is important because it amalgamates the convergence of various risk and protective factors in the life trajectory of a woman and in the important transitional phases, which can be either stressful or rewarding based on a combination of factors.

To the above list, I would add the newer challenges that women in the contemporary world are facing. The role of increasing technology including reproductive and diagnostic technologies, the impact of globalisation which contributes to tenuous family ties and disparity in wealth, accompanied by the changing world of women's working lives all add to the ways in which pregnancy, childbirth, menopause, fertility and reproductive health problems are perceived and dealt with by women the world over.

Among the various risk factors, two areas have emerged consistently as being the most important, in all the three chapters in this section. First, is the role of positive relationships and support as a protective factor and second is the powerful negative effect of an experience of sexual and physical violence either in childhood and adulthood on the mental health of women [2]. The experience of violence, physical, psychological or sexual is often gendered because of the prevailing power equations in most parts of the world. Postpartum mental health problems, menopausal distress, antenatal mental health and conditions such as pelvic pain syndromes all seem to have an experience of violence as a common possible mediating if not causative factor [3–5].

Mental health professionals and reproductive health

In this context, the importance of health professionals evaluating women's sexual health, satisfaction and abuse experiences as part of routine healthcare becomes paramount. Unfortunately, there is not much research on how often mental health professionals discuss these issues with women as part of routine care. In many countries because of the systems of healthcare, only women with severe mental illness are able to approach a trained mental health professional and the management strategies in these systems have become more and more risk oriented. Such approaches may not give the time and space for both patient and professional to discuss and resolve intimate and difficult issues such as violence or abuse and their impact on current mental health problems.

In developing countries where there is a shortage of trained mental health professionals and women often access traditional methods of treatment for reproductive symptoms, again there is a lack of privacy or space to discuss sexual problems or abuse experiences. Much traditional healing happens in the presence of family and in groups at places of worship or is given a religious connotation (in the form of fasting or rituals). There may be several rituals in different cultures which use symbols for healing among women, but while these symbolic healing rituals might serve some purpose, they often do not address or acknowledge any of the above experiences that a woman may be undergoing. Is it a surprise then that women in many cultures often have possession attacks or dissociative episodes that become an idiom of distress related to many of these complex and traumatic experiences?

The paradox related to the divorce between clinical practise and research findings is interesting and disturbing. While on the one hand, research has consistently found that abuse and violent experiences shape many of the experiences of even normal life transitions such as pregnancy, puberty, childbirth and menopause, not to mention sexual dysfunctions and psychosomatic conditions like chronic pelvic pain, these issues are seldom addressed in treatment. Treatment tends to often use a 'medical' model or a traditional healing model, both of which leave the needs of contemporary women unaddressed.

Psychological factors that influence women's sexual health

Psychological factors that influence women's sexual health are only recently being acknowledged. With the advent of the HIV epidemic, world over more attention is being paid to women's control over their sexual lives. In addition, the impact of mental health on risk behaviour and sexual communication is also being acknowledged [6]. The epidemic has forced us to look at the inadequate control women have over safe sex, access to testing, access to treatment, the increased stigma and isolation that women with HIV face and the impact that all this has on their mental health [7, 8]. This is not a challenge just for women but has been equally so for social scientists and policy makers. Interventions that focus on diminishing some of these power differences in couples and also increasing sexual negotiation, are being tested, but with little success.

War and civil unrest are often associated with breakdown of social systems and violence towards women. Recent research from war affected zones in Liberia [9] has focused on the role of combat related sexual violence and its impact on mental health. Uniformly, women faced more sexual violence than men in this study and the psychological effects were also found to be more among women.

However, more research is needed to study both the short and long term impact of wars and civil strife on women's sexual and reproductive health and eventually on their mental health.

Another issue that many women face world over is the lack of vocabulary and language to talk about sexual issues with their healthcare providers even if they do get an opportunity. While women maybe able to talk about vaginal discharge, reproductive tract infections or even dysperunia, they may lack the language to talk about low sexual satisfaction, orgasmic problems, arousal problems or sexual abuse. In fact these discussions are even taboo in some cultures. Sexual health problems in many parts of the world may have to take recourse to a label of reproductive health problems. It is therefore very important that health professionals in the area of women's health are sensitised and have training in mental health issues and mental health professionals have training in reproductive and sexual health issues.

What involuntary childlessness means to women

Satyanarayana *et al.* have discussed at length the importance of mental health issues in infertility in Chapter 3. What is evident is that while infertility is a stress for women in all cultures, in some cultures it extends beyond the realm of motherhood and extends to social status, position in society and the role of a wife. Women with infertility in these societies face significant stigma and the condition of childlessness has important religious implications as well. In India, in some regions, women who have been unable to bear children may be called derogatory names and may also not be allowed to participate in religious and social functions. Suicide rates are also high in these cultures related to infertility [10]. Unfortunately regardless of the cause, in many cultures, infertility appears to be the woman's burden.

Contemporary women also have to deal with increasing technological interventions for handling infertility and the stress that these interventions may cause. In cultures where a high premium is set on motherhood and there are large economic disparities, with specialised interventions such as in vitro fertilization IVF being available only to a select few, the inability to access treatment, may add to the stress.

An interface of reproductive, sexual and mental health needs of lesbian women

One area which does not get adequate attention in most studies is related to the interface between sexual, reproductive and mental health, among lesbian women. Literature on the topic, albeit limited, reveals that lesbian women find it difficult to reveal their sexuality to their healthcare providers and hence miss out on several important health messages and screenings. This lack of disclosure hence leads to unmet sexual and reproductive health needs. While studies on mental health issues reveal high rates of suicide and substance use, data on sexual health is limited [11, 12].

Childbirth and its mental health correlates

While postpartum and pregnancy related depression have received a lot of attention, one area which is still not researched adequately is anxiety disorders in pregnancy and the postpartum period. Anxiety states in pregnancy are important as they affect maternal well-being and may influence pregnancy outcomes. Research on anxiety disorders related to childbirth has focused on two main areas – the prevalence and the predictors of labour-related psychiatric morbidity and posttraumatic stress disorders (PTSDs). During the past few years, childbirth-related fear has been a topic of interest for obstetricians and mental health professionals. Previous research indicates that nearly 25% of women report significant fear related to childbirth, which has been identified as a reason for the growing number of women requesting elective caesarean section as well as for negative birth experiences. Knowledge is scanty about how women's experiences of fear are related to the excretion of stress hormones during labour or in utero. Epidural analgesia is still available only to a privileged few in the developing world. How this influences the birth experience and whether this contributes to higher anxiety among women in the developing world compared to their counterparts in the developed world, needs further enquiry [13].

Fisher *et al.* [14] in their chapter on pregnancy and childbirth emphasise the need for studying pregnancy and postpartum related posttraumatic stress disorder and its implications for obstetric and mental health. An interesting study conducted in five health centres in Nigeria [15] assessed the prevalence of PTSD and its association to childbirth-related experiences, marital satisfaction and social support among 876 women. The prevalence of PTSD in this population was 5.9%, higher than those reported by earlier western data. The factors independently associated with PTSD included hospital admission due to pregnancy complications, instrumental delivery, emergency caesarean section, manual removal of the placenta and poor maternal experience of control during childbirth. The above findings indicate the importance of the birth experience and antenatal care in modifying psychiatric morbidity associated with childbirth-related trauma. This is particularly relevant in the developing world, where women often do not have adequate antenatal care and may be psychologically unprepared to face hospitalisation and procedures related to labour. Despite the increasing literature on PTSD related to childbirth, there are few efforts at documenting interventions and studying their efficacy. With violence increasingly affecting women's lives, the role of experienced violence and terror in pregnant women has been another important area of study.

Mother infant relationships and psychiatric morbidity

Mother infant attachment disorders have not been considered a major problem in psychiatric care and not enough attention has been given both clinically and in research studies to this critical condition. Brockington [16] has stressed the need for more research in the area and has also discussed formal methods of assessment of mother infant attachment and bonding disorders. There is literature from Pakistan to suggest that maternal mental health impacts infant health and development [17].

Another important issue is care of infants of women with severe mental illness in the postpartum period. Child protection and social services are active in the developed world, however, in the developing world, women with postpartum psychosis often have to depend on family members such as the mother or mother in law for infant care. Untreated psychosis in mothers can cause risks to the infant and lack of treatment planning can have serious consequences for the mother in the form of suicide or child harm [18, 19]. Lack of milk substitutes, risks of breast feeding in the absence of adequate paediatric monitoring and disruption in immunisation schedules if a mother is seriously mentally ill, are areas that have not received adequate attention. The majority of the births occur in the developing world where support services are not easily available. Local models of care, such as informal foster care of infants by family members and how mothers with mental health issues handle lactation problems need to be described and discussed to inform mental health professionals about adequate care of the mother infant dyad.

Menopause

As longevity increases and more women are active till a late age, an increasing body of research is now focusing on the quality of life of older women. Astbury [1] in the chapter on menopause emphasises the biopsychosocial approach to understanding menopause in different cultures. It is clear from recent research that it is the menopausal transition rather than the postmenopausal period which appears to confer a higher risk for depression in women. Risk factors for depression in the perimenopausal period include a prior history of premenstrual or postpartum depression, life stress, poor health and absence of a partner [20]. The findings of the Women's Health Initiative as mentioned in the chapter, has thrown open a whole set of new questions related to safety and efficacy of Hormone Replacement Therapies HRTs [21]. There is a sense of uncertainty related to treatment of menopausal symptoms and apprehensions related to long-term oestrogen use, with many women looking for alternatives to oestrogen replacement therapy. With a large proportion of the female population being in the perimenopause or menopause, advances have occurred in measurements, definitions of menopausal stages and sampling, including adequate representation of women from all races and ethnicities.

Conclusions

It is quite evident from the contents of the three chapters in this section, that there are several unanswered questions despite there being a large amount of research in the area. The most important of these probably, is the large amount of variations in healthcare delivery, help seeking and health perceptions among women across the world and in different cultures and societies. As a result, what might be meaningful in a setting such as Sweden or Finland loses its significance in the experiences that modify a woman's psychological health in countries like Congo or Nepal. Similarly, technological advances have also increased the disparity in health services for women in the face of globalisation and women are well aware of this. How this inability to access services for purely economic reasons effects women is an important factor to understand. Factors like female feticide or sex selective abortions are shrouded with secrecy. More qualitative research might be needed on the psychological impact of these issues. The section is by no means complete and several areas such as abortion, HIV and STDs, surrogate motherhood, contraception, the influence of war and women's perceptions of reproductive health services, have not been dealt with. What are especially needed are more studies on the efficacy of interventions to prevent or mitigate mental health problems where they interface with reproduction and sexual health, especially those that can be easily adaptable and are low cost.

References

1. Astbury, J. Menopause and Women's Mental Health: The Need for a Multidimensional Approach. Chapter 3, Section 2.
2. Zink, T., Fisher, B.S., Regan, S. and Pabst, S. (2005) The prevalence and incidence of intimate partner violence in older women in primary care practices. *Journal of General and Internal Medicine*, **20**, 884–88.
3. Walker, E.A., Katon, W.J., Hansom, J. *et al.* (1995) Psychiatric diagnoses and sexual victimization in women with chronic pelvic pain. *Psychosomatics*, **36**, 531–40.
4. Varma, D., Chandra, P.S., Thomas, T. and Carey, M.P. (2007) Intimate partner violence and sexual coercion among pregnant women in India:relationship with depression and post-traumatic stress disorder. *Journal of Affective Disorders*, **102** (1–3), 227–35.
5. Leung, W.C., Leung, T.W., Lam, Y.Y.J. and Ho, P.C. (1999) The prevalence of domestic violence against pregnant women in a Chinese community. *International Journal of Gynaecology and Obstetrics*, **66** (1), 32–30.
6. Kermode, M., Devine, A., Chandra, P.S. *et al.* (2008) Some peace of mind: assessing a pilot intervention to promote mental health among widows of injecting drug users in north-east India. *BMC Public Health*, **8**, 294. DOI: 10.1186/1471-2458-8-294.
7. Blake, B.J., Jones Taylor, G.A., Reid, P. and Kosowski, M. (2008) Experiences of women in obtaining human immunodeficiency virus testing and healthcare services. *Journal of the American Academy Of Nurse Practitioners*, **20** (1), 40–46.

8. Chandra, P.S., Satyanarayana, V.A., Satishchandra, P. *et al.* (2009) Do men and women with HIV differ in their quality of life? A study from South India. *AIDS and Behavior*, Feb, **13** (1), 110–7.

9. Johnson, K., Asher, J., Rosborough, S. *et al.* (2008) Association of combatant status and sexual violence with health and mental health outcomes in post conflict Liberia. *Journal of the American Medical Association*, **300** (6), 676–90.

10. Dhaliwal, L.K., Gupta, K.R., Gopalan, S. and Kulhara, P. (2004) Psychological aspects of infertility due to various causes – prospective study. *International Journal of Fertility and Womens Medicine*, **49** (1), 44–48.

11. King, M., Semlyen, J., See Tai, S. *et al.* (2008) A systematic review of mental disorder, suicide, and deliberate self harm in lesbian, gay and bisexual people. *BMC Psychiatry*, **8** (1), 70 (18 August).

12. King, M. and Nazareth, I. (2006) The health of people classified as lesbian, gay and bisexual attending family practitioners in London: a controlled study. *BMC Public Health*, **6**, 127.

13. Chandra, P.S. and Ranjan, S. (2007) Psychosomatic obstetrics and gynecology – a neglected field? *Current Opinion in Psychiatry*, **20**, 168–173.

14. Fisher, J., Cabral M., Izutsu, T. Mental Health Aspects of Pregnancy, Childbirth and the Postpartum Period. Chapter 9, Section 2.

15. Adewuya, A.O., Ologun, U. and Ibiqbami, O.S. (2006) Posttraumatic stress disorder after childbirth in Nigerian women: prevalence and risk factors. *BJOG: An International Journal of Obstetrics and Gynaecology*, **113**, 284–88.

16. Brockington, I.F., Fraser, C. and Wilson, D. (2006) The postpartum bonding questionnaire: a validation. *Archives of Women's Mental Health*, **9** (5), 233–42.

17. Rahman, A., Lovel, H., Bunn, J. *et al.* (2003) Mothers' mental health and infant growth: a case-control study from Rawalpindi, Pakistan. *Child Care Health and Development*, **30**, 21–27.

18. Lindahl, V., Pearson, J.L. and Colpe, L. (2005) Prevalence of suicidality during pregnancy and the postpartum. *Archives of Women's Mental Health*, **8** (2), 77–87.

19. Chandra, P.S., Bhargavaraman, R.P., Raghunandan, V.N. and Shaligram, D. (2006) Delusions related to infant and their association with mother-infant interactions in postpartum psychotic disorders. *Archives of Women's Mental Health*, **9** (5), 285–88.

20. Cohen, L.S., Soares, C.N., Vitonis, A.F. *et al.* (2006) Risk for new onset of depression during the menopausal transition: the Harvard study of moods and cycles. *Archives of General Psychiatry*, **63**, 385–90.

21. Wassertheil-Smoller, S., Hendrix, S.L., Limacher, M. *et al.* WHI Investigators (2003) Effect of estrogen plus progestin on stroke in postmenopausal women: the Women's Health Initiative: a randomized trial. *The Journal of the American Medical Association*, **289**, 2673–84.

9

Mental health aspects of pregnancy, childbirth and the postpartum period

Jane Fisher[1], Meena Cabral de Mello[2] and Takashi Izutsu[3]

[1]Key Centre for Women's Health in Society, WHO Collaborating Center in Women's Health, University of Melbourne, Melbourne, Australia
[2]Child and Adolescent Health and Development, WHO, Geneva, Switzerland
[3]United Nations Population Fund, New York, USA

In the industrialised world, as pregnancy and childbirth have become safer and maternal mortality rates have declined, awareness has grown in the clinical and research communities of psychological factors associated with health in pregnancy, childbirth and the postpartum period. While there are historical references to disturbed behaviour associated with childbirth, it was not until the 1960s that systematic reports were published of elevated rates of admission to psychiatric hospital in the month after parturition [1]. In 1964, Paffenberger and others reported the nature and course of psychoses following childbirth [2] and also described an atypical depression observable in some women following childbirth. These reports stimulated the substantial research of the past four decades into the nosology of psychiatric illness associated with human reproduction. Most research has been conducted in Australia, Canada, Europe and the United States of America; relatively little evidence is available from developing countries.

Contemporary Topics in Women's Mental Health   Edited by Chandra, Herrman, Fisher, Kastrup,
© 2009 John Wiley & Sons, Ltd   Niaz, Rondón and Okasha

9.1 Mental health and maternal mortality

The predominant focus in endeavours to reduce maternal deaths has been on the direct causes of adverse pregnancy outcomes – obstructed labour, haemorrhage and infection – and on the health services needed to address them [3–5]. Much less attention has been paid to mental health as a contributing factor to maternal deaths. In particular, violence – in the form of self-harm or of harm inflicted by others – during pregnancy or after childbirth has been under-recognised as a contributing factor to maternal mortality [6]. The 2001 World Health Report identified a highly significant relationship between exposure to violence and suicide [7].

Despite close investigation, rates and determinants of suicide in pregnancy or after childbirth have proved difficult to determine, because of the extent to which the problem is underestimated or obscured in recording of causes of death or because systematic data are unavailable [8]. Socially stigmatised causes of death are less reliably recorded and probably under-reported [9, 10]. Postmortem examinations after suicide do not always include the uterine examination necessary to confirm pregnancy and studies that have examined primary records in addition to death certificates have identified significant under-recognition [8, 11]. Investigations of suicide in women often fail to report pregnancy status or consider it as an explanatory factor [12–14]. There are substantial apparent intercountry variations in rates of suicide. Maternal mortality data combine records of deaths occurring during pregnancy and up to 42 days after the end of a pregnancy and, in many settings, specific data regarding suicide or parasuicide in pregnancy are unavailable.

Summary reviews have found that suicide in pregnancy is not common; however, when it happens, it is primarily associated with unwanted pregnancy or entrapment in situations of sexual or physical abuse or poverty [6, 8].

Suicide is disproportionately associated with adolescent pregnancy, and appears to be the last resort for women with an unwanted pregnancy in settings where reproductive choice is limited, for example, where single women are not legally able to obtain contraceptives, and legal pregnancy termination services are unavailable [6, 15].

Investigations in three districts in Turkey found that suicide was one of the five leading causes of death among women of reproductive age, and was associated with age under 25 years and being unmarried; pregnancy status was not reported [16]. Ganatra and Hirve [17], in a population survey of mortality associated with abortion in Maharashtra, India, found that death rates from abortion-related complications was disproportionately higher among adolescents, because they were more likely than older women to use untrained service providers. In addition, a number of adolescents had committed suicide to preserve the family honour without seeking abortion.

There has been relatively limited investigation of suicide after childbirth, but in industrialised countries reported rates are lower than expected, and usually associated with severe depression or postpartum psychosis [18]. Attachment to the infant appears to reduce the risk of suicide in mothers of newborns [15], but population-based comparisons indicate that the rate of suicide among women who have just given birth is not significantly different from the general female suicide rate [19]. Maternal suicide is associated with a heightened risk of infanticide [8]. Confining assessment of maternal mortality to the first six weeks postpartum probably leads to underestimation of maternal mortality from suicide, which may occur much later in the postpartum period [20].

Suicide in combination with other deaths attributable to psychiatric problems, particularly substance abuse, accounted for 28% of maternal deaths in the United Kingdom in 1997–1999 – more than any other single cause [21]. In Sweden, teenage mothers aged under 17 years were found to be at elevated risk of premature death, including suicide and alcohol abuse compared with mothers aged over 20 years [22]. The deaths were not only associated with severe mental illness, but were also related to domestic violence and the complications of substance abuse. Two large data linkage studies found that, compared with childbirth, miscarriage and, more strongly, pregnancy termination were associated with increased suicide risk in the following year, especially among unmarried, young women of low socioeconomic status. These findings were attributed to either a risk factor common to both depression and induced abortion, most probably domestic violence or depression associated with loss of pregnancy [23–25].

There have been very few systematic studies of suicide after childbirth in developing countries. In a detailed classification of cause of 2882 deaths in women of reproductive age, in three provinces in Vietnam in 1994–1995, the leading cause (29%) was external events, including accidents, murder and suicide. Overall 14% of the deaths were by suicide [26]. Lal *et al.* [27] reviewed 219 deaths among 9894 women who had given birth in three rural areas of Haryana, India, in 1992, and found that 20% were due to suicide or accidental burns. Granja *et al.* [28], in a review of pregnancy-related deaths at Maputo Central Hospital, Mozambique, in 1991–1995, found that 9 of 27 (33%) deaths not attributable to pregnancy or coincidental illness were by suicide.

Parasuicide is more prevalent in women than men in most countries. It is associated with low education and socioeconomic status, but predominantly with childhood sexual and physical abuse, and sexual and domestic violence [8, 29]. In pregnancy, suicidal ideation and attempts at self-harm are significantly more common in women with a history of childhood sexual abuse than those without such a history [30, 31].

The Edinburgh Postnatal Depression Scale (EPDS), a widely used screening and research instrument, has a specific item assessing the presence and intensity of suicidal ideation [32]. Most studies using this instrument have not presented data specifically related to this item, but one of the scale's developers [33, 34] has reported that women who are severely depressed commonly have a positive score on it. There is a small emerging body of literature on postpartum parasuicide in developing countries, which suggests that it is not uncommon. Rahman and Hafeez [35] report that more than one-third (36%) of mothers caring for young children and living in refugee camps in the North West Frontier Province of

Pakistan had a mental disorder and that 91% of these women had suicidal thoughts. Fisher *et al.* [36] found that, among a consecutive cohort of 506 women attending infant health clinics six weeks postpartum in Ho Chi Minh City, Vietnam, 20% acknowledged thoughts of wanting to die.

In developing countries, intimate partner violence or violence from other family members is associated with increased maternal mortality, although systematic representative international studies are unavailable. Granja *et al.* [37] found that 37% of pregnancy-related deaths in their investigation in Mozambique were by homicide and 22% were accidents. Batra [38], in describing deaths from burning among young married women in India, noted that 47.8% of the deaths were suicide, with torture by in-laws the most common explanatory factor.

In general, these studies concluded that maternal mortality could be accurately ascertained only if causes of death were expanded to include deaths due to violence inflicted by self or others.

9.2 Mental health and antenatal morbidity

In contrast to the substantial investigations of women's psychological functioning after childbirth, relatively little research has been devoted specifically to mental health during pregnancy [39]. Research has generally focused on the risks for the foetus of poor maternal mental health, in terms of adverse alterations to the intrauterine environment, risky behaviours, in particular substance abuse, failure to attend antenatal clinics and increased risk of adverse obstetric outcome. Conventionally, pregnancy has been regarded as a period of general psychological wellbeing for women, with a lower rate of hospital admissions for psychiatric illness [40, 41], reduced risk of suicide [42] and lower rates of panic disorder [43]. However, Viguera *et al.* [44] reported that risk of recurrence of bipolar affective disorder was not diminished in pregnancy.

9.3 Depression in pregnancy

Llewellyn *et al.* [39] suggest that certain symptoms of depression, including appetite change, lowered energy, sleep disturbance and reduced libido, are considered 'normal' in pregnancy and their psychological significance is therefore underestimated. A range of psychosocial factors has been associated with depression in pregnancy, including unwanted conception, unmarried status, unemployment and low income [45, 46]. Three sources of support appear to influence mood in pregnancy; the woman's own parents, in particular her mother, her partner and her wider social group, including same-age peers [45, 47, 48].

Only a few studies of the prevalence of antenatal depression in South and East Asian, African or South American countries are available. Chen *et al.* [49] surveyed pregnant women attending antenatal clinics at a Singapore obstetric hospital, and reported that 20% had clinically significant depressive symptoms. Young women and women with complicated pregnancies were at elevated risk. Lee *et al.* [50] found that 6.4% of 157 Hong Kong Chinese women in advanced pregnancy were depressed. Fatoye, Adeyemi and Oladimeji (2004) found higher rates of depressive and anxious symptoms in pregnant women than in matched non-pregnant women in Nigeria. Depression was associated with having a polygamous partner, a previous termination of pregnancy and a previous caesarean birth. In a small study of 33 low-income Brazilian women, Da Silva *et al.* [51] found that 12% were depressed in later pregnancy, and that depression was associated with insufficient support from the partner and lower parity. Chandran *et al.* [52] interviewed a consecutive cohort of 359 women registered for antenatal care in a rural community in Tamil Nadu, India, and found that 16.2% were depressed in the last trimester. Rahman *et al.* [53] established that 25% of pregnant women attending services in Kahuta, a rural community in Pakistan, were depressed in the third trimester of pregnancy. Risk was increased among the poorest women and those experiencing coincidental adverse life events.

9.4 Anxiety in pregnancy

There has been a widely held belief that anxiety in pregnancy is harmful to the foetus and contributes to adverse obstetric outcomes. The incidence of anxiety disorders is the same in pregnant women and those who are not pregnant [54]. Subclinical levels of anxiety vary normally through pregnancy, with peaks in the first and third trimester, and are specifically focused on infant health and wellbeing and childbirth [55, 56]. Anxiety in pregnancy is higher among younger, less well-educated women of low socioeconomic status [57].

Pregnant women are generally encouraged to modify their self-care and personal habits to ensure optimal maternal and foetal health. This includes advice to alter their diet, avoid alcohol, stop smoking cigarettes, gain a specified amount of weight, exercise (but not to excess), rest, relax and have regular health checks. The evidence for some of this advice is poor, and the recommendations have been criticised for failing to take into account personal circumstances and social realities [58]. It is difficult for women to ensure adequate nutrition for themselves if they are poor or have restricted access to shared resources [59]. Smoking and substance abuse in pregnancy are associated with depression arising from conflict in marital and family relationships, domestic violence and financial concerns [45, 60, 61]. Women who smoke in pregnancy have poorer nutritional intake [62]. Both physical and sexual abuse are predictive of substance abuse in pregnant adolescents [30]. Pregnant women who are dependent on opiates and have a co-morbid diagnosis of post-traumatic stress disorder (PTSD) are more likely than those without PTSD to have history of sexual abuse and to have experienced severe conflict in their family of origin [63]. Poorer health in pregnancy and delay in accessing antenatal care are linked to insufficient social support [64].

In addition to social factors, participation in prenatal genetic screening and diagnosis can also generate anxiety [65]. This occurs independently of the results of the test, and is worse if there is a long interval between the test and the result becoming available [65]. In the past decade, research has focused on the determinants of informed, autonomous decision making and uptake of services, but not on the emotional consequences of participation in prenatal genetic screening and diagnosis. There is currently no evidence of the psychological impact of increased surveillance during pregnancy on the overall experience of pregnancy and the postnatal period. Systematic investigations are difficult because services are changing rapidly.

Termination of pregnancy for foetal abnormality is relatively rare, but can have significant and lasting psychological consequences [65]. Hunfeld *et al.* [66] compared 27 women with a history of late pregnancy loss (after 20 weeks) due to foetal abnormality, who subsequently had a live birth, with 27 mothers of newborns without such a history. Those with prior pregnancy loss had significantly greater anxiety and depression than women without such a history; this was interpreted as re-evoked grief about the previous loss. They also perceived their infants as having more problems and were more anxious about infant care [66, 67]. Prenatal screening and diagnosis can now be carried out early in pregnancy, and little is known about the psychological consequences of first trimester termination of pregnancy for foetal abnormality. Most research on first-trimester abortion has focused on those carried out for social reasons, after which psychological morbidity is low [68]. Decision-making about first-trimester abortion for foetal abnormality is complicated by the fact that many affected pregnancies, if left, will terminate spontaneously [69]. There is no evidence on the psychological aspects of forced termination of pregnancy, or pregnancy termination associated with sex selection, in settings with restrictions on family size and a preference for male children.

9.5 Cultural preferences and mental health in pregnancy

In many cultures, there is a preference for sons rather than daughters; the psychological consequences of this for pregnant women have not been systematically investigated. Country-level sex ratios are skewed in favour of males in China, India and the Republic of Korea [70, 71]. Clinicians can use techniques such as ultrasound, amniocentesis and chorionic villus sampling to determine foetal sex, and female foetuses may subsequently be aborted selectively [72]. Although legislation prohibits this practise, it is known to persist. Women can be blamed for sex determination and may not be able to make a free choice about continuing or terminating a pregnancy [70, 71]. The birth of a daughter was found to contribute independently to postpartum depression in women in India and

Pakistan [52, 73, 74]; it is therefore reasonable to speculate that mental health during pregnancy may also be adversely affected by the family and social reaction to the conception of a daughter.

9.6 Inflicted violence and mental health in pregnancy

Violence is estimated to occur in between 4 and 8% of pregnancies [75], although higher rates have been reported: 11% in South Carolina between 1993 and 1995 [76]; 13.5% in an American prenatal care programme [77]; 15.7% among women attending an antenatal clinic in a hospital in Hong Kong, China [78] and 22% among women attending a routine antenatal clinic in Nagpur, India [79].

Investigations have focused on the links between violence and adverse maternal and neonatal outcomes, with relatively little emphasis to date on mental health [75, 80]. However Muhajarine and D'Arcy [81] found that women who had experienced physical abuse in pregnancy reported higher stress and more coincidental adverse life events, while Webster *et al.* [82] reported that they were more likely to be taking antidepressant medication than women who had not experienced violence. Steward and Cecutti [83] found that abused women in a range of prenatal care settings were significantly more emotionally distressed than non-abused women.

9.7 Mental health and postpartum morbidity

In becoming a mother, a woman often has to relinquish her autonomy, personal liberty, occupational identity, capacity to generate an income and social and leisure activities in favour of caring for the infant. The adaptation to her new required roles, major responsibilities, moving from being in the childless generation to the parent generation, increased unpaid workload and, for some, harm to bodily integrity through unexpected adverse reproductive events places great demands both on individual psychological resources and on existing relationships. Psychological disequilibrium is normal during life transitions and in adapting to change, and there is continuing theoretical consideration of the extent to which perinatal psychological disorder should be regarded as a normal process. However, there is now substantial evidence that women's mental health can be compromised by childbirth and that some women experience psychiatric illness. Debate continues about whether psychiatric illnesses occurring in pregnancy or after childbirth are clinically distinct from those observed at other phases of the life cycle, and of the relative aetiological contributions of biological and psychosocial factors. There is now a consistent view that psychological disturbance following childbirth can be conceptualised as fitting one of three distinct conditions, of differing severity: transient mood disturbance, depression and psychotic illness.

9.8 Postpartum blues or mild transient mood disturbance

Maternity, third day or postpartum blues are a phenomenon occurring in up to 80% of women in the days immediately following childbirth [84, 85]. The syndrome is characterised by a range of symptoms, most commonly a lability of mood between euphoria and misery, heightened sensitivity, tearfulness often without associated sadness, restlessness, poor concentration, anxiety and irritability [86, 87]. Disturbed sleep [88], feelings of unreality and detachment from the baby have also been reported [1]. There have been a small number of specific transcultural studies of the nature and incidence of postpartum blues, which have reported rates in non-Anglophone countries ranging from 13 to 50% [89, 90]. Sutter et al. [91] reported a rate of 42.5% in a sample of French mothers. Very limited evidence is available about postpartum blues in developing countries. Devidson [92] reported that 60% of newly delivered women in Jamaica were tearful or sad, while Ghubash and Abou-Salech [93] found that 24.5% of Arab women met the criteria for a clinical case of psychiatric morbidity using the WHO Self Reporting Questionnaire on the second day after birth. The coincidence of the maternity blues with the major hormonal changes associated with parturition has led investigations to look for a biological basis to the condition, but findings are generally inconsistent [1, 94]. The distress peaks between three and five days postpartum, and usually resolves spontaneously without specialist intervention. However, in some women a more persistent and severe depression develops. There is some evidence that the more severe symptoms of blues, including early self-reports of feeling depressed, having thoughts about death or being unable to stop crying, predict later development of depression [91, 95].

9.9 Postpartum psychotic illness

A very small group of women (approximately 1 or 2 per 1000) develop an acute psychosis within the first month postpartum; this is the most severe psychiatric illness associated with childbirth. Relative lifetime risk and incidence are usually calculated in terms of psychiatric admissions for treatment of psychotic illness after childbirth. The risk for women of experiencing a psychotic illness is highly elevated for the first 30 days postpartum and remains elevated, but at a lower rate, for two years following childbirth [41, 96]. Clinical characteristics include acute onset and extreme affective variation, with mania and elation as well as sadness, thought disorder, delusions, hallucinations, disturbed behaviour and confusion [97–99]. Postpartum psychoses are most accurately construed as episodes of cycloid affective illness; rates of schizophrenic psychotic episodes are not elevated postnatally [41, 90, 98, 100, 101]. Although treatment is similar, there is a divergence of views as to whether puerperal psychotic episodes in an individual with an existing diagnosis of bipolar affective disorder should be understood to be the same as first episodes following childbirth [98]. Risk of recurrence after subsequent pregnancies is between 51 and 69% [98].

There is continuing conjecture about the relative contributions of biological and psychosocial aetiological factors to the development of postpartum psychoses and the possibilities of meta-analysis to elucidate this are restricted by methodological limitations in existing studies [98]. However, the timing of onset of the illness, family history and molecular genetic studies support an underlying biological aetiology, with childbirth as the precipitating factor [98]. Postpartum psychosis has been associated with primiparity, personal or family history of affective psychosis, unmarried status and perinatal death of an infant [41, 102]. The contribution of obstetric factors is not clear, but there is some evidence that caesarean delivery increases the risk of postpartum psychosis and of relapse after subsequent births [96, 103, 104]. Puerperal and non-puerperal episodes of psychosis are predicted most strongly by a history of psychotic episodes and by marital difficulties [97].

Investigations of women admitted to hospital with postpartum mental illness in countries outside Western Europe and North America report higher rates of puerperal psychosis. Schizophrenia is reported more commonly than affective illness in those settings, but these patterns may reflect intercountry differences in diagnostic criteria [89, 90]. Both Howard [89] and Kumar [90] highlighted the higher incidence in developing countries of puerperal psychoses associated with organic illness, including confusional states related to fever from infections or to poor nutrition. Ndosi and Mtawali [105] described a case series of 86 women who developed psychosis within six weeks of giving birth in the United Republic of Tanzania; the incidence rate of 3.2 per 1000 was approximately double that reported in industrialised countries. Most of the women were young and primiparous; co-existing anaemia and infectious illnesses were common and 80% of the illnesses were categorised as organic psychoses.

9.10 Postpartum depression

Over the lifespan, on average, women experience major depression between 1.6 and 2.6 times more often than men. This difference is most apparent in the life phase of caring for infants and young children [106, 107]. Depression arising after childbirth has attracted substantial research interest in the past 40 years, and there is now an extensive literature on its nature, prevalence, prediction, course and associations with risk and protective factors.

Postpartum depression is a clinical and research construct used to describe an episode of major or minor depression arising after childbirth [106, 108, 109]. The International Classification of Diseases (ICD 10) [110] does not have a specific diagnostic category of postpartum depression, and classifies depression after childbirth as a depressive episode of either mild (four symptoms), moderate (five symptoms) or severe (at least five symptoms, with agitation, feelings of worthlessness or guilt or suicidal thoughts or acts).

While there is debate about whether depression following childbirth is a clinically distinct condition, there is consistent evidence that 10–15% of women in industrialised countries will experience non-psychotic clinical depression in the year after giving birth, with most developing it in the first five weeks postpartum [106, 111, 112]. Severe depression, needing inpatient treatment, occurs in 3–7% of women after childbirth [113].

There is also a lack of clarity over how long the postpartum period should be considered to last, and therefore for how long after delivery a depression can be regarded as specifically postnatal in onset [110, 114]. There is a clustering of new cases around childbirth, which is argued to be distinctive [115]. DSM IV specifies within a month of parturition, but Nott [116] found that the highest incidence of new cases occurred three to nine months postpartum. Chaudron *et al.* [117] demonstrated that 5.8% of cases of depression identified at four months postpartum were not apparent at one month. Most conceptualisations take a categorical approach, in which individuals are classified as satisfying the criteria for a clinical case, or are regarded as well. Some authors, however [118–120], argue that adjustment processes, including transient dysphoria and symptoms of depression, can be observed in most women postpartum, and that a continuum of emotional wellbeing or a broad spectrum of adjustment experiences may be a more accurate conceptualisation. Mood in the first year after childbirth is dynamic and determined by multiple factors [121, 122]. In practise, it is common for any episode of depression during this period to be regarded as linked to the birth [99].

The causes of depression in the postpartum period are still the subject of controversy, debate and research. Broadly, the arguments concern the relative contributions of biological and psycho-social factors. Biochemical hypotheses hold that the dramatic hormonal changes that follow childbirth and are involved in lactation may precipitate or maintain depression [106, 123]. Links between postpartum depression and a history of premenstrual mood change or increased familial vulnerability to affective illness and alcohol dependence are cited in support of a biological aetiology [124]. However, summary and systematic reviews have concluded that, although some women may be particularly psychologically vulnerable to hormonal change, a direct link between hormones or other neurochemicals and postpartum depression has not yet been demonstrated [1, 99, 123].

9.11 Psychosocial risk factors for postpartum depression

A personal history of mood disorder, previous psychiatric hospitalisation and anxious or depressed mood in pregnancy are consistently found to be predictive of postpartum depression [95, 99, 112, 125–127].

A poor relationship between the woman and her partner is now regarded as a major predictor of depression after childbirth [99, 112, 114, 119, 127]. The problems in this relationship have been variously conceptualised as: increased marital conflict [128]; men being less available after delivery, and providing insufficient practical support [129] or poor emotional support [130]; poor adjustment or unhappiness [125]; low satisfaction [127]; insufficient involvement in infant care [119] and holding rigid traditional sex role expectations [126]. The relationship with the partner also appears to significantly affect the time taken to recover [121]. Very similar findings have emerged from transcultural studies. A poor quality of marital relationship – variously described as inability to confide in an intimate partner or lack of support, or arguments and tension in the relationship – is centrally related to women's mental health postpartum, and has been found to distinguish depressed from non-depressed women in Hong Kong, China [131], India [52, 132], Pakistan [74] and Vietnam [133].

Unfortunately, most research on the aetiology of postpartum depression has not assessed the effect of coercion, intimidation and violence by the intimate partner. A prospective cohort study of 838 parturient Chinese women in Hong Kong, China [134], using the Abuse Assessment Screen, found that 16.6% had been abused in the previous year. Among women who had experienced domestic violence, higher scores on the EPDS were reported two to three days after delivery, one to two days after discharge from hospital and six weeks postpartum than among those with no experience of violence. There was no difference between the two groups of women in terms of sociodemographic factors, although the abused women were more likely to report that their pregnancy had been unplanned.

Broader social factors are also associated with depression after childbirth. Poor social support, including having few friends or confiding relationships and lack of assistance in crises, is related to postpartum depression. General dissatisfaction with available support, rather than specific characteristics or number or quality of relationships, appears to be relevant [99, 127, 135]. Postpartum depression has been found to be more common among young mothers and single women [125, 130, 136].

Social disruption associated with recent immigration or relocation, especially if compounded by being unable to speak the local language and understand and obtain local services, also heightens the risk of difficulties in adjusting to parenthood [89, 125, 137, 138].

International studies have also found that a lack of practical assistance from family, including dedicated care during the early postpartum period, is more commonly reported by women who are depressed than those who are not depressed [50, 52, 74, 132, 133, 139, 140]. If this practical dedicated support is available from a supportive and uncritical person, it is psychologically protective [74, 133, 141]. Problematic relationships with the partner's family, especially critical coercion from the mother-in-law, have been found to be more common among women who are depressed in both qualitative [132] and survey investigations [52, 74, 133, 140, 141].

However, there is consistent evidence that maternal mental health is directly affected by poverty in resource-poor countries [142]. Limited education reduces women's access to paid occupations and secure employment. Women living in poverty and experiencing economic difficulties, who have low education and no access to employment that allow them time to care for their infant, are more likely to be depressed [52, 132, 133, 140, 143].

In developing countries, bereavement or serious illness in the family, the partner not having an income, housing difficulties, crowded living conditions and lack of privacy are associated with higher rates of maternal depression [52, 74, 133].

9.12 Infant factors and maternal mental health

Cross-sectional cohort comparisons have found that mothers who are depressed are significantly more likely to report excessive infant crying and disturbed infant sleep and feeding than mothers who are not depressed [144–146]. Some authors have interpreted this as indicating that the behaviour of depressed mothers increases the likelihood of disturbed infant behaviour [144, 146]. However, others acknowledge that the care of an unsettled, crying infant, who resists soothing and has deregulated sleep, undermines maternal confidence and wellbeing and may be relevant to the onset of maternal depression and to disturbances in mother-infant interaction. These inter-relationships have not yet been well conceptualised and are generally under-investigated, but evidence is emerging that they may be more significant than has previously been acknowledged [115, 147, 148].

Hopkins *et al.* [149] compared 25 depressed mothers of six-week-old babies with 24 non-depressed mothers of the same age, socioeconomic status and religious affiliation. They found that the infants of the depressed mothers had more neonatal complications and were less adaptable and fussier than those of the mothers who were not depressed.

Mothers can feel ineffective and helpless caring for an inconsolable infant. Confidence can diminish rapidly and they are less likely to experience their infants as a source of positive reinforcement [150]. Excessive infant crying is associated with earlier cessation of breastfeeding, frequent changes of infant formula, maternal irritability, poor mother-infant relationship, deterioration in the familial emotional environment and heightened risk of infant abuse [151, 152].

9.13 Cultural specificity of postpartum mood disturbance

It has been argued that culturally prescribed ritual forms of peripartum care for women are psychologically protective [89, 153–155]. Socially structured peripartum customs are characterised as providing dedicated care, an honoured status, relief from normal tasks and responsibilities and social seclusion for the mother and her newborn [89, 90, 155].

More recent studies have used validated screening and diagnostic tools to investigate whether postpartum depression is a culture-bound condition. While there is still debate about appropriate methods of measurement, it appears that – if the complexities of translation, literacy levels and familiarity with test-taking are taken into account-structured interviews and screening instruments, such as the EPDS, can be used cross-culturally [156–158].

A number of studies have compared peripartum experiences, rates of depression and risk factors in groups of different ethnicity living in industrialised countries. Fuggle *et al.* [159] examined small groups of Bangladeshi women living in London and Dhaka with English women, and found an overall rate of depression of 11.5%, with no difference between groups. Matthey *et al.* [160] reported that there were no differences in scores in the clinical range on the EPDS between Vietnamese, Arabic and Anglo-Celtic women living in south-west Sydney. Despite some variation in the ranking of the contribution of different risk factors by ethnic group [161], the risk factors identified as relevant to all groups were highly consistent. They were: inability to confide in the partner and insufficient practical support from the partner [160, 161] or from parents or the wider social circle [159].

Studies using structured clinical interviews or screening questionnaires have been conducted in a range of non-English-speaking countries, to establish the incidence and correlates of clinically significant depressive symptoms in the early postpartum period. In Europe, the following incidence rates were found: 8.7% in Malta [162]; 14% in Iceland [163]; 9% in Italy and 11% in France [164]; 11.4% in Sweden and 14.5% in Finland [165] and 29.7% in Spain (based on clinical case criteria in the General Health Questionnaire (GHQ)) [166]. In Singapore, 3.5% of postpartum women satisfied the criteria for a clinical case, but 86% had some depressive symptoms three months postpartum [167]; in Hong Kong, China, 13.5% of postpartum women had a diagnosable psychiatric illness [168] and in Japan the incidence was 17% [169]. In Israel, Glasser *et al.* [170] found that 22.6% of women had EPDS scores in the clinical range at six weeks postpartum.

There is little evidence to support the notion that women in developing countries do not experience depression [133, 171, 172]. The finding of high rates of postpartum depression in developing country contexts challenges the anthropological view that ritual postpartum care protects women. It appears that this assertion may be an oversimplification and warrants more comprehensive and detailed investigation. Even where it is culturally prescribed, ritual may not be available to all women [133, 140]. Observation of postpartum rituals, including lying over heat, wearing warm clothes and using cotton swabs in the ears to protect the body against 'cold', and taking herbal preparations, was no less common among Vietnamese women who were depressed than among those who were not [133].

Wider family relationships are also implicated, but as yet the evidence available is limited. However, problematic relationships with the partner's family, especially critical coercion from a mother-in-law, have been reported to be more common among women who are depressed in both qualitative investigations [132] and survey investigations [52, 74, 133, 140]. In addition, a lack of practical assistance from the family, including dedicated care during the early postpartum period, is more commonly reported by women who are depressed than those who are not depressed [52, 74, 132, 133, 139, 140]. If practical dedicated support is available, it is psychologically protective [74, 133].

There is consistent evidence that maternal mental health is also influenced by socioeconomic factors [142]. Limited education reduces womens' access to paid occupations and secure employment. Women living in poverty and experiencing economic difficulties, who have low education and no access to employment that allows them time to care for their infant are more likely to be depressed [52, 132, 133, 140, 143].

A comprehensive assessment of the links between reproductive experiences and mental health in developing countries is not yet available, However, evidence is emerging that women who have adverse obstetric experiences, including operative birth, poor postpartum health and difficulties in breastfeeding, are more likely to report depressive symptoms in the immediate postpartum period [133, 139, 143].

The focus on postpartum depression has excluded consideration of other relevant expressions of psychological distress in women after childbirth. In particular, relatively little attention has been devoted to the nature and prevalence of postnatal anxiety disorders, despite evidence of substantial co-morbidity with depression [173, 174]. The relevance of PTSDs to mental health in pregnancy, and the potential of childbirth and other reproductive events to evoke post-traumatic stress reactions, remain under explored [175–177].

9.14 Maternal mental health, infant development and the mother-infant relationship

Depression after childbirth, through its negative impact on the mother's interpersonal functioning, disrupts the quality and sensitivity of the mother-infant interaction. This can have adverse effects on the emotional, cognitive and social development of the infant. Postnatal depression reduces the sensitivity, warmth, acceptance and responsiveness of the mother to her infant [178].

Examinations of the behaviour of infants in face-to-face interactions with their depressed mothers have reported fewer positive facial expressions, more negative expressions and protest behaviour, higher levels of withdrawal and avoidance, more fussing and an absence of positive affect [179]. Two-month-old infants whose mothers were depressed had higher rates of disrupted behaviour and were more likely to avoid contact with their mothers than comparison infants [178].

Independently of the adverse effects of poverty, crowded living conditions and infectious diseases, maternal depression contributes to infant failure to thrive in resource-poor settings [180]. Patel *et al.* [181] examined the impact of maternal depression six to eight weeks postpartum on the subsequent growth and development of infants in Goa, India. Compared with controls, infants of depressed mothers were more than twice as likely to be underweight at six months of age (30% versus 12%) and three times more likely to be short for age (25% versus 8%). They also had significantly lower mental development scores, even after adjustment for birth weight and maternal education [181], in a case-control study in a rural community in Tamil Nadu, India, found that infants whose weight was 50–80% of the expected weight for age were significantly more likely to have a mother who was depressed than infants of normal weight.

These effects do not necessarily remit when maternal mood improves. There is consistent evidence of poorer cognitive development in preschool-age children of mothers who were depressed postnatally [178, 182, 183]. Young boys whose mothers were depressed postnatally were found to have poorer cognitive development and to display more antisocial behaviour, over activity and distractibility compared with boys whose mothers were not postnatally depressed [184–186].

Hay *et al.* [187] examined the long-term consequences of maternal depression in a community sample of 132 11-year-old children from south London, whose mothers had completed psychiatric interviews three months postpartum. Children, especially boys, whose mothers had been depressed had significantly lower intelligence scores, and a higher rate of special educational needs, including difficulties in mathematical reasoning and visuomotor performance, and more attentional problems than those whose mothers had been well [187].

Luoma *et al.* [188] assessed a group of school-age children whose mothers had been depressed, according to the EPDS, antenatally, postnatally or currently. They found that depression present both during pregnancy and after childbirth was strongly predictive of behavioural problems in the children at eight to nine years of age. The worst child outcomes were predicted by a combination of prenatal and recurrent maternal depression [188].

A meta-analysis of nine studies [189] found small but significant adverse effects of maternal postpartum depression on the cognitive and emotional development of children older than one year. However, other investigators have found no association between postnatal depression and adverse child development in women who are socially advantaged [185]. When social adversity is taken into account, statistical differences between depressed and non-depressed groups often disappear [190].

The sensitivity of fathers is also a crucial mediating factor. Sensitive fathers reduce the impact of maternal depression and reduced responsiveness, especially for temperamentally reactive infants. Conversely, maternal sensitivity is reduced and risk of depression is increased if the partner behaves aggressively either during pregnancy or postpartum [78, 191]. In general, the long-term adverse effects of maternal depression on child cognitive outcomes are mostly confined to socioeconomically disadvantaged groups, and are worse for boys.

Most of the research into the impact of maternal postnatal depression on child development has been done in developed countries. The recent findings in developing countries of the close relationship between the mental health of mothers and the physical and mental development of their children are of vital importance to both child health and maternal and reproductive health programmes, especially in areas with high rates of poor infant growth.

9.15 Prevention and treatment of maternal mental health problems

Most mild depression in the postpartum year resolves as mothers gain more experience and their confidence grows. However, more severe depression can persist, becoming chronic or recurring from time to time [192].

A range of interventions to prevent the development of depression have been tested in randomised controlled trials; most have had only a modest or negligible effect. Screening questionnaires administered during pregnancy to identify women at risk of becoming depressed after childbirth have low positive predictive values, and reviewers have concluded that there is insufficient evidence to introduce screening as part of routine antenatal care [193]. 'Preparation-for-parenthood' groups for women during pregnancy did not prevent postpartum depression, except when partners were included in at least one session [56, 194]. Although the quality of a woman's relationships, in particular with her partner, is central to her emotional wellbeing during pregnancy and after childbirth, most interventions have not involved family members.

Two recent systematic reviews have concluded that the research base on preventive interventions is extremely limited, and there is currently no compelling evidence to support the introduction of any of the interventions that have been tested in primary prevention trials [99, 193].

There have been a number of randomised controlled trials of treatments for postnatal depression, but many are limited because of high rates of loss to follow-up, a short follow-up period or potential bias because most eligible respondents refused to participate [195, 196]. Both pharmacological and psychological treatments have been found to reduce the severity of symptoms and the duration of depression [197]. Decisions about prescribing pharmacological treatments – usually antidepressant medication – have to be weighed against the potential harm to the foetus or infant, as the drug may be transmitted through the placenta and in breast milk. Most women prefer a non-pharmacological approach [112]. Psychological approaches, combining problem-solving strategies, supportive empathic listening and opportunities to focus on past and present relationships, either in groups or individually, are more effective than routine care in reducing depression. A randomised trial comparing non-directive counselling, cognitive behavioural therapy, psychodynamic therapy and routine primary care found short-term improvements in maternal mood with all treatments; however, only psychodynamic therapy significantly reduced depression [198].

In Taiwan, China, women who attended weekly support group meetings had lower scores on the Beck Depression Inventory, less perceived stress and improved perception of interpersonal support than controls who did not attend group meetings [199]. It is generally agreed that a team approach, involving primary care providers, allied health workers and specialist mental health practitioners, as well as a range of health facilities, is needed [101, 200].

While there have been a number of trials of treatments for postnatal depression, relatively few have been designed to improve developmental outcomes for the child. Murray *et al.* [190], in a comparison of home visits by professional health visitors trained to provide one of three psychotherapies to depressed mothers of newborns, found that non-directive counselling fostered more sensitive mother-infant interactions among those who were experiencing social adversity than psychodynamic or cognitive behavioural therapies. At four months, mothers who received counselling reported fewer difficulties in various aspects of their relationship with their infant, such as play, separation and management of infant needs for attention, compared received routine primary care.

9.16 Summary

Future research

1. Research attention has focused disproportionately on mental health after childbirth, compared with mental health during pregnancy, which warrants more comprehensive investigation.

2. There is increasing evidence about the predictors, prevalence and correlates of poor postpartum mental health in developing countries, but investigations have yet to be conducted in some of the poorest countries.

3. The contribution of maternal mental health to maternal mortality should be ascertained, covering events up to one year postpartum.

4. Interventions to prevent the development of psychopathology after childbirth have focused almost exclusively on women. Emerging evidence suggests that strategies involving partners may be more effective, but these need to be designed and appropriately evaluated.

5. Randomised controlled trials are needed of treatments for depression, during pregnancy and after childbirth that are suitable for use in primary care settings.

6. Investigations of infant development following maternal depression should ascertain and control for the contribution of social adversity.

7. The contribution of intimate partner violence and coercion to women's perinatal mental health has been neglected and warrants inclusion in future investigations.

Policy

1. Risk factors for poor mental health should be ascertained as part of routine primary perinatal healthcare.

2. Mental health is integral to safe motherhood, and should be included in all future initiatives, programmes and recommendations for standard care.

Services

1. All health professionals in perinatal and maternal and infant services should have the skills needed to assess psychological well-being and provide comprehensive, psychologically informed care.

2. Assessment of risk factors for poor reproductive mental health should be routine in perinatal healthcare. These include: past personal or family history of psychiatric illness or substance abuse; past personal history of sexual, physical or emotional abuse; current exposure to intimate partner violence or coercion; current social adversity; coincidental adverse life events and unsettled infant behaviour or developmental difficulties.

3. Specialist perinatal mental health services require an understanding of the contribution of denial of human rights to poor mental health.

References

1. Robinson, G.E. and Stewart, D.E. (1993) Postpartum disorders, in *Psychological Aspects of Women's Health Care: The Interface Bewteen Psychiatry and Obstetrics and Gynecology* (eds N. Stotland and D. Stewart), American Psychiatric Press, Washington, DC.

2. Paffenberger, R. (1964) Epidemiological aspects of postpartum mental illness. *British Journal of Preventive and Social Medicine*, **18**, 189–95.

3. Stokoe, U. (1991) Determinants of maternal mortality in the developing world. *Australian and New Zealand Journal of Obstetrics and Gynaecology*, **31** (1), 8–16.

4. Maine, D. and Rosenfield, A. (1999) The safe motherhood initiative: why has it stalled? *American Journal of Public Health*, **89** (4), 480–82.

5. Goodburn, E. and Campbell, O. (2001) Reducing maternal mortality in the developing world; sector-wide approaches may be the key. *British Medical Journal*, **322** (7291), 917–20.

6. Frautschi, S., Cerulli, A. and Maine, D. (1994) Suicide during pregnancy and its neglect as a component of maternal mortality. *International Journal of Gynaecology and Obstetrics*, **47**, 275–84.

7. WHO (2001) The World Health Report 2001. Mental Health: New Understanding, New Hope, World Health Organization, Geneva.

8. Brockington, I. (2001) Suicide in women. *International Clinical Psychopharmacology*, **16**, S7–19.

9. Radovanovic, Z. (1994) Mortality patterns in Kuwait: inferences from death certificate data. *European Journal of Epidemiology*, **10** (6), 733–36W.

10. Graham, W.J., Flilippi, V.G.A. and Ronsmans, C. (1996) Demonstrating programme impact on maternal mortality. *Health Policy and Planning*, **11** (1), 16–20.

11. Weir, J. (1984) Suicide during pregnancy in London 1943–1962, in *Suicide in Pregnancy* (eds G. Kleiner and W. Greston), Wright, Boston, pp. 40–62.

12. Hjelmeland, H., Hawton, K., Nordvik, H. *et al.* (2002) Why people engage in parasuicide: a cross-cultural study of intentions. *Suicide and Life-Threatening Behaviour*, **32**, 380–93.

13. Pearson, V., Phillips, M.R., He, F. and Ji, H. (2002) Attempted suicide among young rural women in the People's Republic of China: possibilities for prevention. *Suicide and Life-Threatening Behaviour*, **32**, 359–68.

14. Hicks, M. and Bhugra, D. (2003) Perceived causes of suicide attempts by UK South Asian women. *The American Journal of Orthopsychiatry*, **73**, 455–62.

15. Appleby, L. (1991) Suicide during pregnancy and in the first postnatal year. *British Medical Journal*, **302** (6769), 126–27.

16. Tezcan, S. and Guciz Dogan, B. (1990) The extent and causes of mortality among reproductive age women on three districts of Turkey. *Nufusbilim Dergisi*, **12**, 31–39.

17. Ganatra, B. and Hirve, S. (2002) Induced abortion among adolescent women in rural Maharashtra, India. *Reproductive Health Matters*, **10**, 76–85.

18. Appleby, L., Mortensen, P.B. and Faragher, B. (1998) Suicide and other causes of mortality after postpartum psychiatric admission. *The British Journal of Psychiatry*, **173** (9), 209–11.

19. Oates, M. (2003a) Suicide: the leading cause of maternal death. *The British Journal of Psychiatry*, **183**, 279–81.

20. Yip, S-K., Chung, T.K-H. and Lee, T-S. (1997) Suicide and maternal mortality in Hong Kong. *Lancet*, **350** (9084), 1103.

21. Oates, M. (2003b) Perinatal psychiatric disorders: a leading cause of maternal morbidity and mortality. *British Medical Bulletin*, **67**, 219–29.

22. Otterblad Olausson, P., Haglund, B., Ringback Weitoft, G. and Cnattingius, S. (2004) Premature death among teenage mothers. *BJOG: An International Journal of Obstetrics and Gynaecology*, **111**, 793–99.

23. Gissler, M. and Hemminki, E. (1999) Pregnancy-related violent deaths. *Scandinavian Journal of Public Health*, **27** (1), 54–55.

24. Gissler, M., Hemminki, E. and Lonnqvist, J. (1996) Suicides after pregnancy in Finland, 1987–1994: register linkage study. *British Medical Journal*, **313**, 1431–34.

25. Reardon, D.C., Ney, P.G., Scheuren, F.J., Cougle, J.R, Coleman, P.K. and Strahan, T. (2002) Deaths associated with pregnancy outcome: a record linkage study of low income women. *Southern Medical Journal*, **95** (8), 834–41.

26. Hieu, D.T., Hanenberg, R., Vach, T.H., Vinh, D.Q. and Sokal, D. (1999) Maternal mortality in Vietnam in 1994–1995. *Studies in Family Planning*, **30** (4), 329–38.

27. Lal, S., Satpath, Khanna, *et al.* (1995) Problem of mortality in Women of reproductive age in rural area of Haryana, India. *Journal of Maternal Child Health*, Jan-Mar (1), 17–21.

28. Granja, A., Zacarias, E., Bergstrom, S. (2002) Violent deaths: the hidden face of maternal mortality, *BJOG: an International Journal of Obstetrics and Gynaecology*, **109**, 5–8.

29. Stark, E. and Flitcraft, A. (1995) Killing the beast within: woman battering and female suicidality. *International Journal of Health Services*, **25** (1), 43–64.

30. Bayatpour, M., Wells, R.D. and Holford, S. (1992) Physical and sexual abuse as predictors of substance use and suicide among pregnant teenagers. *The Journal of Adolescent Health*, **13**, 128–32.

31. Farber, E.W., Herbert, S.E. and Reviere, S.L. (1996) Childhood abuse and suicidality in obstetrics patients in a hospital-based urban prenatal clinic. *General Hospital Psychiatry*, **18**, 56–60.

32. Cox, J.L., Holden, J.M. and Sagovsky, R. (1987) Detection of postnatal depression. Development of the 10-item Edinburgh Postnatal Depression Scale. *The British Journal of Psychiatry*, **150**, 782–86.

33. Holden, J. (1991) Postnatal depression: its nature, effects, and identification using the Edinburgh postnatal depression scale. *Birth*, **18** (4), 211–20.

34. Holden, J. (1994) Can non-psychotic depression be prevented? in *Perinatal Psychiatry. The Use and Misuse of the Edinburgh Postnatal Depression Scale* (eds J. Cox and J. Holden), Gaskell, London, pp. 55–81.

35. Rahman, A., Hafeez, A. (2003) Suicidal feelings run high among mothers in refugee camps: a crosssectional survey. *Acta Psychiatrica Scandinavica*, **108**, 392–93.

36. Fisher, J.R.W., Morrow, M.M., Nhu Ngoc, N.T. and Hoang Anh, L.T. (2004) Prevalence, nature, severity and correlates of postpartum depressive symptoms in Vietnam. *BJOG: An International Journal of Obstetrics and Gynaecology*, **111**, 1353–60.

37. Granja, A., Zacarias, E., Bergstrom, S. (2002) Violent deaths: the hidden face of maternal mortality, *BJOG: an International Journal of Obstetrics and Gynaecology*, **109**, 5–8.

38. Batra, A. (2003) Burn mortality: recent trends and sociocultural determinants, *Burns*, **29**, 270–5.

39. Llewellyn, A.M., Stowe, Z.M. and Nemeroff, C.B. (1997) Depression during pregnancy and the puerperium. *The Journal of Clinical Psychiatry*, **58** (15), 26–32.

40. Oppenheim, G.B. (1985) Psychological disorders in pregnancy, in *Psychological Disorders in Obstetrics and Gynaecology* (ed. R. Priest), Butterworths, London, pp. 93–146.

41. Kendell, R.E., Chalmers, J.C. and Platz, C. (1987) Epidemiology of puerperal psychosis. *The British Journal of Psychiatry*, **150**, 662–73.

42. Marzuk, P.M., Tardiff, K., Leon, A.C., Hirsch, C.S., Portera, L., Hartwell, N. and Iqbal, M.I. (1997) Lower risk of suicide during pregnancy. *The American Journal of Psychiatry*, **154** (1), 122–23.

43. Sharma, V. (1997) Effects of pregnancy on suicidal behaviour. *The American Journal of Psychiatry*, **154** (10), 1479–80.

44. Viguera, A.C. *et al.* (2002) Managing bipolar disorder during pregnancy: weighing the risks and benefits. *Canadian Journal of Psychiatry*, **47** (5), 426–37.

45. Pajulo, M., Savonlahti, E., Sourander, A., Helenius, H. and Piha, J. (2001) Antenatal depression, substance dependency and social support. *Journal of Affective Disorders*, **65**, 9–17.

46. Zuckerman, B., Amaro, H., Bauchner, H. and Cabral, H. (1989) Depressive symptoms during pregnancy: relationship to poor health behaviours. *American Journal of Obstetrics and Gynaecology*, **160** (5), 1107–11.

47. Berthiaume, M., David, H., Saucier, J.F. and Borgeat, F. (1996) Correlates of gender role orientation during pregnancy and the postpartum. *Sex Roles*, **35** (11/12), 781–800.

48. Brugha, T.S., Sharp, H.M., Cooper, S.A. *et al.* (1998) The Leicester 500 project. Social support and the development of postnatal depressive symptoms, a prospective cohort survey. *Psychological Medicine*, **28** (1), 63–79.

49. Chen, H., Chan, Y.H., Tan, K.H. and Lee, T. (2004) Depressive symptomatology in pregnancy. A Singaporean perspective. *Social Psychiatry and Psychiatric Epidemiology*, **39**, 975–9.

50. Lee, D.T.S., Chan, S.S.M., Sahota, D.S., Yip, A.S.K., Tsui, M. and Chung T. (2004a) A prevalence study of antenatal depression among Chinese women. *Journal of Affective Disorders*, **82**, 93–99.

51. Da-Silva, V.A., Moraes-Santos, A.R., Carvalho, M.S., Martins, M.L. and Teixeira, N.A. (1998) Prenatal and postnatal depression among low income Brazilian women. *Brazilian Journal of Medical and Biological Research*, **31**, 799–804.

52. Chandran, M., Tharyan, P., Muliyil, J. and Abraham, S. (2002) Post-partum depression in a cohort of women from a rural area of Tamil Nadu, India. Incidence and risk factors. *The British Journal of Psychiatry*, **181**, 499–504.

53. Rahman, A., Iqbal, Z. and Harrington, R. (2003) Life events, social support and depression in childbirth: perspectives from a rural community in the developing world. *Psychological Medicine*, **33**, 1161–7.

54. Diket, A.L. and Nolan, T.E. (1997) Anxiety and depression: diagnosis and treatment during pregnancy. *Obstetrics and Gynecology Clinics of North America*, **24** (3), 535–58.

55. Lubin, B., Gardener, S. and Roth, A. (1975) Mood and somatic symptoms during pregnancy. *Psychosomatic Medicine*, **37** (2), 136–46.

56. Elliott, S.A. *et al.* (1983) Mood change during pregnancy and after the birth of a child. *The British Journal of Clinical Psychology*, **22**, 295–308.

57. Glazer, G. (1980) Anxiety levels and concerns among pregnant women. *Research in Nursing and Health*, **3** (3), 107–13.

58. Lumley, J. and Astbury, J. (1989) Advice for pregnancy, in *Effective Care in Pregnancy and Childbirth* (eds I. Chalmers, M. Enkin and M. Keirse), Oxford University Press, Oxford.

59. Nga, D. and Morrow, M. (1999) *Nutrition in Pregnancy in Rural Vietnam: Poverty, Self-Sacrifice and Fear of Obstructed Labour*, Blackwell Science, Oxford (Reproductive Health Matters, special edition).

60. Kitamura, T., Sugawara, M., Sugawara, K. and Toda, M.A. *et al.* (1996) Psychosocial study of depression in early pregnancy. *The British Journal of Psychiatry*, **168** (6), 732–38.

61. Bullock, L.F.C., Mears, J.L.C., Woodcock, C. and Record, R. (2001) Retrospective study of the association of stress and smoking during pregnancy in rural women. *Addictive Behaviors*, **26**, 405–13.

62. Haste, F.M., Brooke, O.G., Anderson, H.R., Bland, J.M., Shaw, A., Griffin, J., Peacock, J.L. *et al.* (1990) Nutrient intakes during pregnancy: observations on the influence of smoking and social class. *The American Journal of Clinical Nutrition*, **51** (1), 29–36.

63. Moylan, P.L., Jones, H.E., Haug, N.A., Kissin, W.B., Svikis, D.S. *et al.* (2001) Clinical and psychosocial characteristics of substance-dependent pregnant women with and without PTSD. *Addictive Behaviors*, **26**, 469–74.

64. Webster, J.W.J., Linnane, L.M., Dibley, D.A.S., Hinson, J.K.M. *et al.* (2000) Measuring social support in pregnancy: can it be simple and meaningful? *Birth: Issues in Perinatal Care*, **27** (2), 97–101.

65. Green, J. (1990a) Prenatal screening and diagnosis: some psychological and social issues. *British Journal of Obstetrics and Gynaecology*, **97**, 1074–76.

66. Hunfeld, J.A.M., Taselaar, A.K.G., Agterberg, G., Wladimiroff, J.W. and Passchier, J. (1997) Trait anxiety, negative emotions, and the mothers' adaption to an infant born subsequent to late pregnancy loss: a case-control study. *Prenatal Diagnosis*, **17** (9), 843–51.

67. Hunfeld, J., Wladimiroff, J. and Passchier, J. (1994) Pregnancy termination, perceived control, and perinatal grief. *Psychological Reports*, **74**, 217–18.

68. Adler, N.E. (2000) Abortion and the null hypothesis. *Archives of General Psychiatry*, **57**, 785–86.

69. McFadyen, A., Gledhill, J., Whitlow, B. and Economides, D. (1998) First trimester ultrasound screening: carries ethical and psychological implications. *British Medical Journal*, **317** (7160), 694–95.

70. Fathalla, M. (1998) The missing millions. *People and the Planet*, **7**, 10–11.

71. Bandyopadhyay, M. (2003) Missing girls and son preference in rural India: looking beyond popular myth. *Health Care for Women International*, **24**, 910–26.

72. Kristof, N. (1993) China: ultrasound abuse in sex selection. *Women's Health Journal*, **4**, 16–17.

73. Patel, V., Rodrigues, M. and Desouza, N. (2002) Gender, poverty and postnatal depression: a study of new mothers in Goa, India. *The American Journal of Psychiatry*, **59**, 43–47.

74. Rahman, A., Lovel, H., Bunn, J. *et al.* (2003) Mothers' mental health and infant growth: a case-control study from Rawalpindi, Pakistan. *Child Care Health and Development*, **30**, 21–27.

75. Petersen, R., Gazmararian, J., Spitz, A., Rowley, D.L., Goodwin, M.M., Saltzman, L.E., *et al.* (1997) Violence and adverse pregnancy outcomes: a review of the literature and directions for future research. *American Journal of Preventive Medicine*, **13** (5), 366–73.

76. Cokkinides, V., Coker, A., Sanderson, M., Addy, C. and Bethea, L. (1999) Physical violence during pregnancy: maternal complications and birth outcomes. *Obstetrics and Gynecology*, **93** (5), 661–66.

77. Covington, D.L., Hage, M., Hall, T. and Mathis, M. (2001) Preterm delivery and the severity of violence during pregnancy. *The Journal of Reproductive Medicine*, **46** (12), 1031–39.

78. Leung, W.C., Leung, T.W., Lam, Y.Y.J. and Ho, P.C. (1999) The prevalence of domestic violence against pregnant women in a Chinese community. *International Journal of Gynaecology and Obstetrics*, **66** (1), 23–30.

79. Purwar, M., Jeyaseelan, L., Varhadpande, U., Motghare, V. and Pimplakute, l. (1999) Survey of physical abuse during pregnancy GMCH, Nagpur, India. *Journal of Obstetrics and Gynaecology Research*, **25** (3), 165–71.

80. Shumway, J., O'Campo, P., Gielen, A. *et al.* (1999) Preterm labour, placental abruption, and premature rupture of membranes in relation to maternal violence or verbal abuse. *The Journal of Maternal-Fetal Medicine*, **8** (3), 76–80.

81. Muhajarine, N., D'Arcy, C. (1999) Physical abuse during pregnancy: prevalence and risk factors. *Canadian Medical Association Journal*, **160** (7), 1007–111.

82. Webster, J., Chandler, J., Battistutta, D. (1996) Pregnancy outcomes and health care use: Effects of abuse. *American Journal of Obstetrics and Gynaecology*, **174** (2), 760–7.

83. Stewart, D., Cecutti, A. (1993) Physical abuse in pregnancy. *Canadian Medical Association Journal*, **149** (9), 1257–63.

84. Pitt, B. (1973) Maternity blues. *The British Journal of Psychiatry*, **122** (569), 431–33.

85. Kennerley, H. and Gath, D. (1986) Maternity blues reassessed. *Psychiatric Developments*, **1**, 1–17.

86. Yalom, I.D., Lunde, D.T., Moos, R.H., and Hamburg, D.A. (1968) "Postpartum blues" syndrome. A description and related variables. *Archives of General Psychiatry*, **18**, 16–27.

87. Stein, G. (1982) The maternity blues, in *Motherhood and Mental Illness* (eds R. Kumar and I.F. Brockington), Academic Press, London, pp. 119–53.

88. Wilkie, G. and Shapiro, C.M. (1992) Sleep deprivation and the postnatal blues. *Journal of Psychosomatic Research*, **36** (4), 309–16.

89. Howard, R. (1993) Transcultural issues in puerperal mental illness. *International Review of Psychiatry*, **5**, 253–60.

90. Kumar, R. (1994) Postnatal mental illness: a transcultural perspective. *Social Psychiatry and Psychiatric Epidemiology*, **29**, 250–64.

91. Sutter, A-L., Leroy, V., Dallay, D., Verdoux, H. *et al.* A French Cross Sectional Study (1997) Post-partum blues and mild depressive symptomatology at days three and five after delivery. *Journal of Affective Disorders*, **44**, 1–4.

92. Devidson, J. (1972) Post-partum mood change in Jamaican women: a description and discussion on its significance. *British Journal of Psychiatry*, **121**, 659–63.

93. Ghubash, R., Abou-Saleh, M.T. (1997) Postpartum psychiatric illness in Arab culture: prevalence and psychosocial correlates. *British Journal of Psychiatry*, **171**, 65–68.

94. Steiner, M. (1998) Further needs in clinical assessment – perinatal mood disorders: position paper. *Psychopharmacology Bulletin*, **34** (3), 301–7.

95. O'Hara, M.W., Schlechte, J.A., Lewis, D.A. *et al.* (1991) Controlled prospective study of postpartum mood disorders: psychological, environmental, and hormonal variables. *Journal of Abnormal Psychology*, **100** (1), 63–73.

96. McNeil, T. and Blenow, G. (1988) A prospective study of postpartum psychoses in a high-risk group. Relationship to birth complications and neonatal abnormalities. *Acta Psychiatrica Scandinavica*, **78** (4), 478–84.

97. Marks, M.N., Wieck, A., Checkley, S.A. and Kumar, R. (1992) Contribution of psychological and social factors to psychotic and non-psychotic relapse after childbirth in women with previous histories of affective disorder. *Journal of Affective Disorders*, **29**, 253–64.

98. Pfuhlmann, B., Stoeber, G. and Beckmann, H. (2002) Postpartum psychoses: prognosis, risk factors, and treatment. *Current Psychiatry Reports*, **4**, 185–90.

99. Scottish Intercollegiate Guidelines Network (2002) *Postnatal Depression and Puerperal Psychosis. A National Clinical Guideline*, Royal College of Physicians, Edinburgh.

100. Brockington, I., Winokur, G. and Dean, C. (1982) Puerperal psychosis, in *Motherhood and Mental Illness* (eds I. Brockington and R. Kumar), Academic Press, London, pp. 37–69.

101. Brockington, I.F. (1992) Disorders specific to the puerperium. *International Journal of Mental Health*, **21** (2), 41–52.

102. Kendell, R. (1985) Emotional and physical factors in the genesis of puerperal mental disorders. *Journal of Psychosomatic Research*, **29** (1), 3–11.

103. Kendell, R., McGuire, R.J., Connor, Y. and Cox, J.L. (1981) Mood changes in the first three weeks following childbirth. *Journal of Affective Disorders*, **3** (4), 317–26.

104. Nott, P.N. (1982) Psychiatric illness following childbirth in Southampton: a case register study. *Psychological Medicine*, **12**, 557–61.

105. Ndosi, N., Mtawali, M. (2002) The nature of puerperal psychosis at Muhimbili National Hospital: its physical co-morbidity, associated main obstetric and social factors. *African Journal of Reproductive Health*, **6** (1), 41–49.

106. Epperson, N. (1999) Postpartum major depression: detection and treatment. *American Family Physician*, **59** (8), 2247–54.

107. Astbury, J. (2001) Gender Disparities in Mental Health, in Mental Health: A call for action by World Health Ministers, World Health Organization, Geneva, pp. 73–92.

108. Cox, J.L. (1994) Introduction and classification dilemmas, in *Perinatal Psychiatry: Use and Misuse of the Edinburgh Postnatal Depression Scale* (eds J.L. Cox and J. Holden), Gaskell, London.

109. Paykel, E.S. (2002) Mood disorders: review of current diagnostic systems. *Psychopathology*, **35** (2/3), 94–99.

110. WHO (1992) International Statistical Classification of Diseases and Related Health Problems, Tenth Revision, World Health Organization, Geneva.

111. Cox, J., Murray, D. and Chapman, G. (1993) A controlled study of the onset, duration and prevalence of postnatal depression. *The British Journal of Psychiatry*, **163**, 27–31.

112. O'Hara, M.W. and Swain, A.M. (1996) Rates and risk of postnatal depression – a meta-analysis. *International Journal of Psychiatry*, **8**, 37–54.

113. O'Hara, M. and Zekoski, E. (1988) Postpartum depression: a comprehensive review, in *Motherhood and Mental Illness* (eds R. Kumar and I.F. Brockington), Butterworth & Company, London, pp. 17–63.

114. Cooper, P.J. and Murray, L. (1997) Prediction, detection, and treatment of postnatal depression. *Archives of Disease in Childhood*, **77**, 97–98.

115. Cramer, B. (1993) Are postpartum depressions a mother-infant relationship disorder? *Infant Mental Health Journal*, **14** (4), 283–97.

116. Nott, P. (1987) Extent, timing and persistence of emotional disorders following childbirth. *British Journal of Psychiatry*, **151**, 523–7.

117. Chaudron, L.H., Klein, M.H., Remington, P. *et al.* (2001) Predictors, prodromes and incidence of postpartum depression. *Journal of Psychosomatic Obstetrics and Gynaecology*, **22** (2), 103–12.

118. Green, J.M. (1998) Postnatal depression or perinatal dysphoria? Findings from a longitudinal community-based study using the Edinburgh Postnatal Depression Scale. *Journal of Reproductive and Infant Psychology*, **16**, 143–55.

119. Romito, P. (1989) Unhappiness after childbirth, in *Effective Care in Pregnancy and Childbirth*. Childbirth, vol. **2** (eds I. Chalmers, M. Enkin and M.J.N.C. Keirse), Oxford University Press, Oxford, pp. 1434–46.

120. Fisher, J.R.W., Feekery, C.J. and Rowe-Murray, H.J. (2002) Nature, severity and correlates of psychological distress in women admitted to a private mother baby unit. *Journal of Paediatrics and Child Health*, **38**, 140–45.

121. Gjerdingen, D.K. and Chaloner, K.M. (1994) The relationship of women's postpartum mental health to employment, childbirth, and social support. *The Journal of Family Practice*, **38** (5), 465–73.

122. Evans, J., Heron, J., Francomb, H., Oke, S. and Golding, J. (2001) Cohort study of depressed mood during pregnancy and after childbirth. *British Medical Journal*, **323** (7307), 257–60.

123. Hendrick, V., Altshuler, L. and Suri, R. (1998) Hormonal changes in the postpartum and implications for postpartum depression. *Pychosomatics*, **39** (2), 93–101.

124. Stowe, Z.N. and Nemeroff, C.B. (1995) Women at risk for postpartum onset major depression. *American Journal of Obstetrics and Gynecology*, **173**, 639–45.

125. Webster, M.L., Thompson, J.M.D., Mitchell, E.A. and Werry, J.S. (1994) Postnatal depression in a community cohort. *The Australian and New Zealand Journal of Psychiatry*, **28** (1), 42–49.

126. Wilson, L.M., Reid, A.J., Midmer, D.K. and Biringer, A. (1996) Antenatal psychosocial risk factors associated with adverse postpartum family outcomes. *Canadian Medical Association Journal*, **154** (6), 785–99.

127. Beck, C.T. (2001) Predictors of postpartum depression: an update. *Nursing Research*, **50** (5), 275–85.

128. Kumar, R. and Robson, K. (1984) A prospective study of emotional disorders in childbearing women. *The British Journal of Psychiatry*, **144**, 35–47.

129. O'Hara, M. (1986) Social support, life events and depression during pregnancy. *Archives of General Psychiatry*, **43**, 569–73.

130. Paykel, E., Emms, E.M., Fletcher, J., and Rassaby, E.S. (1980) Life events and social support in puerperal depression. *The British Journal of Psychiatry*, **136**, 339–46.

131. Chan, S.W., Levy, V., Chung, T.K.H., Lee, D. *et al.* (2002) A qualitative study of the experiences of a group of Hong Kong Chinese women diagnosed with postnatal depression. *Journal of Advanced Nursing*, **39**, 571–79.

132. Rodrigues, M., Patel, V., Jaswal, S. and de Souza, N. (2003) Listening to mothers: qualitative studies on motherhood and depression from Goa, India. *Social Science and Medicine*, **57**, 1797–806.

133. Fisher, J., Morrow, M.M., Ngoc, N.T. *et al.* (2004) Prevalence, nature, severity and correlates of postpartum depressive symptoms in Vietnam. *BJOG: An International Journal of Obstetrics and Gynaecology*, **111**, 1353–60.

134. Leung, W.C., Kung, F., Lam, J. *et al.* (2002) Domestic violence and postnatal depression in a Chinese community. *International Journal of Gynecology and Obstetrics*, **79** (2), 159–66.

135. Boyce, P., Harris, M., Silove, D. *et al.* (1998) Psychosocial factors associated with depression: a study of socially disadvantaged women with young children. *Journal of Nervous and Mental Diseases*, **186** (1), 3–11.

136. Feggetter, G., Cooper, P. and Gath, D. (1981) Non-psychotic psychiatric disorders in women one year after childbirth. *Journal of Psychosomatic Research*, **25** (5), 369–72.

137. Fisher, J.R.W., Feekery, C.J., Amir, L.H. and Sneddon, M. (2002) Health and social circumstances of women admitted to a private mother baby unit. *Australian Family Physician*, **31**, 39–58.

138. Parvin, A., Jones, C.E. and Hull, S.A. (2004) Experiences and understandings of social and emotional distress in the postnatal period among Bangaldeshi women living in Tower Hamlets. *Family Practice*, **21**, 254–60.

139. Mills, E.P., Finchilescu, G. and Lea, S.J. (1995) Postnatal depression – an examination of psychosocial factors. *South African Medical Journal*, **85**, 99–105.

140. Inandi, T., Elci, O.C., Ozturk, A. *et al.* (2002) Risk factors for depression in the postnatal first year, in eastern Turkey. *International Journal of Epidemiology*, **31**, 1201–7.

141. Lee, D.T., Yip, A.S., Leung, T.Y. and Chung, T.K. (2004b) Ethnoepidemiology of postnatal depression. Prospective multivariate study of sociocultural risk factors in a Chinese population in Hong Kong. *The British Journal of Psychiatry*, **184**, 34–40.

142. Cooper, P.J., Landman, M., Tomlinson, M., Molteno, C., Swartz, L. and Murray, L. (2002) Impact of a mother-infant intervention in an indigent peri-urban South African context. *The British Journal of Psychiatry*, **180**, 76–81.

143. Fatoye, F., Adeyemi, A. and Oladimeji, B. (2004) Emotional distress and its correlates among Nigerian women in late pregnancy. *Journal of Obstetrics and Gynaecology*, **24**, 504–9.

144. Milgrom, J., Westley, D. and McCloud, P. (1995) Do infants of depressed mothers cry more than other infants? *Journal of Paediatric and Child Health*, **31**, 218.

145. Armstrong, K., O'Donnell, H. and McCallum, R. *et al.* (1998a) Childhood sleep problems: association with prenatal factors and maternal distress/depression. *Journal of Paediatrics and Child Health*, **34**, 263.

146. Righetti-Veltema, M., Conne-Perréard, E., Bousquet, A. *et al.* (2002) Postpartum depression and mother-infant relationship at three months old. *Journal of Affective Disorders*, **70**, 291–306.

147. Murray, L. and Cooper, P. (1997) *Postpartum Depression and Child Development*, The Guilford Press, London.

148. Armstrong, K., Van Haeringen, A.R., Dadds, M.R. and Cash, R. (1998b) Sleep deprivation or postnatal depression in later infancy: separating the chicken from the egg. *Journal of Paediatrics and Child Health*, **34**, 260.

149. Hopkins, J., Campbell, S., Marcus, M. (1987) Role of infant-related stressors in postpartum depression. *Journal of Abnormal Psychology*, **96** (3), 237–41.

150. Beebe, S., Casey, R. and Pinto-Martin, J. (1993) Association of reported infant crying and maternal parenting stress. *Clinical Pediatrics*, **32**, 15–19.

151. Wolke, D., Gray, P. and Meyer, R. (1994) Excessive infant crying: a controlled study of mothers helping mothers. *Pediatrics*, **94** (3), 322–32.

152. Lehtonen, L. and Barr, R. (2000). 'Clinical pies' for etiology and outcome in infants presenting with early increased crying, in *Crying as a Sign, a Symptom and a Signal* (eds R. Barr and J. Green), MacKeith Press, London.

153. Cox, J. (1996) Perinatal mental disorder – a cultural approach. *International Review of Psychiatry*, **8**, 9–16.

154. Manderson, L. (1981) Roasting, smoking and dieting in response to birth: Malay confinement in cross-cultural perspective. *Social Science and Medicine*, **15B**, 509–20.

155. Stern, G. and Kruckman, L. (1983) Multi-disciplinary perspectives on post-partum depression: an anthropological critique. *Social Science and Medicine*, **17**, 1027–41.

156. Clifford, C., Day, A., Cox, J. and Werrett, J. (1999) A cross-cultural analysis of the use of the Edinburgh Postnatal Depression Scale (EPDS) in health visiting practice. *Journal of Advanced Nursing*, **30** (3), 655–64.

157. Laungani, P. (2000) Postnatal depression across cultures: conceptual and methodological considerations. *International Journal of Health Promotion and Education*, **38** (3), 86–94.

158. Small, R. (2000) *An Australian Study of Vietnamese, Turkish and Filipino Women's Experiences of Maternity Care and of Maternal Depression After Childbirth*, LaTrobe University, Melbourne.

159. Fuggle, P., Glover, L., Khan, F., and Haydon, K. (2002) Screening for postnatal depression in Bengali women: preliminary observations from using a translated version of the Edinburgh Postnatal Depression Scale (EPDS). *Journal of Reproductive and Infant Psychology*, **20** (2), 71–82.

160. Matthey, S., Barnett, B.E. and Elliot, A. (1997) Vietnamese and Arabic women's responses to the Diagnostic Interview Schedule (depression) and self-report questionnaires: cause for concern. *The Australian and New Zealand Journal of Psychiatry*, **31**, 360–69.

161. Stuchbery, M., Matthey, S. and Barnett, B. (1998) Postnatal depression and social supports in Vietnamese, Arabic and Anglo-Celtic mothers. *Social Psychiatry and Psychiatric Epidemiology*, **33**, 483–90.

162. Felice, E., Saliba, J., Grech, V. and Cox, J. (2004) Prevalence rates and psychosocial characteristics associated with depression in pregnancy and postpartum women in Malta. *Journal of Affective Disorders*, **82**, 297–301.

163. Thome, M. (2000) Predictors of postpartum depression in Icelandic women. *Archives of Women's Mental Health*, **3**, 7–14.

164. Romito, P., Saurel-Cubizolles, M. and Lelong, N. (1999) What makes new mothers unhappy: psychological distress one year after birth in Italy and France. *Social Science and Medicine*, **49**, 1651–61.

165. Affonso, D., De, A.K., Horowitz, J., and Mayberry, L. (2000) An international study exploring levels of postpartum depressive symptomatology. *Journal of Psychosomatic Research*, **49** (3), 207–16.

166. Escriba, V., Mas, R., Romito, P. and Saurel-Cubizoles, M.J. (1999) Psychological distress of new Spanish mothers. *European Journal of Public Health*, **9**, 294–99.

167. Kok, L.P., Chan, P.S.L. and Ratnam, S.S. (1994) Postnatal depression in Singapore women. *Singapore Medical Journal*, **35**, 33–35.

168. Lee, D.T., Yip, S.K., Chiu, H.F., (2001) A psychiatric epidemiological study of postpartum Chinese women. *The American Journal of Psychiatry*, **158** (2), 220–26.

169. Yamashita, H., Yoshida, K., Nakano, H. *et al.* (2000) Postnatal depression in Japanese women. Detecting the early onset of postnatal depression by closely monitoring the postpartum mood. *Journal of Affective Disorders*, **58**, 145–54.

170. Glasser, S., Barell, V., Boyko, V., Ziv, A. and Lusky, A. (2000) Postpartum depression in an Israeli cohort: demographic, psychosocial and medical risk factors. *Journal of Psychosomatic Obstetrics and Gynecology*, **21**, 99–108.

171. Moon Park, E.-H. and Dimigen, G. (1995) A cross-cultural comparison: postnatal depression in Korean and Scottish mothers. *Psychologia*, **38**, 199–207.

172. Patel, V. and Andrew, G. (2001) Gender, sexual abuse and risk behaviours in adolescents: a cross-sectional survey in Goa. *The National Medical Journal of India*, **14** (5), 263–67.

173. Barnett, B. and Parker, G. (1986) Possible determinants, correlates and consequences of high levels of anxiety in primiparous mothers. *Psychological Medicine*, **16**, 177–85.

174. Stuart, S., Couser, G., Schilder, K., O'Hara, M. and Gorman, L. (1998) Postpartum anxiety and depression: onset and comorbidity in a community sample. *Journal of Nervous and Mental Diseases*, **186** (7), 420–24.

175. Fisher, J., Astbury, J. and Smith, A. (1997) Adverse psychological impact of operative obstetric interventions: a prospective study. *The Australian and New Zealand Journal of Psychiatry*, **31**, 728–38.

176. Wijma, K., Soderquist, J. and Wijma, B. (1997) Posttraumatic stress disorder after childbirth: a cross sectional study. *Journal of Anxiety Disorders*, **11** (6), 587–97.

177. Boyce, P. and Condon, J.T. (2001) Psychological debriefing: providing good clinical care means listening to women's concerns. *British Medical Journal*, **322** (7291), 928.

178. Murray, L., Fiori-Cowley, A., Hooper, R. and Cooper, P.J. (1996a) The impact of postnatal depression and associated adversity on early mother infant interactions and later infant outcome. *Child Development*, **67**, 2512–16.

179. Field, T., Healy, B., Goldstein, S., *et al.* (1990) Behavior state matching and synchrony in mother-infant interactions in non-depressed versus depressed dyads. *Developmental Psychology*, **26**, 7–14.

180. Patel, V., Rahman, A., Jacob, K.S. and Hughes, M. (2004) Effect of maternal mental health on infant growth in low income countries: new evidence from South Asia. *British Medical Journal*, **328**, 820–23.

181. Patel, V., Desouza, N. and Rodrigues, M. (2003) Postnatal depression and infant growth and development in low income countries: A cohort study from Goa, India. *Archives of Disease in Childhood*, **88**, 34–37.

182. Lyons-Ruth, K., Easterbrooks, M.A. and Cibelli, C.D. (1986) The depressed mother and her one year old infant: environment, interaction, attachment and infant development, in *Maternal Depression and Infant Disturbance. New Directions for Child Development* (eds E.Z. Tronick and T. Field), Jossey-Bass, San Francisco.

183. Murray, L. (1992) The impact of postnatal depression on infant development. *Journal of Child Psychology and Psychiatry*, **33**, 543–61.

184. Cogill, S., Caplan, H., Alexandra, H., Robson, K. and Kumar, R. (1986) Impact of postnatal depression on cognitive development in young children. *British Medical Journal*, **292**, 1165–67.

185. Murray, L., Hipwell, A., Hooper, R. *et al.* (1996b) The cognitive development of 5 year old children of postnatally depressed mothers. *Journal of Child Psychology and Psychiatry*, **37**, 927–35.

186. Sinclair, D. and Murray, L. (1998) Effects of postnatal depression on children's adjustment to school teacher's reports. *The British Journal of Psychiatry*, **172**, 58–63.

187. Hay, D.F. *et al.* (2001) Intellectual problems shown by 11-year-old children whose mothers had postnatal depression. *Journal of Child Psychology and Psychiatry*, **42** (7), 871–89.

188. Luoma, I. *et al.* (2001) Longitudinal study of maternal depressive symptoms and child well-being. *Journal of the American Academy of Child and Adolescent Psychiatry*, **40**, 1367–74.

189. Tatano Beck, C. (1998) The effects of postpartum depression on child development: a meta analysis. *Archives of Psychiatric Nursing*, **1**, 12–20.

190. Murray, L. *et al.* (2003) Controlled trial of the short and long term effect of psychological treatment of post partum depression. *The British Journal of Psychiatry*, **182**, 420–27.

191. Crockenberg, S.C. and Leerkes, E.M. (2003) Parental acceptance, postpartum depression and maternal sensitivity: mediating and moderating processes. *Journal of Family Psychology*, **17**, 80–93.

192. Cooper, P.J. and Murray, L. (1995) Course and recurrence of postnatal depression: evidence for the specificity of diagnostic concept. *The British Journal of Psychiatry*, **166** (2), 191–95.

193. Lumley, J. and Austin, M-P.V. (2001) What interventions may reduce postpartum depression. *Current Opinion in Obstetrics and Gynecology*, **13**, 605–11.

194. Gordon, R.E. and Gordon, K.K. (1960) Social factors in prevention of postpartum emotional problems. *Obstetrics and Gynecology*, **15**, 433–37.

195. Hoffbrand, S., Howard, L. and Crawley, H. (2001) Antidepressant drug treatment for postnatal depression. *Cochrane Database of Systematic Reviews*, 2 (Art. No.: CD002018).

196. Ray, K.L. and Hodnett, E.D. (2001) Caregiver Support for Postpartum Depression (Cochrane Review), The Cochrane Library, Issue 4, 2002, Update Software, Oxford.

197. Appleby, L., Koren, G. and Sharp, D. (1999) Depression in pregnant and postnatal women: an evidence-based approach to treatment. *The British Journal of General Practice*, **49** (447), 780–82.

198. Cooper, P.J. *et al.* (2003) Controlled trial of the short and long term effect of psychological treatment of post-partum depression. Impact on maternal mood. *The British Journal of Psychiatry*, **182**, 412–19.

199. Chen, C.H. *et al.* (2000) Effects of support group intervention in postnatally distressed women. A controlled study in Taiwan. *Journal of Psychosomatic Research*, **49**, 395–99.

200. Barnett, B. and Morgan, M. (1996) Postpartum psychiatric disorder: who should be admitted to which hospital? *The Australian and New Zealand Journal of Psychiatry*, **30**, 709–14.

10

Psychosocial issues and reproductive health conditions: An interface

Veena A. Satyanarayana[1], Geetha Desai[2] and Prabha S. Chandra[2]

[1]*Department of Psychiatry, Washington University School of Medicine, St. Louis, MO, USA*
[2]*Department of Psychiatry, National Institute of Mental Health and Neuroscience, Bangalore, India*

10.1 Introduction

Clinicians and researchers worldwide are recognising the association between gynaecology and psychiatry. The study of the association between reproductive health and mental health has therefore evolved into a subspecialty within the health science, and has attracted increased research attention in the last decade. This chapter focuses on some important gynaecological conditions and procedures that have psychological consequences. The chapter intends to appraise the reader of the relevance of reproductive health in the psychological well-being of women, and vice versa. More specifically, the section on infertility details with psychosocial consequences of childlessness, mental health outcomes following assisted reproductive treatments and the effectiveness of psychological interventions in alleviating distress associated with infertility. Women's experience of loss of the 'uterus', mental health consequences and psychological outcomes following surgical interventions are discussed in the section on hysterectomy.

Contemporary Topics in Women's Mental Health Edited by Chandra, Herrman, Fisher, Kastrup,
© 2009 John Wiley & Sons, Ltd   Niaz, Rondón and Okasha

The immediate and long term impact of some important acute and chronic gynaecological conditions on women's mental and sexual health are described in the section on gynaecological infections. The impact of diagnosis and treatment of gynaecological cancers on mental health has also been discussed. Attempts have been made to include both quantitative and qualitative studies from across the globe, to illustrate socio-cultural underpinnings of the above conditions and procedures.

10.2 Infertility – a psychosocial appraisal

Definition – The difficulties of measuring infertility are compounded by its multiple definitions. The World Health Organization (WHO), using a two-year reference period, defines primary infertility as the lack of conception despite cohabitation and exposure to pregnancy. Secondary infertility is defined as the failure to conceive following a previous pregnancy despite cohabitation and exposure to pregnancy (in the absence of contraception, breastfeeding or postpartum amenorrhoea) [1]. Infertility is a condition that affects 8–12% of couples worldwide at some point in their lives, thus affecting 50–80 million people [2]. Prevalence rates are also found to vary across countries, and correspond to the incidence of preventable conditions that lead to infertility. In Sub Saharan Africa for instance, up to one third of couples are infertile. The prevalence of secondary infertility tends to be higher than primary infertility. Male and female factors are each believed to account for 40% of cases of infertility, the remaining 20% are either unexplained or of shared etiology [3].

Different definitions of infertility are used in clinical practise as well as in epidemiological and demographic research thus affecting prevalence estimates [4–6]. For the purpose of the present chapter, the terms infertility and involuntary childlessness are used interchangeably. An attempt has been made to include studies on both genders so that the differential effects can be discussed. Studies focusing on women with voluntary childlessness have been excluded. Although male and female factors equally contribute to infertility, studies have largely focused on women for reasons that will be clear from the discussion that follows.

Socio-cultural factors

The impact of infertility on an individual and/or couple depends to a large extent on the socio cultural context in which it occurs. In developing countries, infertility is associated with greater stigma than in developed countries [7]. Female infertility has received greater research attention and social blame than male infertility. The experience of infertility causes harsh, poignant and unique difficulties: economic hardship, social stigma and blame, social isolation and alienation, guilt, fear, loss of social status, helplessness and, in some cases, violence [8]. An infertility study in India, reported that approximately 70% of women with infertility were punished for their 'failure' through some form of physical violence and nearly 20% experienced severe violence [9].

A study from Dhaka, in Bangladesh, revealed that people continue to attribute the primary cause of infertility to the spirit world and also reported gender politics in the harsh environment of urban slums [10]. On the other hand, even in countries like Sweden, infertility had a strong impact on women's lives and was a major life theme. It had ramifications across personal, interpersonal and social levels [11]. The role of cultural factors in evaluating the mental health of infertile women has been discussed in a study from Turkey [12]. This study and another which compared Turkish women with Dutch women, examined cultural differences in the effects of infertility on emotional distress. The levels of emotional distress were higher for Turkish women, including migrant women than they were for Dutch women [13]. Infertility can impact both psychological wellbeing and social status of women in the developing world. The delivery of good infertility care in a community requires awareness of the implications of infertility and insight into the context in which these occur [14]. While women feel the brunt of the psychosocial implication, a study among men showed that infertile men also suffered from stigmatisation, verbal abuse and loss of social status [15].

Mabasa [16] observed that for many African women and men, blood ties defined the family and the persona. Thus, failure to have a blood child resulted in courtship and marital break up, extra-sexual relationships, polygamy, divorce and remarriage [17]. Upkong and Orji [18] found that the prevalence of psychiatric morbidity was 46.4% among Nigerian women with infertility. Women with infertility in Kuwait exhibited significantly higher psychopathology in the form of tension, hostility, anxiety, depression, self-blame and suicidal ideation compared to an age-matched pregnant control sample [19]. Researchers have also emphasised the importance of socio cultural issues in the appraisal of infertility and its treatment through newer reproductive technologies [20].

While there is some literature on the psychosocial impact of infertility, the impact of contextual factors on the experience, diagnosis and treatment of infertility is relatively less researched. The above studies illustrate how our understanding of a medical condition can be enriched by considering the context in which it occurs. Being a woman itself may be a vulnerability in patriarchal cultures. In addition, a diagnosis of infertility can have serious ramifications on a woman's gender identity, social status and acceptance by family and society as a whole. These factors in turn, can influence her psychological health and adjustment.

Psychological correlates

The interface of women's reproductive and mental health is an evolving area of psychiatric practise in the world over [21]. A study in Gambia, West Africa, found that being depressed was significantly associated with infertility [22]. A review of studies pertaining to presentation, course and outcome of depression among women in South Asia showed that reproductive health factors including infertility contribute significantly to depression in women [23].

Similarly, a study among Chinese women found that one third of women who sought infertility treatment had impaired psychological wellbeing. Following failed treatment, there was a further deterioration in mental health [24]. Depression, anxiety, relationship and sexual difficulties appeared central to infertility-related stress in Turkey [25]. Anxiety and depression in childless Japanese women were significantly associated with lack of husband's support and feelings of stress [26].

In Africa, a significantly higher proportion (29.7%) of women with infertility was found to have diagnosable psychopathology, mainly in the form of depressive disorder and generalised anxiety disorder. They also experienced poorer marital relationships, had a significant family history of infertility and were more negatively predisposed to child adoption. One important finding was that polygamy had a close association with psychopathology in the sample of infertile women [27].

These findings are not limited to eastern cultures. In Scotland, one third of a sample of women with infertility was found to be at risk for clinically significant psychological disturbances. Distress significantly increased with the number of clinic attendances and decreased as the patient's age increased [28]. A nationally representative sample of American women regardless of fecundity status or treatment status showed consistent positive effects of subfecundity on the odds of fulfilling the diagnostic criteria for anxiety disorders [29].

Differences in the degree of psychopathology between 'organic' and 'functional' infertile subjects and fertile controls in Italy showed that in women, anxiety, depression and tendency towards anger suppression predicted the diagnosis. In men, anger did not emerge as a predictor for diagnosis, whereas anxiety and depression did [30]. In a study from Heidelberg, psychological variables between infertile couples and a representative sample studied indicated that women with infertility showed higher scores on depression and anxiety scales [31].

Studies reviewed above highlight that the internal environment of a woman with infertility is fraught with identity issues and psychological difficulties, with some cultures and contexts posing more challenges than others. Literature has documented a range of psychological problems which may manifest in one or more ways; cognitive, emotional or behavioural. While it seems conclusive that men and women who experience infertility are psychologically distressed, it is important to understand whether this changes in individuals who seek assisted reproductive technology (ART).

Assisted reproductive technology (ART) and psychological outcome

Although the relationship between psychological distress and infertility is supported by empirical studies, a few studies on women seeking ART have found evidence to the contrary. A total of 13 studies were reviewed to investigate the relationship between stress and ART treatment outcomes. Results suggested that stress had a very small negative association with ART treatment outcomes [32]. A study in Sweden found no evidence that psychological stress had any influence on the outcome of in vitro fertilisation (IVF) treatment and suggested that this finding should be made use of, when counselling infertile couples [33]. In another study, a majority reported that marital relationship improved during treatment [34]. In addressing speculations about whether mother child bonding is affected following ART in Sweden, it was found that IVF mothers were attached to their unborn children to the same extent as other mothers [35]. However, the same authors in another study, observed that negative feelings related to infertility were not easily overcome among IVF parents [36].

In Sweden [37] couples displayed a stable relationship from the start and one year after the last failed IVF cycle and majority of the couples had decided to adopt. Interestingly, 73% of the women were interested in more IVF treatment compared to only 33% of the men. A study in Iran found that only 12% of the women seeking infertility treatment reported poor quality of life while nearly 50% reported a good quality of life. Greater economic and psychological pressure from the community and family resulted in lower quality of life [38].

The effects of unsuccessful treatment on marital relationships have been shown to vary depending on several factors. In Finland, several unsuccessful treatment attempts were associated with good dyadic consensus and marital cohesion among ART women. The shared stress of infertility was thought to stabilise marital relationships [39]. A study in Netherlands however, showed that a failure of IVF treatment after a mild treatment strategy resulted in fewer short-term symptoms of depression as compared to failure after a standard treatment strategy [40]. In Germany, it was reported that distress rises significantly only in those patients who were in treatment ≥17 months and experienced treatment failure between the first and the second psychological evaluation [41]. In contrast to the Finland findings, a study from the UK found that women who reported more marital distress required more treatment cycles to conceive than women reporting less marital distress. Hence, it appears that marital life, infertility-related stress and treatment outcome have a complex relationship and distress may be related to the nature, duration and direct and indirect effects of treatment outcome [42–44].

Psychological stress has been shown to affect the outcome of IVF treatment with state anxiety levels being higher among those who did not achieve pregnancy than among those who became pregnant [43]. Psychological functioning among 177 women seeking fertility assistance in Brazil, found that lower age predicted better general health and physical functioning while previous IVF predicted poor psychological health scores [45].

Infertile Chinese women planning to undergo IVF scored significantly higher on all subscales of the symptoms checklist (SCL)-90 and reported unstable relationships than did controls. Age, yearly income, duration of infertility and history of unsuccessful IVF treatment had a negative correlation with psychological health status and marital quality [46]. A study in Netherlands found that differences in emotional status between pregnant and nonpregnant women were present before treatment and became more apparent after the first

IVF cycle [47]. Another study by the same authors found that women showed an increase of both anxiety and depression after unsuccessful treatment and a decrease after successful treatment. Men showed no change in anxiety and depression either after successful or after unsuccessful treatment [48]. Another study on long term psychological adjustment to IVF, found that successful treatment resulted in a more positive long-term emotional status [49].

Inability to conceive children is experienced as stressful by individuals and couples all over the world. The consequences of infertility are manifold and can include societal repercussions and personal suffering. Literature indicates a positive psychological outcome for couples who conceive at the end of treatment, although distress may be apparent prior to and during the process. Couples who fail to conceive following treatment are likely to experience a worsening of symptoms until they come to terms with reality and pursue alternatives. Assisted reproductive technologies, such as IVF, offers hope to many couples, although barriers exist in terms of medical coverage and affordability. The association between distress and fertility outcome, as well as effectiveness of psychosocial interventions merits further study [50]. Several psychological variables seem to predict a favourable outcome and they need to be better identified and studied empirically to ensure better compliance and treatment gains.

Studies have shown both similarities [51] and differences [52–54] in how men and women appraise and cope with infertility and infertility treatments. The diagnosis of infertility in some situations may be as traumatic for men as it is for women [55, 56]. Several contextual, relationship and other psychological variables mediate the level of distress experienced [57–59].

Psychological interventions

Infertility touches all aspects of a person's life [60]. Stress is only one of myriad emotional realities that couples facing infertility deal with, often for extended periods of time. Therefore, mental healthcare appears to be an important component in infertility treatment. Evaluation of a patient education programme for improving communication and stress management skills among couples in fertility treatment showed that intervention participants communicated more with their partner about infertility and its treatment after the intervention. Changes were observed in occurrence, frequency and content of communication with significant others both among men and women. Among women, marital benefit increased significantly, while infertility-related stress was not significantly different. Significantly more intervention participants had contacted support groups, a psychologist and/or agencies for adoption at the 12-month follow-up [61]. In another study, the same authors found that both men (21.1%) and women (25.9%) reported high marital benefit [62, 63].

A randomized controlled trial (RCT) was used to compare the effectiveness of cognitive behavior therapy (CBT) with fluoxetine in the resolution of depression and anxiety in infertile women. Although both fluoxetine and CBT decreased depression significantly, the decrease in the CBT group was significantly more than the fluoxetine group [64, 65]. Women who attended group sessions were significantly less anxious after the IVF treatment than they were before the cycle and men who attended the group sessions were more optimistic but endorsed greater numbers of irrational beliefs [66]. A meta analysis conducted to evaluate the efficacy of group and individual/couple therapies on the reduction of negative emotional symptoms, and the possible promotion of pregnancy found that group and individual/couple psychotherapy led to decreased anxiety [67]. Several couples who failed to achieve conception (despite the use of assisted reproductive techniques and personal psychotherapy) were brought together into a supportive-expressive group which had desirable outcomes [68]. The first clinical impressions about the usefulness of the body-mind group intervention programme in fertility clinics [69] and the effectiveness of yoga and meditation for women experiencing the challenges of infertility [70] seemed promising.

It is evident from the above review that infertility is associated with psychological distress, which persists during treatment and in some cases following unsuccessful treatment. The questions which logically follow is related to what can be done to mitigate the high level of distress. In response to this, different psychological interventions have been proposed which focus on the individual, couple and/or a group. The interventions range from psychoeducational modules to more intensive therapies. Psychological interventions have been found to be beneficial in alleviating distress associated to infertility, therefore, an attempt should be made to integrate psychological interventions with routine care.

Experiential reports

Studies using qualitative methods to understand the experience of infertility are discussed below. Benasutti *et al.* [71] reported nine categories of psychosocial issues that emerged from in-depth qualitative interviews with couples. These were: gender perspectives, emotional reactions, couple decision-making, marital communication, sexual expression, support systems, lessons learned, advice to others and surprises [71]. Another study revealed two novel quality-of-life domains in iatrogenic multiple birth families: social stigma and compounded losses. An unexpected finding was the potential for increased marital solidification as parents coped with the inordinate stresses of multiple births [72]. Finnish women's experiences of infertility treatment showed that two-thirds had sought help from private gynaecologists. Less than half of the women were satisfied with the infertility treatment. The subsequent birth of a baby was the most common reason for satisfaction. Importantly, the most positive treatment experience was respectful, empathic and personal care from the doctor [73].

The association of socio-economic background and infertility indicated that the experience of infertility is different for lower middle/working class women. While all women in the study were profoundly affected by their infertility, the lower middle/working class women were more likely to report a sense of loss of purpose in life and to completely reevaluate their lives in light of their infertility struggles [74]. Qualitative analysis highlighted three groups of women experiencing infertility. Women who recovered from the infertility crisis after having a baby as a result of the treatment, women who started a new life: either they stopped the treatment and remained childless, or they chose to adopt, and women who were in the midst of a very upsetting infertility crisis [75]. Women's identity and roles invariably revolve around child bearing, motherhood, child rearing and nurturance. Therefore, women bear the burden of blame for reproductive failing, resulting in stigma, frustration, anxiety, depression, fear, grief, marital duress, dissolution, abandonment, community ostracism and life threatening medical interventions [76]. Major themes that emerged in in-depth interviews were: childlessness, IVF and hope of achieving pregnancy [77].

Allan [78] in a study assessing experiences of women found that the infertility clinic provided a space in which recognition was given to their intensely private experiences of difference from those in the outside fertile world and allowed them to manage these socially unacceptable, culturally taboo and invisible experiences. However, it is clear that marked variability among women in the extent to which they experience infertility exists. Greater experience of difficulties is usually related to greater levels of distress and lower wellbeing [79].

Women's methods of coping with infertility also vary. A qualitative study on women in Botswana showed that women developed personal measures aimed at preventing or reducing harm inflicted by others as a result of one's infertility. Women coped by looking for deeper meaning, working it out, giving in to feelings, getting more involved, getting away and going in for adoption [80].

In some countries, there could be several filial and religious reasons for seeking help related to infertility. Reasons for help seeking among women presenting with primary and secondary infertility in Pakistan were: to carry on the family name, feeling alone and getting up as a parent on judgement day and because they did not have any male offspring. The effects that infertility had on these women ranged from social pressure, coercion by in-laws to social isolation [81].

In the context of research methods in this area, Peddie and Teijlingen [82] draw attention to the relative lack of qualitative research in fertility and reproduction compared to quantitative methods, and the need to promote qualitative methods as a valuable tool in fertility and reproduction related studies.

Qualitative methods of enquiry are an important gateway to be used in research; particularly in those related to sensitive issues and vulnerable samples. Qualitative data can inform subsequent quantitative designs or complement and corroborate the findings from quantitative studies. In depth interviews, focused group discussions and semi structured interviews generate rich information which cannot be obtained through the use of structured assessments. Contextual factors for instance are best tapped through the use of qualitative approaches such as, grounded theory and ethnography. Qualitative research methods also have the advantage of being therapeutic in itself.

Research in the area of psychosocial factors in infertility and consequently assisted reproductive technology is fairly recent. The above literature offers ample evidence to support the strong positive association between infertility and psychological distress. Although infertility is stressful for both men and women, in most eastern cultures, women tend to experience greater blame and are rendered vulnerable in more ways than one. Several individual, relationship and social variables mediate the level of distress experienced by the individual and influence coping behaviour. Appropriate individual, couple and group oriented psychological interventions ought to be offered and integrated with infertility treatments to effectively manage psychological distress. Infertility counselling, whether provided by a psychiatrist or other healthcare professional, involves the treatment and care of patients not only when they are undergoing fertility treatment, but also with their long-term emotional wellbeing [83]. A recent review of psychosomatic obstetrics and gynaecology showed extensive research in some areas and large gaps in others [84]. Infertility is a complex and sensitive issue which merits clinical and research attention. However, it is important that practise and research in the area be ethically informed. Fertility treatments are expensive and therefore, individuals in resource limited settings have poorer access to them [85]. Individuals and couples need to be educated about the options available to them as well as the costs (economic, medical and psychosocial) and benefits it entails. This will not only help them take an informed decision but also enhances their rapport with the treating clinician.

10.3 The psychological implications of hysterectomy

Hysterectomy is the surgical removal of the uterus, and may sometimes involve the removal of the cervix, ovaries and the Fallopian tubes as well. Even historically, a woman's identity was associated with the 'uterus' and 'ovaries'. Is this association still valid for contemporary women?

A study among American women undergoing hysterectomy revealed that women contemplated the meaning of sexual/reproductive organs in the context of a feminine identity, but did not feel diminished as women because they ceased to menstruate. However, a majority of those who were pre-menopausal at the time of surgery, expressed feelings that their loss of fertility did impair their gender identities [86]. Prevalent myths endorsed by women in France [87] were: loss of feminity, perceived frigidity, change in personality, possible change in body appearance ('hollow', 'empty', 'have a hole inside the belly'), interference in the affective and sexual life and a belief that their companion might change in relation to them (hollow, cold, with no sexual attraction). A study in Turkey [88] among women undergoing hysterectomy revealed five major concerns in relation to: feminine identity, husband/family relationships, sexual life, menopause and relatives' opinions. Loss of a uterus continues to be symbolic of a loss of feminity and womanhood in many cultures, thus impacting gender and social identities.

Magnitude

In 2003, 602 457 hysterectomies were performed in the United States [89]. Of the 538 722 hysterectomies for benign disease, the abdominal route was the most common (66.1%). Hysterectomy surveillance in the US between 1997 and 2005 showed that hysterectomy rates significantly decreased 1.9% per year [90]. In India, 51 obstetric hysterectomies performed during a five year period (January 1999 to December 2004) were analysed and the incidence of obstetric hysterectomy was 4.35 per 1000 confinements [91]. A statistically significant threefold increase in the prevalence of emergency postpartum hysterectomies between 1994 and 2003 was found in UK, as compared to the previous 10 years [92]. Hysterectomy is the most common major surgery for benign non-obstetric reasons in pre-menopausal women.

Psychological consequences

With an increase in both emergency and elective hysterectomy, concerns regarding the immediate and long term consequences of this surgical procedure on one's physical and mental health are on the rise.

Psychological distress appears to vary in different contexts. In a sample of 105 Chinese women, only 1.9% of the participants experienced anxiety, while 4.8% experienced depression following hysterectomy [93]. This may be related to the one child norms in China and loss of the ability to have another child may not be too distressful. However, of 1140 American women undergoing hysterectomy, 10.5% (n = 120) reported that they wanted a/another child before being told that they needed a hysterectomy. Those who desired a (another) child were younger and had higher levels of depression, anxiety, anger and confusion; and were more than twice as likely to have seen a mental health professional for anxiety or depression in the three months prior to their surgery. The differences in psychological distress persisted over the course of the two-year follow-up period [94]. Data from a cohort study of 1249 women [95] showed that women with pelvic pain and depression fared less well 24 months after hysterectomy than women who have either disorder.

Studies have also reported positive effects of hysterectomy, in that, it improves quality of life and decreases psychiatric symptoms among women [96, 97]. A majority of research on the effects of surgical menopause shows improved psychological wellbeing and sexual function after hysterectomy [98]. The overall self-rated health status and physical health showed significant improvements after hysterectomy [99].

In a cross-sectional, population-based study (N = 1177), women reported increased life satisfaction following hysterectomy. It was speculated that the relief from symptoms necessitating hysterectomy may be responsible for this increase [100]. Surgical experience was positive for a majority, with a satisfactory postoperative recovery (70.6%), complete symptom relief (77.9%) and minimal side effects with hormone replacement therapy (5.2%). The benefits included improved physical wellbeing (79.9%), lower depressive symptoms (32.0%) and better sexuality (31.4%) [101]. A comprehensive review of literature on the psychosocial outcomes of hysterectomy published within the past 30 (1986−2005) years suggest that while hysterectomy results in reduced pain, there are no strong effects on sexual or psychological functioning. Nevertheless, some studies reported adverse psychosocial outcomes in a subgroup of 10–20% of women post-hysterectomy [102].

Treatment modalities and psychological outcome

Randomised Controlled Trials have been undertaken to compare the relative effectiveness of different treatment modalities. Hysterectomy was superior to expanded medical treatment for improving health-related quality-of-life after six months in one study [103]. For both total versus subtotal hysterectomy, abdominal pain was significantly reduced post-surgery. There was some evidence for positive effects of hysterectomy on sexual functioning, while psychological functioning did not significantly change [102]. No significant differences between radical hysterectomy patients and controls were found on any of the psychological and health related outcome measures [104].

Few studies have also demonstrated relatively greater complications following hysterectomy. A multicentre prospective study found that complications from treatment were more frequent among patients who had hysterectomy [105] and may be related to chronic pain syndromes and/or posttraumatic stress disorder [106]. Women who had oophorectomy-hysterectomy surgery experienced more negative outcomes compared to the women who had a simple hysterectomy. Sexual functioning was reported as better less than one year since surgery, whereas physical and emotional functioning improved more than a year after surgery. A central complaint with women and their partners was that their physicians had not educated them on the many physical, sexual, emotional side effects of the surgery, but rather emphasised all the positive benefits they would experience after submitting to the surgery [107].

Data collected from 14 072 women aged 45–50 years participating in the baseline survey of the Australian Longitudinal Study on Women's Health showed that compared with women who did not have a hysterectomy, women who had a hysterectomy reported significantly poorer physical and mental health as measured by the short form 36 (SF-36) health survey quality of life profile [108].

Experiential reports

Qualitative data are often a better window to view women's experiences. Women's perception of hysterectomy was explored through focus group discussions and interviews [109]. For many, the choice of hysterectomy was a last resort and was viewed as a technique that could relieve a myriad of symptoms. Most of the women who had a hysterectomy were satisfied with the outcome of surgery, as painful symptoms were relieved. African Americans expressed mistrust of the health providers' motives for recommending surgery, as did several of the Caucasian, non-Hispanic women. Most of the Hispanic participants respected and trusted their providers [110, 111]. Women from three different ethnic groups reported that men perceived women with hysterectomy as less desirable for reasons unrelated to childbearing. All women expressed a strong desire to be involved in elective treatment decisions and would discuss their choice with important others [112].

Seven themes about women's needs related to information and requirements related to hysterectomy were highlighted. These included (i) positive aspects, (ii) hormone replacement therapy, (iii) insufficient information, (iv) changes in sexual feelings and functioning, (v) emotional support, (vi) psychological sequel and (vii) feelings of loss. Women felt that these areas should be addressed by the health professionals prior to surgery [113]. Negative connotations of hysterectomy in the African American community were reported, which caused some women to delay the procedure until they had no choice [114]. It was also noted that a high percentage (80%) of women, particularly those who are young, less educated and black, fear that they will develop cancer if they choose not to undergo the surgery [115]. This emphasises the need for adequate medical education regarding the risk of gynaecological cancer to women contemplating hysterectomy for benign conditions.

The above literature primarily focused on the consequences of hysterectomy for benign conditions. Unlike what was reported in the 1980s and 1990s, literature in the last decade highlights positive outcomes following hysterectomy. These positive outcomes are often in the form of pain reduction, symptom relief, better physical and mental health. Although, few studies have documented negative outcomes following hysterectomy, the psychological disturbances may be either transient or a function of other variables such as, the age of the individual, pre existing mental health problems and presence of biological offspring/s. However, significant variations in the samples recruited, psychological outcome variables studied and measures used, make it difficult to compare findings and draw conclusions.

10.4 Gynaecological infections

Reproductive tract infections include all infections of the genital tract. Some of these infections but not all are sexually transmitted. Poor personal hygiene, poor general health and environmental conditions can lead to higher rates of reproductive tract infections that are not sexually transmitted [116]. An association between reproductive tract infections and mental health has demonstrated that presence of a symptom, most commonly vaginal discharge for more than a month and history of similar symptoms in the past are risk factors for development of common mental disorders like depression, anxiety and somatisation [117, 118].

Some of the reproductive tract infections may be due to overgrowth of the normally present organisms in the reproductive tract and may result in the symptoms like itching, irritation and vaginal discharge. Symptoms of reproductive tract infection are common among low-income women in developing countries [119]. Abnormal or excessive vaginal discharge can be distressing if no cause is found and is not a true indicator of gynaecological morbidity [120]. A community study from India reported higher rates of depression, anxiety and somatisation disorders in women who complained of abnormal vaginal discharge despite low rates of reproductive tract infection [118]. A similar association of depression with reproductive health problems has been reported from a community study in Gambia [121]. It appears, at least in the developing world, that a gynaecological symptom such as vaginal discharge may indicate the presence of psychological problems and may be an idiom of expression of psychosocial distress [122].

Candidiasis is one of the most common causes of vaginal discharge and can be a distressing and recurring condition. In a study conducted among women with chronic vaginal candidiasis, subjects reported dissatisfaction with life, low self-esteem and significant interference with sexual and emotional relationships [123]. Other studies have also reported that women experienced stigmatisation, embarrassment due to the infection [124, 125]. A longitudinal cohort study of bacterial vaginosis has found it to be significantly associated with perceived severity of psychosocial stress [126].

Chronic pelvic pain

Chronic pelvic pain (CPP) is a common gynaecological problem and is also a condition that has been found to have important psychosocial antecedents and consequences. It is defined as cyclic or acyclic pain in the pelvis, persisting for six months or more and severe enough to cause functional incapacity that requires medical or surgical treatments or both [127]. The aetiology of CPP is often not clear as many disorders of reproductive tract, urological system, gastrointestinal tract and musculo skeletal system may be associated with the pain. More than one factor may contribute to the pain.

Prevalence of CPP is reported to be varying, as there is lack of consensus on the definition in the published literature. Studies report prevalence rates of 14–25% in various populations. A systematic review on the prevalence of CPP has been published recently. This study used a definition based on duration of three months and nature of pain (dysmenorrhoea, dyspareunia, noncyclical pelvic pain). The review included studies from the developing and developed world. Wide variation in the geographical distribution of CPP was seen and was attributed not only to the differences in sample characteristics but also to the differences in pelvic inflammatory diseases and availability of certain medical and surgical facilities [128]. CPP also frequently co occurs with another common psychosomatic problem in women, that of irritable bowel syndrome [129]. Because of a poor understanding of the pathogenesis of CPP, many women are subjected to multiple and costly investigations which increase the burden on healthcare systems.

Various psychosocial factors have been linked to CPP. A recent systematic review on the risk factors for CPP included psychological factors such as anxiety, depression, drug/alcohol abuse and childhood sexual abuse [130]. High rates of psychological morbidity have been reported in women with CPP. The common psychological syndromes are depression, anxiety, somatisation, dissociation and drug abuse [131–134]. Posttraumatic stress disorders have also emerged as a commonly occurring syndrome in women with CPP [135].

An important recent and consistent finding is the strong correlation of sexual abuse either in childhood or adulthood with CPP [136]. Various studies have supported this finding [137, 138]. This factor also modulates the experience of pain among women. Quality of life in women with CPP following pelvic inflammatory diseases has been reported to be understandably lower and correlates with the severity of pain.

Recent literature has also focused on sexual functioning among women with CPP. Randolph and Reddy [139] used path analysis to study the contribution of pain experience, depression, mutual support and childhood sexual abuse to sexual functioning and satisfaction among 63 women with CPP. Depression was found to mediate the effect of child sexual abuse and partially mediate the effect of relationship support on sexual satisfaction and functioning. Pain experience in CPP appears to influence sexual functioning mainly through depression.

This finding emphasises the need for screening and treating depression in CPP. Sexual abuse and coercive sexual experiences are common in this group, and women who report physical/sexual abuse also have more psychological distress, depression, anxiety and somatisation in both cyclical and noncyclical pelvic pain.

Endometriosis stands prominent among the causes of CPP in women. The relationship of pain with depression in patients of endometriosis has been recently investigated in a cross-sectional study among outpatients, which revealed depression in 86% of women [140]. There is a dearth of studies reporting psychosocial interventions in the management of CPP, despite the high levels of psychological and sexual morbidity. Longitudinal evaluation of surgical and nonsurgical interventions in CPP has not found any significant difference between the two, with both resulting in a modest improvement in pain as well as an improvement in depression [141].

Polycystic ovarian disease

Polycystic ovarian disease (PCOD) is the most common endocrine disorder affecting women of reproductive age group. It is also one of the common causes for infertility and is characterised by hyperandrogenism with chronic anovulation in the absence of any underlying disease pathology in the adrenal or pituitary glands [142]. The clinical and biochemical features of the syndrome are heterogeneous and the combination and degree of expression of these features vary between individuals.

The symptoms typically associated with polycystic ovary syndrome (PCOS) are amenorrhoea, oligomenorrhoea, hirsutism, obesity, sub fertility, anovulation and acne. In the recent years association of PCOS to long-term health consequences has been reported. It is now clear that PCOS is associated with metabolic disorders and hence at risk for developing cardiovascular diseases [143]. In addition, anovulation of PCOS is associated with increase risk of endometrial cancer. PCOS affects >5% of women of reproductive age [144–146] Its pathophysiology, most likely a combination of genetic disposition and environmental factors, is not completely understood.

Many aspects of the disorder can very conceivably cause a significant amount of emotional stress. Changes in appearance, irregular or absent menstrual periods, difficulties conceiving and possibly disturbances in sexual attitudes and behaviour can result in psychological distress and also influence the feminine identity of patients with PCOS. A recent prospective longitudinal study reported a high rate of depression, anxiety and binge eating disorders in women with PCOS [147]. The determinants of emotional distress were body mass index, age and current wish to conceive [148].

Studies have also looked at sexual functioning in women with PCOS. In a study conducted in Poland, marital sexual dysfunctions were diagnosed in 28.6% of women with PCOS. A negative effect of hirsutism severity on marital sexual life was also observed [149]. Accumulating evidence on the long-term health risks associated with PCOS (e.g. diabetes mellitus) may also have a negative impact on psychosocial wellbeing. Indeed, the diagnosis of PCOS has been found to be associated with feelings of frustration and anxiety.

The impact of symptoms of PCOS on quality of life has been researched using general health quality of life scales as well as specific PCOS quality of life (QOL) scale. PCOS has negative impact on quality of life [149, 150]. The domains affected are those related to general health, physical health, emotion wellbeing and social functioning. When symptoms of PCOS were correlated with QOL dimensions it appeared that weight concerns had a particular negative impact upon health related quality of life (HRQoL) although the role of body mass index in affecting HRQoL scores was inconclusive from the available evidence. Acne was the area least reported upon in terms of its impact upon HRQoL [151]. Issues of hirsutism, being overweight and infertility were also found to be determinants of quality of life and age appeared to mediate these concerns [152]. Most of the quality of life research has focused on adult women with little information about adolescent girls with PCOS.

In one study among adolescents with PCOS, a negative impact was seen on various aspects of health-related quality of life (HRQL) and worries about fertility issues were common [153].

While several studies report reduced quality of life, few have looked at the impact of treatment on QOL. A study on treatment of PCOS with metformin evaluated quality of life and reported improvement in psychosocial, emotional and psychosexual situation of PCOS patients. With treatment [154]. However more data on different treatment methods and their impact on quality of life is needed. It is quite clear however, that women with PCOS be assessed routinely for psychological problems, particularly for depression and body image concerns.

Gynaecological cancers

The comprehensive global cancer statistics from the International Agency for Research on Cancer indicate that gynaecological cancers accounted for 19% of the 5.1 million estimated new cancer cases, 2.9 million cancer deaths and 13 million five-year prevalent cancer cases among women in the world in 2002. Cervical cancer accounted for 493 000 new cases and 273 000 deaths; uterine body cancer for 199 000 new cases and 50 000 deaths; ovarian cancer for 204 000 new cases and 125 000 deaths; cancers of the vagina, vulva and choriocarcinoma together constituted 45 900 cases [155].

Psychosocial factors have an important role in all aspects of gynaecological malignancies. A study which compared the psychosocial and psychosexual concerns of single and partnered women with gynaecologic cancer, suggested that relationship status, whether partnered or single, influences current psychosocial concerns among women with gynaecologic cancer, despite similar levels of illness- and treatment-related intrusions on important life domains [156]. Randomised controlled trials have been conducted to analyse the effect of psychological interventions on psychological symptoms in patients with gynaecological cancer and have provided positive results [157, 158].

Cervical cancer

Cervical cancer is the most common cancer next to breast cancer and accounts for 15% of all cancers in women. There is wide variation of incidence of cervical cancer in developed and developing countries and nearly 80% of the newly diagnosed cases are from developing countries [159]. This difference is due to the lack of awareness of the condition, lack of screening programmes and also poor availability and accessibility of diagnostic facilities.

Human papilloma virus infection has been strongly correlated with cervical caner. Early detection of the cancer is known to improve the outcome and hence, prevention seems to be the best strategy [160].

The commonly used screening test is the PAP smear which can detect premalignant changes is recommended by WHO for population screening, however it may not be feasible in poor countries to due financial constraints. Quite often when the facilities for screening are inadequate, the early changes are detected by visual inspection of the cervix. This examination may not be comfortable for many women and may be a barrier for successful screening programme. Many factors have been associated as being barriers for participation in screening programmes. Low socioeconomic status, women with disabilities, immigrants, lack of knowledge about the risk factors and importance of early detection, fear of having cancer, history of sexual abuse, discomfort about the intimate screening examination and cultural factors have been identified as factors interfering with screening programmes [161–168].

While human papilloma virus (HPV) testing may bring some benefits to the screening programme, testing positive for HPV, a sexually transmitted virus, may have adverse social and psychological consequences for women. In a study conducted in the UK where HPV testing has been part of cervical screening programme, testing positive for HPV was associated with adverse social and psychological consequences, relating primarily to the sexually transmitted nature of the virus and its link to cervical cancer. Women described feeling stigmatised, anxious and stressed, concerned about their sexual relationships and were worried about disclosing their result to others [169].

Women's reactions after disclosure of cervical cancer may mediate further help seeking and coping. In a study that analysed the psychological symptoms experienced by women with a new diagnosis of a gynaecologic cancer at the point of diagnosis and six weeks later, levels of symptomatology remained uniform across the first six weeks following the diagnosis of the cancer regardless of the site of the cancer. Across the spectrum of symptomatology domains, the median scores were all higher in women with poor social supports compared with those with higher social support levels at six weeks. Another study on outpatients with early stage uterine cervical cancer, examined the subjects' mental health and its' relationship with demographic characteristics, clinical characteristics and quality of life. The study suggested that the mental health of outpatients with uterine cervical cancer was influenced by pain and quality of life, rather than the clinical parameters. The presence of a husband or a partner acted as a source of social support and reduced the level of depression [170]. Locus of control and mood were also associated with social support in women with cervical cancer [171].

When the impact of treatment for genital cancer on quality of life and body image was researched before and after surgery, after surgery, both groups indicated their sexual problems were the greatest restriction in terms of quality of life, especially in women with non-reconstructive surgery as well as in women with adjuvant radio and/or chemotherapy. Concerning body image, attractiveness or self-confidence was significantly reduced post operatively compared to the preoperative status in both groups and also worsened with the extent of treatment. Worries about the patient's family and fear of recurrence persisted over time and represented the most important concerns. This study demonstrated the impact not only of the cancer but also the treatment modality on the patient's quality of life, especially related to sexuality and body image [172].

Quality of life in subjects with cervical cancer and long-term psychosocial sequelae of the cancer among women of childbearing age diagnosed with cervical cancer 5–10 years earlier found that the disease-free sample enjoyed good QOL, with physical, social and emotional functioning comparable to or better than comparative norms. However, certain psychological survivorship sequelae and reproductive concerns persisted [173].

Cervical cancer survivors reported significantly more anxiety than endometrial cancer survivors, and more dysphoria, anger and confusion than either endometrial cancer survivors or healthy controls. Greater depression and mood disturbance were reported by unemployed and unmarried cancer survivors. Treatment modality, stage of disease and length of time since diagnosis were not related to quality of life or mood [174].

Treatment modalities of cervical cancer may themselves be associated with poor psychological wellbeing. Even disease free subjects continue to experience psychological reactions following radiotherapy [175]. A study comparing radiotherapy versus surgery for cervical cancer reported poor quality of life and poor sexual functioning in women who received radiotherapy in comparison to women who underwent only surgery [104]. Wellbeing status prior to interventions predicted wellbeing after treatment [176].

Cervical cancers are one of the commonest cancers among women, particularly in developing countries. The psychological implications of the condition start from the time of screening till the time of palliation. However, psychosocial research from the developing world is sparse and one needs more research on interventions that promote early screening and that also alleviate psychological suffering related to the disease and its treatment. More qualitative research may better inform health professional of the real psychosocial needs of women with cervical cancers.

Ovarian, endometrial and other gynaecological cancers

Ovarian cancer is commonly seen in older women. The risk of occurrence is increased in women who have BRCA1/BRCA2 gene mutations. DNA testing for these mutations is available in certain countries. Research is now available related to the psychological impact of genetic testing. A multicentric study conducted in the UK on the impact of predictive genetic testing for breast/ovarian predisposition genes revealed that female carriers who were young continued to experience cancer related worry [177]. However another prospective study of psychosocial consequences following predictive testing for inherited mutations in breast/ovarian and colon cancer susceptibility genes BRCA1, BRCA2, MLH1 and MSH2 was performed. Extensive pre- and post-test information was given. A statistically significant decrease in anxiety mean scores over time was observed among the studied participants and the levels of depression in cancer genes carriers also decreased over time [178].

A study conducted on women who had undergone prophylactic oophorectomy did not report any significant psychological impact on women. Carriers who had undergone prophylactic surgery had a less favourable body image than noncarriers and 70% reported changes in the sexual relationship. A major psychological benefit of prophylactic surgery was a reduction in the fear of developing cancer. Predictors of long-term distress were hereditary cancer-related distress at blood sampling, having young children and having lost a relative to breast/ovarian cancer [179].

Overall it appears that genetic testing may not have serious psychological impact provided adequate support and information is available but there may be issues related to body image and sexuality which need to be addressed [180].

Ovarian cancer presents a range of physical and psychological symptoms during stages of diagnosis, treatment and survival. In a study on prevalence of psychological distress among women with ovarian cancer, approximately one fifth of women reported moderate to severe levels of distress, and more than half reported high stress responses to their cancer and its treatment. Despite the high levels of distress, most participants (60%) were not using any mental health services or psychotropic medications. There was also evidence to suggest that younger patients, patients with more advanced or recurrent disease and patients who had more recently been diagnosed with ovarian cancer experienced greater psychological distress [181].

A prospective study among women with ovarian cancer to determine changes in psychological status in the three months following completion of chemotherapy reported that, social support and intrusive thoughts, rather than physical parameters, were the principal determinants of psychological morbidity in patients with ovarian cancer [182]. In early stage ovarian cancer survivors, quality of life was comparable to same aged non-cancer cohorts [183–185]. However, a majority of the survivors reported problems related to sexual function. In advanced stages of ovarian cancer, limitation of physical activity is the determinant of psychological distress [186].

10.5 Conclusions

Gynaecological conditions have serious psychosocial ramifications, both for the woman and her family. Women from diverse socio-cultural backgrounds endorsed considerable psychological distress secondary to their experience of gynaecological conditions. Women in patriarchal societies however, were rendered relatively more vulnerable due to greater societal stigma and blame. While better psychological functioning and family support act as protective factors which buffer against developing psychiatric disorders, prior psychological vulnerability and lack of support predisposes women to psychiatric disorders, such as depression, anxiety, other stress related conditions and marital/interpersonal difficulties. Further, medical and surgical interventions can often challenge a woman's existing psychological resources, thus emphasising the need for ongoing support from the family and medical staff.

An evaluation of the methodology used in the above literature indicates the use of inconsistent definitions of the constructs, heterogeneous samples, use of a variety of psychological measures and preponderance of quantitative designs. Large numbers of studies have used cross-sectional and co-relational designs. There is a need for longitudinal follow up studies to determine the long term psychological outcome of medical and surgical treatments as well as psychological interventions for individuals with gynaecological conditions. Studies should also identify possible risk factors and focus on prevention and early intervention. Knowledge about demographic and psychosocial predictors of a favourable versus unfavourable outcome is necessary to overcome the latter. It is also equally important and useful to understand positive and negative interactions between psychological variables and physical/physiological parameters during medical and surgical interventions.

Further, several studies have also highlighted the communication gap between the healthcare provider and the consumer, which needs to be overcome in practise. It is the ethical responsibility of every treating clinician to offer accurate and adequate information to the woman and her significant others. In addition to education and information that is made available routinely to all patients, some women considered to be at risk may be screened by the treating clinician and referred to mental health professionals for prevention or management of psychological distress. Also in resource poor settings where psychological help is considered a luxury, integration of group based psycho-educational interventions with minimum supportive work focusing on management of distress, enhancing communication with spouse, accessing support and fostering adaptive coping, with routine care in infertility/gynaecological clinics, will prove to be cost effective.

Acknowledgement

Fogarty International Center ICOHRTA Training Program in Behavioral Disorders (Grant No. TW05811-08; VA Satyanarayana, Fellow; LB Cottler, PI).

References

1. World Health Organization (2008) Infertility. http://www.searo.who.int/LinkFiles/Reproductive_Health_Profile_infertility.pdf.1991 (accessed 10 March 2008).
2. World Health Organization (2002) Current Practices and Controversies in Assisted Reproduction. Report of a Meeting on "Medical, Ethical and Social Aspects of Assisted Reproduction" held at WHO Headquarters in Geneva, Switzerland, 17–21 September 2001 (eds E. Vayena, P.J. Rowe and P.D. Griffin), WHO, Geneva.
3. Program for Appropriate Technology in Health (PATH) (2002) Infertility. Overview/Lessons Learned. Reproductive Health Outlook, Available online (accessed 14 March 2008).
4. Johnson, M.H. and Everitt, B.J. (2000) *Essential Reproduction*, Blackwell Science, Oxford.
5. Habbema, J.D.F., Collins, J., Leridon, H. *et al.* (2004) Towards less confusing terminology in reproductive medicine: a proposal. *Human Reproduction*, **19**, 1497–501.
6. Larsen, U. (2005) Research on infertility: which definition should we use? *Fertility and Sterility*, **83**, 846–52.
7. Peddie, V.L. and Porter, M. (2007) Limitations of infertility treatment: psychological, social and cultural. *Therapy*, **4**, 313–22.
8. Papreen, N., Sharma, A., Sabin, K. *et al.* (2000) Living with infertility: experiences among urban slum populations in Bangladesh. *Reproductive Health Matters*, **8**, 33–44.
9. Unisa, S. (1999) Childlessness in Andhra Pradesh, India: treatment seeking and consequences. *Reproductive Health Matters*, **7**, 54–64.
10. Rashid, S.F. and James, P. (2007) Kal Dristi, stolen babies and 'blocked uteruses': poverty and infertility anxieties among married adolescent women living in a slum in Dhaka, Bangladesh. *Journal of Affective Disorders*, **102**, 219–25.
11. Wirtberg, I., Möller, A., Hogström, L. *et al.* (2007) Life 20 years after unsuccessful infertility treatment. *Human Reproduction*, **22**, 598–604.

12. Gulseren, L., Cetinay, P., Tokatlioglu, B. *et al.* (2006) Depression and anxiety levels in infertile Turkish women. *Social Psychiatry and Psychiatric Epidemiology*, **41**, 720–27.

13. Van Rooij, F.B., Van Balen, F. and Hermanns, J.M.A. (2007) Emotional distress and infertility: Turkish migrant couples compared to Dutch couples and couples in Western Turkey. *Journal of Psychosomatic Obstetrics and Gynecology*, **28**, 87–95.

14. Dyer, S.J., Abrahams, N., Hoffman, M. and van der Spuy, Z.M. (2002) 'Men leave me as I cannot have children': women's experiences with involuntary childlessness. *Human Reproduction*, **17**, 1663–68.

15. Dyer, S.J., Abrahams, N., Mokoena, N.E. and van der Spuy, Z.M. (2004) 'You are a man because you have children': experiences, reproductive health knowledge and treatment-seeking behaviour among men suffering from couple infertility in South Africa. *Human Reproduction*, **19**, 960–67.

16. Mabasa, L.F. (2005) The psychological impact of infertility on African women and their families. *Dissertation Abstracts International: Section B: The Sciences and Engineering*, **65** (10-B), 5412.

17. Stotland, N.L. (2002) Psychiatric issues related to infertility, reproductive technologies, and abortion. *Primary Care*, **29**, 13–26.

18. Upkong, D. and Orji, E. (2006) Mental health of infertile women in Nigeria. *Turkish Journal of Psychiatry*, **17**, 259–65.

19. Fido, A. (2004) Emotional distress in infertile women in Kuwait. *International Journal of Fertility and Women's Medicine*, **49**, 24–28.

20. Bos, H.M.W. and Van Rooij, F.B. (2007) The influence of social and cultural factors on infertility and new reproductive technologies. *Journal of Psychosomatic Obstetrics and Gynecology*, **28**, 65–68.

21. Lolak, S., Rashid, N. and Wise, T.N. (2005) Interface of women's mental and reproductive health. *Current Psychiatry Reports*, **7**, 220–27.

22. Coleman, R., Morison, L., Paine, K. *et al.* (2006) Women's reproductive health and depression: a community survey in the Gambia, West Africa. *Social Psychiatry and Psychiatric Epidemiology*, **41**, 720–27.

23. Trivedi, J.K., Mishra, M. and Kendurkar, A. (2007) Depression among women in the South-Asian region: the underlying issues. *The Journal of Analytical Psychology*, **52**, 479–501.

24. Lok, I.H., Lee, D.T., Cheung, L.P. *et al.* (2002) Psychiatric morbidity amongst infertile Chinese women undergoing treatment with assisted reproductive technology and the impact of treatment failure. *Gynecologic and Obstetric Investigation*, **53**, 195–99.

25. Ozkan, M. and Baysal, B. (2006) Emotional distress of infertile women in Turkey. *Clinical and Experimental Obstetrics and Gynecology*, **33**, 44–46.

26. Matsubayashi, H., Hosaka, T., Izumi, S. *et al.* (2004) Increased depression and anxiety in infertile Japanese women resulting from lack of husband's support and feelings of stress. *General Hospital Psychiatry*, **26**, 398–404.

27. Aghanwa, H.S., Dare, F.O. and Ogunniyi, S.O. (1999) Sociodemographic factors in mental disorders associated with infertility in Nigeria. *Journal of Psychosomatic Research*, **46**, 117–23.

28. Souter, V.L., Hopton, J.L., Penney, G.C. and Templeton, A.A. (2002) Survey of psychological health in women with infertility. *Journal of Psychosomatic Obstetrics and Gynaecology*, **23**, 41–49.

29. King, R.B. (2003) Subfecundity and anxiety in a nationally representative sample. *Social Science and Medicine*, **56**, 739–51.

30. Fassino, S., Pierò, A., Boggio, S. *et al.* (2002) Anxiety, depression and anger suppression in infertile couples: a controlled study. *Human Reproduction*, **17**, 2986–94.

31. Wischmann, T., Stammer, H., Scherg, H. *et al.* (2001) Psychosocial characteristics of infertile couples: a study by the 'Heidelberg Fertility Consultation Service'. *Human Reproduction*, **16**, 1753–61.

32. Mumford, K.R. (2005) The stress response, psychoeducational interventions and assisted reproduction technology treatment outcomes: a meta-analytic review. *Dissertation Abstracts International: Section B: The Sciences and Engineering*, **65** (12-B), 6666.

33. Anderheim, L., Holter, H., Bergh, C. and Möller, A. (2005) Does psychological stress affect the outcome of in vitro fertilization? *Human Reproduction*, **20**, 2969–75.

34. Holter, H., Anderheim, L., Bergh, C. and Möller, A. (2006) First IVF treatment – short-term impact on psychological well-being and the marital relationship. *Human Reproduction*, **21**, 3295–302.

35. Hjelmstedt, A., Widström, A.M. and Collins, A. (2006) Psychological correlates of prenatal attachment in women who conceived after in vitro fertilization and women who conceived naturally. *Birth*, **33**, 303–10.

36. Hjelmstedt, A., Widström, A.M., Wramsby, H. and Collins, A. (2004) Emotional adaptation following successful in vitro fertilization. *Fertility and Sterility*, **81**, 1254–64.

37. Sydsjö, G., Ekholm, K., Wadsby, M. *et al.* (2007) Relationships in couples after failed IVF treatment: a prospective follow-up study. *Human Reproduction*, **22**, 1481–91.

38. Aliyeh, G. and Laya, F. (2007) Quality of life and its correlates among a group of infertile Iranian women. *Medical Science Monitor*, **13**, CR313–17.

39. Repokari, L., Punamäki, R.L., Unkila-Kallio, L. *et al.* (2007) Infertility treatment and marital relationships: a 1-year prospective study among successfully treated ART couples and their controls. *Nursing Inquiry*, **14**, 132–39.

40. de Klerk, C., Macklon, N.S., Heijnen, E.M. *et al.* (2007) The psychological impact of IVF failure after two or more cycles of IVF with a mild versus standard treatment strategy. *Human Reproduction*, **22**, 2554–58.

41. Pook, M. and Krause, W. (2005) The impact of treatment experiences on the course of infertility distress in male patients. *Human Reproduction*, **20**, 825–28.

42. Boivin, J. and Schmidt, L. (2005) Infertility-related stress in men and women predicts treatment outcome 1 year later. *Fertility and Sterility*, **83**, 1745–52.

43. Csemiczky, G., Landgren, B.M. and Collins, A. (2000) The influence of stress and state anxiety on the outcome of IVF-treatment: psychological and endocrinological assessment of Swedish women entering IVF-treatment. *Acta Obstetricia et Gynecologica Scandinavica*, **79**, 113–18.

44. Peterson, B.D., Newton, C.R. and Feingold, T. (2007) Anxiety and sexual stress in men and women undergoing infertility treatment. *Fertility and Sterility*, **88**, 911–14.

45. Chachamovich, J.R., Chachamovich, E., Zachia, S. *et al.* (2007) What variables predict generic and health-related quality of life in a sample of Brazilian women experiencing infertility? *Human Reproduction*, **22**, 1946–52.
46. Wang, K., Li, J., Zhang, J.X. *et al.* (2007) Psychological characteristics and marital quality of infertile women registered for in vitro fertilization-intracytoplasmic sperm injection in China. *Fertility and Sterility*, **87**, 792–98.
47. Verhaak, C.M., Smeenk, J.M., Eugster, A. *et al.* (2001) Stress and marital satisfaction among women before and after their first cycle of in vitro fertilization and intracytoplasmic sperm injection. *Fertility and Sterility*, **76**, 525–31.
48. Verhaak, C.M., Smeenk, J.M., van Minnen, A. *et al.* (2005) A longitudinal, prospective study on emotional adjustment before, during and after consecutive fertility treatment cycles. *Human Reproduction*, **20**, 2253–60.
49. Verhaak, C.M., Smeenk, J.M., Nahuis, M.J. *et al.* (2007) Long-term psychological adjustment to IVF/ICSI treatment in women. *Human Reproduction*, **22**, 305–8.
50. Cousineau, T.M. and Domar, A.D. (2007) Psychological impact of infertility. *Best Practice and Research: Clinical Obstetrics and Gynaecology*, **21**, 293–308.
51. Jordan, C. and Revenson, T.A. (1999) Gender differences in coping with infertility: a meta analysis. *Journal of Behavioral Medicine*, **22**, 341–58.
52. Gibson, D.M. and Myers, J.E. (2000) Gender and infertility: a relational approach to counseling women. *Journal of Counseling and Development*, **78**, 400–10.
53. Mindes, E.J., Ingram, K.M., Kliewer, W. and James, C.A. (2003) Longitudinal analyses of the relationship between unsupportive social interactions and psychological adjustment among women with fertility problems. *Social Science and Medicine*, **56**, 2165–80.
54. Hsu, Y.L. and Kuo, B.J. (2002) Evaluations of emotional reactions and coping behaviors as well as correlated factors for infertile couples receiving assisted reproductive technologies. *The Journal of Nursing Research*, **10**, 291–302.
55. Karlidere, T., Bozkurt, A., Yetkin, S. *et al.* (2007) Is there gender difference in infertile couples with no axis one psychiatric disorder in context of emotional symptoms, social support and sexual function? *Turk Psikiyatri Dergisi*, **18**, 311–22.
56. Peronace, L.A., Boivin, J. and Schmidt, L. (2007) Patterns of suffering and social interactions in infertile men: 12 months after unsuccessful treatment. *Journal of Psychosomatic Obstetrics and Gynecology*, **28**, 105–14.
57. Pooke, M., Krause, W. and Drescher, S. (2002) Distress of infertile males after fertility workup: a longitudinal study. *Journal of Psychosomatic Research*, **53**, 1147–152.
58. Lorber, W. (2007) Efficacy of coping through emotional approach for a working population. *Dissertation Abstracts International: Section B: The Sciences and Engineering*, **67** (11-B), 6740.
59. Morgan, E.M. and Quint, E.H. (2006) Assessment of sexual functioning, mental health, and life goals in women with vaginal agenesis. *Archives of Sexual Behavior*, **35**, 607–18.
60. Hart, V.A. (2002) Infertility and the role of psychotherapy. *Issues in Mental Health Nursing*, **23**, 31–41.
61. Schmidt, L., Tjørnhøj-Thomsen, T., Boivin, J. and Nyboe Andersen, A. (2005) Evaluation of a communication and stress management training programme for infertile couples. *Patient Education and Counseling*, **59**, 252–62.

62. Schmidt, L., Holstein, B., Christensen, U. and Boivin, J. (2005) Does infertility cause marital benefit? An epidemiological study of 2250 women and men in fertility treatment. *Patient Education and Counseling*, **59**, 244–51.

63. Pook, M., Röhrle, B., Tuschen-Caffier, B. and Krause, W. (2001) Why do infertile males use psychological couple counselling? *Patient Education and Counseling*, **42**, 239–45.

64. Faramarzi, M., Alipor, A., Esmaelzadeh, S. *et al.* (2007) Treatment of depression and anxiety in infertile women: cognitive behavioral therapy versus fluoxetine. *Journal of Affective Disorders*, **108** (1–2), 159–64.

65. Tarabusi, M., Volpe, A. and Facchinetti, F. (2004) Psychological group support attenuates distress of waiting in couples scheduled for assisted reproduction. *Journal of Psychosomatic Obstetrics and Gynaecology*, **25**, 273–79.

66. McNaughton-Cassill, M.E., Bostwick, J.M., Arthur, N.J. *et al.* (2002) Efficacy of brief couples support groups developed to manage the stress of in vitro fertilization treatment. *Mayo Clinic Proceedings*, **77**, 1060–66.

67. de Liz, T.M. and Strauss, B. (2005) Differential efficacy of group and individual/couple psychotherapy with infertile patients. *Human Reproduction*, **20**, 1324–32.

68. Christie, G. and Morgan, A. (2000) Individual and group psychotherapy with infertile couples. *International Journal of Group Psychotherapy*, **50**, 237–50.

69. Lemmens, G.M., Vervaeke, M., Enzlin, P. *et al.* (2004) Coping with infertility: a body-mind group intervention programme for infertile couples. *Human Reproduction*, **19**, 1917–23.

70. Khalsa, H.K. (2003) Yoga: an adjunct to infertility treatment. *Fertility and Sterility*, **80**, 46–51.

71. Benasutti, R.D. (2003) Infertility: experiences and meanings. *Dissertation Abstracts International Section B: The Science and Engineering*, **64** (2-A), 677.

72. Ellison, M.A. and Hall, J.E. (2003) Social stigma and compounded losses: quality-of-life issues for multiple-birth families. *Fertility and Sterility*, **80**, 405–14.

73. Malin, M., Hemminki, E., Raikkonen, O. *et al.* (2001) What do women want? Women's experiences of infertility treatment. *Social Science and Medicine*, **53**, 123–33.

74. Loftus, J. (2005) "We Can't Afford It:" Women's Infertility and Social Class. Paper presented at the Annual Meeting of the American Sociological Association, Marriott Hotel, Loews Philadelphia Hotel, August 2005, Philadelphia, Available Online.

75. Malin, M. (2001) How Do Women Use ART Technologies? An Angel Child-Women's Experiences of Childlessness and Infertility Care. Annual Meeting of the International Society of Technology Assessment in Health Care, Helsinki, Finland, p. 17, abstract no. 154.

76. Inhorn, M.C. (1996) *Infertility and Patriarchy. Cultural Politics of Gender and Family Life in Egypt*, University of Pennsylvania Press, Philadelphia.

77. Johansson, M. and Berg, M. (2005) Women's experiences of childlessness 2 years after the end of in vitro fertilization treatment. *Scandinavian Journal of Caring Sciences*, **19**, 58–63.

78. Allan, H. (2007) Experiences of infertility: liminality and the role of the fertility clinic. *Nursing Inquiry*, **14**, 132–39.

79. Benyamini, Y., Gozlan, M. and Kokia, E. (2004) Variability in the Difficulties Experienced by Women Undergoing Infertility Treatments. Presented at the Women, Health and Development Conference, which was held in Jerusalem, on June 8, 2004.

80. Mogobe, D.K. (2005) Denying and preserving self: Botswana women's experiences of infertility. *African Journal of Reproductive Health*, **9**, 26–37.

81. Bhatti, L.I., Fikree, F.F. and Khan, A. (1999) The quest of infertile women in squatter settlements of Karachi, Pakistan: a qualitative study. *Social Science and Medicine*, **49**, 637–49.

82. Peddie, V.L. and Teijlingen, E.V. (2005) Qualitative research in fertility and reproduction: does it have any value? *Human Fertility*, **8**, 263–67.

83. Burns, L.H. (2007) Psychiatric aspects of infertility and infertility treatments. *The Psychiatric Clinics of North America*, **30**, 689–716.

84. Chandra, P.S. and Ranjan, S. (2007) Psychosomatic obstetrics and gynecology – a neglected field? *Current Opinion in Psychiatry*, **20**, 168–73.

85. Indian Council for Medical Research (2000) Need and feasibility of providing assisted technologies for infertility management in resource-poor settings. *ICMR Bulletin*, **3**, 6–7.

86. Elson, J. (2003) Hormonal hierarchy: hysterectomy and stratified stigma. *Gender and Society*, **17**, 750–70.

87. Sbroggio, A.M., Osis, M.J. and Bedone, A.J. (2005) The significance of the removal of the uterus for women: a qualitative study. *Revista da Associacao Medica Brasileira*, **51**, 270–74.

88. Reis, N., Engin, R., Ingec, M. and Bag, B. (2007) A qualitative study: beliefs and attitudes of women undergoing abdominal hysterectomy in Turkey. *International Journal of Gynecological Cancer*, Sep–Oct, **18** (5), 921–8.

89. Wu, J.M., Wechter, M.E., Geller, E.J. *et al.* (2007) Hysterectomy rates in the United States, 2003. *Obstetrics and Gynecology*, **110**, 1091–95.

90. Merrill, R.M. (2008) Hysterectomy surveillance in the United States; 1997 through 2005. *Medical Science Monitor*, **14**, CR24–31.

91. Singh, R. and Nagrath, A. (2005) Emergency obstetric hysterectomy: a retrospective study of 51 cases over a period of 5 years. *Journal of Obstetrics and Gynaecology of India*, **55**, 428–30.

92. Yoong, W., Massiah, N. and Oluwu, A. (2006) Obstetric hysterectomy: changing trends over 20 years in a multiethnic high risk population. *Archives of Gynecology and Obstetrics*, **274**, 37–40.

93. Wang, X.Q., Lambert, C.E. and Lambert, V.A. (2007) Anxiety, depression and coping strategies in post-hysterectomy Chinese women prior to discharge. *International Nursing Review*, **54**, 271–79.

94. Leppert, P.C., Legro, R.S. and Kjerulff, K.H. (2007) Hysterectomy and loss of fertility: implications for women's mental health. *Journal of Psychosomatic Research*, **63**, 269–74.

95. Hartmann, K.E., Ma, C., Lamvu, G.M. *et al.* (2004) Quality of life and sexual function after hysterectomy in women with preoperative pain and depression. *Obstetrics and Gynecology*, **104**, 701–9.

96. Thakar, R., Ayers, S., Georgakapolou, A. *et al.* (2004) Hysterectomy improves quality of life and decreases psychiatric symptoms: a prospective and randomized

comparison of total versus subtotal hysterectomy. *British Journal of Obstetrics and Gynaecology*, **111**, 1115–20.

97. Zobbe, V., Gimbel, H., Andersen, B.M. *et al.* (2004) Sexuality after total vs. subtotal hysterectomy. *Acta Obstetricia et Gynecologica Scandinavica*, **83**, 191–96.

98. Shifren, J.L. and Avis, N.E. (2007) Surgical menopause: effects on psychological well-being and sexuality. *Menopause*, **14**, 586–91.

99. Yang, Y.L., Chao, Y.M., Chen, Y.C. and Yao, G. (2006) Changes and factors influencing health-related quality of life after hysterectomy in premenopausal women with benign gynecologic conditions. *Journal of the Formosan Medical Association*, **105**, 731–42.

100. Kritz-Silverstein, D., Wingard, D.L. and Barrett-Connor, E. (2002) Hysterectomy status and life satisfaction in older women. *Journal of Women's Health and Gender-Based Medicine*, **11**, 181–90.

101. Khastgir, G., Studd, J.W. and Catalan, J. (2000) The psychological outcome of hysterectomy. *Gynecological Endocrinology*, **14**, 132–41.

102. Persson, P., Wijma, K., Hammar, M. and Kjølhede, P. (2006) Psychological well-being after laparoscopic and abdominal hysterectomy – a randomised controlled multicentre study. *British Journal of Obstetrics and Gynaecology*, **113**, 1023–30.

103. Kuppermann, M., Varner, R.E., Summitt, R.L. *et al.* (2004) Effect of hysterectomy vs medical treatment on health-related quality of life and sexual functioning. *Journal of the American Medical Association*, **291**, 1447–55.

104. Frumovitz, M., Sun, C.C., Schover, L.R. *et al.* (2005) Quality of life and sexual functioning in cervical cancer survivors. *Journal of Clinical Oncology*, **23**, 7428–36.

105. Spies, J.B., Cooper, J.M., Worthington-Kirsch, R. *et al.* (2004) Outcome of uterine embolization and hysterectomy for leiomyomas: results of a multicenter study. *American Journal of Obstetrics and Gynecology*, **191**, 22–31.

106. Gardella, C., Johnson, K.M., Dobie, D.J. and Bradley, K.A. (2005) Prevalence of hysterectomy and associated factors in women Veterans Affairs patients. *The Journal of Reproductive Medicine*, **50**, 166–72.

107. Conrad, D.E. (2005) Hysterectomy Outcomes: Evaluating the Quality of Life Factors in Sexual Functioning, Physical and Emotional Health, and Partner-Satisfaction Levels, http://gateway.proquest.com/openurl%3furl_ver=Z39.88-2004%26res_dat=xri:pqdiss%26rft_val_fmt=info:ofi/fmt:kev:mtx:dissertation%26rft_dat=xri:pqdiss:3185663 (accessed on 15 March 2008).

108. Byles, J.E., Mishra, G. and Schofield, M. (2000) Factors associated with hysterectomy among women in Australia. *Health and Place*, **6**, 301–8.

109. Williams, R.D. and Clarke, A.J. (2000) A qualitative study of women's hysterectomy experience. *Journal of Women's Health and Gender-Based Medicine*, **9**, 15–25.

110. Galavotti, C. and Richter, D.L. (2000) Talking about hysterectomy: the experiences of women from four cultural groups. *Journal of Women's Health and Gender-Based Medicine*, **9**, S63–S67.

111. Mingo, C., Herman, C.J. and Jasperse, M. (2000) Women's stories: ethnic variations in women's attitudes and experiences of menopause, hysterectomy, and hormone replacement therapy. *Journal of Women's Health and Gender-Based Medicine*, **9**, S27–38.

112. Groff, J.Y., Mullen, P.D., Byrd, T. *et al.* (2000) Decision making, beliefs, and attitudes toward hysterectomy: a focus group study with medically underserved women in Texas. *Journal of Women's Health and Gender-Based Medicine*, **9**, S39–50.

113. Wade, J., Pletsch, P.K., Morgan, S.W. and Menting, S.A. (2000) Hysterectomy: what do women need and want to know? *Journal of Obstetric, Gynecologic, and Neonatal Nursing*, **29**, 33–42.

114. Augustus, C.E. (2002) Beliefs and perceptions of African American women who have had hysterectomy. *Journal of Transcultural Nursing*, **13**, 296–302.

115. Gallicchio, L., Harvey, L.A. and Kjerulff, K.H. (2005) Fear of cancer among women undergoing hysterectomy for benign conditions. *Psychosomatic Medicine*, **67**, 420–24.

116. Whittaker, M. (2002) Negotiating care: reproductive tract infections in Vietnam. *Women and Health*, **35**, 43–57.

117. Prasad, J., Abraham, S., Akila, B. *et al.* (2003) Symptoms related to reproductive tract and mental health among women in rural southern India. *The National Medical Journal of India*, **16**, 303–8.

118. Patel, V., Weiss, H.A., Kirkwood, B.R. *et al.* (2006) Common genital complaints in women: the contribution of psychosocial and infectious factors in a population based cohort study in Goa, India. *International Journal of Epidemiology*, **82**, 243–49.

119. Jaswal, S. (2001) Gynaecological morbidity and common mental disorders in low-income urban women in Mumbai, in *Mental Health from a Gender Perspective* (ed. B. Davar), Sage Publications, New Delhi, pp. 138–54.

120. Koenig, M., Jejeebhoy, S., Singh, S. and Sridhar, S. (1998) Investigating women's gynecological morbidity in India: not just another KAP survey. *Reproductive Health Matters*, **6**, 84–91.

121. Coleman, R., Morison, L., Paine, K. *et al.* (2006) Women's reproductive health and depression: a community survey in the Gambia, west Africa. *Social Psychiatry and Psychiatric Epidemiology*, **41**, 720–27.

122. Patel, V. and Oomman, N. (1999) Mental health matters too: gynaecological symptoms and depression in South Asia. *Reproductive Health Matters*, **7**, 30–38.

123. Irving, G., Miller, D., Robinson, A. *et al.* (1998) Psychological factors associated with recurrent vaginal Candidiasis: a preliminary study. *Sexually Transmitted Infections*, **74**, 334–38.

124. Chapple, A. and Hassell, K. (2000) You don't really feel you can function normally: women's perceptions and personal management of vaginal thrush. *Journal of Reproductive and Infant Psychology*, **18**, 309–19.

125. Chapple, A. (2001) Vaginal thrush: perceptions and experiences of women of south Asian descent. *Health Education and Research*, **16**, 9–19.

126. Harville, E.W., Hatch, M.C. and Zhang, J. (2005) Perceived life stress and bacterial vaginosis. *Journal of Women's Health (Larchmt)*, **14**, 627–33.

127. Gelbaya, T.A. and El-Halwagy, H.E. (2001) Focus on primary care: chronic pelvic pain in women. *Obstetrical and Gynecological Survey*, **56**, 757–64.

128. Latthe, P., Latthe, M., Say, L. *et al.* (2006) WHO systematic review of prevalence of chronic pelvic pain: a neglected reproductive health morbidity. *BMC Public Health*, **6**, 177.

129. Walker, E.A., Gelfand, A.N., Gelfand, M.D. *et al.* (1996) Chronic pelvic pain and gynecological symptoms in women with irritable bowel syndrome. *Journal of Psychosomatic Obstetrics and Gynaecology*, **17**, 39–46.

130. Latthe, P., Mignini, L., Gray, R. *et al.* (2006) Factors predisposing women to chronic pelvic pain: systematic review. *British Medical Journal*, **332**, 749–55.

131. Walker, E.A., Katon, W.J., Neraas, K. *et al.* (1992) Dissociation in women with chronic pelvic pain. *The American Journal of Psychiatry*, **149**, 534–37.

132. Walker, E.A., Katon, W.J., Hansom, J. *et al.* (1995) Psychiatric diagnoses and sexual victimization in women with chronic pelvic pain. *Psychosomatics*, **36**, 531–40.

133. Badura, A.S., Reiter, R.C., Altmaier, E.M. *et al.* (1997) Dissociation, somatization, substance abuse and coping in women with chronic pelvic pain. *Obstefrks and Gynecology*, **90**, 405–10.

134. Ehlert, U., Heim, C. and Hellhammer, D.H. (1999) Chronic pelvic pain as a somatoform disorder. *Psychotherapy and Psychosomatics*, **68**, 87–94.

135. Meltzer-Brody, S., Leserman, J., Zolnoun, D. *et al.* (2007) Trauma and posttraumatic stress disorder in women with chronic pelvic pain. *Obstetrics and Gynecology*, **109**, 902–8.

136. Reed, B.D., Haefner, H.K., Punch, M.R. *et al.* (2000) Psychosocial and sexual functioning in women with vulvodynia and chronic pelvic pain. A comparative evaluation. *The Journal of Reproductive Medicine*, **45**, 624–32.

137. Poleshuck, E.L., Dworkin, R.H., Howard, F.M. *et al.* (2005) Contributions of physical and sexual abuse to women's experiences with chronic pelvic pain. *The Journal of Reproductive Medicine*, **50**, 91–100.

138. Randolph, M.E. and Reddy, D.M. (2006) Sexual abuse and sexual functioning in a chronic pelvic pain sample. *Journal of Child Sexual Abuse*, **15**, 61–78.

139. Randolph, M.E. and Reddy, D.M. (2006) Sexual functioning in women with chronic pelvic pain: the impact of depression, support, and abuse. *Journal of Sex Research*, **43**, 38–45.

140. Lorrencatto, C., Petta, C.A., Navaro, M.J. *et al.* (2006) Depression in women with endometriosis with and without chronic pelvic pain. *Acta Obstetricia et Gynecologica Scandinavica*, **85**, 88–92.

141. Lamvu, G., Williams, R., Zolnoun, D. *et al.* (2006) Long-term outcomes after surgical and nonsurgical management of chronic pelvic pain: one year after evaluation in a pelvic pain specialty clinic. *American Journal of Obstetrics and Gynecology*, **195**, 591–98.

142. Franks, S. (1999) Polycystic ovary syndrome. *The New England Journal of Medicine*, **333**, 853–61.

143. Dunaif, A. (1997) Insulin resistance and the polycystic ovary syndrome: mechanism of action and implications for pathogenesis. *Endocrine Reviews*, **18**, 774–800.

144. Knochenhauer, E.S., Key, T.J., Kahsar-Miller, M. *et al.* (1999) Prevalence of the polycystic ovary syndrome in unselected black and white women of the southeastern United States: a prospective study. *The Journal of Clinical Endocrinology and Metabolism*, **83**, 3078–82.

145. Asuncion, M., Calvo, R.M., San Millan, J.L. *et al.* (2000) A prospective study of the prevalence of the polycystic ovary syndrome in unselected Caucasian women from Spain. *The Journal of Clinical Endocrinology and Metabolism*, **85**, 2434–38.

146. Azziz, R., Woods, K.S., Reyna, R. *et al.* (2004) The prevalence and features of the polycystic ovary syndrome in an unselected population. *The Journal of Clinical Endocrinology and Metabolism*, **89**, 2745–49.

147. Kerchner, A., Lester, W., Stuart, S.P. and Dokras, A. (2009) Risk of depression and other mental health disorders in women with polycystic ovary syndrome: a longitudinal study. *Fertility and Sterility*, Jan, **91** (1), 207–12.

148. Elsenbruch, S., Benson, S., Hahn, S. *et al.* (2006) Determinants of emotional distress in woman with polycystic ovary syndrome. *Human Reproduction*, **21**, 1092–99.

149. Drosdzol, A., Skrzypulec, V., Mazur, B. and Pawlińska-Chmara, R. (2007) Quality of life and marital sexual satisfaction in women with polycystic ovary syndrome. *Folia Histochemica et Cytobiologica*, **45** (Suppl 1), S93–97.

150. Coffey, S., Bano, G. and Mason, H.D. (2006) Health related quality of life in women with polycystic ovary syndrome: a comparison with general population using the polycystic ovary syndrome questionnaire (PCOSQ) and the short form-36 (SF-36). *Gynecological Endocrinology*, **22**, 80–86.

151. Jones, G.L., Hall, J.M., Balen, A.H. and Ledger, W.L. (2008) Health-related quality of life measurement in women with polycystic ovary syndrome: a systematic review. *Human Reproduction Update*, **14**, 15–25.

152. Pekhlivanov, B., Akabaliev, V. and Mitkov, M. (2006) Quality of life in women with polycystic ovary syndrome. *Akusherstvo i Ginekologiia (Sofiia)*, **45**, 27–31.

153. Trent, M.E., Rich, M., Austin, S.B. and Gordon, C.M. (2002) Quality of life in adolescent girls with polycystic ovary syndrome. *Archives of Pediatrics and Adolescent Medicine*, **156**, 556–60.

154. Hahn, S., Benson, S., Elsenbruch, S. *et al.* (2006) Metformin treatment of polycystic ovary syndrome improves health-related quality-of-life, emotional distress and sexuality. *Human Reproduction.* **21**, 1925–34.

155. Sankaranarayanan, R. and Ferlay, J. (2006) Worldwide burden of gynaecological cancer: the size of the problem. *Best Practice and Research: Clinical Obstetrics and Gynaecology*, **20**, 207–25.

156. de Groot, J.M., Mah, K., Fyles, A. *et al.* (2007) Do single and partnered women with gynecologic cancer differ in types and intensities of illness- and treatment-related psychosocial concerns? A pilot study. *Journal of Psychosomatic Research*, **63**, 241–45.

157. Monti, D.A., Peterson, C., Kunkel, E.J. *et al.* (2006) A randomized, controlled trial of mindfulness-based art therapy (MBAT) for women with cancer. *Psycho-Oncology*, **15**, 363–73.

158. Petersen, R.W. and Quinlivan, J.A. (2002) Preventing anxiety and depression in gynaecological cancer: a randomised controlled trial. *British Journal of Obstetrics and Gynaecology*, **109**, 386–94.

159. Parkin, D.M., Bray, F., Ferlay, J. and Pisani, P. (2005) Global cancer statistics, 2002. *Cancer Journal Clinics*, **55**, 74–108.

160. WHO (2006) Prevention and Control of Sexually Transmitted Infections: Draft Global Strategy, Secretariat, World Health Organization, Geneva, p. 67.

161. Gupta, S., Roos, L.L., Walld, R. *et al.* (2003) Delivering equitable care: comparing preventive services in Manitoba. *American Journal of Public Health*, **93**, 2086–92.

162. Havercamp, S., Scandlin, D. and Roth, M. (2004) Health disparities among adults with developmental disabilities, adults with other disabilities, and adults not reporting disability in North Carolina. *Public Health Report*, **119**, 418–26.

163. Singh, G.K., Miller, B.A., Hankey, B.F. and Edwards, B.K. (2004) Persistent area socioeconomic disparities in U.S. incidence of cervical cancer, mortality, stage, and survival, 1975–2000. *Cancer*, **101**, 1051–57.

164. Taylor, V.M., Schwartz, S.M., Yasui, Y. *et al.* (2004) Pap testing among Vietnamese women: health care system and physician factors. *Journal of Community Health*, **29**, 437–50.

165. Scarinci, I.C., Beech, B.M., Kovach, K.W. and Bailey, T.L. (2003) An examination of sociocultural factors associated with cervical cancer screening among low-income Latina immigrants of reproductive age. *Journal of Immigrant Health*, **5**, 119–28.

166. Coker, A.L., Davis, K.E., Arias, I. *et al.* (2002) Physical and mental health effects of intimate partner violence for men and women. *American Journal of Preventive Medicine*, **23**, 260–68.

167. Farley, M., Golding, J.M. and Minkoff, J.R. (2002) Is a history of trauma associated with a reduced likelihood of cervical cancer screening? *Journal of Family Practice*, **51**, 827–31.

168. Boonmongkon, P., Nichter, M., Pylypa, J. *et al.* (2002) Women's health in northeast Thailand: Working at the interface between the local and the global. *Women and Health*, **35** (4), 59–80.

169. McCaffery, K.J., Waller, J., Nazroo, J. and Wardle, J. (2006) Social and psychological impact of HPV testing in cervical screening: a qualitative study. *Sexually Transmitted Infections*, **82**, 169–74.

170. Ohara-Hirano, Y., Kaku, T., Hirakawa, T. *et al.* (2004) Uterine cervical cancer: a holistic approach to mental health and it's socio-psychological implications. *Fukuoka Igaku Zasshi*, **95**, 183–94.

171. Lalos, A. and Eisemann, M. (1999) Social interaction and support related to mood and locus of control in cervical and endometrial cancer patients and their spouses. *Supportive Care in Cancer*, **7**, 75–78.

172. Hawighorst-Knapstein, S., Fusshoeller, C., Franz, C. *et al.* (2004) The impact of treatment for genital cancer on quality of life and body image – results of a prospective longitudinal 10-year study. *Gynecologic Oncology*, **94**, 398–403.

173. Wenzel, L., DeAlba, I., Habbal, R. *et al.* (2005) Quality of life in long-term cervical cancer survivors. *Gynecologic Oncology*, **97**, 307–9.

174. Bradley, S., Rose, S., Lutgendorf, S. *et al.* (2006) quality of life and mental health in cervical and endometrial cancer survivors. *Gynecologic Oncology*, **100**, 479–86.

175. Klee, M., Thranov, I. and Machin, D. (2000) Life after radiotherapy: the psychological and social effects experienced by women treated for advanced stages of cervical cancer. *Gynecologic Oncology*, **76**, 3–4.

176. Eisemann, M. and Lalos, A. (1999) Psychosocial determinants of well-being in gynecologic cancer. *Cancer Nursing*, **22**, 303–6.

177. Watson, M., Foster, C., Eeles, R. *et al.* (2004) Psychosocial impact of breast/ovarian (BRCA1/2) cancer-predictive genetic testing in a UK multi-centre clinical cohort. *British Journal of Cancer*, **91**, 1787–94.

178. Arver, B., Haegermark, A., Platten, U. *et al.* (2004) Evaluation of psychosocial effects of pre-symptomatic testing for breast/ovarian and colon cancer pre-disposing genes: a 12-month follow-up. *Familial Cancer*, **3**, 109–16.

179. Meiser, B., Tiller, K., Gleeson, M.A. *et al.* (2000) Psychological impact of prophylactic oophorectomy in women at increased risk for ovarian cancer. *Psycho-Oncology*, **9**, 496–503.

180. van Oostrom, I., Meijers-Heijboer, H., Lodder, L.N. *et al.* (2003) Long-term psychological impact of carrying a BRCA1/2 mutation and prophylactic surgery: a 5-year follow-up study. *Journal of Clinical Oncology*, **21**, 3867–74.

181. Norton, T.R., Manne, S.L., Rubin, S. *et al.* (2004) Prevalence and predictors of psychological distress among women with ovarian cancer. *Journal of Clinical Oncology*, **22**, 919–26.

182. Hipkins, J., Whitworth, M., Tarrier, N. and Jayson, G. (2004) Social support, anxiety and depression after chemotherapy in ovarian cancer: a prospective study. *British Journal of Health Psychology*, **9**, 569–81.

183. Matulonis, U.A., Kornblith, A., Lee, H. *et al.* (2008) Long-term adjustment of early-stage ovarian cancer survivors. *International Journal of Gynecological Cancer*, Nov–Dec, **18** (6), 1183–93.

184. Stewart, D.E., Wong, F., Duff, S. *et al.* (2001) What doesn't kill you makes you stronger: an ovarian cancer survivor survey. *Gynecologic Oncology*, **83**, 537–42.

185. Wenzel, L.B., Donnelly, J.P., Fowler, J.M. *et al.* (2002) Resilience, reflection, and residual stress in ovarian cancer survivorship: a gynecologic oncology group study. *Psycho-Oncology*, **11**, 142–53.

186. Kornblith, A.B., Thaler, H.T., Wong, G. *et al.* (1995) Quality of life of women with ovarian cancer. *Gynecologic Oncology*, **59**, 231–42.

11

Menopause and women's mental health: The need for a multidimensional approach

Jill Astbury

School of Psychology, Victoria University, Melbourne, Australia

11.1 Introduction

By the year 2025, the World Health Organization [1] has predicted that global life expectancy will be 73 years and that no country in the world will have a life expectancy of less than 50 years, the average age of menopause in Asia, Europe, the Americas, Australia and Africa [2].

The remarkable growth in the numbers of people living into extreme old age, the majority of whom are women, is most evident in high income countries such as France, where it is estimated that there will be 150 000 centenarians by 2050 [1]. This marked increase in the size of the population of women living 30, 40 or even 50 years beyond menopause, radically challenges existing notions of middle and old age and draws attention to the importance of continued research to establish an accurate understanding of the risk and protective factors associated with a healthy menopausal transition. Such research will underpin the development of improved interventions to assist women in achieving optimal psychological, sexual, physical and social health during and after the menopausal transition.

Menopause is defined retrospectively as the end of menstruation. During the perimenopausal period, women gradually stop menstruating and become unable to conceive and bear children without assisted reproductive technology. Several factors have been identified that reduce the average age of menopause. In high

Contemporary Topics in Women's Mental Health   Edited by Chandra, Herrman, Fisher, Kastrup,
© 2009 John Wiley & Sons, Ltd   Niaz, Rondón and Okasha

income countries, for example, cumulative socioeconomic disadvantage over a lifetime is strongly predictive of an earlier age at menopause [3–7]. The adverse childhood circumstances associated with an earlier menopause include living in a household without access to a car or a bathroom and having to share a bedroom [7]. Smoking is another risk factor. Women who smoke reach menopause some 18 months earlier than their non smoking counterparts. As there is a strong association between smoking and poor socioeconomic circumstances, women exposed to both risk factors are especially vulnerable to an earlier menopause. In low-income countries, poor socioeconomic circumstances are normative by definition but with regard to a significantly earlier menopause, women who have suffered significantly from malnutrition are at highest risk [8, 9].

Menopause is characterised by simultaneous physical, hormonal and psychosocial changes. Physically, health status may decline and chronic diseases associated with ageing may appear for the first time. Hormonally, the perimenopausal transition is characterised by declining ovarian follicular activity and hormonal fluctuations that result in vasomotor instability. Symptoms include hot flushes, vaginal dryness and sleep problems.

11.2 Social, cultural and contextual factors

Dominant social, medical, media and lay discourses on fertility, ageing, the female body and gender roles all help to shape women's expectations of and attitudes towards menopause, and to some extent determine the social status accorded to women in midlife. These views inform women's own expectations and subjective experiences, and the meanings they attach to menopause [10–12].

Cultural conceptions of menopause vary considerably, from its being perceived as a normal and unproblematic part of human development and the female life course to its being seen as a hormone-deficiency disease that gives rise to severe, disabling physical and psychological symptoms requiring medical treatment and surveillance.

A comprehensive review of cross-cultural and comparative research concluded that the majority of women do not find menopause a difficult experience [13]. Similar findings on women's attitudes towards natural menopause have been reported in the USA [14]. In the longitudinal Massachusetts Women's Health study, most women did not seek medical help for menopause, and held primarily positive or neutral attitudes towards it [14]. Similarly, few women in the Seattle Midlife Women's Health Survey [15] defined menopause as a time when increased symptoms, disease risk or medical care should be expected. Most women viewed menopause as a normal process in the course of their lives.

11.3 Variation in symptoms and symptom patterns

The prevalence of menopausal symptoms varies considerably even within the same country. For example, Bosworth et al. [16], in a study of perimenopausal

American women (aged 45–54 years) in North Carolina, found high rates of hot flushes (65%), night sweats (56%), difficulty sleeping (45%), mood swings (49%) and memory problems (44%). Woods and Mitchell [15] in another American study, the Seattle Midlife Women's Health Study reported much lower rates of symptoms, with only 17% of women participating in this study reporting hot flushes and night sweats. An Australian longitudinal cohort study documented changes in the level of symptoms over the menopausal transition including an increase in vasomotor symptoms, such as hot flushes, night sweats, breast tenderness and vaginal dryness [17].

Cross-cultural studies have found significant variation between countries in the level and type of menopausal symptoms experienced, what they signify and the degree of physical and psychological distress generated by them [18, 19]. Women in Japan [10] and other Asian countries, including China (Hong Kong SAR and Province of Taiwan), Indonesia, Republic of Korea, Malaysia, the Philippines and Singapore, tend to report fewer menopausal symptoms than those in the United States [12]. Differences in symptom reporting between different cultural groups within a country have also been documented. The US Study of Women's Health Across the Nation (SWAN) [20] identified significant differences between American women from five racial/ethnic groups (Caucasian, African American, Chinese, Japanese and Hispanic). However, two consistent categories of symptoms were found across these five groups. The first comprised hot flushes and night sweats and the second consisted of psychological and psychosomatic symptoms. Overall Caucasian women reported significantly more psychosomatic symptoms and African American women reported significantly more vasomotor symptoms. Interestingly, in a later stage of follow up from the SWAN study, differences in depressive symptoms were identified between the two Asian groups. Compared with white women, Chinese women had significantly reduced odds (odds ratio, OR = 0.51, confidence interval, CI = 0.33–0.79) while Japanese women had significantly increased odds of depressive symptoms (OR = 1.42, CI = 0.93–2.17) [21].

By contrast, a study conducted in Pakistan, identified high levels of menopausal symptoms of a distinctly different kind amongst women living in rural Lahore [22]. The four most common symptoms reported by more than 50% of women included lethargy (65.4%), forgetfulness (57.7%), urinary symptoms (56.2%) and agitation (50.8%). Hot flushes were reported by just over 36% of the participants, considerably lower than the 45% of women who reported flushes in a population based survey in the United Arab Emirates, where flushes were the most common menopausal symptom [23].

Another large study of women from five developed countries, the United States, United Kingdom, Germany, France and Italy, identified six groups of symptoms of which two were related to markers of menopausal hormonal change [24]. The first of these groups consisted of hot flushes and night sweats and the second comprised symptoms of poor memory, sleeping difficulties, aches in the head, neck and shoulders, vaginal dryness and difficulty with sexual arousal.

Lock [13] cautions against dismissing reports of fewer symptoms in Asian societies simply as the expression of learned cultural expectations about menopause. Indeed, Melby *et al.* [25] have concluded that differences in symptom reports between women from different cultural and ethnic groups reflect real differences. They argue for more rigorous research to clarify how biology and culture interact in the production of different symptom patterns across cultures.

Psychosocially, the perimenopausal transition takes place in a social and personal context that may be marked by significant life changes and upheavals. Family composition may change through death or divorce, children may leave or return home and parents may become frailer and more dependent. Women's own psychological health is clearly affected by the behaviours and functioning of other people. For example, women in relationships with men who are heavy drinkers experience higher levels of psychological distress than women whose partners do not engage in risky drinking [26]. Similarly, older women who live with men who perpetrate physical, sexual or emotional violence against them have higher rates of chronic pain and depression than their non abused counterparts and are unlikely to disclose that abuse is occurring to their healthcare providers [27].

Other external factors that may impose greater demands on women's coping abilities during the perimenopausal transition include their work status, level of earnings and participation in paid work, as well as ageist attitudes and difficulties in finding new work if they become unemployed.

A large literature exists on hormones and hormone treatments in relation to menopausal symptoms and the menopausal transition. However, this research is not the focus of the current chapter for a number of reasons. First, current evidence suggests that while associations have been reported between depressive symptoms and menopausal status, symptoms and hormonal levels, the importance of these associations is considerably ameliorated when other psychosocial and health factors are taken into account. In fact, numerous studies have demonstrated that social, psychological and health factors can exert as great or greater influence on the likelihood of a woman being depressed in mid life than the menopausal transition. For example, the large, prospective, longitudinal SWAN study [21] revealed that very stressful life events were the strongest of all the predictors of depressive symptom scores that were considered. In order, the five variables associated with the highest odds ratios of experiencing depressive symptoms were having two or more very stressful life events (OR = 4.46, CI = 3.85–5.16), neutral or negative attitudes towards menopause (OR = 2.96, CI = 2.37–3.70), one very stressful life event (OR = 2.47, CI = 2.12–2.89) finding it very hard to pay for basics (OR = 2.13, CI = 1.59–2.86) and having late menopausal status compared with premenopausal status (OR = 1.71, CI = 1.27–2.30).

Second, findings from the Women's Health Initiative, a large randomised controlled trial involving more than 16 000 women in the USA, indicate that the combination of oestrogen and progestrogen, as a menopausal treatment carries significant health risks. This study, begun in 1997, was initially intended to be completed in 2005. It was terminated three years early on May 31, 2002, because interim analysis revealed that this particular combination of hormones was associated with statistically significant increases in the risks of breast cancer [28], heart disease [29], stroke [30] and poorer cognitive functioning [31]. In other words, even if hormonal treatments were effective in treating depression, the associated risks would argue against their use.

Although the Women's Health Initiative study was criticised on a number of methodological grounds, even before the publication of its findings from 2002, a large scale behavioural change in the use of hormonal therapy was occurring amongst American women. After 2000, the use of hormonal treatments for menopausal symptoms decreased by approximately 75% in the US. More importantly, this change in usage was accompanied by a marked decrease in the incidence of breast cancer. From 2000–2001 to 2003–2004, age adjusted breast cancer incidence rates per 100 000 women decreased by 18% [32].

Third, hormonal treatments not only carry health risks but are only affordable for women in high income countries and menopause research generally has been criticised for being carried out primarily in middle- and high-income countries on samples of middle class white women [33]. In low-income countries, not only are hormonal treatments unaffordable for the majority of women but given the significantly lower life expectancy of women in resource poor settings it can be argued that the hormonal treatment of menopausal symptoms has low public health relevance. In Sub Saharan Africa, for example, life expectancy for women is trending downwards significantly and is predicted to be less than 45 years from 2008 onwards [34]. Women in this setting experience high risks rates of human immunodeficiency virus (HIV) infection, malaria, malnutrition, anaemia and maternal mortality. In consequence, a range of other health conditions are of more concern, and require more urgent attention, than treatments for menopause.

Fourth, while hormonal treatments for menopause carry significant health risks and menopausal difficulties have a low public priority in developing countries, the importance of paying greater research and clinical attention to mental health in general and depression in particular has been recognised in both developing and developed countries [35]. Depression is the most common psychological disorder worldwide, carries a heavy burden of disability and is experienced twice as often by women as it is by men [36]. Consequently, it is critical to identify and attempt to reduce risk factors for depression and increase gender specific protective factors for women's emotional wellbeing across the life course and the menopausal transition is no exception.

The remaining part of this chapter will therefore focus on two main issues. First, it will examine evidence that teases out the relative contributions made by physical, hormonal and psychosocial factors to mental health, especially depression, during the menopausal transition. Second, it will consider what this evidence indicates in terms of counselling approaches that could provide meaningful assistance to women's needs, concerns and emotional priorities at this stage of their lives.

11.4 The research evidence

The literature on the psychological dimensions of menopause, like much other health research, suffers from a significant high income, developed country bias. Most large scale research studies on the determinants of psychological wellbeing in midlife have been conducted in high-income countries. The validity of these findings for women in different socio cultural and resource-poor settings remains largely unknown. Caution in extrapolating findings from high-income countries is especially warranted with regard to studies from the USA, where rates of gynaecological surgery (hysterectomy) and hormone replacement therapy (HRT) are high, and hence natural menopause is by no means a universal experience.

11.5 Is menopause a time of increased risk for women's mental health?

Evidence from national surveys permits comparison of population-based rates of depression over the lifespan. Throughout their reproductive years, when many women carry the triple burden of paid work, unpaid household work and heavy caring responsibilities, they also experience significantly higher rates of depression than men [37]. This gender difference first emerges in puberty [38, 39] and declines from midlife onwards, although evidence on the age when the sex difference ceases to be important varies from one study and one country to another. For Australian women aged between 45 and 54 years, the rate of depression was 7%, considerably lower than that for women aged 18–24 years (11%) [40]. Two national surveys in the USA have indicated a U-shaped relationship between age and depression, with the lowest rates occurring in the age group 45–49 years [41]. The United Kingdom National Survey of Psychiatric Morbidity found that the sex difference in the prevalence of depression disappeared after the age of 55 years [42]. Similarly, a Canadian study reported that the lowest rate of depression (4.3%) and the smallest gender difference in rates of depression occurred in the age group of 75 years and older [43]. By contrast, one US study found that there was an increase in the rate of depression in older people but only amongst the oldest old people [44].

11.6 The relationship between menopause and depression in midlife

Three main hypotheses have been proposed regarding the relationship between menopause and depression for women in midlife. The first argues that a close relationship exists between hormones and mood, and consequently that changes in hormonal status during the menopausal transition exert direct effects on mood and the likelihood of women developing depression.

The second view repudiates the idea that a simple cause-effect relationship exists between hormonal change and the occurrence of depression. Instead, this view postulates a 'domino' hypothesis. It argues that depression comes about in response to troublesome menopausal symptoms such as night sweats, poor sleep and hot flushes.

The third hypothesis asserts that menopause and its associated hormonal changes are largely irrelevant in explaining depression among women in midlife. Depression during menopause can be primarily accounted for by the classical determinants of depression over the life course, and menopausal status and symptoms make no meaningful additional contribution. Implicit in this view is a criticism of other research on menopause that does not take account of previously identified predictors of depression.

Despite the fact that the gender difference in depression is most marked during the reproductive years, experiences related to changes in sex hormones, such as pregnancy, the use of oral contraceptives, HRT and menopause, do not appear to account for this difference [39, 45].

Large-scale epidemiological surveys of mental health have found no substantial increase in rates of depression among women in midlife. Yet researchers remain interested in identifying the factors that distinguish between women who do and do not experience depression at this time. These include the role of hormonal changes, menopausal status and menopausal symptoms, such as hot flushes and disturbed sleep, psychosocial, socioeconomic and physical health factors and a history of depression [16].

To establish whether menopause has a direct or an indirect effect on depression, prospective, longitudinal research is necessary to elucidate whether depression is a cause or consequence of high levels of symptoms, including hot flushes, insomnia and vaginal dryness. Over the past decade or so, an increasing number of such studies have been carried out in high-income countries, including Australia, Canada, the United Kingdom and the United States [15, 20, 46–49].

Most longitudinal studies have used multidimensional models to investigate why some, but not all, women experience depression during the menopausal transition. As well as menopausal symptoms and menopausal status, these studies have been designed to assess the contributions of sociocultural factors, attitudes towards and expectations of menopause, health status and health behaviours, a history of depression and the influence of age. A stress model of depression is congruent with a multidimensional approach to understanding the pathways to depression in midlife [15]. Stress, as a highly important mediating factor linked to depression, may arise from a number of different sources: from the menopausal transition itself, because of changes in menstrual patterns and the appearance and persistence of vasomotor symptoms; from the woman's life context, which can have a direct impact on mood but is also influenced by negative socialisation experiences and attitudes to menopause and poor health; and from acute or chronic health conditions and thus the woman's physical and psychological health status and history.

The stressors investigated so far include menopausal status, age, life context factors such as psychosocial adversity, marital difficulties, difficulties with children and demands from those within one's social network, negative life events, negative socialisation and attitudes towards menopause, as well as general physical health status and health behaviours.

Overall, there is little evidence that menopausal or hormonal status exerts a strong or direct effect on depression. Rather, the evidence supports a 'domino' hypothesis that an increased level of distressing symptoms can be a cause of depression. Avis *et al.* [20], in a longitudinal study, found that depression was positively associated with symptoms such as hot flushes, night sweats and difficulty sleeping, but not with menopausal status or change in oestradiol levels. Oestradiol had no direct effect on depression independent of symptoms. Glazer *et al.* [46], in the longitudinal Ohio Midlife Women's Study, also found that menopausal status did not significantly predict depression in midlife. Loss of resources and low level of education – both classical determinants of depression – were, however, strongly predictive of depression in this cohort. Anxiety was also predicted by loss of resources but the effectiveness of women's coping strategies and education were important too. The researchers concluded that stress, as indicated by loss of resources, was a better predictor of poor health outcomes than menopausal status.

Bosworth *et al.* [16] conducted a cross-sectional study of a random sample of women aged 45–54 years residing in Durham County, North Carolina. Variables included depression (measured by the abbreviated Centre for Epidemiologic Studies–Depression Scale (CES-D), perceived menopausal stage, climacteric symptoms, health behaviour and markers of socioeconomic status. Overall 164 women (28%) were using HRT, and 236 (41%) reported ever using HRT. Almost one-third (29%) of women in the sample had CES-D scores indicating significant depressive symptoms, but there was no significant difference in menopausal status between depressed and non-depressed women. Depressed women had higher rates of night sweats, hot flushes, insomnia, memory loss/forgetfulness and mood swings. Maartens *et al.* [50] found that stage of menopausal transition in Dutch women was significantly and independently related to depression, after other risk factors were taken into account. Rates of depression, as measured by the Edinburgh Depression Scale, significantly increased from pre- to perimenopause, and again from peri- to postmenopause. In this study depression was also associated with unemployment, inability to work, financial problems, death of a partner or child and a previous episode of depression. More importantly, these factors contributed more to an increased risk of depression than any stage of the menopausal transition and two – unemployment and the death of a child – conferred particularly high risks of depression in midlife.

Dennerstein *et al.* [49] reported that menopausal symptoms exerted no demonstrable effect on Australian women's wellbeing over time. Instead, they observed an improvement in wellbeing from early to late phases of the menopausal transition. Psychosocial variables were most significant in determining this, particularly when a woman formed a new marriage or partnership and experienced increased satisfaction in work.

In population-based longitudinal studies in Massachusetts, USA [51] and Manitoba, Canada [47], stressful life events and circumstances were found to be strongly associated with depression persisting or occurring for the first time in midlife. Sources of stress included marital and relationship problems, difficulties with children, and demands from friends and family. Woods and Mitchell [15] reported that a stressful life context and poor health status had significant direct effects on depressed mood. Stressful life context was significantly associated with having more severe vasomotor symptoms. Women who experienced more menopausal changes tended to have more negative expectations for midlife and poorer health status.

The major explanatory role assigned to attitudes and expectations of menopause in the development of depression presupposes that the majority of women formed these attitudes earlier in life. Avis and McKinlay [52], in a longitudinal study, found that negative attitudes towards menopause predicted both subsequent symptom reporting during menopause and depression. However, in an interview-based study of more than 500 premenopausal women with a median age of 41 years, participating in the Seattle Midlife Women's Health Study, Woods and Mitchell [15] found that most were uncertain about their expectations of their own menopause.

Another possible risk factor for depression during menopause is sexual functioning and changes in the frequency of sex or in the level of sexual pleasure and satisfaction. Some studies have reported a decrease in sexual functioning with age, which becomes more marked in midlife [53–55]. An obvious difficulty for research in this area is separating the effect of increasing age from menopausal status. One longitudinal Swedish study disentangled the effects of these two factors and reported that menopausal status, rather than age, was the important factor for explaining decreased sexual functioning [56]. In addition to age and menopausal status, decreased sexual desire was associated with the lack of a sexual partner, a poor, non-confiding relationship with the sexual partner, insufficient support, alcohol dependence and the partner's own sexual difficulties. Stressors, employment, negative attitudes towards menopause, previous level of sexual functioning and poor physical or psychological health also contribute to decreased sexual desire and functioning in midlife [54–56]. These factors are also predictive of depression. Difficulties or dissatisfaction with sexual functioning can add to stress during the menopausal transition.

11.7 The need for a life course perspective

Schieman *et al.* [44] analysed data from the 1996 to 1998 General Social Surveys in the US to explore the factors associated with age related changes in psychological distress. They also identified several factors in midlife that were related to lower levels of distress, namely having greater control, less shame and greater religious attendance.

The importance of control to emotional wellbeing has been repeatedly reported in studies of workplace wellbeing. An analysis of data from the Canadian Community Health Survey [57] revealed that women with high levels of decision making authority at work were less likely to have major depressive episodes in the past year than their counterparts with low decision making authority. Conversely, women in a manual socio-economic position, indicative of low control, at 42 years of age were significantly more likely to have a depressive disorder at 45 years of age, although the strength of this association was ameliorated when childhood socioeconomic position and childhood psychological disorders were taken into account [58].

Dennerstein *et al.* [59] noted a small decline in self-rated health with increasing age. This decline was not attributable to the menopausal transition, rather it was related to a change in weight and a change in libido and feelings for the partner. Interestingly, women who reported a decline in self-rated health and were in paid employment were significantly more likely than other women to have had an operation or procedure in the previous year.

Kuh *et al.* [49] also found that women who were obese had the highest rates of psychological symptoms, while women who were of normal weight had lower levels of self-reported symptoms than women who were under- or overweight. Other studies have reported that a history of depression prior to the menopausal transition is a powerful predictor of depression during or after the transition [60, 61].

As these studies illustrate, factors preceding menopause, including a history of depression, exert a strong influence on the likelihood of poor mental health at the time of menopause. In general, longitudinal studies of menopause recruit women who are approaching or are already experiencing the perimenopausal transition. This means that potentially important risk factors for depression that have occurred earlier in the life course can only be assessed retrospectively and are susceptible to recall bias. A notable exception is the prospective, cohort study by Kuh *et al.* [49], who investigated the links between earlier experiences (in childhood, adolescence or earlier adult life) and mental health in midlife. Participants in this research were part of the larger Medical Research Council National Survey of Health and Development (MRCNSHD), and were drawn from a representative sample of the British population born in 1946 and assessed repeatedly over subsequent decades. Data on midlife were collected over a six-year period when participants were aged between 47 and 52 years and this was combined with data on risk factors gathered at earlier stages of the study. Risk factors were grouped into six clusters: family background, characteristics of the child, adult health, adult socioeconomic circumstances, social support, lifestyle and current life stress. Pathways through which risk factors determined psychological distress in midlife included cumulative losses, social adversity and negative events and experiences over the course of the women's lives. The importance of negative life events, such as adverse changes in family and work life, for mental health was confirmed in this study. No variation was found in psychological symptoms in midlife according to menopausal stage, in keeping with the results of a number of other studies.

Family background variables were significantly associated with symptoms of psychological distress. Psychologically distressed women were more likely to have lived in council housing, had parents who divorced, and had mothers who had high scores on a measure of neuroticism. Certain characteristics of the women during childhood and adolescence were also associated with adult psychological symptom scores. These included level of neuroticism and antisocial behaviour in adolescence. Women with higher psychological symptom scores in midlife were significantly more likely to have had health problems earlier in adult life. Of particular note were psychological illness between 15 and 32 years, anxiety and depression at 36 years, reported health problems at 36 years and physical disability at 43 years. In other words significant relationships were found between adult circumstances, social relationships, health behaviour and current life stress and high psychological symptom scores.

A significant inverse relationship was found between psychological symptoms and low social class and educational qualifications. Specifically, women living in households where the income was earned by manual labour, or who were themselves on a low income, had higher symptom scores than those from non-manual-labour households or with higher income. Divorced or separated women had a higher symptom score than those who were married or single and women whose children were teenagers or younger also had more psychological symptoms. On the other hand, higher levels of social support, including emotional support, good social networks and access to help in a crisis were associated with low symptom scores. However once all other risk factors were statistically controlled in the analysis, social networks were no longer independently associated with midlife symptoms. Some health risks, such as smoking and weight, were related to symptom scores in midlife. Smokers had the highest symptom scores, lifelong non-smokers the lowest and ex-smokers had intermediate scores. Women of normal weight had lower scores than women who were under- or overweight, while obese women had the highest scores. Alcohol intake and past physical activity were not systematically related to symptom scores.

The researchers concluded that markedly different life course trajectories were associated with psychological distress in midlife, and argued that the relationship between the woman's parents may be even more important than their findings on parental divorce suggested. No measures of parental conflict, parental indifference, or physical, sexual or psychological abuse were included in their study. They commented further that a retrospective question, asked when the women were 42 years old, identified a small number who may have suffered abuse or serious neglect of some kind in childhood. This limited measure of parental maltreatment was strongly associated with midlife psychological distress after adjusting for all other early experiences, and was mediated by mental health status in adult life.

Other research has confirmed the importance of different forms of adversity in childhood, including sexual abuse, for multiple health outcomes in adult life [62]. In addition, there is a well documented link between childhood sexual abuse and intimate partner violence in adult life and increased rates of a number of adverse mental health outcomes, including depression, anxiety and post-traumatic stress disorder [37]. When women in the sixth year of follow-up for the Melbourne Women's Midlife Health Project completed a questionnaire on lifetime experience of violence, 28.5% (101/362) reported having experienced some form of domestic violence – physical, sexual or emotional – during their lifetime.

11.8 Methodological difficulties

Research into the relationship between depression in midlife and possible risk factors, including menopausal and hormonal status and symptoms, faces a number of methodological challenges. While prospective studies minimise reliance on recall for contemporary events and experiences, bias still remains a problem for more distant events and past experiences. Only the life course prospective study by Kuh *et al.* [49] avoided recall bias altogether, but such longitudinal studies are extremely costly to run. As a result, the comparison of findings across studies is limited by differences in methodological approach, ranging from the research design, the method of sample selection, differences in recruitment strategies and choice of instruments for measuring risk factors and outcome variables.

Studies also vary in the choice of methods for defining, detecting and measuring outcome variables, such as depression. Some studies have measured symptoms of depression, some have used standardised measures that permit diagnostic criteria to be applied, and others have used non-standardised self-report measures. There are differences in the age groups of women recruited to the studies, not all important covariates are taken into consideration, and most studies do not consider the impact of cultural factors.

The sample in a longitudinal study is not necessarily representative of the general population, especially if there is a low response rate to the initial invitation to participate. For example, the response rate to the invitation to participate in the Melbourne Women's Midlife Health Project was only 56% [49]. As further attrition in prospective samples occurs with time, sample bias is compounded. It may be that those participating in a cross-sectional study, where only one attempt to recruit participants is needed, are more similar to the general population than those who remain in a longitudinal study. However, cross-sectional studies cannot disentangle cause from effect or capture temporal changes.

Prospective, longitudinal studies are needed to document time-related changes in indicators of health, including recent hormonal, social and psychological changes. All of these may influence and help to explain variations in menopausal symptoms and depressive symptoms between individual women. In addition, significant social and cultural changes can occur over a single generation. Changes in social organisation and gender roles, including increased rates of divorce, decreased fertility rates and increased participation by women in paid work, raise new issues that can affect women's sense of wellbeing in midlife. Recent cohorts of women might differ from earlier cohorts in the significance they assign to work and personal achievement in their lives [15].

In summary, multidimensional models are needed to explain depression in midlife. Depression is more likely to be a consequence of distressing menopausal symptoms than a cause of them. The classical social and contextual determinants of depression, such as unemployment, socioeconomic adversity, negative life events, lack of social support, loss of partner through bereavement or separation or lack of a confiding relationship with a partner, continue to exercise a powerful influence during menopause. Obesity, smoking and depression in midlife are related. Health promotion programmes that seek to reduce these high-risk behaviours among women in midlife will be successful only if they simultaneously address the causes of depression.

11.9 Therapeutic approaches in mid life

Existential and woman centred therapy

The plethora of risk factors associated with depression in midlife cautions against any single 'one size fits all' approach to the counselling and treatment of women with depressive symptoms. The available research highlights the fact that women's emotional wellbeing in mid life is multiply determined by factors operating at the level of the individual, family and relationships, community and broader society.

Depression may be a singular, identifiable outcome, a readily made diagnosis but its determinants including the pathways through which they operate are neither singular nor may they be readily apparent. Different trajectories for the development of depression, its chronicity and its treatability may be related to the specific kinds of negative events experienced from childhood onwards. Furthermore, the patterns of depressive symptoms, a critical consideration in determining appropriate symptom focused treatment, appears to vary according to the particular categories of adverse events encountered.

A recent population based prospective, longitudinal study in the US confirmed that there was an important link between exposure to specific categories of adverse life events and the subsequent pattern of depressive symptoms. Keller *et al.* [63] recruited a sample of 4856 individuals (53% were women) who had experienced depressive symptoms in the 12 months prior to the study and followed them up on four occasions over a maximum of 12 years. On each occasion, participants reported the severity of 12 symptoms that were disaggregated from the nine diagnostic and statistical manual (DSM) 111-R criteria for major depression. Participants were asked to identify whether there was any perceived cause of their symptoms and these causes were classified into nine different categories of adverse life events. For events associated with significant loss such as the death of loved ones and relationship break ups, participants reported high levels of sadness, lack of pleasure, appetite loss and where the event was a romantic break up, high levels of guilt. Where the adverse events involved chronic stress and failures, increased symptoms of fatigue and hypersomnia were more apparent. For the group of participants who reported their depression came 'out of the blue' and were unable to identify any specific cause, symptoms of fatigue, weight gain and thoughts of self harm were more dominant. The researchers concluded that depression is a pathoplastic syndrome and argued there was a causal link between type of adverse events and the particular symptom profile that developed. While this study did not report on gender differences in symptom profiles and the participants were adults in their 30s, the strength of the findings related to adverse life events, together with other findings on adverse events and their impact on psychological functioning in midlife, suggests that this relationship warrants special attention.

Accumulating evidence suggests that specific adverse life events from childhood onwards including psychosocial adversity [48], physical, sexual or emotional abuse, significant losses or people, roles or cherished ideas, chronic stress and experiences of failure, humiliation and defeat [62–64] are linked not only to the likelihood of becoming depressed but configures discrete symptom profiles. Further support for the existence of different symptom profiles comes from an analysis of data from the Canadian Community Health Survey [65]. In this research, men and women were compared in relation to their depressive symptoms. A number of gender differences emerged with women being significantly more likely than men to report symptoms of 'increased appetite', to being 'often in tears' and to having 'thoughts of death'. These findings have significant implications for counselling depressed women in midlife. In particular, it indicates the need to take a 'woman centred approach' that carefully considers depressed symptoms in the context of women's lives as a whole.

Evidence on the characteristics of the events and experiences that give rise to depression, both inform and contextualise the likely meanings a woman will attach to her menopausal symptoms, her attitudes towards ageing, her sexual and gendered identity, her value as a human being and her perceived purpose in life. Further, the meanings attributed to these specific issues will reflect and shape women's responses to more general existential concerns.

Yalom [66] identified four main existential concerns namely death, freedom, existential isolation and meaninglessness. It might be argued that such concerns are especially likely to surface during life transitions that are socially and culturally marked as times of critical change in women's lives. If the sheer volume of published papers is any guide, then menopause is regarded by medical researchers, endocrinologists, sociologists, psychologists and others as just such a critical period in women's lives. Using 'menopause' as a search term, a Medline search yielded more than 39 000 papers in February, 2008. Books, magazine articles and other lay publications on the subject of menopause further reinforce the sense that the menopausal transition is a critical time in women's lives, personally, sexually, socially and relationally.

Woman centred counselling

A woman centred approach to counselling is well placed to offer a safe psychological space in which women can explore their perspectives in relation to the general existential and other more specific concerns noted above. A safe and private space is a critical priority when working with women who have experienced violence and abuse. High lifetime prevalence rates and the link between violence and high rates of depression and other psychological disorders indicates that skills in trauma focussed counselling are necessary for all counsellors and therapists working with women [37].

By working to establish an equal power relationship between client and therapist and placing women's needs and priorities at the centre of therapeutic attention, a woman centred approach is designed to foster a woman's sense of autonomy and control in decision making within the therapeutic context and to promote her dignity as a human being. As noted earlier, being able to exercise control and autonomy contributes to positive psychological outcomes.

It is essential to provide adequate time and scope for exploring the menopausal and psychological symptoms of most concern to the woman herself and working to contextualise them within a life course perspective, including possible relationships with earlier adverse experiences and events. Research on the specific depressive symptoms profiles also suggests that the elucidation of a client's dominant symptoms is an important step towards the development of symptom specific treatment. These activities support undertaking a psychological stocktaking at this important life stage and of identifying treatment plans that can be 'owned' and seen as meaningful by clients.

A more existential, woman centred approach can utilise many of the methods of cognitive behavioural therapy (CBT), while overcoming criticisms that have been levelled at CBT such as that it is victim blaming, ignores social and gendered realities, adverse events and the traumatic experiences and prefers to see depression primarily as the outcome of distorted cognitions by the depressed person.

There is no doubt that the various forms of CBT including Rational Emotive Therapy, Cognitive Therapy, Rational Emotive Behaviour Therapy and Insight Focused Therapy are based on the assumption that there is an inextricable link between cognition and emotion [67]. If a client changes how she thinks it is argued that a corresponding change will occur in how that client feels and behaves. Exploring the link between cognition and emotion does not have to done in a way that invalidates the reality of or repudiates the psychological significance of life events and experiences that have triggered depressed and anxious thoughts or seeks to deny that these thoughts can be seen as a 'realistic' response to the adversities experienced. A more woman centred approach will identify the contextual origins of these thoughts and seek to develop alternative interpretations with the client based on evidence of previously unacknowledged personal strengths including courage, resistance and resilience. Recognition of these strengths provides solid ground for countering a negative, deprecating view of self and allows a different life narrative to emerge. This additional work will undoubtedly lengthen the duration of counselling but is supported by evidence that underlines the critical, highly salient role of negative life events in the development of many psychological disorders including depression, anxiety and Post Traumatic Stress Disorder (PTSD). Being able to make sense of the links between past experience and present feelings counters the negative view that such feelings are unreasonable and personally discrediting.

CBT has proven efficacy with diverse client groups as a short term treatment in reducing a number of psychological disorders including depression and anxiety [67]. However, very little research has focused specifically on women going through the menopausal transition. One small Swiss study of 30 women suffering from climacteric symptoms who received a CBT intervention consisting of psychoeducation, group discussion and coping skills training, did report a significant improvement from pre to post intervention on measures of depression, anxiety, sexuality, hot flushes and cardiac complaints but no positive changes in reported sexual satisfaction or the stressfulness of menopausal symptoms [68]. Similarly, Keefer and Blanchard's [69] study of 19 women reported that a cognitive behavioural group treatment was associated with a significant decrease in the frequency of vasomotor symptoms but in this study no significant improvement was found in psychosocial functioning. Another even smaller study consisting of case reports on two women also found that an individualised CBT treatment had beneficial effects on depression, anxiety, quality of life and reduced the number of hot flushes [70]. Given the small sample sizes of these studies, their findings are suggestive at best and large randomised controlled trials are necessary before the efficacy of CBT for a range of psychological disorders in women experiencing the menopausal transition can be accurately established.

The psycho educational component of CBT can be expanded and aligned to the objectives of a woman centred approach to include the provision of accurate and understandable information about menopausal changes and to canvas the therapeutic options from conventional as well as complementary medicine, that are available to deal with distressing menopausal symptoms when these co exist with depressive symptoms. Accurate information is indispensable in supporting women to make informed choices about how best to optimise their psychological health and at the same time fosters their participation in treatment decisions thus enhancing their sense of control over their lives and health. Patient participation in decision making has been shown to improve adherence to treatments for depression and can thus indirectly relate to better clinical outcomes [71].

Participation, control and responsibility for improving one's emotional well-being are characteristics that fit the goals and assumptions of a woman centred and a CBT approach. Both stress the importance of a collaborative relationship between client and therapist. Similarly, taking an active role in devising the tasks that will support her emotional wellbeing, practising the behavioural strategies best suited to accomplishing these tasks and creating alternative, more empowering interpretations of herself that counter anxious and depressing thoughts and interpretations, are all compatible with the tenets of CBT, while firmly advancing the objectives of a woman centred approach.

However as CBT argues increased awareness alone is insufficient to bring about positive emotional change. Awareness must be augmented by action. For this reason, clients need to take an active role in confronting or being exposed in a gradual manner to the very situations (after adequate skills acquisition and rehearsal), that have previously caused them to feel stressed, anxious and afraid. These situations do not have to be 'in vivo' but can be imagined (imaginal exposure) and involve role playing. Only by confronting these anxiety provoking situations in some form does it become possible to reduce their negative power by successfully applying newly acquired skills and provide experiential evidence for alternative and more positive, interpretations of self.

As well as being effective in the treatment of depressive and anxiety disorders, CBT is an effective therapy for PTSD. This is important because, like depression, there is a significant gender disparity in rates of PTSD with women experiencing PTSD at twice the rate of men. PTSD is one of the commonest psychological consequences of gender based violence (GBV) especially intimate partner violence and sexual violence [36]. Although the incidence of GBV decreases with age and women in mid life have significantly lower rates than younger women, it must be kept in mind that the symptoms of PTSD can persist over many years and PTSD is often comorbid with depression and anxiety. Sleeping difficulties are a common complaint of women in the menopausal transition and affect daytime functioning. Typically these difficulties are considered in relation to vasomotor instability including night sweats and frequent wakening. However, a range of sleeping difficulties are also a common feature of PTSD including difficulties going to sleep and staying asleep, breathing and movement disorders and recurrent nightmares and CBT is effective in treating trauma related sleep problems [72].

11.10 Conclusion

Research to date strongly supports the view that healthcare providers including therapists and counsellors must look beyond menopausal status, hormone levels and menopausal symptoms to adequately explain depressed mood in women at midlife. In fact, there is ample evidence that it is the 'classical' social determinants of depression (low socioeconomic status, lack of social support and a confiding relationship with a partner, unemployment, previous history of depression, adverse life events and high levels of past or current stress), together with distressing somatic symptoms, poor health, high risk health behaviours and decreased sexual functioning and pleasure that make the most sizeable contribution to dysphoria and depression.

To make sense of the complex nature of interconnected risk and protective factor involved in the production of psychological health in mid life, research underlines the need to employ a life course, multidimensional perspective.

In considering psychosocial adversity, past and present, it is necessary to evaluate the sources and impact of stress and their links with specific depressive symptom profiles in women at midlife. Social support can function as a powerful protective factor for emotional wellbeing but it does need to kept in mind that not all social networks are supportive and some may function as conduits of stress.

For women who experience distressing symptoms of depression, anxiety and PTSD in midlife, it is argued that a woman centred, existential approach to counselling is warranted but that this approach can make use of many of the techniques of CBT. While evidence on the efficacy of CBT for the psychological problems experienced by women in midlife is meagre and needs to be increased, the fact that CBT has been effective with other client groups in addressing all three common disorders as well as a range of trauma related sleeping difficulties, makes it a relevant and appropriate therapeutic choice.

References

1. World Health Organization (1998) The World Health Report, World Health Organization, Geneva.
2. Morabia, A. and Costanza, M.C. (1998) International variability in ages at menarche, first livebirth and menopause. World Health Organization Collaborative Study of Neoplasia and Steroid Contraceptives. *American Journal of Epidemiology*, **148**, 1195–205.
3. McKinlay, S.M., Brambilla, D.J. and Posner, G.J. (1992) The normal menopause transition. *Maturitas*, **14** (2), 103–15.
4. Luoto, R., Kaprio, J. and Uutela, A. (1994) Age at menopause and sociodemographic status in Finland. *American Journal of Epidemiology*, **139**, 64–76.
5. Shinberg, D. (1998) An event history of age at last menstrual period: correlates of natural and surgical menopause among midlife Wisconsin women. *Social Science and Medicine*, **46**, 1381–96.
6. Wise, L.A., Krieger, N., Zierler, S. and Harlow, B.C. (2002) Lifetime socioeconomic position in relation to onset of perimenopause. *Journal of Epidemiology and Community Health*, **56**, 851–60.
7. Lawlor, D.A., Ebrahim, S. and Smith, G.D. (2003) The association of socio-economic position across the life course and age at menopause: the British Women's Heart and Health Study. *British Journal of Obstetrics and Gynaecology*, **110**, 1078–87.
8. Khaw, H.T. (1992) Epidemiology of the menopause. *British Medical Bulletin*, **48**, 249–61.
9. Leidy, L.E. (1994) Biological aspects of menopause across the lifespan. *Annual Review of Anthropology*, **23**, 231–53.
10. Lock, M. (1994) Menopause in cultural context. *Experimental Gerontology*, **29**, 307–17.
11. McMaster, J., Pitts, M. and Poyah, G. (1997) The menopausal experiences of women in a developing country: there is a time for everything, to be a teenager, a mother and granny. *Women and Health*, **26**, 1–13.
12. Boulet, M.J., Oddens, B.J., Lehert, P. *et al.* (1994) Climacteric and menopause in seven south east Asian countries. *Maturitas*, **19**, 157–76.
13. Lock, M. (2002) Symptom reporting at menopause: a review of cross cultural findings. *The Journal of the British Menopause Society*, **8**, 132–36.
14. Avis, N.E. and McKinlay, S.M. (1995) The Massachusetts Women's Health Study: an epidemiologic investigation of the menopause. *Journal of the American Medical Women's Association*, **50**, 45–49.
15. Woods, N.F. and Mitchell, E.S. (1997) Pathways to depressed mood for midlife women: observations from the Seattle Midlife Women's Health Study. *Research in Nursing and Health*, **20**, 119–29.

16. Bosworth, H.B., Bastian, L.A., Kuchibhatia, M.N. *et al.* (2001) Depressive symptoms, menopausal status, and climacteric symptoms in women at midlife. *Psychosomatic Medicine*, **63**, 603–8.

17. Dennerstein, L. *et al.* (2000) Life satisfaction, symptoms, and the menopausal transition. *Medscape Women's Health*, **5** (4), E4.

18. Punyahotra, S. and Dennerstein, L. (1997) Menopausal experiences of Thai women. Part 2: the cultural context. *Maturitas*, **26**, 9–14.

19. Fu, S.Y., Anderson, D. and Courtney, M. (2003) Cross-cultural menopausal experience: comparison of Australian and Taiwanese women. *Nursing and Health Sciences*, **5**, 77–84.

20. Avis, N.E., Stellato, R., Crawford, S. *et al.* (2001) Is there a menopausal syndrome? Menopausal status and symptoms across racial/ethnic groups. *Social Science and Medicine*, **52**, 345–56.

21. Bromberger, J.T., Matthews, K.A., Schott, L.L. *et al.* (2007) Depressive symptoms during the menopausal transition: the Study of Women's Health across the nation (SWAN). *Journal of Affective Disorders*, **103**, 267–72.

22. Yahya, S. and Rehan, N. (2002) Age, pattern and symptoms of menopause among rural women of Lahore. *Journal of Ayub Medical College, Abbottabad*, **14**, 9–12.

23. Rizk, D.E., Bener, A., Ezimokhai, M. *et al.* (1998) The age and symptomatology of natural menopause among United Arab Emirates women. *Maturitas*, **29**, 197–202.

24. Dennerstein, L., Lehert, P., Koochaki, P.E. *et al.* (2007) A symptomatic approach to understanding women's health experiences: a cross-cultural comparison of women aged 20 to 70 years. *Menopause*, **14**, 688–96.

25. Melby, M.K., Lock, M. and Kakufert, P. (2005) Culture and symptom reporting at menopause. *Human Reproduction Update*, **11**, 495–512.

26. Tempier, R., Boyer, R., Lambert, J. *et al.* (2006) Psychological distress among female spouses of male at-risk drinkers. *Alcohol*, **40**, 41–49.

27. Zink, T., Fisher, B.S., Regan, S. and Pabst, S. (2005) The prevalence and incidence of intimate partner violence in older women in primary care practices. *Journal of General Internal Medicine*, **20**, 884–88.

28. Chlebowski, R.T., Hendrix, S.L., Langer, R.D. *et al.* (2003) Influence of estrogen plus progestin on breast cancer and mammography in health postmenopausal women. *The Journal of the American Medical Association*, **289**, 3243–53.

29. Pradhan, A.D., Gupta, V., Mukhopadyay, A. *et al.* (2002) Inflammatory biomarkers, hormone replacement therapy, and incident coronary heart disease. *Journal of the American Medical Association*, **288**, 980–87.

30. Wassertheil-Smoller, S. *et al.* (2003) Effect of estrogen plus progestin on stroke in postmenopausal women. *The Journal of the American Medical Association*, **289**, 2673–84.

31. Rapp, S.R. *et al.* (2003) Effect of estrogen plus progestin on global cognitive function in postmenopausal women. The Women's Health Initiative Memory Study: a randomized controlled trial. *The Journal of the American Medical Association*, **289**, 2663–72.

32. Glass, A.G., Lacey, J.V. Jr., Carreon, J.D. and Hoover, R.N. (2007) Breast cancer incidence, 1980–2006: combined roles of menopausal hormone therapy, screening mammography and estrogen receptor status. *Journal of the National Cancer Institute*, **99**, 1152–61.

33. Standing, T.S. and Glazer, G. (1992) Attitudes of low income clinic patients toward menopause. *Health Care for Women International*, **13**, 271–80.

34. UNDP (2003) *Human Development Report 2003. Millennium Development Goals: A compact among nations to end human poverty*. New York, Oxford, Oxford University Press.

35. World Health Organization (2001) Mental Health: New Understanding, New Hope. The World Health Report 2001, World Health Organization, Geneva.

36. Astbury, J. (2001) Gender Disparities in Mental Health, Ministerial Round Tables, 54th World Health Assembly. Mental Health: A call for action by World Health Ministers, World Health Organization, Geneva, pp. 58–73.

37. Astbury, J. and Cabral de Mello, M. (2000) Women's Mental Health: An Evidence Based Review, World Health Organization, Geneva.

38. Wade, T.J., Cairney, J. and Pevalin, D.J. (2002) Emergence of gender differences in depression during adolescence: national panel results from three countries. *Journal of the American Academy of Child and Adolescent Psychiatry*, **41**, 190–98.

39. Kessler, R.C. (2003) Epidemiology of women and depression. *Journal of Affective Disorders*, **74**, 5–13.

40. Andrews, G. *et al.* (1999) The Mental Health of Australia, Commonwealth Department of Health and Aged Care, Canberra.

41. Kessler, R.C. *et al.* (1992) The relationship between age and depressive symptoms in 2 national surveys. *Psychology and Aging*, **7**, 119–26.

42. Bebbington, P. *et al.* (2003) The influence of age and sex on the prevalence of depressive conditions: report from the National Survey of Psychiatric Morbidity. *International Review of Psychiatry*, **15**, 74–83.

43. Akhtar-Danesh, N. and Landeen, J. (2007) Relation between depression and sociodemographic factors. *International Journal of Mental Health Systems*, **1**, 4.

44. Schieman, S., Van Gundy, K. and Taylor, J. (2001) Status, role and resource explanations for age patterns in psychological distress. *Journal of Health and Social Behavior*, **42**, 80–96.

45. Stephens, C. and Ross, N. (2002) The relationship between hormone replacement therapy use and psychological symptoms: no effects found in a New Zealand sample. *Health Care for Women International*, **23**, 408–14.

46. Glazer, G. *et al.* (2002) The Ohio Midlife Women's Study. *Health Care for Women International*, **23**, 612–30.

47. Kaufert, P.A., Gilbert, P. and Tate, R. (1992) The Manitoba Project: a re-examination of the link between menopause and depression. *Maturitas*, **14** (2), 157–60.

48. Kuh, D.L., Wadsworth, M. and Hardy, R. (1997) Women's health in midlife: the influence of the menopause, social factors and health in earlier life. *British Journal of Obstetrics and Gynaecology*, **104** (8), 923–33.

49. Dennerstein, L., Lehert, P. and Guthrie, J. (2002) The effects of the menopausal transition and biopsychosocial factors on well being. *Archives of Women's Mental Health*, **5**, 15–22.

50. Maartens, L.W., Knottnerus, J.A., Pop, V.J. (2002) Menopausal transition and increased depressive symptomataology: a community based prospective study. *Maturitas*, **42**, 195–200.

51. Avis, N.E. *et al.* (1994) A longitudinal analysis of the association between menopause and depression. *Annals of Epidemiology*, **4**, 214–20.

52. Avis, N.E., McKinlay, S.M. (1991) A longitudinal analysis of women's attitudes toward the menopause: results from the Massachusetts Women's Health Study. *Maturitas*, **13** (1), 65–79.

53. Palacios, S. *et al.* (1995) Changes in sex behaviour after menopause: effects of tibolone. *Maturitas*, **22** (2), 155–61.

54. Avis, N.E. (2000) Sexual function and aging in men and women: community and population-based studies. *The Journal of Gender-Specific Medicine*, **3** (2), 37–41.

55. Dennerstein, L., Dudley, E. and Burger, H. (2001) Are changes in sexual functioning during midlife due to aging or menopause? *Fertility and Sterility*, **76**, 456–60.

56. Hallstrom, T. and Samuelsson, S. (1990) Changes in women's sexual desire in middle life: the longitudinal study of women in Gothenburg. *Archives of Sexual Behavior*, **19**, 259–68.

57. Blackmore, E.R., Stansfeld, S.A., Weller, I. *et al.* (2007) Major depressive episodes and work stress: results from a national population survey. *American Journal of Public Health*, **97**, 2088–93.

58. Stansfeld, S.A., Clark, C., Rodgers, B. *et al.* (2008) Childhood and adulthood socio-economic position and midlife depressive and anxiety disorders. *The British Journal of Psychiatry*, **192**, 152–53.

59. Dennerstein, L., Dudley, E., Guthrie, J. (2003) Predictors of declining self rated health during the transition to menopause. *Journal of Psychosomatic Research*, **54**, 147–53.

60. Amore, M., Di Donato, P., Paplini, A. *et al.* (2004) Psychological status at the menopausal transition: an Italian epidemiological study. *Maturitas*, **48**, 115–24.

61. Bromberger, J.T., Kravits, H.M., Wei, H.L. *et al.* (2005) History of depression and women's current health and functioning during midlife. *General Hospital Psychiatry*, **27**, 200–8.

62. Felitti, V.J. *et al.* (1998) Relationship of childhood abuse and household dysfunction to many of the leading causes of death in adults. The Adverse Childhood Experiences (ACE) Study. *American Journal of Preventive Medicine*, **14**, 245–58.

63. Keller, M.C., Neale, M.C. and Kendler, K.S. (2007) Association of different adverse life events with distinct patterns of depressive symptoms. *The American Journal of Psychiatry*, **164**, 1521–29.

64. Brown, G.W., Harris, T.O. and Hepworth, C. (1995) Loss, humiliation and entrapment among women developing depression: a patient and non-patient comparison. *Psychological Medicine*, **25**, 7–21.

65. Romans, S.E., Tyas, J., Cohen, M.M. and Silverstone, T. (2007) Gender differences in the symptoms of major depressive disorder. *The Journal of Nervous and Mental Disease*, **195**, 911.

66. Yahya, S., Rehan, N. (2002). Age, pattern and symptoms of menopause among rural women of Lahore. *Journal of the Ayub Medical College Abbottabad*, **14**, 9–12.

67. Corey, G. (2005) *Theory and Practice of Counseling and Psychotherapy*, 7th edn, Thompson/Brooks-Cole, Belmont.

68. Alder, J., Eymann, B.K., Armbruster, U. *et al.* (2006) Cognitive behavioural group intervention for climacteric syndrome. *Psychotherapy and Psychosomatics*, **75**, 298–303.

69. Keefer, L. & Blanchard, E.B. (2005). A behavioural group treatment program for menospausal hot flashes: results of a pilot study. *Applied Psychophysiology and Biofeedback*, **30**, 21–30.

70. Allen, L.A., Dobkin, R.D., Boohar, E.M. and Woolfolk, R.L. (2006) Cognitive behavior therapy for menopausal hot flushes: two case reports. *Maturitas*, **54**, 95–99.

71. Loh, A., Leonhart, R., Wills, C.E. *et al.* (2007) The impact of patient participation on adherence and clinical outcome in primary care of depression. *Patient Education and Counseling*, **65**, 69–78.

72. Krakow, B., Johnston, L., Melendrez, D. *et al.* (2001) An open-label trial of evidence-based cognitive behavior therapy for nightmares and insomnia in crime victims with PTSD. *The American Journal of Psychiatry*, **158**, 2043–47.

SECTION 3

Service delivery and ethics

Marta B. Rondón

Cayetano Heredia University, Lima, Peru

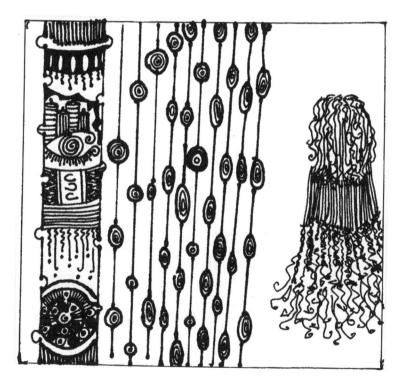

Contemporary Topics in Women's Mental Health   Edited by Chandra, Herrman, Fisher, Kastrup,
© 2009 John Wiley & Sons, Ltd   Niaz, Rondón and Okasha

Commentary

How to give a woman, throughout her life cycle, access to quality mental health-care that conforms with current recommendations and addresses the expectations of both informed providers and users is the subject matter of this section. The delivery of safe, quality healthcare depends on the personal qualifications of the providers, including both technical and ethical competence and personal features such as empathy and warmth, the existence of health establishments that are well accredited, with normalised procedures, well equipped and staffed (human resources are a critical factor in healthcare) and the quality of the environment, which includes policy, laws and regulations, as well as provisions for dignified settings, that insure privacy and comfort.

Gender and ethnic equity, accessibility, availability, efficiency, efficacy, safety and accountability as well as respect for human rights and cultural differences are also important components of the concept of 'quality' in healthcare. Whether a woman approaches or not the mental health services and whether this contact is beneficial or detrimental to her personal wellbeing and development are determined by these various dimensions of quality healthcare.

Technical aspects of our specialty, with a clear gender focus, are the subject matter of this book. In this section, we deal with the ethical and political concerns of mental healthcare for the girl child and the woman and with the appropriateness of services, from a gender and human rights perspective, as it is one of the main concerns of the World Psychiatric Association (WPA) Section on Women's Mental Health as expressed in the International Consensus on Women's Mental Health that the section prepared [1].

Sarabia's chapter discusses the immense contribution of psychopharmacology to the care of mental disorders. Without psychopharmacological interventions, we would still be at the stage where seriously mentally ill women were considered a 'thing of the devil' and separated for life from the family and community.

Without psychopharmacology, we would not have to worry about drug exposure *in utero* and about which medications show up in breast milk. There would be no need for adjustment in contraceptive medication as our female patients would be locked away or their behaviour would be so openly deviant that their chances for normal family life (including having a partner and children) would be nil.

However, we have found out that women's bodies are different from men's bodies in certain respects and Sarabia exposes deftly the need to include women in clinical trials and to examine gender differences in all biomedical research, especially in drug development.

We have also learned that women are more easily prescribed psychoactive drugs than their male counterparts, partly because it is common knowledge that women are more prone to depression and anxiety. We have learned that they receive more diagnoses of anxiety and depressive disorders and that sometimes organic life threatening conditions are missed. We, therefore, have discovered that there has to be consideration given to the impact of psychosocial stress on women's mental health and that drugs, no matter how well chosen and how carefully monitored the adverse effects, are not the answer to the ill feelings of women.

Lack of power, discrimination, segregation and poverty are more common for women than for men. The Women, Gender and Equity Knowledge Network of the World Health Organization (WHO) Commission on the Social Determinants of Health has argued [2] with an impressive array of evidence, that gender is one the strongest social determinants, its weight being such that it can ultimately determine life or death, health or insanity, hospital or community centre.

Interpersonal violence, physical, psychological and sexual, is frequent, accounts for a big proportion of the morbidity and mortality in the world and it affects women disproportionately, not only at home and on the streets, but also at the hands of the states and other political actors and, unfortunately, in health services [3].

In this light, Benjet and Rondón present recommendations, based on current literature, for gender sensitive mental healthcare. Benjet discusses the issues of barriers to care for children and adolescents, highlighting the importance of the family. However, in our present context, the increase in monoparental families and in the number of divorces has complicated the issues of informed consent, home care, medication adherence and supervision of the youngster under treatment.

Corina Benjet also discusses the need for health services to be ready to attend to the different presentations of violence. Latin America has been paradigmatic in the way the Pan American Health Organization and the member states have joined together to respond to the challenge of having some of the highest rates of interpersonal and gender based violence in the world. Legislation has been enacted in most countries to counter violence inside the home. Judges and law enforcement agencies have received hours and hours of specific education on the topic, with the participation of non government organisations and state agencies. Unexpectedly, the health sector has been slow in joining the movement and the response to violence has been stronger in the reproductive health sector rather than in the mental health sector (response).

Benjet's recommendations are thus very timely and can be extrapolated to the care of adult and older adult women. The preparedness of a mental healthcare service to deal with violence includes, of course, space for the personnel to discuss their own experiences with violence and opportunity for mutual support and intervention. One of the reasons that have been invoked in the slow reaction against violence in the health sector has to do with the emotional difficulties experienced by personnel who have witnessed, experienced or perpetrated violence in their private lives, when dealing with victims [4].

Respect for the person's autonomy, protection of the privacy and safety of the victim and the provider are important steps in the care for violence victims. Revictimisation has to be prevented. Quick, informed and effective referral allows for integral care of the victim and should reduce the percentage of persons who become demoralised upon seeking help from health or other state services [5].

'One step' schemes for integral care have been implemented in several sites, but in their absence, clear guidelines for referral are a must.

One of the many things that women expect from their health services is the integration of mental healthcare into primary care. This has been done in the developed world, with Coordinated Centers and Centers of Excellence for women's health in several sites. The satisfaction of users attests to the usefulness of this scheme. Highly centralised health systems, with deficits in human and material resources and many vested interests impinging on how scarce financial resources are utilised are not eager to embrace primary care, although there is great evidence of its efficiency.

Chile is an example of the integration of mental healthcare into primary services, following the recommendations in the Declaration of Caracas. Graciela Rojas and Enrique Jadresic describe the basis of the impulse for psychiatric services in their country: scientific evidence and political decision. The political will came from the democratic governments that replaced Pinochet and that gave great impulse to education and health. The evidence came, among other papers, from the studies of Araya and his group which showed that low education, female gender, unemployment, separation, low social status and lone parenthood were associated with a higher prevalence of common mental disorders in Santiago and the work of Rojas, Araya and Lewis, comparing the affective symptoms of Chilean and British women. The fact that low education has a huge impact on the risk for common emotional symptoms is highlighted in these studies with utmost clarity.

From then on, Chile has tried and implemented a stepped up programme for the treatment of depression, established the National Program for the Detection, Diagnosis and Treatment of Depression and has included treatment of Depressive Episode, Recurrent Depressive Disorder and Depressive Episode of Bipolar Disorder has been included as Explicit Warranty of Health (GES) as of 2006.

The results obtained so far in this innovative system seem to emphasise the importance of equity in health. Equity is a fundamental component of the right to health, as it insures that resources are allocated according to need and not according to financial capacity or equality. States have to guarantee the right to health of citizens, and in this sense, it is up to them to devise the policy, plans, programmes and legislation to insure that gender mainstreaming occurs at all levels of the healthcare system.

Professionals on the other hand, are responsible for the ethical aspects of their work. Psychiatrists deal with certain groups of patients whose judgement may be impaired at times due to their mental illness or who are unable to look after themselves. Such patients, at times, may also become a danger to either themselves or others but may still refuse any medical help. This raises various ethical and human rights issues that have been debated extensively and are still unresolved.

Additionally, in no other medical specialty do patients share with their doctor so many intimate details about their personal, emotional, social or even sexual life.

The doctor-patient relationship in psychiatry is one of great power asymmetry and deep emotional dependence, which result in several risks for the patient and the provider. This raises many ethical issues depending on how the psychiatrist handles the relationship [6].

Roberts and Kristen present a very enriching discussion of ethics in research, including the need to exclude pregnant women from trials, the limitations on patient selection imposed by reproductive hormonal changes and the research on trauma related disorders in combat veterans. Ethical controversies in psychiatry are varied; the advancement of our profession requires that we reflect on these issues and arrive at consensual ethical guidelines that make the benefits of modern psychiatry available to everybody, while the vulnerable and powerless are protected.

Significant progress in women's mental health can only be obtained if careful consideration is given not only to the provision of services that protect and empower women, but also to the strong influence of gender inequity as a social determinant of health.

References

1. Stewart, D.E. (2006) The international consensus statement on women's mental health and the WPA consensus statement on interpersonal violence against. *Women World Psychiatry*, **5** (1), 61–64.

2. Sen, G., Ostlin, P. and George, A. (2007) Women, Gender, Equity Knowledge Network: Unequal, Unfair, Ineffective and Inefficient. Gender Inequity in Health: Why It Exists and What We Can do to Change It. Final Report to the WHO Commission on the Social Determinants of Health.

3. Velzeboer, M., Ellsberg, M., Arcas, C.C. and Garcia-Moreno, C. (2003) Violence Against Women: The Health Sector Responds, Pan American Health Organization.

4. García-Moreno, C. *et al.* (2005) Multi Country Study on Women's Health and Domestic Violence: Initial Results on Prevalences, Health Outcomes and Women's Responses, World Health Organization, Geneva.

5. Feder, G.S., Hutson, M., Ramsay, J. and Taket, A.R. (2006) Women exposed to intimate partner violence: expectations and experiences when they encounter health care professionals: a meta-analysis of qualitative studies. *Archives of Internal Medicine*, **166**, 22–37.

6. Radden, J. (2002) Notes towards a professional ethics for psychiatry. *Australian and New Zealand Journal of Psychiatry*, **36** (1), 52–59. Retrieved October 16, 2008, from http://www.informaworld.com/10.1046/j.1440-1614.2002.00989.

Further reading

Krug, E.G., Dalhberg, L.L., Mercy, J.A., Zwi, A.B. and Lozano, R. (eds) (2002) *World Report on Violence and Health*, World Health Organization, Geneva.

12

Ethics in psychiatric research among women

Laura Roberts[1] and Kristen Prentice[2]

[1]Department of Population Health, Medical College of Wisconsin, Milwaukee, Wisconsin, USA
[2]Maryland Psychiatric Research Center, University of Maryland School of Medicine, Baltimore, Maryland, USA

12.1 The scientific imperative to include women in psychiatric research

Psychiatric illness accounts for about 11% of all disease worldwide and more than 1% of deaths [1], and women are differentially affected by certain of these diseases. Sex differences in the prevalence of some mental illnesses start early in life; for example, girls have higher rates of anxiety than boys but lower rates of attention deficit and conduct disorders. After puberty, girls surpass boys in the incidence of depression and eating disorders and boys surpass girls in drug and alcohol use and dependence. Epidemiological studies show that, worldwide, women are twice as likely as men to have a diagnosis of depression, anxiety disorder or posttraumatic stress disorder (PTSD) and nine times more likely to have eating disorders [2]. Some estimate that as many as a quarter of women will experience clinical depression during their lifetimes, and 10–15% of mothers will have depression during pregnancy and the postpartum period [1, 3]. Women with mood disorders are more likely than men to have co-occurring phobias and panic disorders [4]. Later in life, women of peri-menopausal age are more likely than men of the same age to develop late-onset schizophrenia and bipolar

Contemporary Topics in Women's Mental Health   Edited by Chandra, Herrman, Fisher, Kastrup,
© 2009 John Wiley & Sons, Ltd   Niaz, Rondón and Okasha

disorder [5, 6], and some studies have shown that women comprise the majority of adult psychiatric inpatients aged 50 years or older [7, 8].

The burden of mental illness for women is influenced by society, women's roles as mothers and caretakers and women's physiological changes over time. Globally, women comprise a majority of those who live in poverty and have lower education and literacy rates than men, circumstances which limit their access to care [9]. Women with mental illnesses are more likely than women with other chronic diseases to become disabled and they reach disability earlier [2]. Because mental illnesses tend to emerge in women during early adulthood, critical life stages are interrupted, such as education, job attainment and development of a supportive social and family network [2]. Mentally ill women who become pregnant may face decisions about how and whether to continue psychopharmacological treatment given the known and unknown foetal risks and must cope with illness in addition to the typical challenges of motherhood.

The International Consensus Statement on Women's Mental Health [10] describes the need for appropriate evidence-based mental health services for all women – adolescent, peripartum, midlife, older, immigrant, disabled and others [1]. The statement further asserts that the quality of women's mental healthcare 'should be assessed by indicators that are consistent with the best current knowledge, informed by gender-sensitive research' [10].

The imperative for gender-sensitive and even gender-specific research has earned broad, but not universal, support in contemporary medicine [11]. There has been disagreement on when women's mental health should be considered a specialty and when it should be moved into mainstream psychiatric medicine [12, 13]. A great deal of attention has been paid recently to the underrepresentation of women in clinical research, especially research that is not sex specific. Following decades of staunch opposition to the practise of clinical research in women, methodological and scientific advances have been slow but significant.

As the leading financial supporter of biomedical research in the United States, the National Institutes of Health (NIH) has made a concerted effort to increase the number of women participating in clinical research studies and the amount of research funding in women's health. In the mid 1980s, NIH established a policy encouraging the inclusion of women and minorities in clinical research. After a 1990 investigation by the Government Accounting Office found widespread failure to implement this inclusion policy, Congress passed the NIH Revitalization Act of 1993 to force adherence and formally established the NIH Office of Research on Women's Health. But the policy stopped short of imposing a mandate requiring the inclusion of women and minorities in clinical research. Subsequently, in 1994 [14], NIH revised its policy to require that women and minorities be included in all NIH-funded clinical research studies and that phase III studies be designed to allow analyses of group differences by sex. Since the establishment of inclusion requirements, NIH has seen a significant improvement in the recruitment of women into clinical research studies. In 1997, more than half of clinical research participants were women [15]. There has been less success, however, in the effort to ensure that phase III studies allow for the analysis of intervention effects' differences by sex [15]. One review of papers published between 1993 and 1998 found that no more than one third of non-sex-specific studies included analysis by sex [16].

NIH also has seen significant growth in spending on research in women's health. During the 1990s spending on women's health increased at a rate that surpassed overall spending growth, particularly for some diseases more prevalent in women, including mood disorders and depression, where the spending increased by more than 70% [15]. In U.S. fiscal year 2006, the 4.1 million women participating in women-only NIH-funded studies accounted for 28% of NIH's total reported research enrolment [17].

Nevertheless, even if investigators reach an ideological consensus on the need to include women in their research, the question of how to do so introduces ethical challenges faced by researchers and by the women who might participate in their studies. In the next sections, we will discuss the fundamental tenets of ethically sound clinical research and the unique challenges of including women as participants.

12.2 The ethical challenges of psychiatric research

Ethically sound clinical research embodies the three ethics principles articulated in the 1979 landmark Belmont Report [18]: respect for persons, honouring the dignity and promoting the autonomy of research participants; beneficence, the duty to seek maximal good and to do minimal harm through the conduct of research; and justice, ensuring that the segment of the population bearing the greatest burden of research also benefits from it and that special groups are not exploited as a result of individual, interpersonal or societal attributes or powerlessness.

The practical application of such abstract concepts in the development of a scientific research protocol can be difficult and requires special consideration of critical study design elements and ethical safeguards. One of the primary criteria is that every clinical study should be based on a clear research question that is scientifically valuable, significant and timely and should yield meaningful and interpretable results. In other words, the study's design must guarantee that its anticipated contribution to science justifies the involvement of human participants. Additionally, a study's design should pose the absolute minimal necessary risk to participants and not be so complex that prospective participants cannot understand it.

Roberts [19] has proposed the Research Protocol Ethics Assessment Tool (RePEAT) to help those responsible for writing and reviewing research protocols. RePEAT, a kind of checklist, incorporates scientific merit and design; expertise, commitment and integrity of the research team; risks and benefits to study participants; confidentiality; participant selection and recruitment issues; informed consent procedures, voluntarism and questions of decisional capacity, especially in potentially vulnerable populations; incentives for participation and issues of coercion; scientific and ethical review by institutional and peer/professional bodies and data presentation and disclosure.

In some controversial study designs, such as placebo trials, medication washouts and deception studies, adherence to these guidelines is debated. But scientific innovation requires methodological innovation, and researchers face a constantly changing ethical landscape. For example, advances in genetics research and human brain imaging have created new sets of ethical challenges. Consequently, the research community relies on standard ethics safeguards to provide reliable protection for research participants, such as institutional review and data monitoring, expert and peer review processes and confidentiality protections.

Among the most critical ethics safeguards is the requirement that, before enrolling in a clinical research study, individuals must provide their informed consent. A common myth is that the purpose of informed consent is to indemnify the investigator or institution if something goes wrong. In fact, from an ethical perspective, informed consent is important in establishing a balance between science (study design and methods) and respectful, beneficent and just regard for the individual [20]. It has three main components: information sharing, decisional capacity and capacity for voluntarism [20, 21].

The information sharing component ensures that the prospective participant has every opportunity to hear and fully understand the details of the study, including the purpose of the research, the study procedures, alternatives to participation and potential risks and benefits. The length of this interactive process, during which participants should be invited to ask questions, depends on the complexity of the protocol under consideration.

The decisional capacity component relates to whether the individual is capable of making an independent decision about participating in the specific study. Adequate capacity depends on the individual's ability in four primary domains: understanding the information relevant to the decision, reasoning rationally with that information by weighing risks and benefits, expressing a clear decision about whether to participate and appreciating the personal consequences of that decision. Whether an individual has adequate capacity is a clinical judgement, although in the United States it is assumed that adults are capable of consent unless there is a specific threat to this ability.

The final component of informed consent is the capacity for voluntarism. A genuinely voluntary decision is not coerced, and it is true to one's beliefs about what is right in a given situation [22]. For every prospective research participant, internal and external pressures and biases can affect the decision about whether to participate, not all of which rise to the level of coercion, per se, but carry some measure of influence.

Because of their roles in families and societies, women face distinct challenges to their capacity to make genuinely voluntary decisions about research participation. For example, women may be more likely than men to subscribe to an interdependent approach to health-related decisions, because they tend to prefer a more collaborative decision-making style than men, who often display a more assertive, self-reliant style. Roberts *et al.* [23] asked women and men whether they would agree to participate in a hypothetical clinical trial and found that women believed the decision was more difficult than the men did and desired more study information, opportunities for discussion, time and support. A study assessing attitudes about clinical research among African American women [24, 25] found a general belief that clinical research was designed to help primarily the Caucasian community and that African American women would be more likely to participate in clinical research if investigators made efforts to become involved in their community, gain their trust and ensure cultural diversity in the research team. Compatibility between clinical researchers and prospective women study participants may also be a factor in consent decisions when women view researchers, who are often doctors, as strong authority figures or when women prefer female clinicians [26]. Power relationships between women and researchers can leave some women feeling intimidated or pressured, sometimes because the researchers are doctors, sometimes because they are men and sometimes both.

Women who are pregnant or of childbearing age also approach consent decisions with unique perspectives and values. They weigh potential risks and benefits with respect to their immediate and long-term personal health and may fear potential effects on future pregnancies. Women may be prohibited from participating in clinical research that carries known or unknown risks to foetuses and are often required to submit to a pregnancy test prior to enrolling (an issue addressed in greater depth later in the chapter). Young women research participants also commonly are required to use at least one form of contraception while enrolled in the study, which may violate their personal beliefs and values and is very rarely applied to male participants [27].

Nicholson *et al.* [28] reported that when mothers with psychiatric illness face health-related decisions, the instinct to put the needs of their children ahead of their own often drives their choices. Some women see the opportunity to seek treatment or pursue new therapeutic avenues as a chance to become healthier and therefore better mothers. Others feel compelled to ignore their own needs and fear that new or different treatment would disrupt their lives and compromise their routines and sense of control.

12.3 Unique challenges of psychiatric research in women

Epidemiology, as discussed in the first part of this chapter, confirms the scientific imperative to include women in psychiatric research. Equally important is the ethical imperative to do so. The Belmont [18] principles of respect for persons, beneficence and justice demonstrate the need for clinical research to consider the experience of being a woman in society and the psychiatric community across the developmental arc. Proponents of the inclusion of women in psychiatric research argue that women deserve the attention of medical science and should not be forced to settle for treatments based on knowledge extrapolated from research carried out predominantly in men.

The under-inclusion of women in psychiatry research, and clinical research in general, stems from a perceived inability to provide ethically and scientifically acceptable solutions to the problems posed by ethical principles and guidelines. For example, is it scientifically necessary to test psychotropic medications in women specifically? Or is the risk too great, especially to those who are or may become mothers? How does the potential risk to a relatively small sample of women research participants compare with the potential risk to the larger population of women who might later take the untested drug? A common theme is the question of whether and how to impose the known and unknown burdens of psychiatric research participation on women, given their unique roles in families and societies. Indeed, federal regulations identify pregnant women and women of childbearing age as groups whose capacity to make independent decisions is made vulnerable by the potentially competing interests of the woman and the foetus.

In the remaining sections we will illustrate three special topics in the debate over the involvement of women in psychiatric research: the exclusion of pregnant women from clinical research, reproductive hormonal changes and the need to be gender- and age-specific in clinical research, and researching PTSD and trauma-related mental illness in women veterans.

The exclusion of pregnant women from clinical research

Although the research community has made great strides in improving women's involvement in clinical studies, there is still widespread apprehension about including women of childbearing age and, especially, pregnant women. Much of clinical research in women's health has lapsed into a 'better safe than sorry' approach. As a result, pregnant and potentially pregnant women are still often excluded from drug trials with unknown or minimal toxicity for the foetus [27, 29]. So pervasive is the protectionism that pregnant women have been excluded from studies in which the 'risky' protocol elements were not pharmacological at all, but extended to activities such as vigorous exercise [27].

The participation of women in psychiatric clinical research typically involves a minimum of two potentially vulnerable populations: the mentally ill and women of childbearing age. In the event of pregnancy during participation, the woman moves into the vulnerable pregnant category and the embryo or foetus introduces a third vulnerable category. If the woman gives birth during the study, she may move into the nursing category and the foetus moves into the minor child category. At every step, a new set of potential vulnerabilities emerges. Protective measures, safety monitoring and contingency plans must be laid out with meticulous detail [30].

In many areas of clinical research, non-pregnant women of childbearing age are excluded altogether or required to use birth control or prove sterility while participating in drug trials [27, 31]. Contraceptive requirements introduce a number of scientific and ethical ramifications. Hormonal contraceptives carry known and unknown risks of their own. Their use also prevents critical analyses of drug effects on normally cycling women, which is especially problematic in psychiatry research, because women metabolise some psychotropic drugs differently across menstrual phases. Also, study samples are biased against women whose personal or religious beliefs obviate the use of contraceptives, because abstinence and celibacy are rarely considered acceptable preventative measures and homosexuality does not negate the contraceptive requirement [27].

Another issue is the disproportionate application of these requirements to women relative to men. In one review of the literature, men participating in studies of drugs with known teratogenicity were asked to agree to take precautions such as 'condoms or the use of birth control pills, diaphragm, tubal ligation or hysterectomy *by my partner*' ([27], emphasis added, page 864). Although women were excluded from the study altogether because of foetal risk, there was no mention of abstinence, vasectomy or sterility by male participants. This apparent double-standard supports the implied need to control reproductive choice for women but not for men. The result of these uneven requirements is that women are disproportionately denied the opportunity to independently evaluate information about research-related risks, whether to themselves or to potential future offspring, and to make autonomous decisions. Advocates for women in research suggest that with a strong consent process, in which risks to the woman and an existing or potential foetus are made clear, this imbalance could be reduced to support women's self-determination [9].

The relative absence of women in clinical research has clear and direct consequences for advancing the mental healthcare available to them. Healthcare providers frequently treat pregnant women without adequate information about drug safety or dosing, and pregnant women are denied the opportunity to access drugs with direct clinical benefit. Research on the teratogenic foetal risks associated with maternal use of psychotropic drugs has yielded mixed results, leaving crucial gaps in the knowledge of how to treat mental illness in women [32]. Although the U.S. Food and Drug Administration (FDA) [33] recently proposed new guidelines for expanded foetal risk information on drug labels, few, if any, psychotropic drugs remain with sufficient empirical evidence to warrant FDA approval for use by pregnant women or, consequently, to convince expectant mothers and their clinicians of their safety [34, 35]. Psychiatric illnesses typically emerge in women during peak childbearing years. Many women who become pregnant are already taking psychotropic medications [32, 36]. Because of the lack of data, many women and doctors are hesitant to continue psychotropic medications during pregnancy, weighing risks to the mother against risks to the foetus, which are largely unknown. However, women who choose to discontinue treatment are about twice as likely to experience a relapse during pregnancy than those who continue treatment [34], and such relapses have been associated with poor neonatal outcome, resulting from factors like poor maternal nutrition and medical care and increased use of alcohol, tobacco and drugs [32, 34, 37].

Consequently, treatment discontinuation is not necessarily the safest option, though it is frequently chosen by even the most well-intentioned women and doctors.

Reproductive hormonal changes and the need to be more gender- and age-specific in clinical research

Although the notion of 'women's health' is less centred on issues of reproduction than in years past, it is crucial for the development of women's healthcare to understand the relationships between women's natural reproductive transitions and the course of their illnesses, especially in psychiatry and psychiatric research. The variety of mood disorders observed in women during different stages of life illustrates the need to ask very specific questions about the role of hormonal change in the occurrence of mental illness in women and in its treatment. The onset of many depressive disorders (e.g. premenstrual syndrome, premenstrual dysphoric disorder, postpartum depression, postmenopausal depression) appears to be triggered by natural hormonal changes that occur over the course of a woman's lifespan or by abnormal reactions to those changes [38, 39]. Similar hormonal triggers have been observed in schizophrenia and bipolar disorder [2].

The ethical principle of justice is highlighted here; a one-size-fits-all approach to treating women's mental illness is not tenable. As a result of complex and fluctuating interactions between women's ovarian hormones and neurotransmitters and the consequent effects on the metabolism of psychotropic drugs, generalisation of results from studies of other populations is not optimal for women's care. Not only are studies conducted in largely male samples inadequate sources of evidence-based medicine for women, but studies with women participants also are not necessarily applicable to women across a broad range of ages.

Hormonal changes also influence the pharmacodynamics and pharmacokinetics of psychotropic drugs and vice versa. For example, oestrogen is known to interact with serotonin function to influence mood and affect [38]. On one hand, this makes oestrogen a potential treatment option for depressive disorders, although possible secondary risks to cardiac and other functions are noted. On the other hand, the constant fluctuation of women's oestrogen levels means that selective serotonin reuptake inhibitors, the most common treatment for depressive disorders, behave differently in women in different hormonal phases, such as pre and post menopause [38]. Because most women live a third of their lives after menopause [35], the optimal evidence-based treatment for depressive disorders in older women, for example, should not be based on studies of younger women.

Even short-term hormonal fluctuations across menstrual phases are related to the function of psychotropic medications [35]. Antipsychotic drugs used to treat bipolar disorder and schizophrenia can interfere with a woman's menstrual cycle, cause elevated prolactin, affect fertility and increase the risk of ovarian diseases (e.g. polycystic ovarian syndrome, endometrial hyperplasia) [40]. Similar side effects are seen in women taking certain anticonvulsant medications, which are used more and more to treat illnesses other than epilepsy, such as bipolar disorder [41]. These risks make researchers wary of enrolling women in drug studies. They also emphasise the need for more research on how to safely treat psychiatric illness in women.

Researching PTSD and trauma-related mental illness in women veterans

As the number of women serving in the military increases, so does the need for research into the mental health consequences of their military duty [42, 43]. Between combat-related trauma and sexual assault, the issues facing women veterans are particularly charged. Research is needed on how to provide adequate mental healthcare to women veterans, because these women are infrequent users of existing care structures and often improperly diagnosed.

Among women, a leading cause of PTSD is sexual assault. Sexual assault victims are more likely to commit suicide, suffer depression or anxiety and use drugs and alcohol. Sexual assault has also been linked to increased risk of heart attacks and asthma, as well as breast cancer [44]. Women in the military have higher rates of lifetime sexual assault than civilian women [45]. In one survey, a third of women veterans experienced sexual assault while on active military duty, of whom more than half met criteria for depressive disorder and more than 40% for PTSD [45]. Compared with peers with no history of assault, these veterans were nine times more likely to have PTSD. The personal experience and mental health consequences of military sexual assault can be very different from those of non-military sexual assault. For example, in the military, the perpetrator is likely to be a coworker or person of higher rank with whom the victim must continue working. Only 5% of the women veterans surveyed had civilian assailants.

The high rates of PTSD in women veterans are not reflected in their utilisation of mental health services, particularly from providers based at the Veterans Administration (VA). One reason is that women veterans are significantly less likely than their male counterparts to be 'service connected' for PTSD; that is, they are less likely to collect disability benefits for the illness. Research suggests that this service connection discrepancy does not reflect lower symptom severity in women veterans but, rather, the difficulty of proving their illness is the result of a service-related event. Combat-related trauma, which accounts for the vast majority of PTSD cases in male veterans, is a comparatively straightforward case to make [44].

12.4 Summary

Mental illness among women poses an enormous public health burden and immeasurable suffering for women and their families. Mental illnesses affect women uniquely and are subject to both internal and external influences. Much of what is known about how to treat mental illness in women is extrapolated from research carried out in men. The under-representation of women in clinical research, especially those who are pregnant or of childbearing age, often results in residual exclusion, where care providers, faced with insufficient data on side effects and proper medication administration for women, are reluctant to offer medications to their women patients. Consequently, women are denied access to potentially helpful treatment options or, alternatively, offered potentially unsafe treatment options. In order to resolve these problems, we must decide which poses the greater risk, enrolling a small sample of women in a controlled research study or marketing and prescribing an untested medication to vast numbers of women.

In many cases an investigator's decision about whether to enrol women in a clinical trial is difficult, given the tension between the two primary duties of medicine: to protect individuals made vulnerable by illness and to study their illnesses with the goal of advancing treatment options. As part of these decisions, objective consideration and application of the primary ethical principles of respect for persons, beneficence and justice must continue. Only then can appropriate evidence-based mental health treatment be available for all women.

Acknowledgement

The authors wish to thank Ann Tennier for her editorial assistance. Ms. Tennier and Dr Roberts are funded through the Research for a Healthier Tomorrow-Program Development Fund, a component of the Advancing a Healthier Wisconsin endowment at the Medical College of Wisconsin.

References

1. Stewart, D.E., Ashraf, I.J. and Munce, S.E. (2006) Women's mental health: a silent cause of mortality and morbidity. *International Journal of Gynaecology and Obstetrics*, **94** (3), 343–49.
2. Blehar, M.C. (2003) Public health context of women's mental health research. *The Psychiatric Clinics of North America*, **26** (3), 781–99.
3. Kessler, R.C. (2003) Epidemiology of women and depression. *Journal of Affective Disorders*, **74** (1), 5–13.
4. Blehar, M.C. and Oren, D.A. (1997) Gender differences in depression. *Medscape Women's Health*, **2** (2), 3.
5. Sajatovic, M., Sultana, D., Bingham, C.R. *et al.* (2002) Gender related differences in clinical characteristics and hospital based resource utilization among older adults with schizophrenia. *International Journal of Geriatric Psychiatry*, **17** (6), 542–48.
6. Sajatovic, M., Bingham, C.R., Campbell, E.A. and Fletcher, D.F. (2005) Bipolar disorder in older adult inpatients. *The Journal of Nervous and Mental Disease*, **193** (6), 417–19.

7. Davidson, M., Harvey, P.D., Powchik, P. *et al.* (1995) Severity of symptoms in chronically institutionalized geriatric schizophrenic patients. *American Journal of Psychiatry*, **152** (2), 197–207.

8. Sajatovic, M., Donenwirth, K., Sultana, D. and Buckley, P. (2000) Admissions, length of stay, and medication use among women in an acute care state psychiatric facility. *Psychiatric Services*, **51** (10), 1278–81.

9. Eckenwiler, L.A. (1998) Attention to difference and women's consent to research. *IRB*, **20** (6), 6–11.

10. Stewart, D.E. (2006) The international consensus statement on women's mental health and the WPA consensus statement on interpersonal violence against women. *World Psychiatry*, **5** (1), 61–64.

11. Corbie-Smith, G.M., Durant, R.W. and St George, D.M. (2006) Investigators' assessment of NIH mandated inclusion of women and minorities in research. *Contemporary Clinical Trials*, **27** (6), 571–79.

12. Kimerling, R.E., Ouimette, P.C. and Cronkite, R.C. (1998) Women's health needs. *Psychiatric Services*, **49** (11), 1493–94.

13. Satel, S.L. (1998) Are women's health needs really "special"? *Psychiatric Services*, **49** (5), 565.

14. National Institutes of Health (1994) NIH guidelines on the inclusion of women and minorities as subjects in clinical research. *NIH Guide*, **23** (11). Available at: http://grants.nih.gov/grants/guide/notice-files/not94-100.html (accessed 2 june 2009).

15. United States General Accounting Office (2000) Report to Congressional Requestors: Women's Health: NIH Has Increased Its Efforts to Include Women in Research, GAO/HEHS-00-96. Available at: http://www.gao.gov/archive/2000/he00096.pdf (accessed 20 May 2008).

16. Vidaver, R.M., Lafleur, B., Tong, C. *et al.* (2000) Women subjects in NIH-funded clinical research literature: lack of progress in both representation and analysis by sex. *Journal of Women's Health and Gender-based Medicine*, **9** (5), 495–504.

17. Pinn, V.W., Roth, C., Bates, A.C. *et al.* (2007) Monitoring Adherence to the National Institutes of Health Policy on the Inclusion of Women and Minorities as Subjects in Clinical Research. Comprehensive Report: Tracking of Human Subjects Research Reported in Fiscal Year 2005 and 2006.

18. National Commission for the Protection of Human Subjects of Biomedical and Behavioral Research (1979) The Belmont Report: Ethical Principles and Guidelines for the Protection of Human Subjects of Research.

19. Roberts, L.W. (1999) Ethical dimensions of psychiatric research: a constructive, criterion-based approach to protocol preparation. The research protocol ethics assessment tool (RePEAT). *Biological Psychiatry*, **46** (8), 1106–19.

20. Dunn, L.B. and Roberts, L.W. (2004) Informed consent, in *Encyclopedia of Women's Health* (eds S. Loue, M. Sajatovic and K.B. Armitage), Kluwer Academic/Plenum Publishers, New York, pp. 333–35.

21. Roberts, L.W. and Dyer, A.R. (2004) *Concise Guide to Ethics in Mental Health Care*, American Psychiatric Publishing, Washington, DC.

22. Roberts, L.W. (2002) Informed consent and the capacity for voluntarism. *The American Journal of Psychiatry*, **159** (5), 705–12.

23. Roberts, L.W., Warner, T.D., Nguyen, K.P. *et al.* (2003) Schizophrenia patients' and psychiatrists' perspectives on ethical aspects of symptom re-emergence during psychopharmacological research participation. *Psychopharmacology*, **171** (1), 58–67.

24. BeLue, R., Taylor-Richardson, K.D., Lin, J. *et al.* (2006) African Americans and participation in clinical trials: differences in beliefs and attitudes by gender. *Contemporary Clinical Trials*, **27** (6), 498–505.

25. Smith, Y.R., Johnson, A.M., Newman, L.A. *et al.* (2007) Perceptions of clinical research participation among African American women. *Journal of Women's Health*, **16** (3), 423–28.

26. Hussain-Gambles, M. (2004) South Asian patients' views and experiences of clinical trial participation. *Family Practice*, **21** (6), 636–42.

27. Cain, J., Lowell, J., Thorndyke, L. and Localio, A.R. (2000) Contraceptive requirements for clinical research. *Obstetrical and Gynecological Survey*, **95** (6Pt 1), 861–66.

28. Nicholson, J., Sweeney, E.M. and Geller, J.L. (1998) Mothers with mental illness: I. The competing demands of parenting and living with mental illness. *Psychiatric Services*, **49** (5), 635–42.

29. Grover, S., Avasthi, A. and Sharma, Y. (2006) Psychotropics in pregnancy: weighing the risks. *The Indian Journal of Medical Research*, **123** (4), 497–512.

30. Committee on Ethics, American College of Obstetricians and Gynecologists (1999) ACOG committee opinion. Ethical considerations in research involving pregnant women. Number 213, November 1998. *International Journal of Gynaecology and Obstetrics*, **65** (1), 93–96.

31. Schonfeld, T.L. and Gordon, B.G. (2005) Contraception in research: a policy suggestion. *IRB*, **27** (2), 15–20.

32. Pearlstein, T. (2008) Perinatal depression: treatment options and dilemmas. *Journal of Psychiatry and Neuroscience*, **33** (4), 302–18.

33. United States Food and Drug Administration (2008) FDA Proposes New Rule to Provide Updated Information on the Use of Prescription Drugs and Biological Products During Pregnancy and Breast-Feeding. Available at: http://www.fda.gov/bbs/topics/NEWS/2008/NEW01841.html (accessed 2 August 2008).

34. Lamberg, L. (2005) Risks and benefits key to psychotropic use during pregnancy and postpartum period. *The Journal of the American Medical Association*, **294** (13), 1604–8.

35. Worell, J. and Goodheart, C.D. (2006) *Handbook of Girls' and Women's Psychological Health*, Oxford University Press, New York.

36. Lee, B., Ratnasiri, A., Curtis, M. and Ahmad, S. (2006). Psychotropic Medication Use Among Women Initiating Prenatal Care in the California Medicaid Program, 2003. 12th Annual CDC MCH Epidemiology Conference, Atlanta, Georgia December 6, 2006.

37. Bonari, L., Pinto, N., Ahn, E. *et al.* (2004) Perinatal risks of untreated depression during pregnancy. *Canadian Journal of Psychiatry*, **49** (11), 726–35.

38. Shors, T.J. and Leuner, B. (2003) Estrogen-mediated effects on depression and memory formation in females. *Journal of Affective Disorders*, **74** (1), 85–96.

39. Steiner, M., Dunn, E. and Born, L. (2003) Hormones and mood: from menarche to menopause and beyond. *Journal of Affective Disorders*, **74** (1), 67–83.

40. Joffe, H. (2007) Reproductive biology and psychotropic treatments in premenopausal women with bipolar disorder. *Journal of Clinical Psychiatry*, **68** (Suppl 9), 10–15.

41. Kaplan, P.W. (2004) Reproductive health effects and teratogenicity of antiepileptic drugs. *Neurology*, **63** (10 Suppl 4), S13–23.

42. Murray, P. (2008) Senators Introduce Legislation to Improve Care for Women Veterans. Available at: http://murray.senate.gov/news.cfm?id=295394 (accessed 2 August 2008).

43. Schnurr, P.P., Friedman, M.J., Engel, C.C. *et al.* (2005) Issues in the design of multisite clinical trials of psychotherapy: VA Cooperative Study No. 494 as an example. *Contemporary Clinical Trials*, **26** (6), 626–36.

44. Murdoch, M., Hodges, J., Hunt, C. *et al.* (2003) Gender differences in service connection for PTSD. *Medical Care*, **41** (8), 950–61.

45. Suris, A., Lind, L., Kashner, T.M. *et al.* (2004) Sexual assault in women veterans: an examination of PTSD risk, health care utilization, and cost of care. *Psychosomatic Medicine*, **66** (5), 749–56.

13

Integrating mental health into women's health and primary healthcare: The case of Chile

Graciela Rojas[1] and Enrique Jadresic[2]

[1]*Departamento de Psiquiatría y Salud Mental; Hospital Clínico de la Universidad de Chile, Santiago, Chile*
[2]*Departamento de Psiquiatría y Salud Mental, Universidad de Chile, Santiago, Chile*

13.1 Introduction

In Chile, a middle income nation, with a population of 15 million inhabitants, the public system of health provides care to nearly 70% of the population. During the last 18 years, great achievements incorporating mental health to public policies have been made. This is evidenced by the development, during these years, of several mental health programmes for primary care, by the emergence of psychiatric services in general hospitals and community services; by the increased coverage in the treatment of psychiatric disorders available to the population and by the augmented budget for mental health. Among other factors, political will and scientific evidence have probably been determinant factors explaining this accomplishment.

Contemporary Topics in Women's Mental Health   Edited by Chandra, Herrman, Fisher, Kastrup,
© 2009 John Wiley & Sons, Ltd   Niaz, Rondón and Okasha

13.2 Integrating mental health into primary healthcare

At the end of the 1980s, psychiatric epidemiology showed significant advances in Chile: instruments were validated and extensive and rigorous epidemiological studies were conducted, both in the general population and in primary care. These investigations found that common mental disorders affected approximately one of every four people living in the community and one of every two people who consulted in primary care clinics [1–5].

Two important prevalence studies of psychiatric disorders were carried out in the general population. The study of common mental disorders conducted in the city of Santiago – 1995–1998 – used the clinical interview schedule-revised (CIS-R) and reported 25% of common mental disorders cases (25%) and a weekly prevalence of 'depressive episode' – according to ICD-10 criteria – of 5.5% (men 2.7% and women 8.0%) [1]. In turn, the Chile Prevalence Study, carried out in four cities of Chile – including Santiago – used DSM-III R criteria with CIDI and reported a six month prevalence of 19,7% of any mental disorder and of 4.7% for Major Depressive Disorder (men 3.0%; women 6.2%) [5]. Those two studies found that female sex and poverty were risk factors for common mental disorders. Thus, the study of common mental disorders conducted in the city of Santiago showed that low education, female gender, unemployment, separation, low social status and lone parenthood were associated with a higher prevalence of common mental disorder (Tables 13.1 and 13.2) [1].

A later study used the data base of the Chilean study about Common Mental Disorders and that of a similar cross-sectional psychiatric household survey carried out in Great Britain to compare the sex differences for common affective disorders in the two countries. It found that women in both nations reported more common affective disorders than men but Chilean women had an increased risk in comparison to their British counterparts (Table 13.3) [6].

Among all the variables examined (education, employment and marital status, children at home, social support) education was the only one that showed a statistically significant interaction that could account for the increased risk of the Chilean women. In fact, as the educational level attained in Chilean women decreased there was an increasingly greater risk of developing a common mental disorder, something that did not happen among British women [6].

Epidemiological studies conducted in primary care showed that one out of every two people who attended primary care clinics had a psychiatric disorder and that primary care professionals had to face mental health problems for which they were not prepared [2–4, 7].

The WHO multicentre collaborative study on Psychological Problems in General Health Care that was carried out in 14 different countries showed Chile was the country with the highest prevalence rates of any mental disorders – 52.5% – and that women that attended primary care clinics in Santiago had nearly three times the prevalence rates observed throughout the world (36.8% versus 12.5%) [4]. Other studies have been carried out at the primary care level. One of them reported a point prevalence of Depressive Disorders of 29.5% (DSM-III R)

Table 13.1 One-week prevalence of common mental disorders by gender, age, marital status and family type I

Variable	% Prevalence	Adjusted odds ratio (95% CI)[a,b]
Gender		
Male	15.7	1.00
Female	33.6	2.37 (1.84–3.07)
Age (years)		
16–24	22.4	1.00
25–39	29.5	1.41 (0.87–2.27)
40–54	23.1	0.82 (0.52–1.29)
55–64	23.6	0.61 (0.37–1.01)
Marital status		
Never married	21.9	1.00
Married	24.3	1.08 (0.72–1.62)
Separated	36.6	1.83 (1.14–2.92)
Widowed	37.3	1.65 (0.88–3.11)
Cohabiting[c]	39.2	1.76 (1.00–3.09)
Family type		
Couple with children	24.8	1.00
Couple without children	26.8	1.26 (0.94–1.68)
Young single	20.7	0.93 (0.55–1.56)
Adult single	23.6	1.06 (0.73–1.54)
Lone parent	39.4	1.61 (1.12–2.32)

[a]Weighted sample.
[b]Adjusted by age, gender, marital status, education level, social class, employment status, family type and household size.
[c]Living together for longer than one year without being married.

among individuals attending primary care clinics [2]. In turn, a cross sectional study carried out – 1993–1995 – in five randomly selected primary care clinics in northern Santiago assessed 815 consecutive patients – those aged over 50 or with a chronic illness were excluded – seen by 11 primary care physicians. It showed a prevalence of common mental disorders of 49% (95% CI: 46–53%) [3]. Additionally, a logistic regression analysis was performed, which demonstrated that female gender, severe social problems, important income loss, a personal accident or illness, a poor education and having only one close person at home significantly increased the probability of developing a psychiatric disorder [3]. This study also assessed the detection rates of common mental disorders by primary care physicians and found that doctors identified correctly 63% (95% CI: 55–70%) of those patients who attributed their consultation to psychological causes and 34% (95% CI.: 28–41%) of those patients who attributed their consultation to physical causes. After adjustment for confounders, three

Table 13.2 One-week prevalence of common mental disorders by education, social class and employment status

Variable	% Prevalence	Adjusted odds ratio (95% CI)[a,b]
Educational level[c]		
Higher	14.6	1.00
Secondary	24.3	1.34 (1.01–1.78)
Primary	37.0	2.56 (1.71–3.84)
Social class		
Highest	12.6	1.00
Middle	23.4	23.4 (23.3–23.5)
Low	28.6	1.65 (1.11–2.44)
Unstable	34.7	1.80 (1.15–2.83)
Employment status		
Full-time employed	19.5	1.00
Economically inactive	29.2	1.30 (0.95–1.78)
Self-employed	31.9	1.46 (0.87–2.44)
Unemployed	37.7	2.29 (1.27–4.11)

[a]Weighted sample.
[b]Adjusted by age, gender, marital status, education level, social class, employment status, family type and household size.
[c]Primary education is equivalent to less than eight years, secondary education between 8 and 12 years and higher education is more than 12 years.

Table 13.3 Common affective disorders and sex by country[a]

		Common affective disorders[b]	
		Prevalence % (95% CI)	Adjusted odds ratio[c] (95% CI)
Chile	Men	6.8	1.00
	Women	15.3	2.16 (1.64–2.85)
Great Britain	Men	8.2	1.00
	Women	11.3	1.29 (1.04–1.62)

[a]Un-weighted data.
[b]ICD-10 depressive, generalised anxiety, panic and phobia disorders.
[c]Adjusted by age, marital status, education, employment status, children under 15, social support, physical disease, alcohol consumption and household size.

variables showed significant independent associations with detection: a spontaneous psychological reason for consultation, a psychological causal attribution for the presenting problems and an increased severity of the mental disorder (Table 13.4) [7].

Table 13.4 The association between patients' causal attribution of the reason for consultation and the detection of common mental disorders by primary care doctors*

	Adjusted odds ratio* (95% CI)
Reason for consultation[b]:	
Physical	1
Ambiguous	1.33 (0.72–2.48)
Psychological	6.24 (1.27–30.6)
Patients' causal attribution:	
Physical	1
Psychological	2.31 (1.43–3.74)
Physical illness:	
Absent	1
Present	0.54 (0.28–1.05)
Disability:	
Absent	1
Present	0.91 (0.55–1.46)
Common somatic symptoms:	
Below median	1
Above median	1.30 (0.74–2.28)
Symptom interpretation questionnaire:	
Psychologising:	
Below median	1
Above median	0.81 (0.36–1.79)
Somatising:	
Below median	1
Above median	1.10 (0.67–1.80)
Normalising:	
Below median	1
Above median	0.75 (0.37–1.52)
Clinical interview schedule – revised score:	
12–20 points	1
>20 points	2.00 (1.15–3.50)

*Only cases diagnosed according to psychiatric interview are included.
[a] Logistic regression involved 291 subjects only, because cases with missing data are automatically omitted from the procedure. Using Huber White Robust Estimator for clustering of doctors and adjusted for all study variables.
[b] Fifteen cases are missing and 55 cases are not included because reasons for consultation were unclear or patients were consulting primarily for administrative reasons (for example, physical check up, to obtain a sickness note, and so on).

During the 1990s these scientific evidences were produced and also the political decision to incorporate mental health in the primary care network was made, allowing for the development of mental health programmes including professionals that could deal with psychosocial aspects of healthcare.

From 2000 to 2002 the first randomised controlled trial in primary care clinics to compare the effectiveness of a stepped care programme with usual care (US) to treat depressed women was carried out. The stepped care programme included a structured psycho educational group lead by social workers and nurses, systematic monitoring of clinical progress and structured pharmacotherapy for patients with severe or persistent depression that was executed by trained general practitioners. A total of 240 adult women participated in this trial and the results showed a large and significant difference in favour of the stepped care programme compared with the UC across all assessed outcomes and this difference remained stable during six months (Figure 13.1) [8]. This programme was more effective and marginally more expensive than UC for the treatment of depressed women in primary care. Women receiving the stepped-care programme had a mean of 50 additional depression-free days over six months relative to patients allocated to UC [9].

The results of this trial were well received by policy makers at the Ministry of Health and contributed to the National Program for the Detection, Diagnosis and Treatment of Depression that started in 2001 in primary care clinics [10]. This nationwide programme consists of an assistance system that combines medical and psychosocial interventions, with activities that include detection, diagnosis, registration, treatment and follow up of each case [10]. A clinical guide has been established that uses an algorithm to determine different steps that professionals should take with respect to depressive patients. The programme began in 2001, and by 2004 it was implemented in primary care clinics throughout the country.

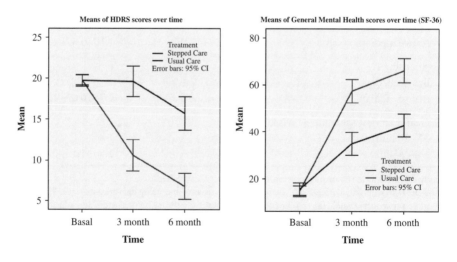

Figure 13.1   HDRS scores and SF-35 scores (general mental health) over time

In 2001, 18 224 people participated in the programme, 29 024 in 2002, 63 067 in 2003, 110 373 in 2004 and approximately 141 000 in 2005 [11, 12]. About 90% of those treated in this programme are women and most of them with a history of previous depressive episodes and low social support network [13].

Worth mentioning is that the programme incorporated psychologists in the primary care clinics to cover its psychosocial demands. Psychologists were not present at primary care clinics until 1990s, and a surge began in 1999. The number of psychologists increased from 120 in 1999 to 247 in 2001 and 452 in 2003 [11, 12]. The primary care guide indicates that severe depression has to be referred to second care level. During the years that the programme has been running, referral to a second level has remained at a level of approximately 7% and the number of mental health interventions at the primary care level has increased. The referral rate was 7% but an evaluation of the programme concluded that there were barriers to secondary level referral. In fact, 79.5% of depression cases treated at primary level were moderate and severe depressions and 60.7% had a history of having a previous depressive episode [13].

Since July 1 2006, within the framework of Chile's current Health Reform, treatment of depressive episode, recurrent depressive disorder and depressive episode of bipolar disorder has been included as explicit warranty of health (GES, Garantías Explícitas en Salud) for all persons of 15 years and older [14]. In other words, health insurances, both public and private, are required by law to provide assistance to depressed people. The GES specifies that mild and moderate depressions may be treated by non-specialised physicians and treatment is guaranteed upon detection; severely depressed patients may be referred to specialised assistance where they must be seen within 30 days from referral [14]. In order to meet these stipulations, the Health Ministry has proposed to increase the number of psychiatrists at the secondary level of the public health system and of psychologists at primary level. Until November 2007, 265 638 depressed persons had been attended at the public health system and around 1000 psychologists work there [11].

13.3 Integrating mental health into women's health

As regards perinatal mental health, several studies have provided important information which will allow progress in proposals concerning its integration to the already existing health programme for women. So far this focuses on mothers and their children.

Some of the available studies demonstrate that at least 1 out of 10 mothers becomes depressed postpartum and 1 out of 7 becomes depressed antenatally [15, 16]. Many more women experience mild depressive and/or anxiety symptoms during the perinatal period. Though Chilean investigators have not found differences in incidence of postpartum depression (PPD) in different socioeconomic groups, they have shown that prevalence does vary depending on socioeconomic status.

Symptoms of depression during pregnancy

In accordance with the international literature [17, 18], three Chilean studies [15, 16, 19] have determined that about 30% of pregnant women experience unspecific, isolated, mild depressive and/or anxiety symptoms (Table 13.1). One study [20] found a lower prevalence rate, probably due to methodological reasons.

Symptoms of depression during the postpartum period

Early puerperium

There has been a trend recently to study women in the early postpartum, two to three days after delivery. First, this may be due to the finding of a higher incidence of postpartum blues among women who later suffer from PPD [21, 22]. Second, the worldwide use and widely accepted validity and reliability of the Edinburgh Postnatal Depression Scale (EPDS) [23] has increased the interest for assessing its potential as an early identifier of mothers at risk. In this way, two Chilean studies [24, 25] have determined the prevalence of depressive/anxiety symptoms early in the puerperium (Table 13.5). Both studies applied a Chilean version of the EPDS [26], which was validated against the research diagnostic criteria (RDC) [27] and used the cut-off point 9/10. This case/non-case threshold score has proved to be the best cut-off point both in middle class [26] and working-class [28] Chilean women.

Likewise, Risco *et al.* [25] have examined the correlation of EPDS scores at day 3 and at 12 weeks postpartum and found that the EPDS completed at two to three days postpartum is useful for detecting those at risk for PPD as was also reported later by a French study [30].

Late puerperium

Three [15, 16, 20] studies that assessed women in mid pregnancy followed them up for several weeks during the postpartum period. In two of them [16, 20], higher prevalence of depressive and/or anxiety symptoms were found during the puerperium. Furthermore, it can be stated, considering all available studies of prevalence of depressive/anxiety symptoms during the postpartum, that in comparison to pregnancy following childbirth a higher percentage of women – up to nearly 50% in three studies –, experience symptoms of depression and/or anxiety (Table 13.5).

Prevalence and incidence of PPD in Chile

Two Chilean studies [15, 16] have determined the frequency of PPD assessing it as a well-defined syndrome. This means applying strictly defined criteria to a constellation of symptoms that are clearly disturbing and interfere with daily functioning and relationship with others.

Table 13.5 Prevalence of depressive and/or anxiety symptoms during mid pregnancy early and late postpartum in Chile

Period	Investigators	Simple size	Instrument	Socioeconomic status	Prevalence
Mid pregnancy	Lemus and Yañez [20]	60	GHQ-30	Middle	16.7%
	Millán et al. [19]	179	GHQ-20	Lower	30.2%
	Jadresic et al. [16]	108	Partial RDC	Middle	35.2%
	Alvarado et al. [15, 28]	125	DSM III-R	Lower	30.4%
Early postpartum	Risco et al. [25]	103	EPDS	Middle-lower and lower	27.2% (3 d)
	Florenzano et al. [24]	88	EPDS	Middle-lower and lower	50.0% (1–10 d)
Late postpartum	Lemus and Yañez [20]	60	GHQ 30	Middle	40.0% (1 mo)
	Jadresic et al. [16]	108	Partial RDC	Middle	48.1% (2–3 mo)
	Alvarado et al. [15]	125	DSM-III-R	Lower	20.5% (8 wk)
	Jadresic and Araya [29]	542	EPDS	Upper, middle and lower	36.7% (2–3 mo)
	Risco et al. [25]	43	EPDS	Middle-lower and lower	48.0% (12 wk)

Jadresic *et al.* applying RDC criteria in a sample of 108 middle class women at two to three month postpartum found 10.2% prevalence and 9.2% incidence rates and Alvarado *et al.* applying DSMIII-R in a sample of 125 lower class women at eight weeks postpartum found 20.5% prevalence and 8.8% incidence rates.

If strictly defined operational criteria are used, no differences of incidence emerge, neither in results obtained in Chile nor with results derived from other countries using the same methodology. Thus, in the USA O'Hara *et al.* [31] found a 10% incidence of PPD at two months postpartum using RDC, and in Japan Aoki *et al.* [32] reported a 9.3% incidence at one month, also using the RDC.

Alvarado, in turn [15], found a 8.8% incidence of PPD in Chile applying DSM-III-R [33], which is very similar to the 9.3% incidence of PPD reported by Aderibigbe *et al.* in Nigeria [34] using the same DSM criteria at six to eight weeks.

Socio-economic associations of PPD

For a long time it has been asserted that there is little evidence that demographic variables, and in particular SES (Socio-economic Status), are associated with an increased risk for PPD [35]. For instance in 1988 O'Hara [35] found that of the 13 studies that reported on the relationship between PPD (diagnosis or symptom level) and SES, only two studies [36, 37] found a significant association. Both studies reported that higher SES was associated with lower levels of depression after delivery. Chilean research supports this connection, showing that women of socially disadvantaged sectors of society are more at risk. For example, if PPD is assessed at the symptoms' level and SES is represented by family income, the data demonstrates that there is an inverse relationship between SES and prevalence of PPD [29].

Mothers with lower incomes had a threefold increase in prevalence of PPD in comparison to mothers with higher incomes [29]. Interestingly, this association between low SES and PPD appears to transcend cultural and regional lines. In fact, we are aware of several later studies showing that mothers from lower socio-economic groups are most at risk for PPD. These studies come from the United States [38], Portugal [39], Spain [40] and other countries – see tables in Halbreich [41].

We would like to highlight the point that methodological difficulties in previous research (i.e. the limitations of demographically homogeneous samples) may have contributed to the absence of an observed relation between SES and PPD.

In keeping with the results of a U.S. study which identified single women with low socio-economic status as being more likely to experience postpartum depressive symptoms [42], Chilean researchers have found that single mothers (unmarried, separated and widows) were twice as likely to be diagnosed with PPD [29]. This may be due to the fact that unstable relationships can lead to a perception of pregnancy as a negative life event which can lead to the development of postpartum depressive symptoms. In addition, stressful life events, marital conflicts or lack of a partner, unwanted pregnancy and having depressive and/or anxiety symptoms during pregnancy are all variables that have been shown by

Chilean investigators to be significantly associated with PPD [15, 25, 43]. This is in accord with reports from the international literature [31, 44–46].

Despite these findings, the National Program for the Detection, Diagnosis and Treatment of Depression does not include pre or PPD in its algorithms.

From the therapeutic standpoint, some relevant contributions have been made. Thus, a Chilean randomised controlled trial carried out in primary care revealed that treatment of depressed postpartum women by non-medical health workers is not only possible but also effective [47]. This study demonstrated that a multi-component intervention can attain better outcome results after three months when compared to a UC control group. The intervention included psycho-educational groups, medical consultations, structured pharmacotherapy and systematic monitoring and maintenance of treatment adherence. At three months recovery was 61% (95% CI 51–71%) in the study group versus 34% (95% CI 25–44%) in the UC group. After adjusting for baseline EPDS, the mean EPDS at three months was approximately one standard deviation lower for the postnatal depression multicomponent intervention group (PND-MCI) compared with UC (Figure 13.2) [47].

In the UC group these proportions were 17% (10–25%) and 11% (6–19%) correspondingly. Amongst those taking antidepressants a larger proportion recovered by three months in the PND-MCI than the UC group (50 and 22% respectively) [47].

Although improvement gained in these first few months declined after a six month period (due mostly to a decrease in usage of antidepressant medication), the percentage of women in the study group who remained on medication and recovered at six months was still higher than that of the UC group (36% versus 11%). The results are promising for acute treatment of socially disadvantaged postpartum depressed women especially in a primary care setting.

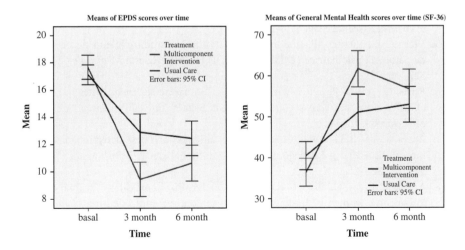

Figure 13.2 EPDS scores and SF-35 scores (general mental health) over time

Overall, this study shows that it is possible to improve the acute treatment of PPD in resource-poor settings, even though many obstacles remain to achieving more lasting improvements. Resource utilisation was similar to a previous trial carried out for depressed women at primary care level in Chile [20] and thus it is possible that incremental costs may be comparable and affordable for a middle-income country such as Chile. Special subgroups may need more support and for longer in order to facilitate adherence to adequate treatment. Equally, alternative modalities for treatment delivery need to be explored further, such as home treatment and follow-up for 'difficult-to-reach' mothers as well as innovative ways to provide longer-term support to improve treatment adherence. Since so many health programmes in developing countries are focused around the perinatal period this provides a great opportunity to find ways of improving the recognition and treatment of PPD and reducing its seemingly harmful impact on children.

References

1. Araya, R., Rojas, G., Fritsh, R. *et al.* (2001) Common Mental Disorders in Santiago, Chile: prevalence and socio-demographic correlates. *The British Journal of Psychiatry*, **178**, 228–33.
2. Florenzano, R., Acuña, J., Fullerton, C. and Castro, C. (1998) Estudio comparativo de frecuencia y características de los trastornos emocionales en pacientes que consultan en el nivel primario de atención en Santiago de Chile. *Revista Médica de Chile*, **126**, 397–405.
3. Rojas, G., Araya, R. and Fritsch, R. (2000) Salud Mental, problemas psicosociales y atención primaria de salud. *Acta – Psiquiatria y Psicologia de América Latina*, **46** (2), 119–26.
4. Sartorius, N., Üstün, T.B., Costa e Silva, J.A. *et al.* (1993) An international study of psychological problems in primary care. Preliminary report from the WHO Collaborative Project on Psychological Problems in General Health Care'. *Archives of General Psychiatry*, **50**, 819–24.
5. Vicente, B., Rioseco, P., Valdivia, S. *et al.* (2002) Estudio chileno de prevalencia de patología psiquiátrica (DSM-III-R/CIDI) (ECPP). *Revista Medica de Chile*, **130**, 527–36.
6. Rojas, G., Araya, R. and Lewis, G. (2005) Comparing sex inequalities in common affective disorders across countries: Great Britain and Chile. *Social Science and Medicine*, **60**, 1693–703.
7. Araya, R., Lewis, G., Rojas, G. *et al.* (2001) Patient knows best: detection of common mental disorders in Santiago, Chile: cross sectional study. *British Medical Journal*, **322**, 79–84.
8. Araya, R., Rojas, G., Fritsch, R. *et al.* (2003) Treating depression in primary care in low-income women in Santiago, Chile: a randomised controlled trial. *Lancet*, **361**, 995–1000.
9. Araya, R., Flynn, T., Rojas, G. *et al.* (2006) Cost-effectiveness of a primary care treatment program for depression in low-income women in Santiago, Chile. *The American Journal of Psychiatry*, **163**, 1379–87.

10. Ministerio de Salud (2001) Guía Clínica Para la Atención Primaria. La Depresión, Detección, Diagnóstico y Tratamiento, Ministerio de Salud, Santiago.

11. Ministerio de Salud (2007) Departamento de Estadísticas e Información de Salud y Unidad de Salud Mental, Ministerio de Salud, Santiago.

12. Minoletti, A. and Sacaría, A. (2005) Plan Nacional de Salud mental en Chile: 10 años de experiencia. *Revista Panamericana de Salud Pública*, **18** (4), 346–58.

13. Universidad de Chile, Facultad de Medicina, Escuela de Salud Pública (2002) *Evaluación de la Efectividad del Programa Para la Detección, Diagnóstico y Tratamiento Integral de la Depresión en Atención Primaria. Informe Final*, Universidad de Chile, Santiago.

14. Ministerio de Salud de Chile (2005) Guía Clínica Para el Tratamiento de Personas con Depresión, Ministerio de Salud, Santiago.

15. Alvarado, R., Rojas, M., Monardes, J. *et al*. (1992) Cuadros depresivos en el postparto y variables asociadas en una cohorte de 125 mujeres embarazadas. *Revista de Psiquiatria*, **3–4**, 1168–76.

16. Jadresic, E., Jara, C., Miranda, M. *et al*. (1992) Trastornos emocionales en el embarazo y el puerperio: estudio prospectivo de 108 mujeres. *Revista Chilena de Neuro-Psiquiatria*, **30**, 99–106.

17. Hrasky, M. and Morice, R. (1986) The identification of psychiatric disturbance in an obstetric and gynaecological population. *The Australian and New Zealand Journal of Psychiatry*, **20** (1), 63–69.

18. Sharp, D.J. (1988) Validation of the 30-item GHQ in early pregnancy. *Psychological Medicine*, **18**, 503–7.

19. Millán, T., Yévenes, R., Gálvez, M. and Bahamonde, M.I. (1990) Encuesta sobre síntomas de depresión en embarazadas de un consultorio urbano de atención primaria. *Revista Médica de Chile*, **118**, 1230–34.

20. Lemus V. and Yañez N. (1986) *Estudio Descriptivo-Comparativo de la Sintomatología Neurótica Depresivo-Angustiosa del pre y Postparto en Mujeres Primíparas. Tesis Para Optar al Título de Psicólogo. Escuela de Psicología*, Universidad Católica de Chile.

21. Fossey, L., Papiernik, E. and Bydlowski, M. (1997) Postpartum blues: a clinical syndrome and predictor of postnatal depression? *Journal of Psychosomatic Obstetrics and Gynaecology*, **18** (1), 17–21.

22. Yamashita, H., Yoshida, K., Nakano, H. and Tashiro, N. (2000) Detecting the early onset of postnatal depression by closely monitoring the postpartum mood. *Journal of Affective Disorders*, **58** (2), 145–54.

23. Cox, J.L., Holden, J. and Sagovsky, R. (1987) Detection of postnatal depression: development of the 10-item Edinburgh Postnatal Depression Scale (EPDS). *The British Journal of Psychiatry*, **150**, 782–86.

24. Florenzano, R., Botto, A., Muñiz, C. *et al*. (2002) Frecuencia de síntomas depresivos medidos con el EPDS en puérperas hospitalizadas en el Hospital del Salvador. *Revista Chilena de Neuro-Psiquiatria*, **40** (Suppl 4), 10.

25. Risco, L., Jadresic, E., Galleguillos, T. *et al*. (2002) Depresión postparto: alta frecuencia en puérperas chilenas, detección precoz, seguimiento y factores de riesgo. *Psiquiatría y Salud Integral*, **2** (1), 61–66.

26. Jadresic, E., Araya, R. and Jara, C. (1995a) Validation of the Edinburgh postnatal depression scale (EPDS) in Chilean postpartum women. *Journal of Psychosomatic Obstetrics and Gynaecology*, **16** 187–91.

27. Spitzer, R.L., Endicott, J. and Robins, E. (1978) Research diagnostic criteria: rationale and reliability. *Archives of General Psychiatry*, **36**, 773–82.

28. Alvarado, R., Vera, A., Rojas, M. *et al.* (1992) La Escala de Edimburgo para la detección de cuadros depresivos en el postparto. *Revista de Psiquiatria*, **3–4**, 1177–81.

29. Jadresic, E. and Araya, R. (1995b) Prevalencia de depresión postparto y factores asociados en Santiago, Chile. *Revista Médica de Chile*, **123**, 694–99.

30. Teissèdre, F. and Chabrol, H. (2004) Detecting women at risk for postnatal depression using the Edinburgh Postnatal Depression Scale at 2 to 3 days postpartum. *Canadian Journal of Psychiatry*, **49**, 51–54.

31. O'Hara, M.W., Neunaber, D.J. and Zekoski, E.M. (1984) A prospective study of postpartum depression: prevalence, course, and predictive factors. *Journal of Abnormal Psychology*, **93**, 158–71.

32. Aoki, M., Kitamura, T., Sinia, S. and Sugawara, M., (1989) Baby blues project, in *Hattatsu*, Vol. 9 (eds K. Okonogi and H. Watanabe), Minerva Shoubou, Tokyo.

33. American Psychiatric Association. (1987) *Diagnostic and Statistical Manual for Mental Disorders*. 3rd Edition Revised. APA, Washington DC.

34. Aderibigbe, Y.A., Gureje, O. and Omigbodun, O. (1993) Postnatal emotional disorders in Nigerian women. A study of antecedents and associations. *The British Journal of Psychiatry*, **163**, 645–50.

35. O'Hara, M.W. (1988) Postpartum depression: a comprehensive review, in *Motherhood and Mental Illness*, Vol. 2 (eds R. Kumar and I.F. Brockington), Wright, London.

36. Feggetter, P. and Gath, D. (1981) Non-psychotic psychiatric disorders in women one year after childbirth. *Journal of Psychosomatic Research*, **25**, 369–72.

37. Playfair, H.R. and Goers, J.I. (1981) Depression following childbirth- a search for predictive signs. *The Journal of the Royal College of General Practitioners*, **31**, 201–8.

38. Holbfoll, S.E., Ritter, C., Lavin, J. *et al.* (1995) Depression prevalence and incidence among inner-city pregnant and postpartum women. *Journal of Consulting and Clinical Psychology*, **63** (3), 445–53.

39. Augusto, A.G., Kumar, R., Calheiros, J.M. *et al.* (1996) Post-natal depression in an urban area of Portugal: comparison of childbearing women and matched controls. *Psychological Medicine*, **26** (1), 135–41.

40. Sierra Manzano, J.M., Carro Garcia, T. and Ladron Moreno, E. (2002) Variables associated with the risk of postpartum depression. Edinburgh Postnatal Depression Scale. *Atencion Primaria*, **30** (2), 103–11.

41. Halbreich, U. (2004) Prevalence of mood symptoms and depressions during pregnancy: implications for clinical practice and research. *CNS Spectrums*, **9** (3), 177–84.

42. Zlotnick, C., Johnson, S.L., Miller, I.W. *et al.* (2001) Postpartum depression in women receiving public assistance: Pilot study of an interpersonal-therapy-oriented group intervention. *Am J Psychiatry*, **158**, 638–40.

43. Jadresic, E., Jara, C. and Araya, R. (1993) Depresión en el embarazo y el puerperio: estudio de factores de riesgo. *Acta Psiquiátrica y Psicológica de América Latina*, **39** (1), 63–74.

44. Brockington, I. (2004) Postpartum psychiatric disorders. *Lancet*, **363**, 303–10.

45. Cooper, P.J. and Murray, L. (1998) Postnatal depression. *British Medical Journal*, **316**, 1884–86.

46. Kumar, R. and Robson, K.M. (1984) A prospective study of emotional disorders in childbearing women. *The British Journal of Psychiatry*, **144**, 35–47.

47. Rojas, G., Fritsch, R., Solis, J. *et al.* (2006) Treatment of postnatal depression among low-income mothers in primary care in Santiago, Chile: a randomised controlled trial. *Lancet*, **370**, 1629–37.

Further reading

Halbreich, U. (2005) Postpartum disorders: multiple interacting underlying mechanisms and risk factors. *Journal of Affective Disorders*, **88**, 1–7.

Spijker, J., de Graaf, R., Bijl, R.V. *et al.* (2002) Duration of major depressive episodes in the general population. Results from the Netherlands Mental health survey and Incidence Study (NEMESIS). *The British Journal of Psychiatry*, **181**, 208–13.

Halbreich, U. and Karkun, S. (2006) Cross-cultural and social diversity of prevalence of postpartum depression and depressive symptoms. *Journal of Affective Disorders*, **91**, 97–111.

Zelkowitz, P. and Milet, T. (2001) The course of postpartum psychiatric disorders in women and their partners. *The Journal of Nervous and Mental Disease*, **189**, 575–82.

Bloch, M., Daly, R.C. and Rubinow, D.R. (2003) Endocrine factors in the etiology of postpartum depression. *Comprehensive Psychiatry*, **44** (3), 234–46.

Kumar, R. (1994) Postnatal mental illness: a transcultural perspective. *Social Psychiatry and Psychiatric Epidemiology*, **29**, 250–64.

14

Gender sensitive psychiatric care for children and adolescents

Corina Benjet

Instituto Nacional de Psiquiatría, México D.F., Mexico

14.1 Mental health services for children and adolescents

Despite the demographic ageing of the developed world, those under age 15 continue to represent almost a third of the total world population [1]. However mental health services for the young across the world trail far behind mental health services for adults in terms of coverage and quality [2]. Many studies have revealed important deficits of treatment adequacy for youngsters with mental health problems [3–8]. However, most such studies were conducted in economically developed regions; there is considerably less known about mental healthcare for children and adolescents in less-developed countries. It has been estimated that only 7% of countries worldwide have a specific child and adolescent mental health policy [9]. Youth mental health regional policy programmes can be found in 0% of low income countries compared with 77.8% of high income countries [10]. Unsurprisingly, the nations with the highest proportion of young people are the least likely to have child and adolescent mental health policies and programmes. Additionally many youngsters with mental health problems are seen in non-healthcare systems such as juvenile justice, educational and social service systems [10]. Because mental health service policies and programmes are so lacking for this population worldwide virtually no attention has been paid to gender sensitive services and care for youngsters.

Gender differences in the prevalence of mental disorders in children and adolescents

The relevance of gender sensitive care begins with gender differences in the prevalence of mental disorders in children and adolescents. While there is no consistent difference in overall prevalence, girls beginning at puberty have higher rates of internalising disorders such as depression and anxiety disorders whereas boys have higher rates of externalising disorders such as conduct disorder, substance use disorders and attention deficit hyperactivity disorder [11, 12]. However, while the adolescent girls of today continue to be much more frequently depressed than adolescent boys [13], the gender gap is narrowing in substance use and abuse, unfavourably for females such that females are using and abusing more than before [14]. Actually, the gender differences in substance use appear to be related to opportunities for use more than the likelihood of using given the opportunity [15–17]. In many countries girls have fewer opportunities to obtain and use substances, but this is quickly changing and substance use in females is highly stigmatising in most societies, even more so than for boys [14]. Another dangerous indicator of mental illness and distress is suicidality. While boys are more likely to die from a suicide attempt (probably due to the methods they employ) females are roughly twice as likely to experience suicidal ideation and to make a suicide attempt [18].

Violence is a major determinant of mental illness in females. While males experience greater assaultive violence outside the home or by non-family members than females, females experience greater violence in the home by family members and are particularly vulnerable to sexual assault; being the victim of assaultive violence for both males and females peaks between the ages of 16 and 20. Higher rates of post traumatic stress disorder in females can be attributed to greater risk following assaultive violence, especially in terms of avoidance and numbing symptoms [19]. Violent and sexual trauma is related to the highest rates of post traumatic stress symptoms [20] and suicidality [21].

Puberty marks a surge in mental health disparities between males and females with an increase in depression and anxiety in the latter. The link between puberty and gender differentiation in mental health symptomatology, or disorder, has been posited to be related in part to an intensification of gender socialisation [22]. Early adolescence may be particularly challenging for females because of sex differences in the timing of pubertal development (female pubertal maturation is on average two years earlier than boys), physiological changes in girls (such as breast development) which are more salient to others and thus generate often undesirable reactions from parents, peers and teachers and in many cultures are inconsistent with cultural ideals of beauty (increased body fat, decrease in shoulder to hip width ratio) [23]. Pubertal development often represents greater restrictions on independence, objectification and increased household responsibilities, for girls.

14.2 Barriers to service use

One of the most important differences for service use among the young as opposed to adults is their reliance on an intermediary for detection of mental health problems and help-seeking. Children do not seek services for themselves; an adult (usually a parent or teacher) must first recognise a problem, take the child or adolescent to services, pay for those services and then follow through with treatment. This can be quite a barrier considering that many parents of children with mental health issues have mental health problems themselves. The most frequent mental health problems in boys (externalising disorders such as conduct problems, hyperactivity, substance abuse) are more easily detected given that they are generally bothersome to adults in the home and at school, whereas disorders more common in girls (internalising disorders such as depression/anxiety) are often overlooked or in some cases such as the school setting, where low energy and passiveness helps control the classroom environment may even be appreciated by teachers. There is some evidence for the greater detection of externalising disorders [24] though the evidence is inconsistent [6]. Some studies find adolescents males to be more likely to receive services than females [7], but others have not [4, 5, 25, 26]. The gender difference in service use appears to be related to age in that males are more likely to receive mental health services in childhood and early adolescence and females in later adolescence [6].

Additional barriers to youth mental health service use are issues related to parental consent requirements and confidentiality. Adolescents are often reluctant to discuss with parents issues related to substance use, sexual activity, suicidal ideation or conduct problems. Services which are limited to adolescents who arrive with a parent or guardian or do not assure adolescents confidentiality are likely to exclude many adolescents. Allowing for a non-parental adult (such as aunt or older cousin) to accompany the adolescent instead of a parent or guardian may help reduce this barrier to some degree. Adolescents need services specific to them separate from child and adult services.

14.3 Recommendations for gender sensitive psychiatric care of children and adolescents

Recommendations for gender sensitive psychiatric services include improving the recognition and treatment of trauma and violence. Improvement requires training of mental health professionals in order to detect and treat victims of violence, to collaborate with social service, justice system and school professionals in this area, to be sensitive to the needs of victims, and to challenge their own ideas regarding violence and gender. Services need to include routine assessment of victimisation, specific guidelines as to how to handle such cases and ideally to include a consultant group of specialists in the area to help professionals with the numerous ethical dilemmas which arise in situations in which the violence is on-going.

Gender sensitive psychiatric services should provide psychological health promotion programmes which integrate issues of gender equality, self-esteem and mental health. Girls would also benefit from health promotion programmes which include early sex education in order to help prevent sexual abuse, sexually transmitted diseases and teenage pregnancy all of which are related to adolescent mental illness and distress. Services for adolescents should assure confidentiality and allow adolescents to receive treatment without parental consent.

To a greater degree than for adult mental health services, child and adolescent mental health services should maintain close interactions with school, justice and social services. Ideally mental health services should be delivered in schools. Because in many parts of the world many adolescents drop out of school early and girls, in particular, have fewer educational opportunities especially in South Asia, Western Asia and sub-Saharan Africa [27], services should also be delivered in other community settings in as flexible a manner as possible given that girls are often burdened with greater responsibilities for care of younger siblings and the home.

Finally, children and adolescents are particularly vulnerable as they do not have the power or autonomy to change adverse situations such as the family or neighbourhood they live in, their school or often employment in informal sectors of society (such as begging or selling products on the street). Minors are dependent upon the decisions their parents make for them. Because of this, parental education is paramount for prevention and treatment of childhood disorders as is family interventions and mental health services for the parent. Child and adolescent mental health begins with parental mental health. Gender sensitive child and adolescent mental healthcare requires gender sensitive education of families, health providers, school, social and justice system professionals as well as those responsible for public health policy planning and implementation.

References

1. Population Reference Bureau 2007 World population Data Sheet, World Population Bureau, Washington, DC.
2. Levav, I., Jacobsson, L., Tsiantis, J. *et al.* (2004) Psychiatric services and training for children and adolescents in Europe: Results of a country survey. *European Child and Adolescent Psychiatry*, **12**, 395–401.
3. Leaf, P.J., Alegria, M., Cohen, P. *et al.* Methods for the Epidemiology of Child and Adolescent Mental Disorders Study (1996) Mental health service use in the community and schools: results from the four-community MECA Study. *Journal of the American Academy of Child and Adolescent Psychiatry*, **35** (7), 889–97.
4. Verhulst, F.C. and van der Ende, J. (1997) Factors associated with child mental health service use in the community. *Journal of the American Academy of Child and Adolescent Psychiatry*, **36** (7), 901–9.

5. Sourander, A., Helstela, L., Ristkari, T. *et al.* (2001) Child and adolescent mental health service use in Finland. *Social Psychiatry and Psychiatric Epidemiology*, **36** (6), 294–98.

6. Kataoka, S.H., Zhang, L. and Wells, K.B. (2002) Unmet need for mental health care among U.S. children: variation by ethnicity and insurance status. *American Journal of Psychiatry*, **159** (9), 1548–55.

7. Zwaanswijk, M., Verhaak, P.F.M., Bensing, J.M. *et al.* (2003) Help seeking for emotional and behaviour problems in children and adolescents: a review of recent literature. *European Child and Adolescent Psychiatry*, **12**, 153–61.

8. Alegria, M., Canino, G., Lai, S. *et al.* (2004) Understanding caregivers' help-seeking for Latino children's mental health care use. *Medical Care*, **42** (5), 447–55.

9. Shatkin, J.P. and Belfer, M.L. (2004) The global absence of child and adolescent mental health policy. *Child and Adolescent Mental Health*, **9** (3), 104–8.

10. World Health Organization (2005) Atlas: Child and Adolescent Mental Health Resources, World Health Organization, Geneva.

11. Costello, E.J., Mustillo, S., Erkanli, A. *et al.* (2003) Prevalence and development of psychiatric disorders in childhood and adolescence. *Archives of General Psychiatry*, **60**, 837–44.

12. Roberts, R.E., Roberts, C.R. and Xing, Y. (2007) Rates of DSM-IV psychiatric disorders among adolescents in a large metropolitan area. *Journal of Psychiatric Research*, **41**, 959–62.

13. Costello, J.E., Erkanli, A. and Angold, A. (2006) Is there an epidemic of child or adolescent depression? *Journal of Child Psychology and Psychiatry*, **47** (12), 1263–71.

14. Poole, N. and Dell, C.A. (2005) Girls, Women and Substance Use, Canadian Centre on Substance Abuse, Ottawa.

15. Benjet, C., Borges, G., Medina-Mora, M.E. *et al.* (2007) Drug use opportunities and the transition to drug use among adolescents in the Mexico Metropolitan Area. *Drug and Alcohol Dependence*, **90** (2–3), 128–34.

16. Van Etten, M.L. and Anthony, J.C. (1999) Comparative epidemiology of initial drug opportunities and transitions to first use: marijuana, cocaine, hallucinogens, and heroin. *Drug and Alcohol Dependence*, **54**, 117–25.

17. Van Etten, M.L., Neumark, Y.D. and Anthony, J.C. (1997) Male-female differences in the earliest stages of drug involvement. *Addiction*, **94** (9), 1413–19.

18. Kessler, R.C., Borges, G. and Walters, E.E. (1999) Prevalence of and risk factors for lifetime suicide attempts in the national comorbidity survey. *Archives of General Psychiatry*, **56** (7), 617–26.

19. Breslau, N., Chilcoat, H.D., Kessler, R.C. *et al.* (1999) Vulnerability to assaultive violence: further specification of the sex difference in post-traumatic stress disorder. *Psychological Medicine*, **29** (4), 813–21.

20. Copeland, W.E., Keeler, G., Angold, A. and Costello, E.G. (2007) Traumatic events and posttraumatic stress in childhood. *Archives of General Psychiatry*, **64**, 577–84.

21. Borges, G., Benjet, C., Medina-Mora, M.E. *et al.* (2008) Traumatic events and suicide related outcomes among Mexico City Adolescents. *The Journal of Child Psychology and Psychiatry*. **49** (6), 654–66.

22. Benjet, C. and Hernández-Guzman, L. (2001) Gender differences in psychological well-being of Mexican early adolescents. *Adolescence*, **36** (141), 47–65.

23. Benjet, C. and Hernández-Guzman, L. (2002) A short term longitudinal study of pubertal change and psychological well-being of Mexican early adolescents. *Journal of Youth and Adolescence*, **31** (6), 429–42.

24. Wu, P., Hoven, C.W., Bird, H.R., Moore, R.E., Cohen, P., Alegria, M., Dulcan, M.K., Goodman, S.H., Horwitz, S.M., Lichtman, J.H., Narrow, W.E., Rae, D.S., Regier, D.A., Roper, M.T. (1999) Depressive and disruptive and mental health service utilization in children and adolescents. *Journal of the American Academy of Child and Adolescent Psychiatry*, **8**, 1081–90.

25. Cohen, P. and Hesselbart, C.S. (1993) Demographic factors in the use of children's mental health services. *American Journal of Public Health*, **83** (1), 49–52.

26. Flisher, A.J., Kramer, R.A., Grosser, R.C. *et al.* (1997) Correlates of unmet need for mental health services by children and adolescents. *Psychological Medicine*, **27** (5), 1145–54.

27. Population Reference Bureau (2006) The World's Youth 2006 Data Sheet, Population Reference Bureau, Washington, DC.

15

Gender sensitive care for adult women

Marta B. Rondón

Universidad Peruana Cayetano Heredia, Department of Psychiatry and Mental Health Hospital Nacional Edgardo Rebagliati Martins, Lima, Peru

15.1 Introduction

It has been shown and discussed elsewhere in this book that women bear an unequal share of the burden of common psychiatric disorders: anxiety and depression, and that depression poses a serious threat to the human development of women. There are studies showing that female divorced, separated or widowed people have more depressive symptoms with a propensity to depression of females after a stressful event accounting for some of the differential [1]. Therefore, the promotion of mental health for girls and women, the prevention of these disorders and the secondary and tertiary prevention services should be a priority in the health agenda of all countries Unfortunately, however, there is evidence that mental healthcare services for women do not adequately respond to their needs, reproducing and even amplifying the inequalities and injustices that mark women's lives in general [2].

The WHO Commission on the Social Determinants of Health has shown that ill health is determined by unequal distribution, on both global and national levels, of power, income, goods and services and by the consequent injustices that affect populations and individuals in an immediate and visible fashion: access to healthcare, schooling, education, working conditions and leisure time, housing. Unequal distribution of experiences that pose a risk for wellbeing and health is not 'natural' but rather the result of a combination of deficient social

Contemporary Topics in Women's Mental Health   Edited by Chandra, Herrman, Fisher, Kastrup,
© 2009 John Wiley & Sons, Ltd   Niaz, Rondón and Okasha

policies and programmes, unfair economic arrangements and poor political administration [3].

Gender describes the economic, social, political and cultural attributes and opportunities associated with being male or female. It is fundamental to our perception of who we are, the roles we adopt and the way in which perceive others and are perceived by others.

Gender is an important determinant of health and disease, and it influences the longevity and the disease burden in very clear ways in different parts of the world. Gender relations of power constitute the roots of gender inequality are some of the most powerful of the social determinants of health. They determine whether a person's health needs are acknowledged, whether they have voice and agency over their lives and their health and whether they can realise their rights [4].

Like other social relations, gender relations are experienced in daily life and in the everyday day business of feeling ill or well, and are based on core structures that govern how power is embedded in social hierarchy. Gender power relations determine who is well and who is ill, but also who gets treated or not, who is exposed to risks, and whose health needs are acknowledged or ignored.

The quality, safety and accessibility of health services is also determined by gender and power relations, and health services, reflect, like education or employment access, the relative position of a group in society. The impact of gender power for physical and mental health of girls, women, gays, lesbian, transgender people and also men and boys is great. Furthermore, the extent to which the health needs of the chronically ill and the older populations have to be met by women due to the crumbling of health systems is increasing, and women have become the 'shock absorbers' of the health systems, expected to act as such in good and bad times, especially during the bumps caused by emergencies, disasters and economic crisis. The higher vulnerability of women to social conditions has been documented before [5, 6].

The Women, Gender and Equity Knowledge Network of the CSDH has recommended that, in order to diminish the negative impact of gender, there is a need to 'transform the gendered politics of health systems by improving their awareness and handling of women's problems, as both producers and consumers of healthcare, improving women's access to health care and making health systems more accountable to women'.

In the same direction, the International Consensus on Women's Mental Health [7] has recommended that 'Women should have access to respectful, knowledgeable mental health care in a timely fashion, in a non-stigmatising, suitable setting within their economic means, by adequately skilled health professionals with access to appropriate treatments....' and 'Treatment settings should be safe and free from breaches of fiduciary trust by health care providers and staff'. The consensus calls for governments and individuals to 'Support safe, respectful, appropriate, gender sensitive comprehensive mental and physical health services for girls and women across the life cycle irrespective of their economic and social status'.

In this framework, this chapter will provide some basic theoretical and practical information on how to make services for adult women more gender sensitive. Empowerment of women who come in touch with mental healthcare is especially considered, in keeping with our framework and with the recommendations in the current literature on the administration and delivery of services for women [8].

It is well documented that services are 'not always sensitive to the needs of women' and consequently there have to be changes to accommodate gender dependent needs as discussed above [9].

Goldberg and Huxley [10] have stated that women are present at different proportions in different levels of services, more women than men present at the General Practitioner level with psychological complaints, but more men get referred to specialist services. Also there is some evidence that women are reluctant to seek help from mental health professionals, especially in deprived areas and in ethnic minorities. Women and fare differently once they have established contact with mental health services: more women attend day services for people with low levels of functioning [11], and older women receive less intensive treatment than men. On the other hand, more men are committed to institutions.

Even in the industrialised countries there are gaps in the services available for women, for instance community based care for eating disorders, drug abuse and forensic outpatient and inpatient facilities.

15.2 Gender sensitive and informed mental healthcare: Basic strategies

Gender runs like a fault line, interconnecting with and deepening the disparities associated with other important socio economic determinants, such as income, employment and social position [12].

Gender roles and the relative power of men and women shape the division of labour, the allocation of responsibilities, attitudes and behaviour related to healthcare and to mental healthcare.

Strategies may:

- Exploit gender inequalities.
- Accommodate differences.
- Integrate gender relations.

When an intervention emphasises or underlines, out of context, a peculiarity of females in detriment of equality, we say it is **exploiting gender inequalitie**s. For example, a legislative initiative to give two days off to all women working for the state, on account of 'premenstrual dysphoria', increases prejudice about the relative lower productivity of women in certain settings. It may reinforce discrimination in the work force. Likewise undue emphasis on menopause and peri menopause as endocrine diseases or hormone-deficient states may result in risky exposure of women to hormone treatment.

There are other interventions, which may make it easier for women to conform to established rules which are based on gender inequities. For instance, changing hours at paediatric clinics to **accommodate** working mothers or giving special training to female staff does not contribute to a more equitable distribution of childcare responsibilities, but allows the woman to attend the clinic without conflicting with her paid work.

Gender integration refers to strategies that take gender into consideration and compensate for gender-based inequalities. Integration of gender relations calls for programmes and activities that encourage critical awareness of rules and norms, promote the position of women relative to men, challenge the imbalance of power, distribution of resources and allocation of duties between men and women and that address the unequal relationships between men and women providers.

The voices of women

Women want more female providers, more emotional support, help with side effects and more information on contraceptive methods [13].

Men often regulate women's access to health services through control of finances, women's mobility, control of transportation, women's decisions and healthcare decisions [14].

Women who access health services face unequal power relations with providers. Female patients tend to keep silent and be passive, letting many questions go unanswered and often feel how services are fragmentary, stigmatising and reproduce the everyday conflicts that have brought emotional distress to their lives.

When asked, women say that the causes of their mental disorders are mostly social: their early experiences of sexual and domestic violence, intimate partner violence and other adverse experiences. This has been corroborated by surveys of severely ill women [15], and in studies of traumatic stress disorder [16].

Women who have experienced contact with the mental health system in diverse settings complain about powerlessness, lack of safety and lack of human warmth. Official and NGO sponsored surveys of inpatient services find 'institutional aimlessness, poor staff-patient relationships and a lack of attention to human and civil rights' [17, 18].

The lack of safety is worrying because it reproduces adverse circumstances in everyday life and increases the feeling of powerlessness of female psychiatric patients. Women would like to be spared the need to deal with disruptive or threatening male patients, (Patiniotis op cit) and it related to complaints about privacy and dignity in mixed sex wards, where women feel paraded in front of both male patients and staff members.

15.3 Principles of gender sensitive care

The principles of gender sensitive mental health services are:

- Equality.
- Knowledge and commitment.
- Relationships [19, 20].

Equality

Equality has to do with the use of power [21], and it is a very sensitive issue when working with women, because social inequalities and the trauma experienced in unequal relationships with people who have power are at the root of many women's mental disorders. Another consideration is that when gender and other inequalities are treated as irrelevant and power is used unfairly the quality and safety of the care suffers. Therefore it is essential to have good partnerships with those who have the power (such as ministry authorities or labour leaders) and with those who use the services (namely patients, women's groups).

Knowledge and commitment

Staff needs to be familiar with the ways in which inequalities cause distressing experiences and can make them worse and also the ways in which inequalities shape the behaviour and symptoms of the women who attend the mental health services. There is also the need for the staff to feel comfortable translating this knowledge into practise, especially in their relationship with women patients. Staff need:

1. Training and education about gender.

2. Listening to women survivors talk about their lives and experiences.

3. Reflection about their personal experiences of gender and other inequalities.

4. Supervision from gender competent staff and the chance to interact with them in everyday practise.

Relationships

It has been documented [22] that women (and men) who use mental health services want to be treated with respect and expect mutuality, and this is central to the process of forming the therapeutic alliance and starting the road to recovery. The centrality of this therapeutic relationship should not get lost in the everyday practise of evidence based medicine. Staff must be able to provide women with a loving, caring and containing relationship even in the most challenging of circumstances.

A respectful relationship is based on the patient's best interest and includes the transparent exercise of power. A respectful relationship is predictable and consistent, and maintains the patient protected from abuse, shame and blame. If tensions and conflict arise in such therapeutic relationships, these are worked out openly, not closed down.

Relational security (which many patients have not enjoyed in their lives) promotes recovery and feelings of self esteem, wellbeing and social inclusion.

In order to foster the capacity to enter this type of relationship, staff should be encouraged to:

1. Learn from stories of women's experiences.

2. Value a woman's strength and resilience.

3. Shift the focus away from diagnosis and problems towards hopes about the patient's future.

4. Validate the woman's choices.

5. Provide opportunities for women using the services to help each other.

6. Take steps to ensure that feedback is given and taken into account in the planning and development of services.

People working in mental health who want to have gender sensitive services have many resources at their disposition, even on the Internet. For example, the courses provided by Inequality agenda (www.inequalityagenda.co.uk), the Medical Women's International Association [23], the Swedish International Development Cooperation Agency [24] and by the Royal College of Nurses [19].

15.4 Characteristics of gender sensitive services

To meet the aim of ensuring that all stages and modalities of mental healthcare are sensitive to the needs of women and respond to their gendered needs, it may be necessary to challenge the traditional ways of solving problems and the values of the institutions and organisations involved: the establishment of services for women only, the involvement of female providers and users in the planning and assessment of the services have to be explicitly supported. It is fundamental to ensure women's voices are heard throughout health and social care organisations, and that we develop services which address the sometimes very specific needs of women [25, 26].

The development of mental healthcare services for women should not occur at the expense of services for men: discrimination and inequalities in health and other social determinants should be addressed for all, both men and women. Better understanding of gendered differences allows for better allocation of resources.

Women's services have to take into account the multiple gender dependent differences in needs which derive from:

1. Differences in life experiences: women are more likely to have experienced interpersonal including sexual violence and to have experience as care takers, while men are more likely to have experienced accidents and have been perpetrators of violence.

2. Differences in socio economic realities: women are more likely to be poor, to work in vulnerable, informal employment and to be the backbone of an organisation and less likely to have a high corporate or leadership position. On the other hand, men are more likely to fully employed and to have benefits.

3. The expressions of mental distress also vary from men to women. The former show higher rates of antisocial personality disorders, higher rates of alcohol and drug consumption and are more likely to present with early onset psychotic disorders, while women show higher rates of depression and anxiety, eating disorders and self harm; also women may experience specific emotional disorders related to the events of the reproductive cycle, with perinatal depression being a frequent cause of concern.

4. There exists a different route or entrance pathway into services for men and women: women come into contact with mental health services through primary and community services, and not infrequently through referral from reproductive health services. In fact, it must be remembered that the reproductive health provider is likely to be the woman's only contact with the health services, especially in deprived areas and when domestic violence is an issue. Men may come in contact with mental health services through the judiciary, or referred from emergency wards or alcohol and drug services.

5. Women tend to prefer services that are included in primary care, where men respond better to early intervention and assertive, specialised services.

Mental health services for women ought to address the issue of stigmatisation, they should promote self esteem and empowerment and build on women's strengths, and they should be safe and confidential, welcoming and supportive and should take a holistic approach to health and wellbeing. They should respond to specific needs, such as access for people with physical limitations, care for children while mother attends [27]. They should also encourage access to other services: community centres, lifelong learning and should be well integrated with primary care and specialist services [28, 29].

The characteristics of mental health inpatient care are: attention to safety, knowledgeable staff and respectful, consistent and non judgemental relationships.

Safety

Although conventional wisdom has it that psychiatric patients are dangerous, quite the contrary is true: there is a vast potential for psychiatric patients to be victims of abuse at home, on the street and within the healthcare system.

Large studies of up to 500 persons with severe mental illness who are served within public-sector mental health clinics have shown high prevalence rates of trauma victimisation (51–98 %) and post traumatic stress disorder (PTSD) (up to 43 %) [30]. Persons with severe mental illness may also be vulnerable to additional traumatic or iatrogenic experiences that occur within psychiatric settings [31]. For example, use of control procedures, such as seclusion and restraint, may recapitulate previous traumatic experiences and thereby exacerbate symptoms of PTSD or other mental illness.

Data from a sample of 142 randomly selected adults revealed high rates of reported lifetime trauma that occurred within psychiatric settings, including physical assault (31%), sexual assault (8%) and witnessing traumatic events (63%). The reported rates of potentially harmful experiences, such as being around frightening or violent patients (54%), were also high. Finally, reported rates of institutional measures of last resort, such as seclusion (59%), restraint (34%), takedowns (29%) and handcuffed transport (65%), were also high. Having medications used as a threat or punishment, unwanted sexual advances in a psychiatric setting, inadequate privacy and sexual assault by a staff member were associated with a history of exposure to sexual assault as an adult [32].

However frequent these incidents may be, there is a lack of empirical data for events that, although they do not meet *DSM-IV* criteria for trauma, involve insensitive, inappropriate, neglectful or abusive actions by mental health staff or authorities and invoke among patients a response of fear, helplessness, distress, humiliation or loss of trust in staff (sanctuary harm).

There are two main safety concerns: dealing with sexual abuse and the use of seclusion and restraint.

Protection from sexual abuse: Sexual safety

A history of physical or sexual abuse can confound treatment for many people diagnosed with a major mental illness, and especially for women. These mentally ill survivors often become high users of mental health services for such related issues as substance abuse, suicidality, self injury, assaultiveness and repeated victimisation.

As a consequence of inadequate assessment and inappropriate treatment, neither hospital-based nor crisis services have been able to meet the needs of these women for more than temporary respite. Indeed, there is growing evidence from both clinicians and consumer/survivors that in some mental health settings, such clients may be retraumatised, leaving them in a continuing cycle of trauma and response.

Sexual abuse of patients is unfortunately common, and other patients as well as staff have been implicated. Results of a study of female patients indicated that most (85%) with a history of abuse reported feeling unsafe in mixed-gender units [33]

Patients tend to have a fatalistic view, as they feel defenceless, and sometimes have been through previous experiences of sexual abuse, so they have a feeling that this is supposed to happen to them in both inpatient and outpatient mental health services as well.

The codes of ethics and other documents of professional associations such as the World Psychiatric Association and the World Medical Association, as well as national psychiatric societies are very clear in their protection of sexual safety of the patients. The World Psychiatric Association has determined in the Declaration of Madrid that sexual misconduct is a grave ethical breach and the International Consensus on Women's Mental Health, which was approved by the WPA General Assembly in 2005 in Cairo asserts that women should have services that are free from sexual or other types of abuse. However, there are many instances in which misuses of power, including sexual exploitation, still occur between patient and staff and there is an acute need to educate patients and staff in this regards, and also to continue dissemination of the pertinent sections of the ethical codes. Staff should know how to react and whom to inform. Patients and their relatives or representatives have to be educated in the right to be free from exploitation and abuse [34–41].

A recent survey has shown that this is not the case in most parts of the world, where leaders at the national level, are not sure of the legislation and the severity of power misuse and boundary violations with patients (Stewart DE, personal communication)

Central to the discussion of sexual activity with patients is consent: the woman needs to have the capacity to consent, and this capacity is diminished by the cognitive manifestations of the mental disorder, the use of medication and by the power differential between mental health provider and patient.

The Use of seclusion and restraint

There is worldwide interest in reducing the incidence of measures of last resort that are used to manage disruptive behaviour on inpatient psychiatric units. The target of these efforts has been seclusion and restraint because of the mounting evidence that these may, because of the associated loss of control, represent a highly distressing experience for patients. Evidence indicates that psychiatric patients in the emergency department prefer psychotropic medication (64%) to seclusion or restraint (36%) [42] Another study found that although psychiatric nurses rated restraint as appropriate in 98% of cases, patients perceived it as being necessary in only 35% of the cases [43]. Also, although patients' perceptions of the necessity for involuntary commitment change from the time of commitment to follow-up, negative perceptions of seclusion and restraint are stable across time (N = 433) [44].

The greatest risks for injury in psychiatric facilities, emergency departments, and elsewhere come about when aides or security guards physically put their hands on an agitated individual rather than trying to de-escalate the situation without use of physical force. Many people, including the majority of women frequently hospitalised for serious psychiatric disabilities, have traumatic histories of physical and sexual abuse [9]. When an individual with PTSD or dissociative identity disorder is touched from behind, grabbed, escorted by physical force or held down, it may trigger memories of intense terror. This terror may, in turn, transform agitation or obstreperous but non dangerous behaviour into panic-stricken flashbacks, triggering surges of adrenaline and a profound need to fight back at all costs. For the patient experiencing the flashback, escaping from the hold feels like a fight for survival. From the point of view of personnel, the transformation of a previously agitated woman into someone who is clearly out of control, with escalating aggression (which is self-defence from the patient's perspective), confirms the needs to restrain the patient. Thus, even though the decision to put hands on the patient to take him or her out of the environment has escalated the crisis, each party's need for control now predominates. The more the aides and/or guards struggle, the more the terrified patient thrashes, especially when the initial terror is combined with an inability to breathe because of pressure on his or her body by the people who are trying to subdue the patient. Indeed, an individual can die within 5 minutes of the initial takedown [45].

Restraint can be dangerous and traumatic for patients and staff alike. Federal and state mental health leaders have called the use of restraint a sign of treatment failure [46]. Nearly all of the places that have substantially reduced or eliminated the use of restraint have achieved significant collateral benefits: patient satisfaction has improved, along with staff morale; staff and patient injuries have declined; and workers' compensation claims and staff turnover have been reduced.

Knowledgeable staff

In a high quality service all people involved should know how gender and other inequities are detrimental to mental health, be able to pinpoint and challenge the inequities that undermine the safety of the service and they should be able and willing to discuss their gendered lives and experiences [47].

Admission to an inpatient ward can feel very threatening for a woman, especially for those from cultural settings where there is little mixing with the opposite sex outside of the family.

Gender and other inequities have the potential to harm mental health, affect how people express and experience mental distress and affect how mental or emotional distress is understood and to affect how mental health services are accessed and experienced.

Respectful relationships

Patients report significant distress associated with a range of staff behaviours, from sanctioned measures of last resort to name-calling and physical assaults.

Some clinic and ward based practises may be changed to insure that women feel respected and protected during their contact with mental health services:

1. *Information gathering procedures*: screening, assessment, record keeping: women need to be reassured by staff that many of the situations that have brought them to the service are common and that their distress in understandable. It is sensible to limit the number of team members who assess the woman and also to devise a record keeping procedure which minimises the need for the woman to repeat private or painful experiences.

2. *Power and control*: staff has to be careful not to perpetuate issues of inequality, such as tolerating low grade sexual harassment in mixed sex wards, not appreciating individual differences in maintaining interpersonal physical and psychological boundaries, using language that is too casual, handing out sanitary wear items instead of making them available.

3. *Use of language*: gender sensitive care invites staff to use language that is respectful and meaningful. Descriptions of behaviour should be preferred to the use of adjectives (for instance 'Mrs A experiences the ward as fearful and feels very unsafe instead' of 'Mrs A is paranoid')

4. *Partnership working*: coercive relationships should be replaced by collaboration. A harm minimisation programme instead of close observation and removal of a woman's possession to reduce risk is a good example. Other examples include shared decision making about medication, opportunities to access therapies and a willingness to keep patients involved in plans.

5. *Relationships*: safe, consistent, transparent and non judgemental.

Keeping in mind that many women who experience mental disorders have histories of manipulative, abusive and profoundly asymmetric relationships, it is important to strive for an atmosphere of acceptance and empowerment.

References

1. Alegría, M., Kessler, R.C., Bijl, R. *et al.* (2000) Comparing data on mental health service use between countries, in *Unmet Need in Psychiatry: Problems, Resources, Responses* (eds G. Andrews and S. Henderson), Cambridge University Press, Cambridge, pp. 97–118.
2. Stewart, D.E., Rondón, M., Damiani, G. and Honikman, J. (2001) International psychosocial and systemic issues in women's mental health. *Archives of Women's Mental Health*, **4** (1), 13–17.

3. World Health Organization (2007) Commission On The Social Determinants Of Health. Final Report.

4. Sen, G., Ostin, P. and George, A. (2007) Women, Gender, Equity Knowledge Network: Unequal, Unfair, Ineffective and Inefficient. Gender Inequity in Health: Why it Exist and What We Can Do to Change It. Final Report to the WHO Commission on the Social Determinants of Health.

5. Bifulco, A., Brown, G.W., Moran, P. *et al.* (1998) Predicting depression in women: the role of past and present vulnerability. *Psychological Medicine*, **28**, 39–50.

6. Cooper, H., Arber, S., Fee, I. *et al.* (1999) The Influence of Social Support and Social Capital on Health, Health Education Authority, London.

7. Stewart, D.E. (2006) The international consensus statement on women's mental health and the WPA consensus statement on interpersonal violence against women. *World Psychiatry*, **5** (1), 61–64.

8. Masterson, S. and Owen, S. (2006) Mental health service user's social and individual empowerment: using theories of power to elucidate far-reaching strategies. *Journal of Mental Health*, **15** (1), 19–34. Retrieved September 13, 2008, from http://www.informaworld.com/10.1080/09638230500512714.

9. Patiniotis, J. (2005) Who's Listening: Gender Sensitive Mental Health Service Provision: Key Issues from the Perspective of Service Users, PPI Forum for Mersey Care, Liverpool.

10. Goldberg, D. and Huxley, P. (1992) *Common Mental Disorders*, Routledge, London.

11. Ramsay, R., Welch, S. and Youard, E. (2001) Needs of women patients with mental illness. *Advances in Psychiatric Treatment*, **7** (2), 85–92.

12. WHO (2001) Gender Disparities in Mental Health, World Health Organization, Geneva.

13. Barnett, B. and Stein, Warningy.J. (1998) Women's Voices, Women's Lives: The Impact of Family Planning, Family Health International, Research Triangle Park, North Carolina.

14. Schuler, R.S., Bates, L.M. and Islam, K. (2002) Paying for Reproductive Health Services in Bangladesh: intersections between cost, quality and culture. *Health Policy and Planning*, **17** (3), 273–280.

15. Lu, W., Mueser, K., Rosenberg, S. and Jankowski, M. (2008) Correlates of adverse childhood experiences in adults with severe mood disorders. *Psychiatric Services*, **59**, 1018–26.

16. Goodman, L.A., Salyers, M.P., Mueser, K.T. *et al.* (2001) Recent victimization in women and men with severe mental illness: prevalence and correlates. *Journal of Traumatic Stress*, **14**, 615–32.

17. Barnes, M., Davis, A. and Rogers, H. (2006) Women's voices, Women's choices: Experiences and creativity in consulting women users of mental health services. *Journal of Mental Health*, **15** (3), 329–41. Retrieved September 13, 2008, from http://www.informaworld.com/10.1080/09638230600700664.

18. Walton, P. (2000) Psychiatric hospital care: a case of the more things change, the more they remain the same. *Journal of Mental Health*, **1**, 77–88.

19. Williams, J. and Paul, J. (2008) *Royal College of Nursing Informed Gender Practice: Mental Health Acute Care that Works for Women*, National Institute for Mental Health in England.

20. Department of Health, Mental Health, Health & Social Standards & Quality Group (2003) The Department of Health Mainstreaming Gender and Women's Mental Health: Implementation Guidance.

21. Keshet, S., Kark, R., Pomerantz-Zorin, L. *et al.* (2006) Gender, status and the use of power strategies. *European Journal of Social Psychology*, **36** (1), 105–17.

22. O'Malley, A.S., Sheppard, V.B., Schwartz, M. and Mandelblatt, J. (2004) The role of trust in use of preventive services among low-income African-American women. *Preventive Medicine*, **38**, 777–85.

23. Medical Women's International Association (2002) Training Manual for Gender Mainstreaming in Health, http://www.mwia.net/gmanual.pdf (accessed 10 September 2008).

24. Swedish International Development Cooperation Agency (1997) Handbook for Mainstreaming: A Gender Perspective in the Health Sector, Swedish International Development Cooperation Agency, Stockholm.

25. Saulnier, C., Bentley, S., Gregor, F. *et al.* (1999) Gender Mainstreaming: Developing a Conceptual Framework for En Gendering Healthy Public Policy, Submitted to the Maritime Centre of Excellence for Women's Health Gender and Policy Paper Series, Halifax.

26. Tudiver, S. (2002) Gender matters: evaluating the effectiveness of health promotion. *Health Policy Research Bulletin*, **1** (3), 22–23.

27. Newbigging, K. and Abel, K. (2006). *Supporting Women Into the Mainstream*. Department of Health. London. Available at: http://www.dh.gov.uk/en/Publicationsand-statistics/Publications/PublicationsPolicyAndGuidance/DH_4131070 (accessed Oct 10, 2008).

28. Anderson, R.T., Weisman, C.S., Scholle, S.H. *et al.* (2002) Evaluation of the quality of care in the clinical care centers of the National Centers of Excellence in Women's Health. *Women's Health Issues*, **12** (6), 309–26.

29. Giardina, E-G.V., Cassetta, J.A., Weiss, M.W. *et al.* (2006) Reflections on a decade of experience in implementing a center for Women's Health at an Academic Medical Center. *Journal of Women's Health*, **15** (3), 319–29.

30. Mueser, K., Goodman, L.A., Trumbetta, S.L. *et al.* (1998) Trauma and posttraumatic stress disorder in severe mental illness. *Journal of Consulting and Clinical Psychology*, **66**, 493–99.

31. Cohen, L.J. (1994) Psychiatric hospitalization as an experience of trauma. *Archives of Psychiatric Nursing*, **8**, 78–81.

32. Frueh, B., Knapp, R., Cusack, K. *et al.* (2005) Special section on seclusion and restraint: Patients' reports of traumatic or harmful experiences within the psychiatric setting. *Psychiatric Services*, **56**, 1123–33.

33. Gallop, R., McCay, E., Guha, M. *et al.* (1999) The experience of hospitalization and restraint of women who have a history of childhood sexual abuse. *Health Care for Women International*, **20**, 401–16.

34. Margison, F. (1996) Boundary violations and psychotherapy. *Current Opinion in Psychiatry*, **9** (3), 204–8.

35. Sarkar, S. (2004) Boundary violation and sexual exploitation in psychiatry and psychotherapy: a review. *Advances in Psychiatric Treatment*, **10**, 312–20.

36. Radeen, J. (2003) The debate continues: unique ethics for psychiatry. *Australian and New Zealand Journal of Psychiatry*, **38**, 115–18.

37. American Psychiatric Association (2008) The Principles of Medical Ethics with Annotations Especially Applicable to Psychiatry, American Psychiatric Association, Washington, DC.

38. Garfinkel, P., Dorian, B., Sadavoy, J. and Bagby, R. (1997) Boundary violations and departments of psychiatry. *Canadian Journal of Psychiatry*, **42**, 764–70.

39. Nadelson, C. and Notman, M. (2002) Boundaries in the doctor-patient relationship. *Theoretical Medicine and Bioethics*, **23**, 191–201.

40. American Academy of Child and Adolescent Psychiatry (1995) American Academy of Child Adolescent Psychiatry Code of Ethics. Annotations to AACAP Ethical Code With Special Reference to Evolving Health Care Delivery and Reimbursement Systems, American Academy of Child and Adolescent Psychiatry, Washington, DC.

41. Galletly, C. (2004) Crossing professional boundaries in medicine; the slippery slope to patient sexual exploitation. *The Medical Journal of Australia*, **181** (7), 380–83.

42. Sheline, Y. and Nelson, T. (1993) Patient choice: deciding between psychotropic medication and physical restraints in an emergency. *Bulletin of the American Academy of Psychiatry and the Law*, **21**, 321–29.

43. Outlaw, F.H. and Lowery, B.J. (1994) An attributional study of seclusion and restraint of psychiatric patients. *Archives of Psychiatric Nursing*, **8**, 69–77.

44. Gardner, W., Lidz, C.H., Hoge, S.K. *et al.* (1998) Patients' revisions of their beliefs about the need for hospitalization. *The American Journal of Psychiatry*, **156**, 1385–91.

45. New York Commission on Quality of Care for the Mentally Disabled (2006) A Case Study On restraint, Traumatic Asphyxia and Investigations, www.cqc.state.ny.us./could_this_happen/caseneillarkin.htm (accessed 29 March 2006).

46. The Substance Abuse and Mental Health Services Administration (2003) Summary Report – A National Call to Action:Eliminating the Use of Seclusion and Restraint, http://alt.samhsa.gov/seclusion/SRMay5report2.htm (accessed 29 March 2006).

47. Levin, B.L., Blanch, A.K. and Jennings, A. (eds) (1998) *Women's Mental Health Services: A Public Health Perspective*, Sage, Thousand Oaks, p. 448.

16
Psychopharmacology

Silvana Sarabia

Asociacion Psiquiatrica Peruana, Lima, Peru

Great progress has been gained in women's health and wellbeing in the last century. Since the 1900, important changes favouring women's health have been obtained, such as, age at death has increased from 48 to 80 years, the average number of children and infant mortality has decreased from 8 to 1.9 and from 124–158 per 1000 to 7 per 1000 respectively. Also, the primary cause of death has changed from tuberculosis and child birth to heart disease and the number of women in workforce has augmented from negligible to 59%. Data indicate that between family, work and community responsibilities, women are often so busy taking care of others that they overlook their own health needs [1]. Mental illnesses affect women and men differently, some disorders are more common in women and some express themselves with different symptoms. Only recently scientists are beginning to distinguish the contributions of various biological and psychosocial factors to mental health and mental illness in both women and men. In addition, researchers are currently studying the special problems of treatment for serious mental illness during pregnancy and the postpartum period [2]. Improving women's mental health is still a challenge and every effort to do so, by studying gender differences and psychopharmacology, will be of assistance.

16.1 History of psychopharmacology

In the past 50 years considerable progress has been made in psychopharmacology. Before that, electroconvulsive therapy (ECT), used since the 1930s was the most effective biological treatment for mental disorders. Use of ECT has diminished since the second half of the twentieth century, but it remains an effective treatment for major depression and life-threatening psychiatric conditions [3]. Unlike the

Contemporary Topics in Women's Mental Health   Edited by Chandra, Herrman, Fisher, Kastrup,
© 2009 John Wiley & Sons, Ltd   Niaz, Rondón and Okasha

therapies of that period, ECT remains in the active treatment folder of modern therapeutics. As the mechanism of action of the drugs was discovered new theories on the physiopathology of psychiatric disorders emerged [4]. These findings have also facilitated rational drug development of new compound and have changed psychiatric treatment from a psychoanalytic to a biological orientation.

Since 1952 when chlorpromazine was first used many drugs have appeared in the market (see Table 16.1). Another important success for psychopharmacology was when clozapine, the first antipsychotic agent with few extrapyramidal symptoms (EPS) and superior efficacy, especially for the treatment resistant schizophrenic patients, became available. EPS diminished significantly after Serotonin-Dopamine Antagonists (Atypical or Second-Generation Antipsychotics) appeared in the market. Nevertheless, other types of adverse events increased considerably, such as, weight gain and the increased risk of diabetes mellitus [5].

Despite the progress that has been made in more than half a century, no antidepressant has exceeded the tricyclic antidepressant (TCA) and monoamine oxidase inhibitors (MAOIs) in efficacy. In spite of this, these drugs did not reach their full potential due to side effects [4]. Progress has been gained greatly in drug tolerability, less so in efficacy. Patients now have many more treatment options and the drugs used are better understood. In spite of all the progress in drug development, it is only in the last 15 years that women have been considered as possible candidates for early phase clinical trials. There is still much information that should be studied with respect to psychopharmacology and gender differences [6].

16.2 Ethics

The ethical requirements in clinical research aim to minimise the possibility of exploitation and ensure that the rights and welfare of subjects, including women, are respected while they contribute to the generation of knowledge. Researchers and patients involved in clinical trials should understand the distinction between clinical practise and clinical research. Clinical practise refers to interventions that are intended solely to enhance the wellbeing of an individual patient who has a reasonable expectation of success [7]. On the other hand, clinical research is an activity planned to test a hypothesis, allow conclusions to be drawn and therefore contribute to generalisable knowledge [8]. Research and practise may be carried on together when research is designed to evaluate the safety and efficacy of a drug. The general rule is that if there is any element of research in an activity, that activity should undergo review for the protection of human subjects [9].

The ethical principles underlying the conduct of research are: respect to persons, beneficence and justice. The inclusion and selection of subjects must be fair. Fair subject selection requires that the scientific goals of the study, not vulnerability, privilege or other factors not related to the hypothesis to be tested by the research, be the primary basis for determining the individuals who will be recruited and enrolled in a study. It is important that the results of research be generalisable to the population that will use the intervention [10]. Until recently,

Table 16.1 The table shows psychotropic name, brand name and the year they appeared in the market. In the last 50 years considerable progress has been made in psychopharmacology. As the mechanism of action of the drugs was discovered new theories on the physiopathology of psychiatric disorders emerged. These findings have also facilitated rational drug development of new compounds [63–77]

Psychotropic drug (brand name)	Year appeared in the market
Phenobarbital (Luminal)	1912 synthesised
Chlorpromazine (Thorazine)	1954
Meprobamate (Equanil)	1955
Imipramine (Tofranil)	1957
Iproniazide (Marsilid)	1957
Haloperidol (Haldol)	1958
Chlordiazepoxide (Librium)	1959
Diazepam (Valium)	1963
Lithium (Eskalith)	1970
Fluvoxamine (Luvox)	1983 (introduced in Switzerland)
Fluoxetine (Prozac)	1987
Bupropion (Wellbutrin)	1989 (approved as antidepressant)
Clozapine (Clozaril)	1958 (discovered)
	1972 (first approved)
	1975 (withdrawn due to agranulocytosis)
	1990 (reintroduced in the market worldwide)
Moclobemide (Manerix)	1992
Risperidone (Risperdal)	1993
Olanzapine (Zyprexa)	1995
Sertraline (Zoloft)	1992
Paroxetine (Paxil)	1993
Tacrine (Cognex)	1993
Venlafaxine (Effexor)	1994
Valproic acid (Depakene)	1995
Mirtazapine (Remeron)	1995
Bupropion (Wellbutrin)	1996 (approved for smoking cessation)
Donepezil (Aricept)	1996
Quetiapine (Seroquel)	1998
Citalopram (Celexa)	1998
Rivastigmina (Exelon)	2000
Ziprasidone (Zeldox)	2001
Galantamine (Reminyl)	2001
Aripiprazole (Abilify)	2002
Escitalopram (Lexapro)	2002
Lamotrigine (Lamictal)	2003
Memantine (Ebixa)	2003
Duloxetina (Cymbalta)	2006
Paliperidona (Invega)	2007

women were not routinely included in many clinical trials to determine whether drugs were safe and effective. The reason usually given was that excluding women protected them, since there was often no way to be sure that a woman would not become pregnant whilst in the study or that the drug might not cause some problem that might interfere with future pregnancies [11]. In addition, it was thought that women's hormonal cycling or other factors characteristic to being female might constitute variables that could skew trial results. This does not mean that every woman must be offered the opportunity to participate in the study; it means that women should have the opportunity to participate and cannot be prejudicially excluded. If a potential drug is likely to be prescribed for women, if proven safe and effective, then they should be included in the study, to be able to learn how the drug affects them. Ethical requirements for clinical research do not end when individuals, women and men, either sign the written informed consent and are enrolled or refuse to participate. Individuals should be treated with respect throughout their participation, even if they refused to participate, and after their participation ends. The restriction on women with childbearing potential implies a lack of respect for their autonomy and decision-making capacity. The ethical principles articulated in the Belmont Report, respect for persons, beneficence and justice; imply that women should have the right to make their own risk-benefit choices [10].

16.3 Sources and interpretation of data

The content of this chapter is based on many sources of information. Information on psychopharmacology come from published randomised, controlled, double blind clinical trials, open label studies, case reports, the opinion of experts as mentioned in review articles and clinical guidelines and direct experience in the clinical setting. Depending on the information and experience that the clinician has, the idea formed of a drug can vary. Evidence-based medicine is not restricted to randomised clinical trials and meta-analyses, it integrates all important evidence found and it is then applied to each individual patient. It is valuable to the extent that it is complete and unbiased. Most of the clinical trials published have positive results; those having negative results are usually not published. It appears that incomplete reporting of outcomes within published articles of randomised trials is common and is usually associated with statistical non-significance. Therefore, the medical literature regarding clinical trials represents only a fraction of the information actually studied. Recently, Turner *et al.* reported that according to the published literature, it appeared that 94% of the trials conducted were positive. By contrast, the Food and Drug Administration (FDA) analysis showed that only 51% were positive [12]. This selective reporting denies physicians the complete information to estimate accurate results.

The purpose of research is to confirm or refute evidence that a drug has a therapeutic effect. A study, to demonstrate efficacy, must proof that the new agent is more effective than placebo or as effective as a proven treatment, and risks should not outweigh its benefit. Fairness requires that women be included in the research, unless there is a good reason, such as excessive risks. Despite adequate participation by both women and men in the last 20 years, however, few analyses of the data have been conducted to detect possible differences in effectiveness or safety between genders. The data should be examined for sex differences in the effectiveness, adverse-event rates and dose response of drugs. If the analyses suggest differences between the sexes, or if the presence of such differences could be important, as in the case of drugs with a low therapeutic index, additional studies may be needed. All new drug applications should include appropriate analyses by sex.

16.4 Women in clinical trials

Clinical trials are tested in three phases. Phase 1 studies are the initial studies in humans and generally involve a small number of healthy volunteers or patients treated over a short period of time. These studies assess individual tolerance of the drug and examine its metabolism and short-term pharmacokinetics. They may also provide preliminary pharmacologic information related to clinical effectiveness. Phase 2 studies, which normally involve a few hundred patients, are the earliest controlled trials designed to demonstrate effectiveness and relative safety. During phase 3, the final testing phase, as many as several thousand patients are studied [10]. These studies provide additional evidence regarding safety and effectiveness, including data on long-term exposure; improve information on dose-response and concentration-response relations and identify relatively rare adverse effects.

FDA guidance recommended against including women of child bearing potential in the early phases of drug testing except for life-threatening illnesses in 1977 (see Table 16.2). It was only until 1993, that the restriction on women of child bearing potential was lifted, and permitted them in early phase clinical trials. At present, most of the research protocols involve both women and men; and there are only a limited number of single sex protocols. Such single sex studies are appropriate, as the exclusion of either women or men may be allowed, if based on convincing scientific justification. Of the studies in which women are enrolled exclusively, most deal with questions of female reproductive health, whereas others focus on disorders more prevalent in women [13, 14].

During a five-year period examined by the FDA from 1995 to 1999, women participated in clinical trials at nearly the same rate as men. Overall, women appear to participate in the clinical trials at nearly the same rate as men even when gender-specific products were excluded. Labelling for two-thirds of the products contained some statement about gender, although only 22% described actual gender effects. Ninety per cent of the effects discussed in the labelling were pharmacokinetic, 12% were safety and 5% were efficacy. Despite these findings no product recommended a change in dosage for women. Possible pharmacokinetic differences between women and men should be assessed either by formal studies or with the use of pharmacokinetic screening. The number of women that should

Table 16.2 The participation of women in clinical trials has changed throughout the years due to recommendations of the different regulation agencies. In 1977 FDA recommended against including women of child bearing potential in the early phases of drug testing restriction that was lifted in 1993

Participation of women in clinical trials	Year
Food and Drugs Act and its enforcement. Required dangerous ingredients to be labelled on all drugs, and allowed for seizure of illegal foods and drugs.	1906
Food, Drug and Cosmetic Act. Mandated pre-market approval of all new drugs, such that a manufacturer would have to prove to FDA that a drug were safe before it could be sold.	1938
Spurring drug reforms to prevent birth defects. Required a drug to be tested in animals before being tested on people.	1961
Politics on protection of human rights.	1966
FDA guidance recommended against including women of child bearing potential in the early phases of drug testing except for life-threatening illnesses.	1977
Guideline for the study and evaluation of gender differences in the clinical evaluation of drugs. Allowed the restriction on women of child bearing potential to be lifted and allowed them in early phase clinical trials. Emphasised the need for representation of both women and men in clinical trials to allow detection of clinically significant gender/sex differences.	1993
Final rule on investigational new drug applications and new drug applications (demographic rule). Requires that analyses of effectiveness and safety data for important demographic subgroups, including gender [78].	1998

be included will depend on the hypothesis to be tested in a particular study and the prevalence of the disorder. The total number enrolled will vary on a case by case basis. The number of women and men included, in every clinical trial, should allow enough representation of both sexes so that significant gender differences will be detected. Generalising results to the entire population must not be done unless sex differences are sought [15].

16.5 Pharmacodynamics and pharmacokinetics in women

Heterogeneity of response characterises most psychotropic drugs. Genetic and environmental factors influence individual response to and tolerability of psychotropic drugs. The characteristics of each drug, combined with the characteristics of each individual patient account for the profile of efficacy, tolerability and safety. All these variables make it difficult to predict a drug's effect [16]. The clinical effects of the drugs are best understood in terms of pharmacokinetics which describes what the body does to a drug and, pharmacodynamics which describes what the drug does to the body [17, 18]. Research reveals sources of variability in the amount of drug available for therapeutic action after administration, therapeutic properties and adverse effects of medication. An important aspect that should be considered when assessing pharmacokinetics and pharmacodynamics of a drug is gender.

Possible gender differences regarding pharmacokinetics include absorption. The amount of a drug that is absorbed from the gastrointestinal tract depends on the acid-base and lipophilic properties. It is suggested that women secrete less gastric acid and empty both solids and liquids more slowly than men. The distribution of a drug is determined by its physical and chemical properties. Females have a lower ratio of lean body mass to adipose tissue mass. Over time, the potential for storage of medication in adipose tissue is higher, therefore, half-life may become prolonged and serum levels could be greater in patients with less body mass [16, 19].

There are other important pharmacokinetic issues that may provide evidence of differences between the sexes, such as, the effects of the menstrual cycle [20] and menopausal status [21]; the effects of concomitant oestrogen supplementation or use of systemic contraceptives, including both oestrogen-progestin combinations and long-acting progesterone and the influence of a drug on the effectiveness of oral contraceptives.

There are several possible menstrual phase specific changes, for example, some women experience water retention. An increase in fluid retention may dilute the concentration of medication; the amount of fluid retained would have to be large, to result in lower plasma levels. Also, changes in the activity of monoamine oxidase may occur during menstrual cycle, it may be decreased by oestrogens and increased by progesterone [22]. All this highlights the importance of establishing menstrual cycle phase when investigating pharmacokinetic and pharmacodynamic properties of a new drug. Therefore, the inclusion of women, with childbearing potential, in all age groups early in drug development must be encouraged. Women should participate in the earliest phases of clinical trials.

16.6 Psychotropic treatments in women

Treating women with psychotropic drugs require a special consideration. Although there are no specific doses established for women when using psychotropic medications (see Table 16.3), some articles have been published regarding different treatment response between women and men. The majority of the studies recognise that the difference found is not clinically significant, but advise further research. Some even suggest treating women with selective serotonin reuptake inhibitors (SSRIs) and men with a serotonin-norepinephrine reuptake inhibitor (SNRI) or a TCA [23].

Table 16.3 Recommended doses of psychotropic drugs are shown; it should be noted that no specific doses are established for women when using psychotropic medications

Psychotropic drug (brand name)	Total daily dose (mg)
Antipsychotics	
Aripiprazole (Abilify)	10–30
Chlorpromazine (Thorazine)	200–800
Clozapine (Clozaril)	100–800
Haloperidol (Haldol)	5–10
Risperidone (Risperdal)	1–16
Olanzapine (Zyprexa)	5–20
Paliperidona (Invega)	6–12
Quetiapine (Seroquel)	25–800
Ziprasidone (Zeldox, Geodon)	40–160
Antidepressants	
Amitriptiline (Elavil)	150–300
Bupropion (Wellbutrin)	150–450
Citalopram (Celexa)	20–60
Escitalopram (Lexapro)	10–20
Duloxetina (Cymbalta)	30–120
Fluoxetine (Prozac)	20–60
Fluvoxamine (Luvox)	50–300
Mirtazapine (Remeron)	15–45
Moclobemide (Aurorix, Manerix)	300–600
Paroxetine (Paxil)	20–50
Sertraline (Zoloft)	50–200
Venlafaxine (Effexor)	150–375
Mood stabilisers	
Carbamazepine (Tegretol)	400–1600
Lithium (Eskalith)	900–1800
Lamotrigine (Lamictal)	300–500
Valproic acid (Depakene)	750–1500
Cholinesterase inhibitors and similarly acting compounds	
Tacrine (Cognex)	10–40
Donepezil (Aricept)	5–10
Rivastigmina (Exelon)	3–12
Galantamine (Reminyl)	16–32
Memantine (Ebixa)	5–20

Modified from: Newport, D.J., Fisher, A., Graybeal, S., Stowe, Z.N. Psychopharmacology during pregnancy and lactation. In: Schatzberg, A.F. and Nemeroff, C.B., editors. *Textbook of Psychopharmacology*. 3rd edn. Arlington (VA): American Psychiatric Publishing, Inc; 2004. pp. 1109–46 [45].

Another important aspect, which should be considered because of the reproductive risks associated with specific psychotropic drugs and drug interaction with hormonal contraceptives; is treating women during their reproductive years [24].

This section of the chapter will reflect on treatment response in women, reproductive years and psychotropic drugs and; pregnancy, breastfeeding and drugs.

Treatment response in women

As mentioned above, no specific doses have been established for women when using psychotropic drugs. Despite this, several researchers have found differences with regard to treatment response between women and men.

Antipsychotics

Higher antipsychotic plasma levels and lower dose requirements have been found in female patients [25]. These findings lead, in some cases, to a better efficacy in women [26, 27]. Due to this finding, some authors have hypothesised that the enhanced efficacy could be due to an antidopaminergic effect of oestrogens [28]. Another plausible explanation could be associated with differences in pharmacokinetics between women and men, as previously mentioned. Some of these studies did not control for smoking or contraceptive use [16].

Szymanski et al., found that female first-episode schizophrenic patients had later onset, a better response, greater levels of prolactin and plasma homovanillic acid than men [29]. These results are consistent with the gender difference in degree of symptom improvement with medication. Other studies have not found differences between gender and antipsychotic use.

Antidepressants

As with other psychotropic drugs, results regarding gender differences and treatment response with antidepressants are controversial.

Thirty randomised, placebo-controlled trials that included 3886 patients (1555 men and 2331 women) submitted to obtaining marketing authorisation between 1979 and 1991 examined gender differences in response to TCA [30]. This study pointed to no gender difference in the efficacy of TCA. Another study that included 96 men and 196 women with major depression treated with clomipramine, citalopram, paroxetine and moclobemide found that both genders had similar remission rates when treated with clomipramine, and had significantly higher remission rates with clomipramine than with comparable treatments. This was despite significantly higher plasma concentrations of clomipramine found in women than in men. No gender differences were found in post treatment Hamilton depression scales, nor did the therapeutic effects on treatment depend on gender. Also, rates of drop-outs and side effects were similar for men and women. It was concluded that there was no relationship between plasma concentrations, gender and therapeutic outcome [31].

Kornstein *et al.*, found that women were significantly more likely to show a favourable response to sertraline than imipramine, and men were significantly more likely to show a favourable response to impramine than sertraline. In this study, women and men with chronic depression showed a significantly different response to a selective SSRI and TCA. The differing response rates between drug classes in women were observed primarily in premenopausal women. The authors' conclusion was that female sex hormones may enhance response to SSRIs or inhibit response to tricyclics [32].

A total of 125 Japanese patients with major depression were included in a study to assess gender differences in the treatment response to fluvoxamine and milnacipran SNRI [33]. The results suggest that fluvoxamine is more effective in younger female patients than older female patients and male patients, while milnacipran is generally effective irrespective of gender or age.

The effect on menopause and treatment response has also been studied. Overall some studies suggest that menopause is related to a worse treatment response, while others found that neither sex nor menopausal status may be relevant for antidepressant treatment of adult depressed patients [34]. Further research elucidating gender differences in response to antidepressant treatment is needed. Some studies report that the pharmacokinetics of antidepressants may vary between men and women. Therefore, clinicians should be aware that potential differences in antidepressant pharmacokinetics may exist, and a dosage adjustment may be necessary for women to ensure favourable drug response, compliance and decreased incidence of adverse events [35, 36]. Both gender and menopausal status should be taken into account when deciding on an antidepressant.

Lithium

Data from 17 studies published from 1967 to 1998, involving 1548 patients (1043 women and 505 men) found no differences between sexes in response to lithium [37].

Reproduction and psychotropic drugs

Some psychotropic drugs can alter the menstrual cycle, modify pregnancy potential and enhance the risk for chronic conditions associated with hormone changes, such as, prolactin elevation and polycystic ovarian syndrome (PCOS). When the menstrual cycle is changed, fertility is reduced and osteoporosis and endometrial hyperplasia may appear. Also, some drugs used to treat psychiatric patients can alter the hypothalamic-pituitary-gonadal (HPG) axis; this alteration can change women's menstrual cycle.

Due to this, it is important to determine the patient's menstrual cycle before starting any psychotropic medication to know if that medication is responsible for the changes, if they occur, or if the patient already had those menstrual cycle irregularities [38]. Irregular menses are common, one out of five women have irregular menstrual cycles. Abnormal reasons for menstrual irregularities are prolactin elevation and PCOS; both of these syndromes can be associated with psychotropic medication. Joffe *et al.*, has reported PCOS in women taking valproate. Manifestations of PCOS are hirsutism, acne, male pattern balding, obesity, high serum levels of free testosterone or dehydroepiandrosterone sulfate (DHEAS) and the abnormal polycystic ovarian pattern. The prevalence of PCOS in women taking valproate for bipolar disorder varies from 8 to 10%. Early intervention, such as, changing valproate for another mood stabiliser or directly treating PCOS can diminish the health risks associated with PCOS, that include, insulin resistance, diabetes mellitus, endometrial hyperplasia, reduced fertility and possible cardiovascular disease [39, 40].

Another complication associated with psychotropic medication, especially antipsychotic drugs, is hyperprolactinaemia. Hyperprolactinaemia affects both women and men. Prolactin is normally inhibited by dopaminergic neurons from the hypothalamus acting on dopamine 2 (D_2) receptors. Antipsychotics that have a high affinity for D_2, such as, classical antipsychotics and risperidone, block these receptors, increasing prolactin secretion and producing hyperprolactinaemia. Symptoms related to hyperprolactinaemia are: galactorrhoea, sexual dysfunction, irregular menses or amenorrhoea, which can lead to osteoporosis and infertility [41]. Management of hyperprolactinaemia should be considered, even if asymptomatic, due to the recent data that suggest an association between high levels of prolactin and breast cancer [42].

Another important aspect, which should be considered to avoid an expected pregnancy, is drug interactions between hormonal contraceptive and some psychotropic drugs. Other birth control methods, such as barrier methods or intrauterine devices, should be recommended to women taking carbamazepine, oxcarbazepine, topiramate and modafinil, these medications lower the efficacy of oral contraceptives via induction of hepatic cytochrome P450 isoenzymes [38].

Pregnancy and psychotropic drugs

Historically, it was assumed that pregnancy protected women, making them less susceptible to psychiatric disorders. This assumption was based on a study that reported a low rate of hospitalisation during pregnancy, rate that increased dramatically during the postpartum period. Another study that measured the rates of recurrence was similar between pregnant (52%) and nonpregnant (58%) patients after discontinuing lithium therapy, suggesting that pregnancy is risk neutral. That is, pregnancy neither protects, nor is a risk factor for relapse [43].

Every woman with childbearing potential should be informed, when first prescribed a psychotropic drug, of the possible risks, to the foetus, of becoming pregnant while taking psychotropic drugs. Patients should be informed because most women learn they are pregnant at five to eight weeks of gestation and therefore may be past the window of risk for foetal abnormalities associated with psychotropic medications [24]. Ideally, pregnancy in women with psychiatric disorders should always be planned. Planned pregnancies allow time for thoughtful treatment choices; thus physicians ought to encourage their female patients to plan their pregnancies. However, even if planned; pregnancy poses a complex problem for the patient, foetus and psychiatrist.

Eventually, risk-benefit decisions are made that should consider the risk of symptom relapse for the mother, against the risk of foetal exposure to the drug with the hazard of teratogenicity. No clinical decision is free of risk and patients with similar risk benefit information of treatment options could make different decisions. Nonetheless, awareness of all the available information regarding psychotropic drugs and pregnancy will allow the patient, well up-dated by her psychiatrists, to make the best informed decision. The clinician should be able to provide as much current data as possible, on the benefits and risks of psychotropic drugs during pregnancy, to inform the patient and support her in making the decision [44]. The patient ought to understand that no decision is free of risk, nor is ideal. The decision should be specific to each pregnant woman and must be done in a case by case basis. Psychiatrists should work jointly with the patient to weigh risk of relapse if drugs are discontinued and the possible risk to the foetus if the drugs are continued.

When considering the use of medications during pregnancy, the decision-making process should evaluate three types of possible risks to the foetus, which are: teratogenesis or organ malformation, neonatal toxicity or withdrawal syndrome and potential long-term neurobehavioural sequelae. A teratogen is any agent that increases the risk for foetal malformation, usually due to exposure during the first trimester. The prevalence of major malformations in women not taking any medication ranges from 2 to 4%. In order to evaluate whether a drug is teratogenic, it has to be compared to the risk of a control group ideally matched to as many variables as possible [24].

The decision-making process must also consider the potential risks that may increase if psychiatric symptoms go untreated in the pregnant patient. Risks of clinical worsening include severe psychological distress, suicidal ideation, social and occupational dysfunction, an inability to plan for and successfully cope with the future life transitions and poor infant care. Also, some evidence indicates that untreated depression in mothers can impair the neurocognitive development of the child. In general, maintenance treatments for psychiatric disorders have proved to be protective against relapse, signifying that the patient and her psychiatrists are obliged to be attentive of various treatment options during pregnancy, being the fundamental goal to minimise the risk for recurrence of illness during pregnancy [44].

Pharmacological treatment may be continued during pregnancy when the risk to the foetus and mother outweighs the teratogenic risks of pharmacotherapy. When the decision is made to use a psychotropic drug, the objective is to maximise efficacy so that the mother's exposure to mental illness can be reliably eliminated, while avoiding offspring's exposure to risky medications [24]. Some authors consider that the most important factor when choosing a medication is treatment history. That is, if a patient has a history of a positive response to a specific medication a new drug should not be started, unless the agent being used is contraindicated during pregnancy. If a patient was taking a particular medication earlier in gestation and it was efficacious, continuing or restarting that medication is preferable to changing to a new medication. Switching medications automatically may extend the duration of maternal illness and increases the number of medications the child is exposed to. In addition to the treatment history when choosing a drug other factors should be considered, such as, medications with some published pregnancy safety data, drugs that have been available in the market for a longer time usually have more information accessible [45]. New drugs in the market do not have enough, if any, information of its use during pregnancy and probably are not the best choices for pregnant women. Data regarding these agents during pregnancy are usually sparse, with most postmarketing observations frequently limited to case reports or small series. Medications with conflicting data should be avoided. Also, medications with lower FDA risk category (see Table 16.4), few or no metabolites, fewer side effects and drug interactions are preferable.

Over the last decade pregnancies registries, associated to antiepileptic drugs (AEDs), also used as mood stabilisers, have emerged around the world making data collection on foetal risk possible. Information demonstrates that the malformation rate increases with the use of two or more antiepileptic drugs. The rate of major infant malformation, defects recognised within the first five days of neonatal life, for valproate was approximately 10%, including spina bifida, heart defects and multiple anomalies. The relative risk (RR) of malformation for infants exposed to valproate was sevenfold. The RR of malformation for infants exposed to lamotrigine varied from 11- to 24-fold [46]. Adverse neurobehavioural outcomes are additional, potentially important risks to consider when prescribing AED during pregnancy. Children exposed to valproic acid in utero had three times greater risk of developing difficulties requiring special educational interventions than children without the exposure. Children exposed to carbamazepine or other AED, on monotherapy, had no superior risk of developing difficulties than children not exposed [43, 46, 47].

The goal of treatment during pregnancy is adequate treatment of symptom remission. Partial treatment only increases risk by continuing to expose mother and infant to both illness and medication. The minimum effective dose should be maintained during treatment, having in mind that dosage requirements may change during pregnancy.

It is highly recommended that the psychiatrist discuss the medication prescribed with the patient's obstetrician and her infant's paediatrician [48].

Table 16.3 shows FDA categories for drug used during pregnancy and drug examples in each category. It should be noted that most of the drugs are listed in Category C, that is, human studies are lacking. It should be kept in mind that no psychotropic drug is approved for use during pregnancy by the FDA.

Breastfeeding and psychotropic drugs

The postpartum period has a greater susceptibility than before for new onset and worsening of symptoms of psychiatric disorders. Usually, these patients

Table 16.4 FDA categories for drug used during pregnancy and drug examples in each category. No psychotropic drug has been approved for use during pregnancy

Category	Definition	Drugs
A	No foetal risk in controlled studies	
B	Foetal risk in animal studies but no risk in controlled human studies or no foetal risk in animal studies but no controlled human studies.	Clozapine Bupropion Maprotiline Buspirone
C	No human data available and adverse foetal effects in animals.	SSRIs (except paroxetine) Classical antipsychotics Atypical antipsychotics (except clozapine) Mirtazapine Venlafaxine Oxcarbazepine Lamotrigine Gabapentin Topiramate Trihexiphenidyl
D	Positive evidence of risk.	Paroxetine TCA Lithium Valproic acid Carbamazepine Benzodiazepines
X	Contraindicated in pregnancy	Flurazepam Temazepam Estazolam Triazolam

Modified from: Berga, S.L., Parry, B.L., Cyranowski, J.M. Psychiatry and reproductive medicine. In: Sadock, B.J. and Sadock, V.A., editors. *Kaplan & Sadock's Comprehensive Textbook of Psychiatry*. 8th edn. Philadelphia (PA): Lippincott Wiliams & Wilkins; 2005. p. 2309 [21].

would benefit from pharmacological treatment. Despite this, many physicians are cautious about prescribing medications for women who decide to breastfeed.

Women faced with this decision should be well-informed about potential side effects in her infants. Before beginning maternal medication, the newborn should be assessed by a paediatrician, to determine baseline behaviour, such as, sleep, feeding and alertness. It is recommended that the mother take the medication just after nursing and before the baby's longest sleep interval. Plasma concentrations of antidepressant drugs are usually low in the breast-fed infant, and most studies demonstrate that certain antidepressants can be used during lactation without any important adverse effects on the infant [49, 50]. The amount of medication in breast milk varies according to when the drug is taken and what part of breast milk is assayed, but usually maternal use does not lead to substantial levels in the child. Neonates should be constantly monitored for difficulty feeding, weight gain, sleep or state changes if the mother is undergoing psychotropic treatment while breastfeeding. The choice of medication should minimise accumulation of the drug in milk and infant serum, this depends on diagnosis, past history of the mother, side effect reports, dose flexibility and pharmacokinetic characteristics. Dosage should be as low as possible but should achieve psychiatric remission. Ineffective doses represent needless exposure by infant to medication. It is important to weigh the risks and benefits of exposing the newborn baby to maternal mental illness against the exposure to psychotropic medications. The impact of drug exposure through breast milk is still limited. Infant drug exposure is, however, generally higher during pregnancy through placental passage than through breast milk. Women with postpartum disorders have need of efficient management to provide symptom relief for the suffering mother while simultaneously ensuring the baby's safety [51–53].

16.7 Treatment of postpartum disorders

Notably, the postpartum period has an increased susceptibility for both, new onset and worsening of symptoms of psychiatric disorders (see Table 16.5).

Postpartum blues

Many women, up to 85%, experience the postpartum blues (PPB), characterised by mild depressive symptoms, tearfulness, often for no apparent cause, anxiety, irritability, mood lability and fatigue. The PPB peak three to five days after delivery, may last hours to days and are usually resolved by the 10th postnatal day. Evidence suggests that women who experience severe symptoms of postpartum blues have an increased risk for postpartum depression (PPD) later in the postpartum period. Women, who met criteria for PPD six weeks after delivery, were found to have had two thirds of them PPB. Likewise, women who experience the mild euphoria and increased energy, within the first few days of delivery are more likely to be depressed several months later. Therefore, mild mood symptoms after delivery should be an indication for further follow-up later in the postpartum period [21].

Table 16.5 Prevalence, onset and symptoms of the most frequent postpartum disorders are shown. Blues is the most frequent PPD, depression and psychosis is less frequent but symptoms are more severe

Disorder	Prevalence	Onset	Symptoms
Blues	50–80%	From day 3. Time limited, usually lasts until day 10 postpartum.	Rapid mood shifts, tearfulness, irritability, anxiety, insomnia, lack of energy, loss of appetite.
Depression	10–15%	From 24 hours to several months after delivery	Indistinguishable from major depressive disorder. Frequent anxiety symptoms.
Psychosis	0.1–0.2%	Within the first month of delivery	Auditory and visual hallucinations, paranoid and grandiose delusions, impulsivity.

Postpartum depression

The aetiology of PPD is unknown; it is probably multifactorial, with biological factors, including hormonal changes, psychological factors and social factors, such as poor social support and stressful life events. One of 10 childbearing women has PPD and it is frequently underdiagnosed. PPD may begin anywhere from 24 hours to several months after delivery. When its onset is abrupt and symptoms are severe, women are more likely to seek help early in the illness. In cases with an insidious onset, treatment is often delayed, if it is ever sought [21]. Women who had a previous history of mood disorders, both puerperal and nonpuerperal, are at increased risk of relapse after delivery. At least one third of the women who have had PPD have a recurrence of symptoms after a subsequent delivery. PPD is relatively frequent in women with bipolar disorder. It is not clear what proportion of women presenting with a first episode of PPD will have symptoms that progress to a bipolar disorder. Women with no history of mood disorder that present with PPD should always be screened for personal and family history of hypomania or mania. Education about signs and symptoms of hypomania and mania should be provided since antidepressant treatment may cause symptom switching [54–56].

If PPD is left untreated, the disorder can have serious adverse effects on the mother and on the child's emotional and psychological development. PPD has shown to have damaging consequences for the infants of affected mothers. Impaired bonding has been associated with attachment insecurity in the child. Children of depressed mothers have impaired emotional and language development, as well as impaired attention and cognitive skills. Also, they are more likely to develop long-term behavioural problems. Impairment in the mother can lead to impairment in the children [57].

Table 16.6 Treatment of PPD is based on that of nonpuerperal depression. Some studies have been published, many more are needed to establish specific treatments for PPD

Authors	Type of study	Indication	Treatment	Conclusion
Appleby et al. [61]	Randomised-controlled	Postpartum depression	Fluoxetine vs placebo plus 1 or six sessions of cognitive behavioural counselling	Both fluoxetine and cognitive-behavioural counselling given as a course of therapy are effective.
Cohen et al. [60]	Open-label	Postpartum depression	Venlafaxine	Effective treatment.
Suri et al. [59]	Open-label	Postpartum depression	Fluvoxamine	Effective treatment.
Wisner et al. [56]	Double-blind	Prevention of postpartum depression	Sertraline vs placebo	Sertraline conferred preventive efficacy for postpartum-onset major depression beyond that of placebo.
Misri et al. [58]	Randomised-controlled	Postpartum depression and anxiety	Paroxetine vs CBT	Antidepressant monotherapy and combination therapy with antidepressants and CBT were both efficacious in reducing depression and anxiety symptoms.
Nonacs et al. [79]	Open-label	Postpartum depression	Bupropion SR	Effective and well-tolerated.
Wisner et al. [50]	Double-blind	Postpartum depression	Sertraline vs nortriptyline	The proportion of women who responded and remitted did not differ between drugs Breast-fed infant serum levels were near or below the level of quantifiability for both agents.

CBT = Cognitive behavioural therapy.

To date, the treatment of PPD is based on that of nonpuerperal depression, that is, antidepressant therapy, alone or in combination with psychotherapy [50, 58–62]. Some studies have been published on the treatment on PPD (see Table 16.6).

Postpartum psychosis

Postpartum psychosis occurs in 0.2% of childbearing women. Most puerperal psychosis has its onset within the first month of delivery. Women present sleep difficulties for several nights, agitation, expansive or irritable mood and avoidance of the infant. When delusions or hallucinations are present, they often involve the infant. Postpartum psychosis is considered a medical emergency, because the woman is at risk of harming herself, her baby or both. Little is known about which predictors of maternal filicide programmes focused on reliable markers for maternal filicide are needed to better prevent these events. Most patients with puerperal psychosis need to be hospitalised and treated with antipsychotics [21, 63].

References

1. Centers for Disease Control and Prevention. Achievements in Public Health. 1900–1999: Healthier mothers and babies. Morbidity and mortality weekly report. Atlanta, GA, U.S. Government Printing Office, 1999; 48: 848–859.
2. Sussman, N. (2005) Biological therapies, in *Kaplan and Sadock's Comprehensive Textbook of Psychiatry*, 8th edn (eds B.J. Sadock and V.A. Sadock), Lippincott Wiliams & Wilkins, Philadelphia, pp. 2676–99.
3. Prudic, J. (2005) Electroconvulsive therapy, in: *Kaplan & Sadock's Comprehensive Textbook of Psychiatry*, 8th edn (eds B.J. Sadock and V.A. Sadock). Philadelphia (PA): Lippincott Williams & Wilkins; pp. 2968–83.
4. Domino, E.F. (1999) History of modern psychopharmacology: a personal view with an emphasis on antidepressants. *Psychosomatic Medicine*, **61**, 591–98.
5. Kammen, D.P. and Marder, S.R. (2005) Serotonin-dopamine antagonists (atypical or second-generation antipsychotics), in *Kaplan and Sadock's Comprehensive Textbook of Psychiatry*, 8th edn (eds B.J. Sadock and V.A. Sadock), Lippincott Wiliams & Wilkins, Philadelphia, pp. 2914–38.
6. Hayunga, E.G. and Pinn, V.W. (2002) NIH Policy on the inclusion of women and minorities as subjects in clinical research, in *Principles and Practice of Clinical Research* (ed. J.I. Gallin), Elsevier, San Diego, pp. 145–60.
7. The Belmont Report (1979) Ethical Principles and Guidelines for the Protection of Human Subjects, The National Commission for the Protection of Human Subjects of Biomedical and Behavioral Research.
8. Eisenberg, L. (1977) The social Imperatives of medical research. *Science*, **198**, 1105–10.
9. Emanuel, E.J., Wendler, D. and Grady, C. (2000) What makes clinical research ethical? *The Journal of the American Medical Association*, **283**, 2701–11.
10. Gallin, J.I. (2002) (ed). *Principles and Practice of Clinical Research*. Elsevier, California.

11. Chan, A.W. and Altman, D.G. (2005) Identifying outcome reporting bias in randomized trials on PubMed: review of publications and survey of authors. *British Medical Journal*, **330**, 753.

12. Turner, E.H., Matthews, A.M., Linardatos, E. *et al.* (2008) Selective publication of antidepressant trilas and its influence on apparent efficacy. *The New England Journal of Medicine*, **358**, 252–60.

13. Merkatz, R.B., Temple, R., Sobel, S., Feiden, K. and Kessler, D.A. (1993) Women in clinical trials of new drugs – A change in Food and Drug Administration Policy. *N Engl J Med* , **329**, 292–6.

14. Kirschstein, R.L. (1991) Research on women's health. *Am J Public Health*, **81**, 291–3.

15. Evelyn, B., Toigo, T., Banks, D., Pohl, D., Gray, K., Robins, B. and Ernat, J. (2001) Participation of racial/ethnic groups in clinical trials and race-related labeling: a review of new molecular entities approved 1995–1999. *J Natl Med Assoc*, **93**, 18–24.

16. Yonkers, K.A., Kando, J.C., Cole, J.O. and Blumenthal, S. (1992) Gender differences in pharmacokinetics and pharmacodynamics of psychotropic medication. *The American Journal of Psychiatry*, **149**, 587–95.

17. Greenblatt, D.J. and von Moltke, L.L. (2005) Pharmacokinetics and drug interaction, in *Kaplan and Sadock's Comprehensive Textbook of Psychiatry*, 8th edn (eds B.J. Sadock and V.A. Sadock), Lippincott Wiliams & Wilkins, Philadelphia, pp. 2699–706.

18. Stahl, S.M. (2008) Synaptic Neurotransmission and the anatomically addressed nervous system, in *Stahl's Essential Psychopharmacology. Neuroscientific Basis and Practical Applications*. Cambridge University Press, pp. 21–51.

19. Abernethy, D.R., Greenblatt, D.R., Divoll, M. *et al.* (1982) Impairment of diazepam metabolism by low-dose estrogen-containing oral- contraceptive steroids. *The New England Journal of Medicine*, **306**, 791–92.

20. Wald, A., Van Thiel, D.H., Hoechstetter, L. *et al.* (1981) Gastrointestinal transit: the effect of the menstrual cycle. *Gastroenterology*, **80**, 1497–500.

21. Berga, S.L., Parry, B.L. and Cyranowski, J.M. (2005) Psychiatry and reproductive medicine, in *Kaplan and Sadock's Comprehensive Textbook of Psychiatry*, 8th edn (eds B.J. Sadock and V.A. Sadock), Lippincott Williams & Wilkins, Philadelphia, pp. 2293–2315.

22. O'Malley, K., Crooks, J., Duke, E. and Stevenson, I.H. (1971) Effect of age and sex on human drug metabolism. *British Medical Journal*, **3**, 607–9.

23. Scheibe, S., Preuschhof, C., Cristi, C. and Bagby, R.M. (2003) Are there gender differences in major depression and its response to antidepressants? *J Affect Disord*, Aug **75** (3), 223–35.

24. Cohen, L.S. (2007) Treatment of bipolar disorder during pregnancy. *The Journal of Clinical Psychiatry*, **68**, 4–9.

25. Simpson, G.M., Yadalam, K.G., Levinson, D.F. *et al.* (1990) Single dose pharmacokinetics of fluphenazine after single dose fluphenazine decanoate administration. *Journal of Clinical Psychopharmacology*, **10**, 417–21.

26. Chouinard, G., Annable, L., Ross-Chouinard, A. and Nestoros, J.N. (1979) Factors related to tardive dyskinesia. *The American Journal of Psychiatry*, **136**, 79–83.

27. Seeman, V.M. (1983) Interaction of sex, age and neuroleptic dose. *Comprehensive Psychiatry*, **24**, 125–28.

28. Fields, J.Z. and Gordon, J.H. (1982) Estrogen diminishes the dopaminergic super-sensitivity induced by neuroleptics. *Life Sciences*, **30**, 229–34.

29. Szymanski, S., Lieberman, J.A., Alvir, J.M. *et al.* (1995) Gender differences in onset of illness, treatment response, course and biological indexes, in first-episode schizophrenic patients. *The American Journal of Psychiatry*, **152**, 698–703.

30. Wohlfarth, T., Storosum, J.G., Elferink, A.J.A. *et al.* (2004) Response to tricyclic antidepressants: independent of gender? *The American Journal of Psychiatry*, **161**, 370–72.

31. Grubbe Hildebrandt, M., Willem Steyerberg, E., Bjerregaard Stage, K. *et al.* (2003) Are gender differences important for the clinical effects of antidepressants? *The American Journal of Psychiatry*, **160**, 1643–50.

32. Kornstein, S.G., Shatzberg, A.F., Thase, M.E. *et al.* (2000) Gender differences in treatment response to sertraline versus imipramine in chronic depression. *The American Journal of Psychiatry*, **157**, 1445–52.

33. Naito, S., Sato, K., Yoshida, K. *et al.* (2007) Gender differences in the clinical effects of fluvoxamine and milnacipran in Japanese major depressive patients. *Psychiatry and Clinical Neurosciences*, **61**, 421–27.

34. Pinto–Meza, A., Usall, J., Serrano-Blanco, A. *et al.* (2006) Gender differences in response to antidepressant treatment prescribed in primary care. Does menopause make a difference? *Journal of Affective Disorders*, **93**, 53–60.

35. Quitkin, F.M., Stewart, J.W., Mc Grath, P.J. *et al.* (2002) Are there differences between women's and men's antidepressant responses? *The American Journal of Psychiatry*, **159**, 1848–54.

36. Frackiewicz, E.J., Sramek, J.J. and Cutler, N.R. (2000) Gender differences in depression and antidepressant pharmacokinetics and adverse events. *The Annals of Pharmacotherapy*, **34**, 80–88.

37. Viguera, A.C., Tondo, L. and Baldessarini, R.J. (2000) Sex differences in response to lithium treatment. *The American Journal of Psychiatry*, **157**, 1509–11.

38. Joffe, H. (2007) Reproductive biology and psychotropic treatments in premenopausal women with bipolar disorder. *The Journal of Clinical Psychiatry*, **68**, 10–15.

39. Joffe, H., Cohen, L.S. and Supess, T. (2006) Valproate is associated with new-onset oligoamenorrhea with hyperandrogenism in women with bipolar disorder. *Biological Psychiatry*, **59**, 1078–86.

40. Isojarvi, J.L., Laatikainen, T.J. and Pakarinen, A.J. (1993) Polycystic ovaries and hyperandrogenism in women taking valproate for epilepsy. *The New England Journal of Medicine*, **329**, 1383–88.

41. Haddad, P.M. and Wieck, A. (2004) Antipsychotic-induced hyperprolactinaemia: mechanisms, clinical features and management. *Drugs*, **64**, 2291–314.

42. Wang, P.S., Walker, A.M. and Tsuang, M.T. (2002) Dopamine antagonists and the development of breast cancer. *Archives of General Psychiatry*, **59**, 1145–54.

43. Viguera, A.C., Koukopoulus, A., Muzina, D.J. and Baldessarini, R.J. (2007) Teratogenicity and anticonvulsants: lessons from neurology to psychiatry. *The Journal of Clinical Psychiatry*, **68**, 29–33.

44. Cohen, L.S., Atshuler, L.L. and Harlow, B.L. (2006) Relapse of major depression during pregnancy in women who maintain or discontinue antidepressant treatment. *The Journal of the American Medical Association*, **295**, 499–507.

45. Newport, D.J., Fisher, A., Graybeal, S. and Stowe, Z.N. (2004) Psychopharmacology during pregnancy and lactation, in *Textbook of Psychopharmacology*, 3rd edn (eds A.F.

Schatzberg and C.B. Nemeroff), American Psychiatric Publishing, Inc., Arlington, pp. 1109–46.

46. Viguera, A.C., Cohen, L.S. and Bouffard, S. (2002) Reproductive decisions by women with bipolar disorder after prepregnancy psychiatric consultation. *Am J Psychiatry*, **159**, 2102–4.

47. Wyszynsky, D.F., Nambisan, M. and Surve, T.(2005) Increased rate of major malformations in offspring exposed to valproate during pregnancy. *Neurology*, **64**, 961–5.

48. Schatzberg, A.F., Cole, J.O. and De Battista, C. (2007) *Manual of Clinical Psychopharmacology*, 6th edn, American Psychiatric Publishing, Inc., Arlington.

49. Wisner, K.L., Hanusa, B.H., Perel, J.M. *et al.* (2006) Postpartum depression: a randomized trial of sertraline versus nortriptyline. *Journal of Clinical Psychopharmacology*, **26**, 353–60.

50. Yonkers, K.A. (2007) The treatment of women suffering from depression who are either pregnant or breastfeeding. *The American Journal of Psychiatry*, **164**, 1457–59.

51. Stowe, Z.N. (2007) The use of mood stabilizers during breastfeeding. *The Journal of Clinical Psychiatry*, **68**, 22–28.

52. Burt, V.K., Suri, R., Altshuler, L. *et al.* (2001) The use of psychotropic medications during breast-feeding. *The American Journal of Psychiatry*, **158**, 1001–9.

53. Eberhard-Gran, M., Eskild, A. and Opjordsmoen, S. (2006) Use of psychotropic medications in treating mood disorders during lactation: practical recommendations. *CNS Drugs*, **20**, 187–98.

54. Payne, J.L. (2007) Antidepressant use in the postpartum period: practical considerations. *The American Journal of Psychiatry*, **164**, 1329–32.

55. Sharma, V. (2006) A cautionary note on the use of antidepressants in postpartum depression. *Bipolar Disorders*, **8**, 411–14.

56. Wisner, K.L., Perel, J.M., Peindl, K.S. *et al.* (2004) Prevention of postpartum depression: a pilot randomized clinical trial. *The American Journal of Psychiatry*, **161**, 1290–92.

57. Kendrick, M.S. (2207) Treatment of perinatal mood and anxiety disorders: a review. *Canadian Journal of Psychiatry*, **52**, 489–98.

58. Misri, S., Reebye, P., Corral, M. and Milis, L. (2004) The use of paroxetine and cognitive-behavioral therapy in postpartum depression and anxiety: a randomized controlled trial. *The Journal of Clinical Psychiatry*, **65**, 1236–41.

59. Suri, R., Burt, V.K., Altshuler, L.L. *et al.* (2001) Fluvoxamine for postpartum depression. *The American Journal of Psychiatry*, **158**, 1739–40.

60. Cohen, L.S., Viguera, A.C., Bouffard, S.M. *et al.* (2001) Venlafaxine in the treatment of postpartum depression. *The Journal of Clinical Psychiatry*, **62**, 592–96.

61. Appleby, L., Warner, R., Whitton, A. and Faragher, B. (1997) A controlled study of fluoxetine and cognitive-behavioural counselling in the treatment of postnatal depression. *British Medical Journal*, **314**, 932–36.

62. Epperson, C.N. (1999) Postpartum major depression: detection and treatment. *American Family Physician*, **59**, 2247–54.

63. Kendell, R.E., Chalmers, J.C. and Platz, C. (1987) Epidemiology of puerperal psychosis. *The British Journal of Psychiatry*, **150**, 662–73.

64. Marder, S.R. and van Kammen D.P. (2005) Dopamine receptor antagonists (typical antipsychotics), in *Kaplan and Sadock's Comprehensive Textbook of Psychiatry*, 8th edn

(eds B.J. Sadock and V.A. Sadock), Lippincott Wiliams & Wilkins, Philadelphia, pp. 2817–38.

65. Post, R.M. and Frye, M.A. (2005) Anticonvulsants, in *Kaplan and Sadock's Compre-hensive Textbook of Psychiatry*, 8th edn (eds B.J. Sadock and V.A. Sadock), Lippincott Wiliams & Wilkins, Philadelphia, pp. 2732–46.

66. Ketter, T.A. (2005) Lamotrigine, in *Kaplan and Sadock's Comprehensive Textbook of Psychiatry*, 8th edn (eds B.J. Sadock and V.A. Sadock), Lippincott Wiliams & Wilkins, Philadelphia, pp. 2749–53.

67. Frye,M.A. and Post, R.M. (2005) Valproate, in *Kaplan and Sadock's Comprehensive Textbook of Psychiatry*, 8th edn (eds B.J. Sadock and V.A. Sadock), Lippincott Wiliams & Wilkins, Philadelphia, pp. 2756–66.

68. Nemeroff, C.B. and Putnam, J.S. (2005) Barbiturates and similarly acting substances, in *Kaplan and Sadock's Comprehensive Textbook of Psychiatry*, 8th edn (eds B.J. Sadock and V.A. Sadock), Lippincott Wiliams & Wilkins, Philadelphia, pp. 2775–81.

69. Dubovsky, S. (2005) Benzodiazepine receptor agonists and antagonists, in *Kaplan and Sadock's Comprehensive Textbook of Psychiatry*, 8th edn (eds B.J. Sadock and V.A. Sadock), Lippincott Wiliams & Wilkins, Philadelphia, pp. 2781–91.

70. Rush, A.J., Hudziak, J. and Rettew, D.C. (2005) Bupropion, in *Kaplan and Sadock's Comprehensive Textbook of Psychiatry*, 8th edn (eds B.J. Sadock and V.A. Sadock), Lippincott Wiliams & Wilkins, Philadelphia, pp. 2791–97.

71. Jann, M.W. and Small, G.W. (2005) Cholinesterase inhibitors and similarly acting compounds, in *Kaplan and Sadock's Comprehensive Textbook of Psychiatry*, 8th edn (eds B.J. Sadock and V.A. Sadock), Lippincott Wiliams & Wilkins, Philadelphia, pp. 2808–17.

72. Jefferson, J.W. and Greist, J.H. (2005) Lithium, in *Kaplan and Sadock's Comprehensive Textbook of Psychiatry*, 8th edn (eds B.J. Sadock and V.A. Sadock), Lippincott Wiliams & Wilkins, Philadelphia, pp. 2839–51.

73. Thase, M.E. (2005) Mirtazapine, in *Kaplan and Sadock's Comprehensive Textbook of Psychiatry*, 8th edn (eds B.J. Sadock and V.A. Sadock), Lippincott Wiliams & Wilkins, Philadelphia, pp. 2851–54.

74. Kennedy, S.H., Holt, A. and Baker, G.B. (2005) Monoamine oxidase inhibitors, in *Kaplan and Sadock's Comprehensive Textbook of Psychiatry*, 8th edn (eds B.J. Sadock and V.A. Sadock), Lippincott Wiliams & Wilkins, Philadelphia, pp. 2854–63.

75. Thase M.E. (2005) Selective serotonin-norepinephrine reuptake inhibitors, in *Kaplan and Sadock's Comprehensive Textbook of Psychiatry*, 8th edn (eds B.J. Sadock and V.A. Sadock), Lippincott Wiliams & Wilkins, Philadelphia, pp. 2881–87.

76. Kelsey, J.E. (2005) Selective serotonin reuptake inhibitors, in *Kaplan and Sadock's Comprehensive Textbook of Psychiatry*, 8th edn (eds B.J. Sadock and V.A. Sadock), Lippincott Wiliams & Wilkins, Philadelphia, pp. 2887–914.

77. Nelson, J.C. (2005) Tricyclics and tetracyclics, in *Kaplan and Sadock's Comprehensive Textbook of Psychiatry*, 8th edn (eds B.J. Sadock and V.A. Sadock), Lippincott Wiliams & Wilkins, Philadelphia, pp. 2956–67.

78. 100 years of protecting and promoting women's health. [Online]. (2006) [cited 2008 Jan 16]; [14screens]. Available from: http://www.fda.gov/womens/milesbro.html.

79. Nonacs, R.M., Soares, C.N., Viguera, A.C., Pearson, K., Poitras, J.R. and Cohen, L.S. (2005). Bupropion SR for the treatment of postpartum depression: a pilot study. *Int J Nueripsychopharmacol*, **8**, 445–9.

SECTION 4

Impact of violence, disasters, migration and work

Unaiza Niaz[1] and Marianne Kastrup[2]

[1]*The Psychiatric Clinic & Stress Research Center, Karachi; University of Health Sciences, Lahore, Pakistan*
[2]*Transcultural Psychiatry, Psychiatric Department of Rigshospitalet, Copenhagen, Denmark*

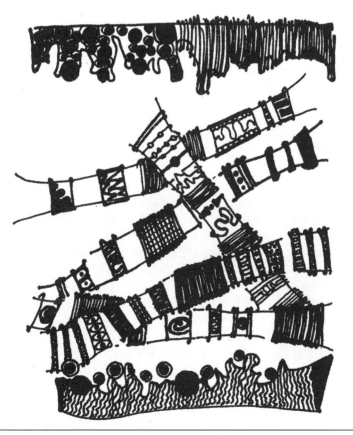

Contemporary Topics in Women's Mental Health   Edited by Chandra, Herrman, Fisher, Kastrup,
© 2009 John Wiley & Sons, Ltd   Niaz, Rondón and Okasha

Commentary

Impact of work on women's mental health
(Saida Douki)

In the past few decades, extensive, socially relevant and significant research on women's mental health issues has been published [1–5]. The research, however, has not only paid insufficient attention to social factors, but also ignored discrimination and gender specific negative life events in favour of the role of reproductive life and endocrinology. Consequently, these biological factors have – to a large degree – been considered as the major explanations for high rates of psychiatric illnesses in women.

It is necessary that research pays due attention to social forces that commonly impinge on women's mental health and emotional wellbeing, such as sexual and physical trauma, stiff gender roles, workplace discrimination and the pressure for physical beauty.

Furthermore, many aspects of war and collective violence affect the health of women and girls disproportionately through societal changes that subordinate women and under prioritise their life and health. Also, WHO has stressed the serious health consequences for women of collective violence, including war, and violent political conflict [6].

Poverty is now recognised to be one factor particularly relevant to women's mental health, in the global scenario. Approximately 60% of US children living in mother-only families are poor, compared with only 11% of two-parent families [7]. The rate of poverty is even higher in African-American single-parent families, in which two out of every three children are poor [8].

Until recently, research studies on the relation between work and health, have focused on men's experiences. Saida Douki, in her chapter 20 discusses the impact of psychosocial factors, stress and strains on working women. Even in the most traditional societies, women have entered the workforce. Also among women in western countries with a high percentage working full time we see increased stress, and studies from OECD have demonstrated that it is among women aged 35–65 exposed to the stresses and risks of working life that we find the excess mortality [9].

Women at the top, often face a hostile work environment, and a Danish study of stress found that female physicians had more than twice the risk of being daily stressed compared to their male colleagues, even when controlling for stressors in relation to daily life, working life and health [10].

The impact of women's multiple roles on their wellbeing was initially assumed to add to the stress in their lives and, consequently, it would be linked to negative health outcomes [11]. Several other research findings conflict with these views. At present, a number of studies point out that multiple roles may grant benefits to women's physical and mental health [12, 13]; other research studies in fact have identified the protective benefits of multiple roles, in women. The effects on women of combining paid employment and family roles clearly depend on characteristics of the individual, her family and her job situation. In general, however, occupying more than one role appears to buffer women from the stress [14]. For instance, longitudinal data have indicated that declines in job quality were associated with increased psychological distress for single women and women without children; however, changes in job quality were unrelated to psychological distress for women with partners and women with children [15, 16]. These studies suggest that women who encounter problems in their jobs are more likely to feel depressed and anxious if they are single than if they are married or parents.

Impact of culture on women's mental health (Marianne Kastrup and Unaiza Niaz)

Historically, culture, customs, traditions and beliefs have in their own way fostered various forms of violence against women. Women's roles have primarily been as wives and mothers with the main responsibility to reproduce the next generation [17].

The former UN Secretary General Kofi Annan [18] once called violence against women the most pervasive, yet least recognised, human rights abuse in the world. In some regions of South East Asia, violence has reached staggering levels; in a recent population-based study from India, nearly half of women reported physical violence [19]. Annually an estimated one million pregnant Pakistani are physically abused at least once during pregnancy [20].

In China when the Communist government came to power in 1949, discrimination against women was institutionalised within all the usual structures of society: family, the economy, education, culture and the political system.

In the Arab world, women experience what Deniz Kandiyoti [21] has called a 'double jeopardy'. The resulting 'intersection' of patriarchies [22] created a historically specific momentum of increasing control exercised over women by men, families, communities and the state.

In Muslim countries, several customary practises that allow violations of women's human rights in the region – honour crimes, stoning, female genital mutilation (FGM) or virginity tests – have no Quranic basis, as women researchers and activists in the region point out.

There is a clear rise of NGOs focusing on women's status, of the creation by governments of national commissions for women, and there is increase in women entering the workforce in countries where women's participation in paid labour was previously negligible [23].

The significance of women in Arab societies become obvious with the access to the Internet, and to TV channels, such as Al-Jazeera's handling of programmes about women's status [24].

Also in the European region women face violence and according to Amnesty International [25] domestic violence is the major cause of death and disability for European women aged 16–44.

Effects of globalisation on women's mental health (Unaiza Niaz)

Women's struggles for human rights generally, have been more pronounced with regard to violence against women than they have been concerning their economic rights. It is equally important for women to struggle for economic independence, as economic empowerment in turn would give women a chance for independent, violence free existence (e.g. in victims of domestic violence, who continue to suffer due to lack of education or skills for job procurement).

Women's physical and mental health is inextricably linked with social, cultural and economic factors that influence all aspects of their lives, and it has consequences also for the wellbeing of their children, the functioning of households and the distribution of resources. The greatest challenge is to minimise or offset the damage resulting from impacts of globalisation and consolidate the benefits. This could be achieved by enabling women to take power and control over their life situation and redefining ways of giving women the power to utilise the globalisation process to their own advantage, economically, socially as well as politically.

Globalisation also produces new forms of commoditisation, to the extent of making human life itself a commodity. One of the consequences is human trafficking, the two groups most affected being women and children. Human trafficking involves 'moving men, women and children from one place to another and placing them in conditions of forced labour' [26]. Women from Africa, and Asia are most commonly trafficked across international borders for commercial sex work in Europe. Besides that, many women and young children from South-East Asian regions are trafficked and forced into prostitution, undesired marriages and bonded labour.

In South Asia an increase in women's employment is thought to modify the balance of power within the household. However, increasing female wages do not always result in positive benefits for women. No women's movement in any country or community can be studied and understood without taking global influences into account. Though globalisation may be beneficial in many ways, one must bear in mind the massive mental health and financial cost, when it affects women in a negative way.

Women and disasters (Unaiza Niaz)

In both natural and man made disasters women are particularly left behind in receiving help in crises and later in the rehabilitation phase of disaster management programmes. Niaz discusses these issues in her chapter on Women in Disasters.

The plight of displaced women is particularly difficult. Armed conflict displaces people from their homes and livelihoods. The first WHO World Report on Violence and Health states 'More than 85% of the major conflicts since the second world war have been in poor countries... Between 1986 and 1996, a major proportion of those dying as a result of armed conflicts were civilians, particularly women and children . . . '.

The rise in the proportion of civilian, and notably women's and children's deaths, in twentieth century warfare is attributed to changes in war technology and war tactics. Women are now documented to be the most vulnerable to the mental health consequences of war. In all recent wars, like the Afghan War, the war in Bosnia, the ongoing Iraq war and so on women bear the brunt postwar, distressed by multiple social and mental health problems. Women now make up 15% of active duty forces, four times more than in the 1991 Gulf War.

Globally women are also known to suffer more difficulties in natural disasters [27]. The Pakistan Earthquake in 2005 killed 70 000 people mostly school children and women, rendering about four million homeless. This disaster has left many women and children disabled. There were no adequate facilities to help them in their helpless condition. Relatives themselves were struggling to rehabilitate themselves and often did not have the energy or motivation to help these women.

In wars, and natural disasters, the only feasible solution is a quick rehabilitation and re-organisation of the fractured society at all levels. The support system needs to be strengthened as early as possible. Quick rehabilitation would be an effective ameliorating factor particularly for the vulnerable women. The frustration, anger, sense of deprivations and helplessness, should be channelled and transformed into positive energies and constructive activities. The need for large-scale therapeutic procedures focusing on the particular needs of high risk groups (women, children and elderly) cannot be over emphasised.

Female mutilation (Amira Eldin)

FGM has been practised for more than a 1000 years, and despite the general perception there is no basis that FGM is prescribed by any religion.

FGM is a public health issue of global concern, today practised particularly in Africa and the Middle East, as well as in immigrant communities. Of the countries that demonstrate the highest prevalence there is no evidence of change in prevalence over time [28] In spite of increasing concern for the practise of FGM evidence suggests that it still occurs more frequently than previously thought. It is estimated that approximately 5500 girls every day are exposed to FGM, and FGM should be seen as an urgent human rights violation, requiring further interventions [28].

It is today well known that the consequences of FGM are extensive both from a physical and a psychological perspective.

Particular focus has been paid to the physical sequels that ultimately may lead to death when FGM is carried out under unsanitary conditions; bleeding; chronic infections of bladder and vagina; or reproductive problems.

Less focus has been paid to the psychological consequences and research is needed to elucidate the mental health effects of FGM. According to Eldin, many girls report psychological distress such as depression, nightmares, passivity and feelings of betrayal, and FGM may result in long-lasting mental health consequences as reported in many case studies [29]

FGM, as reported in a study by Behrendt and Moritz [30], may lead to psychological distress and ultimately to psychiatric disorders, especially PTSD, in up to 30%, which is similar to what is reported in children who have been victims of early childhood abuse.

The practise has till recently been characterised by a conspiracy of silence and the affected girls tend not to report the distress which is further supported by the fact that expressing feelings of psychological distress may in some cultures not be socially acceptable.

As mental health professionals we should be aware that the use of trained personnel rather than traditional practitioners in carrying out the FGM is on the rise. This may reflect the impact of campaigns where the health risks are described, but as pointed out by Eldin fail to address the underlying motivations for its perpetuation. Unless effective interventions are found to convince communities to abandon the practise, FGM will continue. There is an increasing recognition among many campaigners, and health workers in settings practising FGM for the need to change, but no suggestion of ways to achieve such an extensive social transformation [31].

Migration and mental health in women (Solvig Ekblad)

The mental health of migrant women is closely associated with their integration in the new society as described by Ekblad in her chapter. But unfortunately the magnitude of human rights violations towards women shows no decline [32] and furthermore migrant and refugee women run a relatively higher risk of family and domestic violence [33], which may pamper the integration as interpersonal violence is documented to lead to poorer integration [34].

In a recent study of Somali and Oromo refugees it is shown that women are as likely to have been exposed to torture as men, Jaranson et al. [35], which is in contrast to the general perception that men are the primary target of human rights violations and may reflect that many of the atrocities women are experiencing go unnoticed, hidden from the public eye.

A number of factors have an impact on women's mental health including premigratory traumatic events, events taking place during the migration, as well as postmigratory stressors. It is well documented that the stressors may act independently of each other and all contribute to the distress.

But there is an increasing awareness that it is not only important to consider the individual vulnerability factors but also bear in mind the protective factors that may facilitate the differentiation between those who are resilient and those who may be in need of help [36].

Of the factors that are clearly linked with better mental health, one important factor is access to economic opportunities Porter and Haslam [37]. Unemployment is documented as a significant stress factor in the integrative process [38], which makes women's lives difficult as many of them do not have the option to transfer their competences to a new environment, and a life in poverty is a major contributory factor in predicting psychological problems in migrant women.

A major task for mental health professionals globally is to develop strategies in order to work for the empowerment of migrant women [39]. This is a long process in which we need among other things to ensure their access to information on their own rights and set their own priorities in order for them to realise their capacities and skills.

As pointed out by Ekblad there is a tendency to overlook the association between mental health and human rights and a lack of recognition that, to recover from a traumatic experience, is not only a personal and public health issue, but also a matter of social justice.

Interventions for intimate partner violence (Krishna Vaddiparti and Deepthi S. Varma)

Intimate partner violence (IPV) is widely reported and in a survey from 10 countries physical or sexual violence from a partner was reported among 15–71% of women [40]. It is well documented that women who have been exposed to systematic abuse have a greater likelihood for developing depressive symptoms, post traumatic stress disorder, anxiety disorders, somatoform disorders or substance use. Over time many intervention projects have been developed aiming to prevent, treat or reduce the consequences of IPV. Some have focused on the primary preventive aspects – like public awareness campaigns or empowerment of women programmes, others have been directed towards ending further partner violence; some have in their approach been victim focused, others have focused on interventions with the perpetrators/batterers of violence.

It is characteristic that the interventions directed towards the victims have had their origin primarily in the health sector, where, for example, WHO have developed strategies to increase the health system's ability to identify and deal with the consequences of IPV [41]. Programmes directed towards the batterers have, on the other hand, predominantly been developed by the criminal justice system aiming to reduce further abuse and to rehabilitate the batterers.

Despite the increasing concern for IPV and the awareness of its magnitude, the mental health consequences hereof for those abused, as well as the ever-growing variety of intervention programmes, there is still a lack of evidence on the effectiveness of such interventions. As pointed out by Vaddiparti and Sharma, hitherto the scientific evidence of their effectiveness has been inconsistent. We still lack randomised control studies documenting the effect of interventions towards the abused women. But the interventions aiming at the abusive partners also have restrictions regarding their stringency. The participation of the batterers may not be voluntary and the effectiveness of the programmes has not been sufficiently assessed.

IPV is documented in all parts of the world and in all cultural settings. Yet we know that certain groups of women are particularly vulnerable. In this section we have amply reported that, for example, refugee women, and immigrant women are less likely to seek the police in case of partner violence either due to a fear of discrimination or due to the fact that they may directly risk being deported. Furthermore, in some parts of the world women are at risk of either neglect by the police or experiencing abusive behaviour from the police force if reporting partner violence. In certain parts of the world violence is very prevalent due to war or societal dissolution and it is essential that the socio-cultural context is kept in mind when developing treatment programmes, as well as when assessing the outcome. Only if this is the case may interventions be used on a global level.

References

1. Niaz, U. (1997) Contemporary Issues of Pakistani Women: A Psycho-social Perspective, Publication of Pakistan Association Of Women's Studies, Karachi University, Pakistan ISBN: 969-8400-00-1.
2. Niaz, U. (2004) Women's mental health around in Pakistan. *World Psychiatry*, **3**, 60–61.
3. Kessel, B., Gise, L., Milgrom, J. *et al.* (2003) Women's mental health around the world (culture). *Journal of Psychosomatic Research*, **55**, 119–19.
4. Ekblad, S., Kastrup, M., Eisenman, D. and Arcel, L. (2007) Interpersonal violence towards women: an overview and clinical directions, in *Immigrant Medicine* (eds P. Walker and E. Barnett), Saunders, Elsevier, Philadelphia.
5. Arcel, L. and Kastrup, M. (2004) War, women and health. *Nordic Journal of Women's Study*, **12**, 40–47.
6. Krug, E.G., Mercy, J.A., Dahlberg, L.L. *et al.* (2002) World report on violence and health. WHO. *Lancet*, **360**, 1083–88.
7. Olson, S.L. and Banyard, V. (1993) Stop the world so I can get off for a while: sources of daily stress in the lives low-income single mothers of young children. *Family Relations*, **42**, 50–56.
8. McLoyd, V.C., Jayaratne, T.E., Ceballo, R. and Borquez, J. (1994) Unemployment and work interruption among African American single mothers: effects on parenting and adolescent socio emotional functioning. *Child Development*, **65**, 562–69.
9. (2006) http://www.oecd.org/october.
10. Hargreave, M., Petersson, B. and Kastrup, M. (2007) Kønsforskelle i stress blandt læger (gender differences in stress among physicians). *Ugeskr Læg*, **169**, 2418–22.
11. Sears, H.A. and Galambos, N.L. (1993) The employed mother's well-being, in *The Employed Mother and the Family Context* (ed. J. Frankel), Spring, New York.
12. Barnett, R.C. (1993) Multiple roles, gender, and psychological distress, in *Handbook of Stress: Theoretical and Clinical Aspects*, 2nd edn (eds L. Golderger and S. Breznitz), The Free Press, New York.
13. Green, B.L. and Russo, N.F. (1993) Work and family roles: selected issues, in *Psychology of Women: A Handbook of Issues and Theories* (eds F.L. Denmark and M.A. Paludi), Greenwood Press, Westport.

14. Crosby, F.J. (1991) *Juggling: The Unexpected Advantages of Balancing Career and Home For Women and Their Families*, The Free Press, New York.

15. Barnett, R.C., Marshall, N.L. and Singer, J.D. (1992) Job experiences over time, multiple roles, and women's mental health: a longitudinal study. *Journal of Personality and Social Psychology*, **62**, 634–44.

16. Amato, P.R. (1993) Children's adjustment to divorce: theories, hypotheses, and empirical support. *Journal of Marriage and Family*, **55**, 23–58.

17. Papic, V. (1994) Nationalism, patriarchy and war in ex-Yugoslavia. *Women's History Review*, **3**, 115–17.

18. Annan, K. (2004) Review of the Implementation of the Beijing Platform for Action and Women 2000: Gender, Equality, Development and Peace for the 21st Century, E/CN.6/2005/2, p. 22.

19. Jejeebhoy, S. (1999) Wife battering in rural India; husband's right? Evidence from survey data. *Economic Political Weekly*, **33**, 855–62.

20. Fikree, F.F., Jafarey, S.N., Korejo, R. *et al.* Intimate Partner Violence Before and During Pregnancy: Experiences of Postpartum Women in Karachi, Pakistan, Health Communications Population Reference Bureau, Washington, DC.

21. Kandiyoti, D. (1995) Reflections on the politics of gender in Muslim societies: from Nairobi to Beijing, in *Faith and Freedom: Women's Human Rights in the Muslim World* (ed. M. Afkhami), I. B. Tauris, London.

22. Suad, J. and Slyomovics, S. (2001) Introduction, in *Women and Power in the Middle East* (eds J. Suad and S. Slyomovics), University of Pennsylvania Press, Philadelphia.

23. Abdel-Wahab al-Afifi, N. and Abdel-Hadi, A. (eds) (1996) The Feminist Movement in the Arab World, Dar Al-Mostaqbal Al-Arabi/New Woman Research and Study Center, Cairo.

24. Sakr, N. (2001) *Satellite Realms: Transnational Television, Globalization and the Middle East*, I. B. Tauris, London.

25. Amnesty International http://web.amnesty org.

26. Orhant, M. (2001) Trafficking in Persons: Myths, Methods and Human Rights, Population Reference Bureau, Washington, DC, in a 2001 report published by Amnesty 42-UNICEF, 2001, p. 6–11.

27. Niaz, U. (2007) Gender perspectives in psycho-trauma, the Pakistan earthquake 2005, in *The Day The Mountains Moved* (ed. U. Niaz), Sama Books, Karachi.

28. UNICEF (2004) UNICEF Global Consultation on Indicators, NYHQ, Child Protection.

29. Kagondu, G. (2002) Female Genital Mutilation Eradication Project: Pilot Project in Four Districts of Kenya, mid-term evaluation report, Maendeleo Ya Wanake Organization (MYWO) and Program for Appropriate Technology in Health (PATH).

30. Behrendt, A. and Moritz, S. (2005) Post traumatic stress disorder and memory problems after female genital mutilation. *American Journal of Psychiatry*, **162**, 1000–2.

31. World Health Organization (2001) Female Genital Mutilation: Policy Guidelines for Nurses and Health Workers.

32. Jaranson, J., Ekblad, S., Kroupin, V. and Eisenman, D.P. (2007) Epidemiology and risk factors. Section 7: mental health and illness in immigrants, in *Immigrant Medicine* (eds P.F. Walker, E.D. Barnett and J. Jaranson), Saunders, Elsevier, St. Louis, pp. 627–32.

33. Rees, S. and Pease, B. (2007) Refugee Settlement, Safety and Wellbeing: Exploring Domestic and Family Violence in Refugee Communities, Paper Four of the Violence Against Women Community Attitudes Project. VicHealth, Immigrant Women's Domestic Violence Service Inc.

34. Ekblad, S., Kastrup, M.C., Eisenman, D.P. and Arcel, L.T. (2007) Interpersonal violence towards women \warning. Section 7: mental health and illness in immigrants, in *Immigrant Medicine* (eds P.F. Walker, E.D. Barnett and J. Jaranson), Saunders, Elsevier, St. Louis, pp. 665–71.

35. Jaranson, J.M., Butcher, J., Halcon, L. *et al.* (2004) Somali and Oromo refugees, correlates of torture and trauma history. *American Journal of Public Health*, **94**, 591–98.

36. Silove, D., Ekblad, S. and Mollica, R. (2000) Health and human rights. The rights of the severely mentally ill in post-conflict societies. *Lancet*, **355** (9214), 1548–49.

37. Porter, M. and Haslam, N. (2001) Forced displacement in Yugoslavia: a meta-analysis of psychological consequences and their moderators. *Journal of Traumatic Stress*, **14**, 817–34.

38. Beiser, M. and Hou, F. (2001) Language acquisition, unemployment and depressive disorder among Southeast Asian refugees: a 10-year study. *Social Science and Medicine*, **53**, 1321–34.

39. UNCHR (2008) Handbook for the Protection of Women and Girls, UNHCR, Geneva.

40. Ellsberg, M., Jansen, H.A.F.M., Watts, C.H. and Garcia-Moreno, C. WHO Multi-Country Study on Women's Health and Domestic Violence against Women Study Team (2008) Intimate partner violence and women's physical and mental health in the WHO multi-country study on women's health and domestic violence: an observational study. *Lancet*, **371**, 1165–72.

41. Ferris, E.L. (2008) Intimate partner violence. Doctors' role should be integrated with the needs of patients and society. *British Medical Journal*, **334**, 706–7.

17

Women and disasters

Unaiza Niaz[1,2]

[1]*The Psychiatric Clinic & Stress Research Center, Karachi, Pakistan*
[2]*University of Health Sciences, Lahore, Pakistan*

Worldwide, women are known to be the worst sufferers in all adversities. Women generally are marginalised in society, and crises situations often exacerbate gender gaps. In disasters, they are subjected to further stress and strains of coping with traumatic, unpredictable and life threatening situations. In both natural and man-made disasters women are particularly left behind in receiving help, both in the acute crises and later in the rehabilitation phase of disaster management programmes.

Certain vulnerabilities in women enhance their miseries in crises situations, as compared to men. Women are often considered particularly vulnerable in conflict situations. Conflicts have a different impact on men, women, children and the elderly. Understanding the specific needs of women displaced by war, is vital in relief operations, if they are to be helped appropriately. Many war widows became sole wage earners, often going hungry to feed their children; about 60% suffer from psychological problems, with physical manifestations such as weight loss and difficulty in breast-feeding [1]. Recent research studies had alarming results, in that there is a strong correlation between mothers' distress and child's mental health, thus contributing to an inter-generational transmission of psychological trauma, further reinforcing the long-term impact of war [2].

Eighty per cent of the world's refugees and internally displaced persons are women and children [3]. This new phenomenon, disturbing women's mental health, is the displacement of people within their own countries due to war or natural disasters. The plight of displaced women is particularly complex and difficult to understand by inexperienced relief workers. Overall a total of 72

Contemporary Topics in Women's Mental Health   Edited by Chandra, Herrman, Fisher, Kastrup,
© 2009 John Wiley & Sons, Ltd   Niaz, Rondón and Okasha

million people are believed to have lost their lives during the twentieth century due to conflict, with an additional 52 million lives lost through genocides [4].

17.1 Wars and women's mental health

You can't treat war any differently from other risks to health. We are... developing a much wider debate in the health community about the serious implications of war on public health.

Richard Horton, Editor, The Lancet

Since the Second World War more than 145 conflicts amounting to wars have occurred and the vast majority of them have taken place in developing countries [5]. First World Report on Violence and Health, World Health Organization (WHO), states 'More than 85% of the major conflicts since the second world war have been in poor countries... During the 1990s the poorest countries of the world became saturated with arms, with brokers often supplying both sides of a conflict... Between 1986 and 1996, a major proportion of those dying as a result of armed conflicts were civilians, particularly women and children... Huge differences in the health of mothers and children exist between the poor countries undergoing conflict and the predominantly rich countries exporting arms to them' [6].

The tragic reality in the world today is that the battlefield for modern conflict and confrontation occurs within civilian domains rather than on separate battlefields. The armed fighters target civilians to kill, rape, terrorise and expel. The rise in the proportion of civilian, and notably women's and children's deaths, in twentieth century warfare is attributed to the changes in war technology and war tactics. Consequently, in most human conflicts, there are interactions between the direct effects of warlike and terrorist actions on local environments resulting in hazardous situations for the health, assets and social welfare of local populations, leading to much greater devastation and catastrophe [7]. Resident and displaced populations, refugees and famine-affected peoples are caught up in conflict [8]. Civilians comprise 80–90% of all who die or are injured in conflicts – mostly children and their mothers [9].

There has been a paradigm shift, through speed of communications and direct involvement, psychological impacts of human-made disasters are now centre point rather than side effects. Terrorism has become an growing concern since 2001. A number of studies and articles on the psychological aspects of terrorism have shown that psychological impacts are the defining hallmark of terrorism and are increasingly recognised as an important constituent of all disasters [10–14].

Women are now documented to be the most vulnerable to the mental health consequences of war. In 2001, the WHO report 'Mental Health: new understanding, new hope' estimated that, in the situations of armed conflicts throughout the world, 10% of the people who experience traumatic events will have serious mental health problems, such as depression, anxiety and psychosomatic problems. People who are socially or economically vulnerable, including children, the elderly and in many cases women, are most susceptible to the mental health consequences of war [15].

Since the Second World War, there has been an increase in the conflicts within countries with the purpose of eradicating an entire population. The Nazis 'final solution' against the Jews has been replicated in recent internal conflicts against Cambodians during the Pol Pot regime, Muslims in Yugoslavia, Tutsis in Rwanda, and Kurds in Iraq. The victims of genocide include not only men and women, but innocent children; women, are also sexually exploited, tortured and killed for their ethnicity. In 1994 in Rwanda, nearly one million people were killed in ethnic conflict during a three month period. An estimated 40–45% of those killed were women; and up to 500 000 women and girls were raped and sexually tortured [16].

Sexual exploitation of women

The world was shocked in the 1990s by the reports of systematic and widespread rape in the former Yugoslavia and Rwanda [17]. *The Lancet* also published several articles about wartime rape and demanded the development of clear strategies against sexual violence in conflict [18–20]. Rape and sexual exploitation in war, were acknowledged and named as war atrocities and crimes until the recent investigations of the genocidal rape of Muslim women in the former Yugoslavia and of Tutsi women in Rwanda. Historical reports reveal that senior officers of war and military occupation have always authorised and normalised the sexual exploitation of local women by military men. Governments have tolerated military brothels under the auspices of 'rest and recreation' for their soldiers, with the secret permission that a controlled system of brothels will contain male sexual aggression, limit sexually transmitted diseases in the military, and boost soldiers' morale for war [21].

The United Nations High Commissioner for Refugees (UNHCR) and Save the Children released a report on their investigation into allegations of sexual abuse of West African refugee children in Guinea, Liberia and Sierra Leone. The interviews of 1500 women, men and child refugees documented that girls between the ages of 13 and 18 were sexually exploited by male aid workers, many of whom were employed by national and international non-governmental agencies (NGOs) and the United Nations (UNs), and also by UN peacekeepers and community leaders [22].

According to United Nations (International) Children's Fund (UNICEF) in 2006, more than 90% of war victims are civilians. Children and women are extremely vulnerable to traumatic experiences in times of war and the risk continues even in post-war-situations [23].

As far as former war-children are concerned, a high prevalence of post-traumatic stress symptoms is apparent even six decades after the Second World War [24].

Sex crimes in Bosnia: The sexual exploitation of girls and women by UN peacekeepers and aid workers in West African refugee camps has been recently revealed. Also the trafficking of women and girls by international police in the post-conflict protected area of Bosnia has cast a spotlight on predatory male peacekeepers, aid workers and police and the particular vulnerability of women and girl refugees reliant on them for food, basic life provisions and physical security [25].

'Comfort women'

This term is fairly well known, but few people have an idea of the bloody stories behind it. 'Although few forced comfort women are still alive, what this event has revealed to us should not be ignored: the way that women were tortured and hurt'. Taipei Women Rescue Foundation "I agree to call Ms. Huang and others 'survivors' rather than 'victims' or simply 'comfort women'. Because only people with strong mentality can survive the suffering that the forced recruitment, war, overseas wandering brought about and live with the pain [26, 27]".

Plight of women in Iraq and Afghanistan

The plight of women in Iraq is of growing concern, with ever-increasing reports of murders, rapes and kidnappings, as well as general intimidation and oppression. Mental Health Professionals must take cognisance of the fact of how different the Iraq war is for women than any other American war in history [28].

More than 160 500 American female soldiers have served in Iraq, Afghanistan and the Middle East since the war began in 2003, which means one in seven soldiers is a woman. Women now make up 15% of active duty forces, four times more than in the 1991 Gulf War. About 450 women have been injured in Iraq, and 71 have died – more female sufferers and deaths than in the Korean, Vietnam and first Gulf Wars collectively [29].

In this war there are no front lines or safe zones. Consequently women soldiers are returning home with missing limbs, mutilating wounds and severe trauma, no different from their male counterparts [30]. The crux of the whole issue is society's failure to accept women as equal partners at an intellectual level. With equality women have unwittingly made it worse for themselves: although they give spouses care, they may not receive it in return when they need it.

Nevertheless, despite the equal risks women are taking, they are still being treated as inferior soldiers and sex toys by many of their male colleagues. Last year, Col. Janis Karpinski caused a stir by publicly reporting that in 2003, three female soldiers had died of dehydration in Iraq, which can get up to 126° in the summer, because they refused to drink liquids late in the day. They were afraid of being raped by male soldiers if they walked to the latrines after dark [31].

Since 1980 Iraq has been through three wars and years of severe economic sanctions which has imprinted its burden on the family and the mother in particular. The mother, in Iraq is regarded as the key person or the primary caregiver in the family, as most of the men are busy at that time in the military services. This was the situation up to 9 April 2003 (the date of the occupation of Iraq). Since then economic sanctions have become worse, added to the steep economic fall in the income with which the mother has to cope with an appalling quality of life. The working mother or housewife still has to face the same daily grind to meet the normal minimal needs of the family, along with maintaining her own healthy maternal, physical wellbeing, relationships with others, social, and her community [32].

For nearly 20 years, the Afghans suffered the health consequences of armed conflict and human rights violations. In the Afghan war against the Soviet Union, women in refugee camps on the borders with Pakistan, Niaz *et al.*, found many pregnant women were malnourished, psychologically traumatised, underweight, exhausted and highly susceptible to disease and infection. Many of them reported symptoms of post traumatic stress disorder (PTSD) including recurrent nightmares of traumatic violence. There were high rates of clinical depression and anxiety in these women refugees. In addition; rape and other sexual crimes were frequently reported by women in war zones [33].

Violence in Kashmir

The militant violence rampant in Jammu and Kashmir since 1989 has precipitated a human crisis of appalling magnitude. It has claimed more than 60 000 lives of innocent civilians; ethnic cleansing and communal hostility has forced thousands of families to run from their homes in the valley and live dislocated lives as refugees in other parts of their own state and country. But the psycho-social vulnerability of women has made them the worst affected victims of the violence; women have suffered as wives, mothers and daughters. Stress, anxiety, hysteria, depression, high blood pressure and other psychiatric illnesses have increased manifold. In addition to many pressures placed on women, the forms of politico-socio-cultural violence have contributed to high distress [34, 35].

Kashmiri women are now suffering from some of the more predictable afflictions of women caught in conflict situations: psychological trauma, destitution and acute poverty that puts them at increased risk of being victims of trafficking.

The Algerian war

During the Algerian war for independence from France (1954–1962), thousands of women were active participants, taking the initiative even on deadly missions. About 2200 *mujahidat* (women combatants) were arrested and tortured [36]. The French military and police did not spare women participants who were captured. A rare study of seven *mujahidat* in Auras (a region from which more than one-third of women fighters came) describes their considerable difficulties reintegrating after the Algerian war [37]. All enlisted when very young and later had marital problems.

The Family Code is by far the most preoccupying women's issue in Algeria. Khalida Messaoudi (1995: 90) calls it a history of 'crimes against women' [38].

The Chadli administration (1979–1991), which was particularly detrimental to women, was known to make compromises with the Islamic opponents to stay in power, and sacrificed women's autonomy. During the civil war in Algeria, several thousand women and girls were the victims of terrorists and were denied not just their womanhood but their humanity [39].

War in the Middle East

For over four decades the Middle East has been in a situation of overt inter-nation armed conflicts as well as long-term low intensity conflicts. Every day the media reports on the horrors of the ongoing war situation in Iraq, Palestine, Israel and Lebanon [40]. Lebanon became the site of a civil war, in 1975. As the Lebanese conflict went on, women became active participants in the war experience: they found themselves confronted with a widespread community violence, faced with the main responsibility for care giving in the family, and as the fate of their husbands was unknown, placed under new and unfamiliar duties [41].

Several areas in the south of Lebanon were under occupation until the year 2000. Events associated with the occupation have affected the psychological and physical health of the population. Results of a study showed that the majority of the population in all towns has experienced at least one war related traumatic event. Levels of PTSD vary, but are consistently higher, even five years after the end of the occupation, than found in studies conducted in countries not suffering from recent armed conflict. Females were six times more likely to have PTSD than males. Also depression, general health (scored on General Health Questionnaire) and PTSD followed the same pattern and were significantly correlated: this reflects the high prevalence of PTSD and the co-morbidity associated with it. The extent of exposure to traumatic events was a positive predictor both for PTSD as well as general psychiatric morbidity in Lebanese women. Some socio-economic and lifestyle factors were also able to partly predict PTSD [42].

Armed conflict in Columbia

Colombia has been ravaged by over four decades of armed conflict. Psycho-social impacts are the defining hallmark of terrorism and are increasingly recognised as prominent detrimental effects of all disasters. Women, especially those bringing up children alone or lacking family support, and children already living in poor circumstances, disabled or lacking strong family support, are most vulnerable to emotional disturbance. Disasters magnify psychological disturbances, already present in vulnerable women and children [43].

Likewise, the war in Sierra Leone displaced hundreds of thousands of victims, the bulk of whom fled to neighbouring Guinea and Liberia. They left behind an excess of humanitarian problems, including pointless destruction of life and property. Post-war, women bore the brunt, distressed by multiple social and mental health problems [44].

Women's mental health issues in post-war Liberia

Women's mental health issues have tremendously increased in recent times. This increase is due to the traumatic and tragic events during the 14 years of civil war. PTSD sufferers presently have no primary care or psychiatric attention. Mentally ill female ex-combatants are patrolling in and around the cities with violent and life-threatening behaviours. Studies have revealed that the continuous abuse of illicit drugs is a prime risk factor for the increase in mental health illness in Liberia. Liberian National Association for Suicide Prevention Inc (LNASP) documents that drug abuse has increased during and after the civil war and that the suicide rate is also increasing [45].

Widows of war

Widows who have survived political and personal crises, are uncounted and unidentified, and are the least likely voices to be heard. 'The poorest widows', concludes the UN, 'are the old and frail, those with young children to shelter and feed, the internally displaced and refugees, and those who have been widowed due to armed conflict [46].'

In Cambodia, 35% of rural households are headed by women, many of whom are widows. Many young widows raising children in poverty have had to turn to prostitution as a way of surviving.

In regions such as Nepal and Bangladesh, where girls are trafficked into Indian brothels, the daughters of widows are often taken out of school to help their mothers and these girls are at increased risk of being trafficked into prostitution. Angola, Bosnia and Herzegovina, Kosovo, Mozambique and Somalia, are recent war-torn countries, where the majority of adult women are widows. Seventy per cent of Rwandan children are supported only by mothers, grandmothers or oldest female children. Girls in Rwanda are heads of family for an estimated 58 500 households. Many war widows live as recluses in refugee camps because they have no male relative to assist in repairing their homes.

Many widows who return from refugee camps have no social safety nets or any advocacy organisations; consequently, they become destitute and socially marginalised. UN studies reveal that the household census in developing countries fails to document the inequality and poverty of widows within intergenerational households and misses completely those who are homeless.

The psycho-social outcomes of the war

An appropriate example of how war can change the psyche and social outlook in women, which is pertinent, touching and vivid in description, is from women in Mozambique. For over a decade from the late 1970s to October 1992, a war raged in Mozambique, resulting in what has been described as one of the 'most terrible genocides in the history of Africa'. The Mozambican women described a constellation of psycho-social consequences of the war. In addition to the clinically documented PTSD symptoms, they also described subjective pain and distress which they explained in terms of their own world view. The trauma hit the core of their being. They said *vavisa e moya* which means 'my spirit is sore' and expressed an injury to the life force. The refugee women identified loss of social belonging and identity, 'spirit damage' and somatic problems, as the most serious outcomes of their traumatic experiences [47]. In fact this is the overriding feeling described by women braving war in any part of the world today.

Death and injury by landmines

Women and children are common casualties in agrarian and subsistence-farming societies where landmines were deliberately placed in agricultural fields and along routes to water sources and markets, intended to starve people by killing its farmers.

Women make up a larger percentage of farmers than men in Asia and Africa, responsible for up to 80% of food produced in many parts of Africa. When maimed, they lose the ability to farm and feed their family; and their husbands often abandon them, leaving them to beg on the streets or be sexually exploited. Nearly one-half of land in Cambodia, where one in every 236 people is an amputee due to landmine injury, is unsafe for cultivation and human use. So as the recovery from war continues, it is likely that an even greater percentage of those injured and killed by landmines will be women and children as they return to peacetime sustenance activities, collecting firewood and water, tending animals and farming [48].

Summary

In 2001, the WHO report 'Mental Health: new understanding, new hope' estimated that, in the situations of armed conflicts throughout the world, 10% of the people who experience traumatic events will have serious mental health problems, such as depression, anxiety and psychosomatic problems. It is those who are socially or economically vulnerable, like children, the elderly, and in most cases women, who are most susceptible to the mental health consequences of war.

Women are especially susceptible to poverty, exclusion and the sufferings caused by armed conflict when they are already subject to discrimination in peace times.

In patriarchal societies, women are the victims of prejudice, injustice and intolerance; they face discrimination at home, at work and within the community at large. In some contexts, this can make women socially and economically vulnerable and it is a feature that must be taken into account in assessing the situation and the woman's needs.

All the same, women show remarkable strength in crisis situations, as can be seen from their roles as combatants or peace activists and the duties and responsibilities they take on in wartime to protect and support their families.

Throughout the world, women affected by conflict can be extremely determined and brave and they often find ingenious ways of coping with the difficulties they face when fulfilling the role as head of household, caring for and earning income for their families or taking part in community life.

Mental health professionals must be aware of the specific risks to the mental health of women in war and work to propagate this knowledge at different forums like healthcare delivery, disaster management and rehabilitation and share their concerns that women bear the brunt of the burden of ensuring the day-to-day survival of their families, both in times of war and peace.

17.2 Natural disasters and women

The past century has witnessed major global disasters, but in the last few decades, the number has increased threefold. Earthquakes have caused more than 1 million deaths in the past 20 years, accounting for one-third of the total mortality by disasters worldwide. About 80% of human loss came from nine countries: China, Japan, Iran, Italy, Peru, Turkey, former Soviet Union and lately Pakistan [49].

There is a dearth of research literature on natural disasters in developing countries as compared to the frequency with which such disasters occur in these countries. With an average of almost 200 incidents annually, Asia dramatically leads the rest of the world in disaster frequency, followed by the Americas with 111 events annually on average [50].

There is little knowledge about how culture shapes the psychological impact of disasters. The research to date strongly suggests that natural disasters in developing countries often produce severe effects on the public's mental health. In fact, the modal sample-level outcome after natural disasters in developing countries was severe, whereas the modal outcome after natural disasters in developed countries was moderate. This general finding from the research studies may reflect the fact that disasters tend to be more destructive when they occur in the developing world.

Fran H. Norris [51] indicates the following risk factors for adults: severe exposure to the disaster, especially injury, threat to life and extreme loss; living in a highly disrupted or traumatised community; female gender; age, particularly those aged between 40–60; little previous experience relevant to coping with the disaster; ethnic minority group membership; poverty or low socioeconomic status; the presence of children in the home; psychiatric history; secondary stress and weak or deteriorating psychosocial resources.

Disaster is hardly ever gender neutral. In the 1995 Kobe, Japan, earthquake, 1.5 times more women died than men; in the 2004 Southeast Asia tsunami, death rates for women across the region averaged three to four times that of men. The gender, class and race dimension of each disaster needs particular explanation. Feminists working in relief agencies, for instance, identified several factors that explain the gender skew in the 2004 tsunami deaths. In some instances, sex differences in physical strength clearly made a difference in the ability of survivors to climb, cling or run to safety. [52].

Gender and disasters

Gender influenced post-disaster outcomes in many research samples; almost always, women or girls have been reported to be affected more adversely than were men or boys. The effects had a wide range of outcomes, but the significant effects noted were for PTSD, for which women's rates often exceeded men's by a ratio of 2 : 1. The effects of gender were marked in the groups who came from traditional cultures and in the context of severe exposure [53].

An Oxfam [54] report on the Asian tsunami in 2005 reiterates that 'disasters, however 'natural,' are intensely discriminatory. Among the differences that determine how people are affected by such disasters is that of gender.' Reports of rapes in the midst of the New Orleans disaster and in the Asian tsunami are documented. Even in conditions of extreme human suffering, no disaster experts assured women that rape-support teams were included in the rescue teams, and even later there were no discussions about the medical and psychological resources that women needed who had survived unimaginable tragedy and stress and had also been raped. The long-term effects of tsunami are expected to hit women particularly hard. International Labour Organisation's research shows that disasters tend to sharpen existing inequalities [55]. Yet, given the chance women have a crucial role to play in post-tsunami rebuilding. They can play an important role in recovery, not just of physical infrastructure, but of families and communities.

Tsunami in South East Asia – 2004

This recent tsunami disaster had devastating impacts, in many countries in South and South-East Asia, causing loss of life, injuries, separation from and loss of loved ones, extreme trauma and loss of security, basic needs and livelihoods. The particular needs of women are always neglected, as stated by one of the few Indonesian women human rights groups which responded to the needs of Banda Aceh women after the Indian Ocean tsunami in December 2004 [56].

Trafficking in women and girls is one of the most scathing forms of the violation of human rights that must be addressed from a gender and a human rights perspective. In addition to immediate efforts to prevent trafficking in the aftermath of the disaster, the rebuilding efforts must explicitly also deal with the root causes of trafficking in women, including poverty, women's inferior status in the family and society, lack of legal protection and of awareness of their rights. Traffickers must be promptly prosecuted and punished, and trafficked women and girls must have access to adequate support and protection [57].

Earthquake 2005, Pakistan Azad Jammu and Kashmir

Based on the latest figures nearly 4 million people in Pakistan and Azad Kashmir were affected; 78 000 dead, 70 000 injured, 3.5 million homeless and an estimated 10 000 children orphaned. The government body Earthquake Relief and Reconstruction Authority (ERRA) has tried to fulfill its mandate. There were serious concerns that the women survivors would not be able to benefit from this, as they have been and were being marginalised from most of the relief packages and operations. There were very few women social workers; it was difficult for the women to articulate their needs: personal needs such as fabric for their clothes, and related needs for lactating mothers, menstruating women and other reproductive health needs.

Most of the female headed families in the 2005 earthquake in Pakistan and Kashmir had no bank accounts, and even for those who had, these accounts were in the names of the men of the house. For those who had lost their husbands and fathers, they had no means to access relief money and compensation; only male heads of the household were recognised. This was the same issue in land ownership: lands were named to men. With these conceptual and structural impediments the survival of women becomes difficult. Women's role in the joint family care must be recognised and supported. Their rights to have access to resources that would improve their lives must be upheld.

This is the moment in time to take this long over-due step to effect genuine and just changes in the disaster areas in the developing countries. Women are often absent from public debate and economic activities. Their workload and stress increases manifold. Policy makers in these situations need to be sensitive to the vulnerabilities of women if they are to help them in their helpless, miserable conditions [58].

Niaz's study of Widows and Destitute Women, in the camp, following the earthquake in Pakistan found that the majority of these widows were housewives and illiterate. The majority of them, 90%, owned their houses which collapsed. Seventy per cent were trapped in rubble, 21% lost their entire families. These destitute women clearly had significant risk factors for PTSD. Results showed 94% had PTSD, 81% reported depression, 82% reported fear and avoidance and 66% reported severe disability [59].

The greatest challenge mental health professionals face presently, is to handle trauma in various forms, as in the prevailing situation, where there is not even a remote possibility of any individualised or collective support or therapy. In these situations the only feasible solution is a quick rehabilitation and re-organisation of the fractured society at all levels. This support system needs to be strengthened as soon as possible.

Quick rehabilitation would be an ameliorating factor for both children and adults. The frustration, anger, sense of deprivation and helplessness, are all the negative emotions. These damaging and disruptive emotions can be channelled and transformed into positive energies and constructive activities. The need for a large-scale psycho-social support network and specific trauma therapies would be valuable in the high risk groups (women, children and elderly).

Prevention from developing chronic psychiatric illnesses by providing early rehabilitation cannot be over emphasised for the sake of a better future. The health of women is well documented to have a positive impact on the general health of all members of a society. Training primary care physicians, nurses and other health workers in the recognition and appropriate referral and/or treatment of mental illness is central to expanding community services to meet needs. Mainstreaming a gender perspective will build on the interests of many women professionals who have entered the field of mental healthcare as psychiatrists, psychiatric nurses, counsellors and social workers [60].

Gender equality and disaster risk reduction

Gender equality is not a separate topic, but rather a cross cutting element that needs to be considered in an integrated manner in all development projects or activities if we are to achieve sustainable development in our societies.

These disasters and their increasing impact is mainly the result of flawed development practises and processes. In the long term, the future disaster profile will very much depend on the daily development decisions that we make; such as where and how do we build our cities and villages, manage our scarce water resources, manage the environment, educate our children and communicate and inform the public on these issues. Both women and men have equally important roles in all these issues.

The importance of gender equality has been recognised recurrently in many global processes. The Beijing Platform for Action has provided a valuable guidance to many international processes. The Second World Conference on Disaster Reduction (WCDR), which took place in Kobe, Japan 18–22 January 2005, also benefited from the Beijing process. The WCDR stressed the fact that gender perspective should be integrated into all disaster management decision-making processes, including those related to risk assessments, early warning, information management, education and training.

Women and men are affected by disasters differently and the response to their needs must take this into consideration. In recognition of the importance of gender and disaster risk reduction, participants from 28 countries met at the East-West Centre in Honolulu August, 2004 to develop a strategy for incorporating gender-fair practises in disaster risk management. One of the outcomes of the Conference was a set of recommendations, prepared by the platform on Gender Equality and Disaster Risk Reduction, in preparation for the WCDR.

These recommendations are all relevant and provide concrete guidelines on how to ensure that gender perspectives are consistently integrated into all aspects of disaster risk reduction:

- *Mainstreaming a gender perspective in all disaster management initiatives*: The civil population and NGOs are encouraged to mainstream a gender perspective in the promotion of sustainable development processes, including disaster reduction, preparedness, response and mitigation strategies. Also one needs to target information and resources to non-traditional leaders of social institutions in the community to facilitate education of disaster issues.

- *Building capacity in women's groups and community-based*: Incorporating culture and traditional knowledge is vital. Ensuring access to information, resources and funding will support women and women's groups to be active in disaster management. Consequently women will take leadership roles and responsibilities. It is also essential to integrate issues of poverty and social vulnerability in designing disaster risk reduction programmes.

- *Gender mainstreaming in communications, training and education*: It is imperative to develop curriculum standards and introduce formal, non-formal and informal education and training programmes at all levels, including in the areas of science, technology and economics. Also there is a need to establish an agenda for gender specific research in risk reduction. Focus on an integrated, gender-sensitive approach to environmentally sound and sustainable resource management and disaster reduction, response and recovery, is needed to change attitudes and behaviour in rural and urban areas. Media can be extremely useful to raise awareness and behaviour change.

- *Gender mainstreaming in implementation, monitoring and evaluation of programmes*: In order to monitor the progress, we need to develop benchmarks and indicators to monitor efforts to integrate gender equality and social vulnerability in national and international disaster reduction activities.

Gender equality is possibly the single most important objective in the field of disaster reduction as without it no risk and vulnerability reduction can be achieved in an effective and sustainable manner. It is condition sine qua non for the achievement of disaster reduction objectives.

These recommendations were prepared by the Platform on Gender Equality, which is composed of international, regional, national, local, community-based, governmental and NGOs, as well as academic and research institutions, disaster risk managers and practitioners. Many of these recommendations are not only valid for the topic of disaster reduction, but also for any other development activity that needs to consider a gender balanced approach.

Gender must be incorporated into disaster training and planning activities. The lessons of Hurricane Katrina and other major disasters indicate that women are at particular mental health risk due to factors such as family responsibilities, women's higher rates of poverty, their greater risk of depression and anxiety disorders and their vulnerability to sexual abuse and domestic violence.

And finally, the importance of trauma, violence and abuse needs to be recognised by providers, researchers, policymakers and the general public. Trauma, violence and abuse are far more prevalent in the lives of girls and women than commonly thought – and they may lead to serious, long-standing physical ailments, co-occurring conditions and risky behaviours that, if left unrecognised and untreated, can compromise women's health [61].

Disaster risk reduction in the united nations programmes

Ironically, the Disaster Risk Reduction remains a low priority programme in the UN. It is entirely dependant on extra-budgetary or voluntary contributions. The High-level Panel made a very minor recognition of the issue in a small paragraph and failed to identify the International Strategy for Disaster Reduction launched in 2000 and the recent second WCDR and its substantive outcome, the Hyogo Framework for Action. Much greater priority continues to be given to conflicts or so called 'complex emergencies' despite the fact that disasters triggered by natural hazards provoke much greater and recurrent damage to communities in many more countries.

As a result, the gap remains enormous and it can only be filled with a resolute action of governments and international organisations, to provide higher priority to these issues, to address them with joint programming exercises and to work in close partnership with non-governmental and community-based organisations, the private sector, the media and other relevant sectors.

In post-disaster reconstruction, countries can benefit from a 'window of opportunity'. Women are seen to be a 'group' that could profit to a significant degree as unequal power relations are revealed and unmasked by the disaster, thus creating a window for civil society and the women's movement to build on women's capacities. However, women are involved in reconstruction only to a certain extent as they constitute a large group of altruistic service providers creating an image not of 'women's rights as human rights' but of a 'feminisation of disaster relief and reconstruction'.

Conclusion

There is ample evidence that women in disasters are the real sufferers, though men also go through similar ordeals. The fact remains that a woman has the accepted role of being a nurturer, care-giver of the family. In disasters this role is highlighted in protecting the family and keeping it together. In the case of loss of the bread earning family member, she has to take over this additional role. A woman is the link between society and the wellbeing of her children, starting from the antenatal period to the attainment of maturity of her offspring. She produces, nurtures and sustains continuity and hence she is the nucleus of society.

Culture is a vital source of resilience but it can also become a barrier to the recognition and acceptance of mental health issues. Girls and women draw great support from cultural connections and identity but also feel the burden of cultural pressures to remain silent about personal issues, not to discuss problems outside the family, or to be strong. Culturally sensitive diagnostic approaches are needed to assess trauma symptoms and associated impairment. Immediate relief operations can start with non-specific interventions to help groups of affected individuals organise around issues of feeling safe and promote perspectives for the future that involve mastery and engagement in rebuilding life [62].

A woman's inherent purpose is to sustain life and society needs to recognise this unique human quality of a woman. This quality is biological, instinctive and intellectual and above all it is the dynamic interplay of her multiple attributes, which in essence is woman. Consequently these multiple roles of a woman increase her vulnerability in disasters. A woman suffers tremendous stress and strain in her endeavours to continue to fulfill her roles in times of disaster. It cannot be emphasised more that in the Disaster Relief Operations, the planners and policy makers must take cognisance of a woman's central role. Disaster relief and rehabilitation activities must support and strengthen women's efforts.

Today at the heart of the current issues on Women's Mental Health in the Face of Disasters, Women's Mental Health and Human Rights – the role of health professionals is the notion that the health professionals must act as principled agents and take action to do what is ethically and professionally right. The World Psychiatric Association has recognised disaster psychiatry as a new specialty.

> We stand at a critical moment in Earth's history, a time when humanity must choose its future. As the world becomes increasingly interdependent and fragile, the future at once holds great peril and great promise. To move forward we must recognize that in the midst of a magnificent diversity of cultures and life forms we are one human family and one Earth community with a common destiny. We must join together to bring forth a sustainable global society founded on respect for nature, universal human rights, economic justice, and a culture of peace. Towards this end, it is imperative that we, the peoples of Earth, declare our responsibility to one another, to the greater community of life, and to future generations.
>
> (del preámbulo de la declaración de The Earth Charter, 2005)

References

1. Snyder, U. (2003). In the Face of War. *Medscape Ob/Gyn and Women's Health*, **8** (1).
2. Krugman, S. (1987) Trauma in the family: perspectives on the intergenerational transmission of violence, in *Psychological Trauma* (ed. B.A. van der Kolk), American Psychiatric Press, Washington, DC, pp. 127–53.
3. Hynes, P. (2003) Widows of War. War And Women, http://www.zmag.org/content/showarticle.cfm?ItemID=3229 (13 March, 2003).
4. Smith, R. (2006) *The Utility of Force. The Art of War in the Modern World*, Penguin Publisher.
5. Williams, R. (2006) The psychosocial consequences for children and young people who are exposed to terrorism, war, conflict and natural disasters. *Current Opinion in Psychiatry*, **19** (4), 337–49.
6. Taylor, S.B. and Eriksson, M. (2002) Major armed conflicts, appendix 1A. In: *SIPRI year book 2002: armaments, disarmaments and international security*. Oxford University Press.
7. Smith, R. (2005) *The Utility of Force: The Art of War in the Modern World*, Allen Lane, London.
8. Tai-Ann Cheng, A. and Chang, J-C. (1999) Mental health aspects of culture and migration. *Current Opinion in Psychiatry*, **12** (2), 217–22.

9. Barenbaum, J., Ruckin, V. and Schwab-Stone, M. (2004) The psychological aspects of children exposed to war, practice and policy initiatives. *Journal of Child Psychology and Psychiatry*, **45**, 41–62.

10. Alexander, D.A. and Klein, S. (2005) The psychological aspects of terrorism: from denial to hyperbole. *Journal of the Royal Society of Medicine*, **98**, 557–62.

11. Alexander, D.A. and Klein, S. (2003) Biochemical terrorism: too awful to contemplate. Too serious to ignore. *The British Journal of Psychiatry*, **183**, 491–97.

12. Baum, A. and Dougall, A.L. (2002) Terrorism and behavioral medicine. *Current Opinion in Psychiatry*, **15**, 617–21.

13. Yehuda, R. and Hyman, S.E. (2005) The impact of terrorism on brain, and behaviour: what we know and what we need to know. *Neuropsychopharmacology*, **30**, 1773–80.

14. Prigerson, H.G., Narayan, M., Slimack, M. *et al.* (1998) Pathways to traumatic stress syndromes. *Current Opinion in Psychiatry*, **11**, 149–52.

15. World Health Organization (WHO) (2001). *World health report 2001 – Mental health: new understanding, new hope*. Geneva: Switzerland.

16. Southall, D.P. and O'Hare, B. (2002) Empty arms: the effect of the arms trade on mothers and children. *British Medical Journal*, **325** (7378), 1457–61.

17. Shanks, L. and Schull, M.J. (2000) Rape in war: the humanitarian response. *Canadian Medical Association Journal*, **163** (9), 1152–6.

18. Shanks, L., Ford, N., Schull, M. and de Jong, K. (2001) Responding to Rape. *The Lancet*, **357**, 304.

19. Hargreaves, S. (2001) Rape as a war crime: putting policy into practice. *Lancet*, **357**, 737.

20. Hargreaves, S. (2004) Recognizing rape as torture: legal and therapeutic challenges. *Lancet*, **363**, 1916.

21. World Health Organization (2002) World Report on Violence and Health: Summary, Geneva.

22. United Nations High Commissioner for Refugees, & Save the Children UK (2002) Note for Implementing and Operational Partners by UNHCR and Save the Children UK on Sexual Violence & Exploitation: The Experience of Refugee Children in Guinea, Liberia, and Sierra Leone, http://www.unhcr.ch.

23. UNICEF (2006) The State of the World's Children.

24. Kuwert, P., Spitzer, C., Träder, A. *et al.* (2007) Sixty years later: post-traumatic stress symptoms and current psychopathology in former German children of World War II, *International Psychogeriatrics*, Vol. 19, Cambridge University Press, pp. 955–61.

25. Hipkins, D. (2008) UN Condones Dyncorp Sex Crimes and Sex Slavery, Conspiracy Planet- An Alternative News & History Network February 23.

26. Yoshimi, Y. (2000) *Comfort Women. Sexual Slavery in the Japanese Military During World War II*, translation Suzanne O'Brien, Asia Perspectives, Columbia University Press, New York, pp. 100–111. isbn 0-231-12033-8.

27. Hicks, G. (1995) *The Comfort Women: Japan's Brutal Regime of Enforced Prostitution in the Second World War*, W.W. Norton & Company, New York, p. 303. isbn 978-0-393-03807-1.

28. Walter, N. (2006) The Plight of Women in Iraq Guardian Newspapers Limited.

29. Cohen, S. (2006) Women Take on Major Battlefield Roles, WASH. POST (online ed.), *Available at* http://washingtonpost.com/wpdyn/content/article/2006/12/02/AR2006120200476.html (2 December, 2006).

30. Linda, W. (2007) The Impact of War: Wounded in War: The Women Serving in Iraq, NPR (National Public Radio).

31. The Vermont Guardian (2006) Rape Fears Lead Women Soldiers to Suicide, Death, editorial@ vermontguardian.com (*February 8, 2006*).

32. Alkaisy, M. (2006) Mental Health Symptoms following wars and repression at Mosul city\Iraq. 23rd Annual Meeting of ARABMED in Europe, Aleppo.

33. Niaz, U. (2007) Introduction, Gender Perspectives in Psycho-trauma, in *The Pakistan Earthquake, 2005: The Day The Mountains Moved* (ed. U. Niaz), Sama Books, Karachi, Pakistan Hard Cover. isbn-060-8784-52-7.

34. Tamheed, A. (2007) The Effects of Violence on Mental Health in Kashmir Deutsche Welle, 04.01.2007, http://dwelle.de/southasia/1.209097.1.html.

35. Hashmi, J.S. (2007) Trauma Of Daily Violence In Jammu And Kashmir, **Telling Upon Mental Health 27 June, 2007** Countercurrents.org.

36. Hessini, L. (1996) Living on a Fault Line: Political Violence against Women in Algeria, Population Council, Cairo.

37. Haddab, Z.. (2000) Les femmes, la guerre de liberation et la politique en Algerie, in *Les Algeriennes, Citoyennes en Devenir*, Instituto per il Mediterraneo, Oran, Editions CMM.

38. Messaoudi, K. (1995) *Une Algeerienne Debout*, J'ai Lu, Paris.

39. Meredeth, T., New School for Social Research Gale Group (2002) Algerian Women in the Liberation Struggle and the Civil War: From Active Participants to Passive Victims? Farmington Hills, Michigan, http://www.encyclopedia.com/doc/1G1-94227145.html (22 September, 2002).

40. Bryce, J.W., Walker, N., Ghorayeb, F. *et al.* (1989) Life experiences, response styles and mental health among mothers and children in Beirut, Lebanon. *Social Science and Medicine*, **28**, 685–95.

41. Cooke, M. (1987) Women write war: the feminization of Lebanese society in the war literature of Emily Nasrallah. *Bulletin British Society for Middle Eastern Studies*, **14** (1), 52–67.

42. Farhood, L.F. (2003) PTSD, depression, and health status in lebanese civilians exposed to a church explosion. *The International Journal of Psychiatry in Medicine*, **33** (1), 39–53.

43. Williams, P. (2004) The West and the War in Sierra Leone, 1991–2002: A Critical Security Studies Perspective. Paper presented at the Annual Meeting of the International Studies Association, Le Centre Sheraton Hotel, March 17, 2004, Montreal.

44. Human Rights Watch (2002) Back to the Brink: War Crimes by Liberian Government and Rebels, May 2002.

45. Jamison, D.T. (2006) Violence and injuries, *Disease And Mortality in Sub-Saharan Africa*, World Bank Publications, p. 363.

46. Bennett, T., Bartlett, L., Olatunde, O.A. and Amowitz, L. (2004) Refugees, forced displacement, and war [conference summary]. *Emerging Infectious Disease*. **10** (11) [serial on the Internet]. http://www.cdc.gov/ncidod/EID/vol10no11/04-0624_03.htm.

47. Sideris, T. (2003) War, gender and culture: Mozambican women refugees. *Social Science and Medicine*, **56** (4), 713–24(12).

48. Stover, E. and McGrath, R., (1991) Land Mines in Cambodia: The Coward's War, New York Physicians for Human Rights and Asia Watch, p. 59.

49. Arun, P.K. (2006) in *Management of Natural Disasters in Developing Countries Centre for Science and Technology of Non-Aligned and Other Developing Countries* (eds H.N. Srivastava and G.D. Gupta). NAM S&T Centre, isbn 81-7035-425-0.

50. IFRC (2000) World Disasters Report 2000.

51. Norris, F.H. (2005) Psychosocial Consequences of Natural Disasters in Developing Countries: What Does Past Research Tell Us About the Potential Effects of the 2004 Tsunami? National Center for Post-Traumatic stress Disorder, Department of Veterans Affairs.

52. Oxfam Report (2007) Gender Mainstreaming During Disasters: The Case of the Tsunami in India, © Oxfam International September 2007.

53. Norris, F., Perilla, J., Ibañez, G. and Murphy, A. (2001) Sex differences in symptoms of post-traumatic stress: does culture play a role? *Journal of Traumatic Stress*, **14**, 7–28.

54. Oxfam (2005). The Asian Tsunami: Three Weeks on Oxfam Briefing Note. 14 January 2005.

55. Overton, L. (2005) Flirting with disaster: gendered impacts of women's access to land and housing in Post-tsunami Sri Lanka. BA Dissertation, Middlesex University. l.r.overton@lse.ac.uk.lisaroseanneoverton@sky.com.

56. United Nations (2004) Women Survivors of Indian Ocean Disaster Face Urgent Needs, Warns UNFPA, UNITED NATIONS, New York, 31 December 2004.

57. Division for Advancement of Women (DAW) (2005). News Tsunami. Policy Guidance on Trafficking in Women and Girls, http://www.un.org/ga/59/documentation/list1.html (23 February 2005).

58. Niaz, U. (2007) *Pakistan Earthquake 2005, The Day The Mountains Moved. International Perspectives in Handling Psycho Trauma*, Sama Books, Karachi, pp. 140–44.

59. Niaz, U., Hassan, S. and Hasan, M. (2007) Post-traumatic Stress Disorder(PTSD), depression, fear and avoidance in destitute women, earthquake survivors of NWFP, Pakistan. *Journal of Pakistan Psychiatric Society*, **4** (1), 44–49.

60. Briceño, S. (2005). Gender Equality and Disaster Risk Reduction The Gender and Disaster Network has Produced a Broadsheet Containing Six Principles for Engendered Relief and Reconstruction, Available at www.unisdr.org/wcdr/preparatoryprocess/inputs/gender-broadsheet.pdf.

61. Enarson, E. (2004). Gender Equality & Disaster Risk Reduction. An Action Workshop for Social Change, August 10–12, 2004, Honolulu.

62. United Nations International Strategy for Disaster Reduction (UNISDR) (2007). Gender Perspective: Working Together for Disaster Risk Reduction Good Practices and Lessons Learned, Negotiating Cultural Roles, Power Patterns through an "Incentive" Approach. Geneva.

18

Intimate partner violence interventions

Krishna Vaddiparti[1] and Deepthi S. Varma[2]

[1]*Department of Psychiatric Social Work, Institute of Human Behaviour and Allied Sciences, Delhi, India*
[2]*Population Council, Golf Links, Delhi, India*

18.1 Mental health consequences of intimate partner violence on women

Violence against intimate partners has existed from time immemorial, and women as compared to men have always been the more vulnerable victims of such violence [1]. A recent report on intimate partner violence (IPV) across 10 countries noted that the physical or sexual violence among women who ever had a partner ranged from 15 to 71% [2]. The same report concluded that there is more awareness regarding the prevalence of IPV compared to 'how to identify, prevent or reduce it' [3].

Several studies have been conducted on the physical and mental health consequences of IPV among clinical as well as non-clinical male and female populations from different parts of the world [4]. Research has also indicated that victims of violence are vulnerable to revictimisation and have a greater chance of perpetrating violence on others. Though both men and women have chances of being victimised, women are more vulnerable to IPV from their spouses than men. Their physical and mental health consequences are also reportedly more traumatic and debilitating as compared to men. Women's emotional and economic dependence have been found to be strong contributing factors towards their increased trauma. The most frequently reported mental health consequences of IPV are depressive symptoms, post traumatic stress disorder (PTSD), anxiety disorders, somatisation and substance use. Research also indicates that women who experience systematic abuse have greater likelihood than men to develop depression and other serious mental health consequences [5].

Several interventions have been developed and implemented across the world to prevent, treat and reduce the physical and psychological impact of IPV on the victim. Though there are some interventions exclusively for the primary prevention of partner violence, almost all interventions discussed here are assumed to serve the dual purpose of primary prevention (by spreading the message in the community and empowering women) as well as ending further partner violence. For the purpose of discussion we have divided the interventions into three broad categories: (i) victim focused interventions, (ii) interventions for batterers or the perpetrators of violence and (iii) other interventions. In addition to a brief description of the intervention, empirical data on their effectiveness is presented wherever available.

18.2 Victim focused interventions

World Health Organization (WHO) has provided a comprehensive strategy which discusses how the health sector can help while dealing with women subjected to IPV [3]. The WHO strongly recommends health services as entry points to identify and help women in abusive relationships. It also recommends adding an 'anti-violence component to ante natal services, parenting classes and to other services that involve men'. WHO also recommends the role of the health sector in dealing with IPV adopting the framework of Canadian Medical Education Directions for Specialists (CanMEDS). This framework gives examples of integrating appropriate responses against IPV into all aspects of clinical care. It has spelt out in detail the multiple roles played by a clinician, as a medical expert, health advocate, collaborator and as a professional in sensitising and training other health professionals and in identifying, preventing and treating the victims of violence [3].

The following are the most common interventions carried out for victims to help them deal with the trauma of violence as well as prevention of further partner violence:

Screening

Routine screening for IPV by the primary physician or in an emergency department (ED) has been one of the most recommended measures to prevent violence in the IPV literature. It has been considered as a 'low-risk, low-cost procedure' when carried out with reliable screening tools [6]. Though there is no research that indicates concretely that routine screening by a health professional can end the violence experienced by a victim, it could definitely detect the existence of violence and initiate a process of discussion regarding the abuse by the victim. These discussions could invariably facilitate the victim's movement towards exiting an abusive relationship [7]. Recent research proposes a trans-theoretical-stages-of-change model, to explain the progress of a woman towards leaving an abusive relationship. The proponents of this model report that movement towards change, that is, leaving an abusive relationship is a multi-step process rather than a distinct one time action [8–10]. These studies also indicate that the response provided by the healthcare workers should match the stage-of-readiness of change for positive outcomes in treatment [10, 11].

Routine screening not only helps in identifying the abuse but also in providing effective treatment for the various mental health consequences such as depression, anxiety and other PTSD symptoms. Screening provides a chance to provide information regarding various resources available for the victim in the neighbourhood that can be accessed whenever the victim is ready to do so. Recent research on interventions for women who attend the ED for treatment of physical assault report that the presence of a well-trained nurse at ED who can recognise and respond to a woman's status of abuse and her readiness to change may go a long way to helping an abuse victim [8].

Shelter stay

Temporary or emergency shelters for women who have been abused along with intense counselling or behavioural therapy have also been reported to be effective in preventing the cycle of abuse. Shelters for battered women are reported to be the response to the 'nowhere to go' rallying call of battered women during the 1970s. Though initially these shelters only provided safe emergency shelter, food and clothing for women who left their abusive homes, soon it developed into an integral part of the movement for the victims of partner violence [12]. Most of them are now actively involved in providing peer counselling, support groups, legal information and referrals. However, the long term benefits of these for mental health or decreasing violence are yet to be established. Several post-shelter programmes are also offered by these shelters as a continuum to a victim's shelter stay, in order to facilitate a smooth transition back into the community. Though shelters do not offer a permanent solution to a victim's problems, they do play a pivotal role in helping the woman to stay away from an abusive relationship at least for a while and provide a safe non-exploitative respite from abuse.

Enhancing social support

Improving the social support system of the victims is one of the key components of most interventions with battered women. Women who are victims of partner violence are often isolated from their family and friends either by themselves (due to their embarrassment over abuse) or by their spouses. Such social alienation can result in a sense of low self-esteem and other psychological problems. Social support provided to such victims in the form of emotional support is found to have a mediating effect on the negative impact of the violence on women. It is also found to enhance the overall well-being of the individual as well as improving her ability to cope better with the stress [13]. Recent research highlights that all support need not be institutionalised, instead it could even be from the spontaneous expressions of support offered by friends, colleagues and healthcare workers [13].

A recent study from South Africa reported that structural intervention that combined a microfinance programme with gender and HIV training had a 55% reduction of IPV in the intervention group as compared to the comparison group [14]. This highlights the significance of economic independence resulting in the empowerment of women in reducing IPV.

Transitional Housing Programme (TSH)

The Transitional Housing Programmes (TSHs) for battered women provides a safe and affordable alternative to living with abusive partners. It also serves as a main support for many poor women who are victims of abuse and have no other resources to free themselves of their abusing partners. As compared to emergency shelters, a victim is allowed to live for a longer period in a TSH. Melbin [15] reports that though there are no standardised procedures of intake, most of them allow the women to stay for a certain period of time till they find their own housing, employment and are able to be on their own. Some of these homes charge a very nominal amount from the woman's income as a rent during their stay in these homes. They also provide several services such as counselling, safety planning, housing and employment assistance to these women. 'Case management' services, support groups and other practical assistance such as transportation vouchers, telephones, referrals to other agencies and advocacy are also made available by these homes.

Advocacy

Advocacy interventions have been found to be effective in improving the overall life quality of the abuse victim by encouraging them to explore and access resources in their own community. Advocacy interventions are primarily provided as a supporting service through emergency shelters or a TSH. Sullivan and Bybee [16] reported the efficacy of an intervention that aimed at reducing violence through an intense community-based advocacy programme with promising results towards the prevention of domestic violence. They adopted a five-phase process of advocacy comprising of assessment, implementation, monitoring, secondary implementation and termination, where the advocate is an active participant along with the client in all the five phases. Assessment involved rapport building and setting the goals for the client. The second phase mainly involved mobilisation of resources followed by the monitoring of the intervention that has been implemented. The secondary implementation is carried out if the earlier one had failed to achieve the set goals. Termination of the services of the advocate and transferring of the skills and knowledge to the client begin at about 7–10 weeks into the intervention. The phases described above are not categorical or routinely need to follow one after the other. They often overlap with the client and the advocates engaged in various phases simultaneously. The advocates were found to act as a 'protective factor' against the ill effects of violence by reducing the intensity of depressive symptoms and enhancing the social support and the victim's access to required resources from the community.

18.3 Interventions with batterers of violence

Interventions with abusers during the last two decades were predominantly developed by the criminal justice system to prevent abuse as well as to rehabilitate the batterers found guilty so that they do not abuse in future. The essential feature of these interventions was to ensure accountability of the batterer to their violent act and impress upon them that it is a criminal offence to perpetrate violence on one's partner. Usually, IPV cases move through a series of criminal justice interventions (Figure 18.1) that start with police enquiry and arrest followed by issue of protection orders, prosecution and finally a court mandated batterers' intervention programme for the abuser in the event of being found guilty [17].

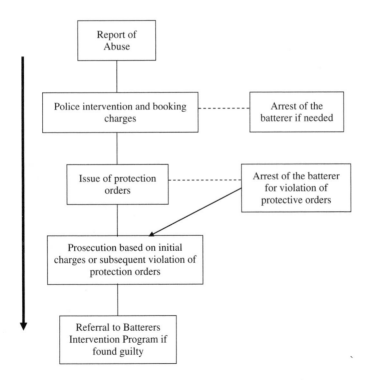

Figure 18.1 Graphic representation of the typical interventions with batterers

Police arrest

Police arrest to a large extent depends on the intervention options available to the personnel, which are relative from place to place. However, in most cases police are empowered to make an arrest of the batterer if it warrants and then prosecute them. Police arrest was found to be an effective deterrent of violence as indicated by subsequent police arrest records [18]. However, this finding could not be established in later replication studies [19, 20]. Hence, it cannot be concluded that arresting a batterer deters further violence. However, in several parts of the world mandatory arrest policies are made to protect victims of violence.

Protection orders

Civil protection orders provide the victim of violence a justice system alternative to the traditional criminal court system. As per civil protection orders, the victim could ask for intervention of the court to stop the ongoing violence. Civil protection orders are designed to provide the victim with an array of solutions and protections that they can enforce, such as, ordering the batterer to refrain from violence, evicting the batterer from the home shared by the victim and abuser, issue stay away orders, property allocation, child custody, court costs and other remedies that could help reduce future violence in the relationship [21, 22]. Violation of protective orders is deemed a criminal offence in several parts of the world.

As far as the effectiveness of protection orders in averting future violence goes, there is some degree of evidence to suggest that protection orders can reduce the chances of abuse and foster the victim's autonomy [23, 24]. Follow-up studies showed that women who received protection orders reported a decrease in violence for up to two years post protection orders [25–27]. Similarly, Dutton [28] studied the effectiveness of civil protection orders in reducing IPV among 153 low-income immigrant women. A significant proportion (68%) of the women filed a protection order against their partner and out of these, 22.7% reported them to be helpful and 65% of them very helpful in reducing violence against them. Although almost all the women (98%) stated that they would recommend another woman who they knew to seek protection orders if needed, a substantial number (36.8%) feared that availing protection would increase their danger of further victimisation as well. Holt [29] compared women with no protection orders versus women with temporary protection orders and women with permanent protection orders and concluded that permanent protection orders, but not temporary, are associated with a significant decrease in violence against women by their partner. Harrell and Smith [30] in their study found that more than half of the women with protection orders reported violations of these orders by their abusers during the year after they were issued.

Prosecution

Victims of violence are not always ready to pursue prosecution against their abuser. Hence, to overcome this obstacle and encourage women to participate in the prosecution the criminal justice system have created several alternative strategies such as, having police file the charges against the abuser instead of the woman, adopting no-drop policies, pursuing victimless prosecution and involving victim advocates to empower the women to take part in the prosecution of the abuser [31]. Prosecution policies that allowed women to drop charges against her abuser were compared with no-drop policies to test their effectiveness in reducing violence. Significant re-abuse occurred in the six months following case settlement in both groups irrespective of the policy [32]. However, the effectiveness in reducing further partner violence has not been fully explored.

Batterer intervention programmes

Batterer intervention programmes (BIPs) emerged in an effort to reduce repeated spousal violence. BIPs came into action in the United States about two and half decades ago and are now increasingly popular in several parts of the world. BIPs are more or less similar in reference to the underlying philosophy and structure; however, they differ with regard to the theoretical approach. Programmes are usually based on Feminist or Family Systems or Psychological Models [33]. Partner violence has been viewed as a consequence of underlying mental health problems and that batterers need help to deal with their mental health problems in order to prevent violence. In addition, it had been found that while victims of violence opposed the violence against them perpetrated by their male partners, they were also not happy about the incarceration of their partners for the violence. In response to this, the criminal justice system, while still holding batterers accountable, made it mandatory and began to refer them to BIPs.

The curricula of mainstream BIPs in the US are largely drawn from the Duluth model, cognitive behavioural therapy (CBT), Emerge and Abusive Men Exploring New Directions (AMEND) models (Table 18.1).

Duluth model

The Duluth Model is based on the feminist theory that patriarchal ideologies cause violence against women. The Duluth Model helps men gain insight into their attitudes about power and control and equips them with alternate strategies to deal with their partners [34]. The Model predominantly follows a classroom or psycho-education approach for intervention. Intervention is focused to help batterers gain insight into their violent behaviour and develop respect, honesty and fairness in a relationship and interpersonal skills to negotiate, communicate effectively and resolve conflicts without resorting to violence.

Table 18.1   Curriculum of batterer intervention programmes

Model	Underlying theory/belief	Format	Goals
Duluth Model	Feminist theory	Psychoeducation/ classroom	Foster critical thinking skills relating to the themes of nonviolence, non-threatening behaviour, respect, support, trust, honesty, partnership, negotiation and fairness in relationship
Cognitive behavioural therapy	Abuse is a result of erroneous thought process	Group	Gain insight, alter thought process and develop behavioural change. Acquire new skills such as empathy, communication, management of anger and jealousy
EMERGE	Multiple causes for battering	Eclectic	Insight into abusive behaviour and control tactics, accept responsibility for their violence, explore and improve relationship between batterer and victim,
AMEND	Multiple causes for battering	Eclectic	Enhance client accountability to their violence, accept violence as unacceptable and illegal, understand the social context of battering and develop new social skills

Cognitive behavioural therapy

This is one of the most commonly used interventions for physically abusive men. CBT views abusive behaviour as a consequence of maladaptive cognitions and assumptions. Thus, the goal of CBT is to bring changes in the way abusive men think about violence and the circumstances that lead to violence, so, breaking the chain of events that lead to partner violence. CBT is delivered either in group, couple or individual formats [35].

EMERGE

EMERGE is a 48 week intervention programme developed in Cambridge, Massachusetts for batterers of their intimate partners. EMERGE adopts a combination of approaches, psycho-educational, skill building and CBT. The goal of EMERGE is to help batterers gain insight into violent acts, take personal responsibility, thereby improving personal accountability and develop skills to deal with conflicts [33].

AMEND

AMEND, a programme in Denver, Colorado, is more or less similar to EMERGE. The programme spans several months and the goals are to improve batterers' personal accountability to violence, enhance their awareness of the social contexts of abusive behaviour and develop new skills. A unique feature of this programme is that the group leaders serve as 'moral guides', who firmly express that violence is unacceptable and illegal [33].

The much talked about and widely used BIPs surprisingly were found to be less than average in their effectiveness in reducing IPV. Over the past two decades several research studies were conducted to test the effectiveness of these programmes and the results yielded from most of these studies were inconclusive about the effectiveness of BIPs. For instance, Rosenfeld [36] examined studies that reported recidivism and found no significant difference in the rates of recidivism between men who were incarcerated and not referred to BIP and men who were incarcerated and also received BIP (39% vs. 36%). Likewise, Babcock [37] found that men who attended BIPs are only 5% less likely to be violent towards their partner compared to men who do not attend BIP. In a randomised control trial (RCT) of 376 men convicted of partner violence in Brooklyn, New York, randomised to an 8 weeks BIP based on Duluth Model, a 26 weeks BIP or a community service control group, assessments at 6 and 12 months follow-up showed a significant reduction of violence in all the three groups as per the police reports of violence recidivism. However, the partner report of violence at 6 and 12 months follow-up did not confirm this reduction [38]. In another RCT conducted in Broward County, Florida, 404 men convicted for IPV were randomised to traditional BIP (Duluth Model) plus probation monitoring, or to a probation monitoring only control group. Six and 12 months follow-up confirmed that violence rates according to police and partner reports were similar for men in both groups [39].

Similarly, the effectiveness of CBT in reducing partner violence could not be confirmed. A review of six RCTs to test the effectiveness of CBT in reducing IPV concluded that the effect size in the reduction of violence in all the studies was small enough to draw conclusions in favour of CBT. These studies could not conclude that CBT is effective in reducing partner violence [35]. For instance, in San Diego, 861 abusive men in the US Navy were randomised to a 26 weeks CBT group, a 26 weeks couple therapy group, a rigorous monitoring group or to a no-treatment group. Follow-up assessments at 6 and 12 months showed no significant difference in the male-to-female violence in the four groups according to the female partners of the men in the study [40].

18.4 Other intervention approaches

Couple focused interventions

Couples therapy views men and women as equal partners in violence in a relationship and attempts to alter interaction patterns that result in violence through communication and problem solving skills training. Couples therapy approaches however, were criticised mainly for holding the victim also responsible for the violence that is perpetrated on them. Stith and colleagues [41] compared the effectiveness of individual couple or multi-couple group treatment in reducing partner violence. Results showed that men in the multi-couple group were more likely to deter from partner violence at six months follow up compared to their counterparts in individual couple intervention. In addition, marital satisfaction increased significantly, and both marital aggression and acceptance of wife battering decreased significantly among individuals in multi-couple group intervention compared to an individual couple group. However, there is a paucity of evidence-based research to conclude on the effectiveness of couple focused intervention in reducing partner violence.

Restorative justice

Restorative Justice (RJ) is an informal criminal justice intervention; the purpose of RJ is to create or recreate meaningful and egalitarian social relationships along with restoration of whatever has been lost such as dignity and property, and so on. RJ mainly uses family group conference approach in order to accomplish offender accountability, victim safety and victim choice [42]. In some instances, supportive friends and family members of the victim and offender are involved in the conferences along with relevant criminal justice members and community leaders in order to facilitate an open and safe dialogue between the abuser and victim. The underlying theory behind the RJ approach is that the family and social networks are capable enough to ensure accountability, reform and rehabilitate the abuser as well as ensure future safety of the victim [43, 44]. The effectiveness of RJ approaches has not been systematically studied. A few studies from the US, Canada and Australia reported higher rates of victim involvement and satisfaction when compared with other traditional approaches [45–47].

Intimate abuse circles

The Intimate Abuse Circles (IACs), based on RJ principles, is an alternate to the criminal justice interventions. The IAC is specifically meant for couples who opted to stay in the relationship even when violence has occurred. IAC is specifically found to be helpful for immigrant, minority and religious families where it is likely that the couple relationship stay intact [48]. The philosophy does not blame the victim, however, recognises that victims do have a power in relationship. It validates that couples in violence usually have complex and conflicting needs that are likely to contribute to violence in their relationship. The goal of IAC is to create concentric circles of support comprising of family, friends, community leaders, and so on within the couple unit in order to help them deal with the conflicting situations that are likely to cause partner violence [49].

Public education and awareness promotion

Public awareness campaigns about partner violence are a widely used strategy to spread the message to end violence against women; they are increasingly becoming popular worldwide and use a range of means such as TV, radio, newspapers, magazines, Internet web sites, posters, and so on to create awareness about human rights violation and dispel myths and stereotypes about IPV. These campaigns usually have a potential to reach a large population. Some of the strategies of these campaigns are public discourses, meetings, support groups and so on. The goals of these campaigns include building awareness about the magnitude of the problem, women's human rights and men's role in stopping violence against women [50]. The effectiveness of these programmes in improving knowledge and behaviour change has not been empirically tested. However, there are programmes and campaigns that are popular worldwide, for instance, the 16 days of Activism Against Gender Violence Campaign is one such movement that calls for the elimination of all forms of violence against women throughout the world by raising awareness, strengthening local work around violence against women, sharing new and effective strategies to curtail violence and pressurising governments to make policies to eliminate violence against women [51]. The White Ribbon Campaign (WRC) is another such campaign, which began in Canada about two decades back and now over 50 countries are involved in this campaign. The campaign was originally initiated by men with a goal to end violence against women. WRC achieves this by raising awareness among the public, especially targeting young men and boys by challenging them to think about their belief systems and behaviour. The campaign works in collaboration with several other women's organisations, corporate sector and media and supports WRCs around the globe [52].

Intervention with men and boys

The objectives of this approach are to enhance awareness among men and boys about partner violence and facilitate change in attitudes and beliefs about gender norms, power, violence and norms about masculinity. The rationale behind this approach is that men are usually the perpetrators of violence and hence they should be targeted to cease violence against women. Boys/adolescents are targeted as a preventive measure of partner violence given that their attitudes and perceptions about gender norms; masculinity, power and control are still in the formative phase and hence are more malleable [50]. The effectiveness of these programmes in stopping partner violence is not yet fully understood due to the lack of long-term follow-up studies. However, working with men and boys to encourage gender equality has become a popular approach in several countries.

School based programmes

Violence in intimate relationships is not an exclusive phenomenon of adulthood; there is enough evidence to suggest that youth and adolescents engage in violence in their dating relationships [53]. School/college based programmes to prevent partner violence have become increasingly popular in several countries. These interventions generally aim at primary prevention of partner violence and the typical curriculum includes training in a range of life skills such as, conflict resolution, interpersonal skills and family relation skills [54]. In addition, issues related to gender relations, masculinity, power and control are addressed as well. Adolescents who participated in a Safe Dates programme in the US, on follow-up reported fewer perpetrations of psychological, sexual violence and moderate physical dating violence, but not of severe physical violence [55]. The gains made by this group were maintained at four years follow-up as well [55]. Review of school based programmes shows that, multi-session, skill building and age appropriate interventions are more effective than single, information providing only sessions [50].

18.5 Conclusion

It is evident that interventions to reduce or prevent IPV are proliferating, but there is not enough evidence on their effectiveness. Research conducted over the past two decades on the effectiveness of interventions with victims and batterers have yielded mixed and inconsistent findings. For instance, interventions with victims such as shelter stay and advocacy counselling were proven effective in a few observational studies, but well designed, randomised control studies fail to conclude if these interventions with victims really help women in the true sense. On the other hand, there is always a debate about the side effects of these interventions and whether these interventions increase the risk of further violence by male partners.

Likewise, intervention programmes with batterers have several limitations. Referral to BIPs to a large extent depends on their availability as well as on the attitude of criminal justice professionals about IPV and perpetrators of this violence. In addition, participation in BIPs is often court mandated and not a voluntary choice by the batterers. Participation by batterers in these programmes to a large extent is to avoid arrest and other penalties rather than the actual need to change and end violence. Moreover, studies conducted on the effectiveness of BIPs have been criticised for lack of methodological rigour. In addition, it is difficult to draw conclusions from these reports unless we have data on batterers or couples who voluntarily participated in BIPs. Interventions with batterers that enhance their motivation to change and relapse prevention are needed. To some extent, the major awareness campaigns and self-help groups by men have these components, but their effectiveness in ending or preventing violence against an intimate partner is not empirically assessed. Similarly, chronic repeat offenders are less likely to respond to conventional BIPs. Intervention with this group should consider the batterer's mental state; personality and substance use behaviours and then tailor intervention accordingly.

The use of other criminal justice interventions such as police involvement and prosecution by victims is determined by several factors. For instance, victims' prior experience with police and prosecution is likely to determine their future utilisation of services in the event of need. In addition, racial and ethnic minority and immigrant women are less likely to involve police in the event of partner violence for fear of discrimination and deporting. Similarly, victims who have familial and financial obligations are less likely to prosecute their partners and are more likely to live in a relationship that is potentially dangerous to them. Another criticism against prosecution policies is that, they are more likely to disempower victims and affect their self-esteem when the victims are coerced to testify against their partner [56, 57].

The impact of culture is often overlooked or minimised in traditional IPV intervention programmes [58]. Participation in treatment programmes and the outcome is likely to vary from individual to individual belonging to different cultures and backgrounds. Interventions that take into consideration these socio-cultural realities are more likely to be accepted and successful. It is essential to note that victims and batterers are unique and the underlying causes for violence are uniquely different in every relationship and hence the 'one size fits all' concept is less likely to work in preventing partner violence. Interventions that are adaptive in nature are to be designed to deal with victims and batterers. Finally, most of the literature on intervention programmes is from the Western world. There are very few success stories or even reports from other parts of the world, about initiatives that focus exclusively on reducing violence. Parts of the world where civil strife, wars, poverty and HIV infection contribute to IPV, locally sustainable interventions need to be developed both for men and women. The next generation of research needs to focus on how some of the initiatives that have worked in the developed world can be culturally adapted and used globally.

References

1. Ramsey, C.B. (2006) Public responses to intimate violence: a glance at the past. *Public Health Reports*, **121**, 460–63.
2. Ellsberg, M., Jansen, H.A.F.M., Watts, C.H. and Garcia-Moreno, C. WHO Multi-Country Study on Women's Health and Domestic Violence against Women Study Team (2008) Intimate partner violence and women's physical and mental health in the WHO multi-country study on women's health and domestic violence: an observational study. *Lancet*, **371**, 1165–72.

3. Ferris, E.L. (2008) Intimate partner violence. Doctors' role should be integrated with the needs of patients and society. *British Medical Journal*, **334**, 706–7.

4. Coker, A.L., Davis, K.E., Arias, I. *et al.* (2002) Physical and mental health effects of intimate partner violence for men and women. *American Journal of Preventive Medicine*, **23**, 260–68.

5. Carbone-Lopez, K., Kruttschnitt, C. and Macmillan, R. (2006) Patterns of intimate partner violence and their association with physical health, psychological distress and substance abuse. *Public Health Reports*, **121**, 382–92.

6. Koziol-McLain, J., Coates, C.J. and Lowenstein, S.R. (2001) Predictive validity for a screen for partner violence against women. *American Journal of Preventive Medicine*, **21**, 93–100.

7. McCloskey, A.L., Lichter, E., Williams, C. *et al.* (2006) Assessing intimate partner violence in health care settings leads to women's receipt of interventions and improved health. *Public Health Reports*, **121**, 435–44.

8. Watt, M.H., Bobrow, E.A. and Moracco, K.E. (2008) Providing support to IPV victims in the emergency department: vignette-based interviews with IPV survivors and emergency department nurses. *Violence Against Women*, **14**, 715–26.

9. Chang, J.C., Dado, D., Ashton, S. *et al.* (2006) Understanding behavior change for women experiencing intimate partner violence: mapping the ups and downs using the stages of change. *Patient Education and Counseling*, **62**, 330–39.

10. Zink, T., Elder, N., Jacobson, J. and Klostermann, B. (2004) Medical management of intimate partner violence considering the stages of change: precontemplation and contemplation. *Annals of Family Medicine*, **2**, 231–39.

11. Chang, J.C., Cluss, P.A., Ranieri, L. *et al.* (2005) Health care interventions for intimate partner violence: what women want? *Women's Health Issues*, **15**, 21–30.

12. Brownwell, P. and Roberts, A.R. (2002) National organizational survey of domestic violence coalitions. Introduction, public policy, research and social action, in *Handbook of Domestic Violence Intervention Strategies* (eds A.R. Roberts and M.D. Fields), Oxford University Press, Oxford.

13. Coker, A.L., Watkins, K.W., Smith, P.H. and Brant, H.M. (2003) Social support reduces the impact of partner violence on health: application of structural equation models. *Preventive Medicine*, **37**, 259–67.

14. Pronyk, P.M., Hargreaves, H.R., Kim, J.C. *et al.* (2006) Effect of a structural intervention for the prevention of intimate partner violence and HIV in rural South Africa: a cluster randomized trial. *Lancet*, **368**, 1973–83.

15. Melbin, A., Sullivan, C.M. and Cain, D. (2003) Transitional supportive housing programs: battered women's perspectives and recommendations. *Affilia*, **1894**, 1–16.

16. Sullivan, C.M. and Bybee, D.I. (1999) Reducing violence using community-based advocacy for women with abusive partners. *Journal of Consulting and Clinical Psychology*, **67**, 43–53.

17. Danis, F.S. (2003) The criminalization of domestic violence: what social workers need to know. *Social Work*, **48**, 237–47.

18. Fagan, J. (1996) *The Criminalization of Domestic Violence: Promises and Limits*, National Institute of Justice, Washington, DC.

19. Sherman, L.W. (1992) The influence of criminology on criminal law: Evaluating arrests for misdemeanor domestic violence. *Journal of Criminal Law and Criminology*, **83**, 1–45.

20. Bowman, C.G. (1992) The arrest experiments: a feminist critique. *Journal of Criminal Law and Criminology*, **83**, 201–8.

21. Klein, C. and Orloff, L.E. (1993) Providing legal protection for battered women: an analysis of state statutes and case law. *Hofstra Law Review: Symposium Issue on Domestic Violence*, **21**, 801.

22. Wilson, K.J. (1997) *When Violence Begins at Home: A Comprehensive Guide to Understanding and Ending Domestic Abuse*, Hunter House, Alameda.

23. Finn, P. (1991) Civil protection orders: a flawed opportunity for intervention, in *Woman Battering: Policy Responses* (ed. M. Steinman), Anderson, Cincinnati.

24. Hart, B. (1992) State Codes on Domestic Violence: Analysis, Commentary and Recommendations, National Council of Juvenile and Family Court Judges, Reno.

25. Gist, J., McFarlane, J., Malecha, A. *et al.* (2001) Protection orders and assault charges: do justice interventions reduce violence against women. *American Journal of Family Law*, **15**, 59–71.

26. Holt, V., Kernic, M., Wolf, M. and Rivara, F. (2003) Do protection orders affect the likelihood of future partner violence and injury? *American Journal of Preventive Medicine*, **24**, 16–21.

27. Malecha, A., McFarlane, J., Gist, J. *et al.* (2003) Applying for and dropping a protection order: a study of 150 women. *Criminal Justice Policy Review*, **14**, 486–504.

28. Dutton, M.A., Ammar, N., Orloff, L. and Terrell D. (2006) Use and Outcomes of Protection Orders by Battered Immigrant Women [On-line], [cited 2008 sep 5], http://www.ncjrs.gov/pdffiles1/nij/grants/218255.pdf.

29. Holt, V.L., Kernic, M.A., Lumley, T. *et al.* (2002) Civil protection orders and risk of subsequent police-reported violence. *Journal of American Medical Association*, **288**, 589–94.

30. Harrell, A. and Smith, B.E. (1996) Effects of restraining orders on domestic violence victims, in *Do Arrests and Restraining Orders Work?* (eds E. Buzawa and C.G. Buzawa), Sage Publications, Thousand Oaks.

31. Mills, L.G. (1998) Mandatory arrest and prosecution policies for domestic violence: a critical literature review and the case for more research to test victim empowerment approaches. *Criminal Justice and Behavior*, **25**, 306–19.

32. Ford, D.A. and Regoli, M.J. (1993) *The Indianapolis Domestic Violence Prosecution Experiment, in Legal Interventions in Family Violence: Research Findings and Policy Implications*, National Institute of Justice, Washington, DC.

33. Healy, K., Smith, C. and O'Sullivan, C. (1998) *Batterer Intervention: Program Approaches and Criminal Justice Strategies*, National Institute of Justice, Washington, DC.

34. Pence, E. and Paymar, M. (1993) *Education Groups For Men Who Batter: The Duluth Model*, Springer, New York.

35. Smedslund, G., DalsbØ, T.K., Steiro, A.K. *et al.* (2007) Cognitive behavioural therapy for men who physically abuse their female partner. *Cochrane Database of Systemic Review* 3 (Art. No.: CD006048).

36. Rosenfeld, B.D. (1992) Court ordered treatment of spouse abuse. *Clinical Psychology Review*, **12**, 205–26.

37. Babcock, J.C., Green, C.E. and Robie, C. (2004) Does batterers' treatment work? A meta-analytic review of domestic violence treatment. *Clinical Psychology Review*, **23**, 1023–53.

38. Taylor, B.G., Davis, R.C. and Maxwell, C.D. (2001) The effects of a group batterer treatment program: a randomized experiment in Brooklyn. *Justice Quarterly*, **18**, 171–201.

39. Feder, L. and Dugan, L. (2002) A test of the efficacy of court mandated counselling for domestic offenders: the Broward experiment. *Justice Quarterly*, **19**, 343–75.

40. Dunford, F.W. (2000) The San Diego Navy experiment: an assessment of interventions for men who assault their wives. *Journal of Consulting and Clinical Psychology*, **68**, 468–76.

41. Stith, S.M., Rosen, K.H., McCollum, E.E. and Thomsen, C.J. (2004) Treating intimate partner violence within intact couple relationships: outcomes of multi-couple versus individual couple therapy. *Journal of Marital Family Therapy*, **30**, 305–18.

42. Edwards, A. and Haslett, J. (2002) Domestic Violence and Restorative Justice: Advancing the Dialogue. [On-line], [cited 2008 Sep 12], http://www.sfu.ca/cfrj/fulltext/haslett.pdf.

43. Zehr, H. (2002) *The Little Book of Restorative Justice*, Good Books Press, Intercourse.

44. Burford, G. and Pennell, J. (1995) Family Group Decision Making: New Roles for "old" Partners in Resolving Family Violence: Implementation Report Summary, Memorial University of Newfoundland, St. John's.

45. Mills, L.G. (2003) *Insult to Injury: Rethinking Our Responses to Intimate Abuse*, Princeton University Press, Princeton NJ.

46. Mills, L.G. (1999) Killing her softly: intimate abuse and the violence of state intervention. *Harvard Law Review*, **113**, 550–613.

47. Presser, L. and Gaarder, E. (2007) Can restorative justice reduce battering? Some preliminary considerations. *Social Justice*, **27**, 175–94.

48. Griffing, S., Ragin, D.F., Sage, R.E. *et al.* (2002) Domestic violence survivor's self identified reasons for returning to abusive relationship. *Journal of Interpersonal Violence*, **17**, 306–19.

49. Grauwiler, P. and Mills, L.G. (2004) Moving beyond the criminal justice paradigm: a radical restorative justice approach to intimate abuse. *Journal of Sociology and Social Welfare*, **31** (1) [serial online] [cited 2008 September 12], http://findarticles.com/p/articles/mi_m0CYZ/is_1_31/ai_n6065939/print?tag=artBody;col1.

50. Harvey, A., Gracia-Moreno, C. and Butchart A. (2007) Primary Prevention of Intimate-Partner Violence and Sexual Violence: Background Paper for WHO Expert Meeting, May 2-3, 2007, [cited 2008 Sep 12], http://www.who.int/violence_injury_prevention/publications/violence/IPV-SV.pdf.

51. About the 16 days (2008) Center for Women's Global Leadership, http://www.cwgl.rutgers.edu/16days/about.html.

52. The White Ribbon Campaign: Men working to end men's violence against women (2008), http://www.whiteribbon.ca/about_us/.

53. Pinheiro, P. (2006) World Report on Violence Against Children, United Nations Secretary General's Study on Violence against Children, Geneva.

54. Smithey, M. and Straus, M.A. (2004) Primary prevention of intimate partner violence, in *Crime Prevention-New Approaches* (eds H. Kury and J. Obergfell-Fuchs), Weisser Ring Gemeinnutzige Verlags-GmbH, Mainz.

55. Foshee, V.A. Bauman, K.E., Ennett, S.T, Linder, G.F., Benefield, T., Suchindran, C. (2004) Assessing the long-term effects of the safe dates program and a booster in

preventing and reducing adolescent dating violence victimization and perpetration. *American Journal of Public Health*, **94**, 619–24.

56. Mills, L.G. (1998) Mandatory arrest and prosecution policies for domestic violence: a critical literature review and the case for more research to test victim empowerment approaches. *Criminal Justice and Behavior*, **25**, 306–19.

57. Hanna, C. (1996) No right to choose: mandated victim participation in domestic violence prosecutions. *Harvard Law Review*, **109**, 1850–910.

58. Ameida, R.V. and Dolan-Delvecchio, K. (1999) Addressing culture in batterers intervention: the Asian Indian community as an illustrative example. *Violence Against Women*, **5**, 654–83.

19

Migration and mental health in women: Mental health action plan as a tool to increase communication between clinicians and policy makers

Solvig Ekblad

Stress Research Institute, Stockholm University, and Karolinska Institutet, Stockholm, Sweden

The involved reader (of the book "Healing Invisible Wounds: Paths to Hope and Recovery in a Violent World" by R. Mollica [1]) may conclude with the author that healing the consequences of mass violence trauma is a social and political as well as a medical responsibility [2, p. 709].

19.1 Definitions: Mental health and health

The World Health Organization (WHO) [5] defines mental health 'as a state of wellbeing in which every individual realises his or her own potential, can cope with the normal stresses of life, can work productively and fruitfully, and is able to make a contribution to her or his community'. In this chapter we use a definition of health developed by Professor Richard F. Mollica [6] at the Harvard Program in Refugee Trauma (HPRT), USA: 'Health is a personal and social state

Contemporary Topics in Women's Mental Health   Edited by Chandra, Herrman, Fisher, Kastrup,
© 2009 John Wiley & Sons, Ltd   Niaz, Rondón and Okasha

of balance and well being in which people feel strong, active, wise and worth while; where their diverse capacities and rhythms are valued; where they may decide and choose, express themselves and move about freely'.

19.2 Introduction

Ten years ago, a WHO European meeting [7] concluded that regardless of social or economic status, equity in healthcare and the social inclusion of members of minority groups, especially women, are of significance for the wellbeing of the whole society. This is supported by the results from 30 years of research in social epidemiology [8]. The health of women is one of the priority issues of WHO in the European Region [9]. On International Women's Day (8 March 2008), United Nations High Commissioner for Refugees (UNHCR) launched a handbook for the protection of women and girls, which replaces UNHCR's 1999 Guidelines on the Protection of Refugee Women. The handbook denounces a massive culture of neglect and denial about violence against women and girls and outlines strategies to answer the protection challenges faced by women and girls of concern. It also sets out international legal standards and responsibilities in this area. The handbook is of particular significance for women in the third world countries/developing countries, but few in those areas have access to it due to lack of resources.

Women and girls as risk groups

The target group in this chapter are women and girls as asylum-seekers, refugees, internally displaced, returnees, stateless and those who have integrated into new communities. Even though the references in the issue are mostly from Western countries, the chapter is concerned with women living in remote areas. Google Earth's new mapping programme, a geospatial tool, takes the reader in front of his or her computer on a virtual reality tour with the UNCHR of some of the world's major displacement crises and the humanitarian efforts aimed at helping the victims. Hopefully, the reader, sitting thousands of kilometres away, hears and develop an emotional understanding of what it is like to be a refugee in the physical context, daily life, education and health (www.unhcr.org/events/47f48dc92.html).

The number of internally displaced persons (IDPs), who now outnumber asylum seekers and refugees, is influenced by the prevalence of armed conflicts mainly in the poorest countries of the world. Such conflicts expose everyone to violence but women and girls are particularly at risk on account of their social status and their sex. According to the UNHCR [10], sexual and gender-based violence (SGBV) – including rape, forced impregnation, forced abortion, trafficking, sexual slavery and the international spread of sexually transmitted infections, including HIV/Acquired Immuno Deficiency Syndrome (AIDS) – is a defining characteristic of contemporary armed conflicts. The primary targets are women and girls.

In general, women have greater difficulties than men in reaching a country where they can seek visa and asylum, due to lack of the means to travel and/or knowledge about their rights and especially the hazards they encounter during flight.

Promotion of social inclusion

According to Arcel and Kastrup [11], interpersonal violence exacerbates discrimination against women. The promotion of social inclusion is therefore both strategically important for public health work and highly significant for forced displaced and immigrant groups, particularly women. According to the UNHCR [10], 'these human rights violations are not only a result of forced displacement, they are directly related to the discrimination and violence women and girls endure in peace time, since women and girls do not enjoy equal status with men and boys in most societies' (p. 2).

The effect on perceived health of adverse life circumstances after migration

Immigrant women's psychological ill health is connected with their introduction to and integration in a new society. A review shows that while patterns of immigration have changed over time, problems with human rights and discrimination persist and have even become worse [12]. Traumatic life events in the home country, in transit, internal displaced and after reception in a host county influence the target group's mental health outcome. According to Silove *et al.* [13], besides considering the most common illnesses and psychopathology, it is instructive to look at the protective and risk factors which differentiate those who are resilient from those who need clinical help. In a meta-analysis focused on the resettlement environment, Porter and Haslam [14] found that assumed economic opportunities – that is, the right to work, access to employment and maintenance of socioeconomic status – were associated with better mental health.

A review of the literature shows that interpersonal violence towards women leads to more health and mental health problems and poorer integration in the reception societies [4].

Unemployment has been identified as one of the most frequent resettlement stress factors experienced by refugees and immigrants [15]. Being employed is not just a matter of economic stability; it also structures time, provides new social contacts, boosts creativity, confers aim and coherence to life and is an important aspect of personal identity [16]. A study shows that, compared with younger immigrants, female immigrants over the age of 50 more often experience gender and ethnic discrimination and lack of access to skill-training programmes [17]. Lindencrona *et al.* [18] stress the importance of exploring how research on perceived reduced working ability is conducted among women from different immigrant groups and how the impairment is originated and developed.

An obstacle to employment is that while newcomers may have general skills, they usually lack the country-specific human capital that employers value (e.g. host-country language and knowledge of work practises, local institutions, cultural norms and behaviour and how organisations are structured and function). Cultural distance is also more relevant for female immigrants than for male. Women's access to the labour market varies with their cultural background and the level of socio-economic development in the country of origin [19]. A stratified study of the Swedish population of immigrants from Bosnia Herzegovina, using the Göteborg Quality of Life instrument, showed that women were associated with higher levels of self-rated symptoms of poor mental health. Women in the urban region were particularly associated with higher levels of symptoms, but no statistically significant difference in the use of medicines was found between men and women [20, 21].

Rodriguez *et al.* [22] show that the relationship between unemployment and mental illness may be weaker among Afro-American population groups in the USA. A possible explanation is that victims of long-term exposure to discrimination develop coping strategies and their mental wellbeing is less dependent on work.

A six-month longitudinal study [23], utilising a detailed semi-structured interview protocol and standardised questionnaires, was conducted with a group of 50 Chinese women who had immigrated to Canada with their spouses during the last decade. The most negative life event was employment-related and the greatest difficulty was the financial strain of living below the poverty line, factors that significantly predicted the women's mental health. Social support was neither a main determinant of mental health nor a buffer between life events and mental health.

High levels of distress may elicit more support from kin and more avoidance from non-kin [24]. Familial ties may not be supportive if they are more obligatory than voluntary [23].

19.3 Risk factors

Interpersonal violence

Interpersonal violence occurs in a variety of forms, such as war-related violence, torture, sexual violence, forced disappearance and extrajudicial killing as mentioned above, and each form may be involved in additive violence. A review of prevalence studies in clinical and community samples shows that the majority of asylum seekers and refugees have experienced significant pre-migration political violence [12]. Usually, men are the primary target of organised violence and experience more psychological problems but in their study of Somali and Oromo refugees in Minnesota, Jaranson *et al.* [25] found that women were as likely to have been subjected to torture as men. An example from clinical and research experience is that male family members are often the first to apply for asylum and that while waiting to reunite the family, their wives and children may have been exposed to horrific traumatic life events.

Loss and separation

Loss and separation can refer to land, climate, culture, social traditions, food and roots in general, family members, friends, dwelling, job and status, self-esteem and material and private belongings. Many female asylum seekers and refugees from the south come from cultures where the primary social unit is the group, family members and other relatives, thus not the individual as in modern societies. The equivalent to our social welfare is the family and refugees accordingly have economic responsibilities for the family members whom they leave behind. This economic burden may influence post-migration stress. Loss and separation may influence mental health and women exposed to loss and separation from significant others and to loss of social status and self-esteem may have difficulty in recovering from the trauma of interpersonal violence.

The literature shows that family separation predicts distress among women but not men. 'The loss of extended family support networks may have a greater impact on women, especially those who have to look after young children alone' [26]. That study highlights the importance of examining the post-arrival life situation of forced migrants, that is, not only trauma before arrival. Using acculturation models for asylum seekers can be misleading because 'such a term disguises the fact that many of the demands (e.g. unemployment and family separation) concern the thwarting of psychological needs that are common to all humans, irrespective of their ethnocultural background' (p. 14).

Socioeconomic factors

It is important to distinguish between psychopathology (diagnose) and expected or specific culture-bound responses which may or may not be deviant in the specific cultural context. In assessment and treatment, excessive reliance on models of cultural determinism would be as unproductive as totally disregarding cultural factors [27]. Further, factors that may impact health status include: '(i) conflict between traditional and new norms and values, such as gender roles for young women, leading to stress between their own aspirations and the values of their parents, (ii) unfamiliarity with the role of women in the host population and (iii) poor employment opportunities or entrapment in unsatisfactory work environments' [28, p. 251].

19.4 Resilience and coping

Antonovsky [29] developed a theory regarding psychological dimensions that affect health – a sense of coherence: (i) 'comprehensibility' or the extent to which a person can make sense of internal or external stimuli; (ii) 'manageability' or the extent to which one perceives that resources are available and (iii) 'meaningfulness' or the perception that life is meaningful and worth living despite its hardships. Jablensky *et al.* [30] identified the following range of factors that provide protective functions in the face of hardships after migration:

1. *Extended family*: the availability of an extended family as a unit of mutual support.

2. *Employment*: Access to employment during the 'transit' phase and upon arrival in a host country.

3. *Human rights organisations*: the visible presence of human rights organisations among refugee populations, especially in camps.

4. *Self-help groups*: The emergence of self-help groups that empower the refugees and provide opportunities for catharsis and shared memories.

5. *Small camps*: The distribution of refugees into small rural camps rather than large agglomerations.

6. *Cultural practises*: The opportunity of refugees to freely practise their traditions, beliefs and customs, as well as to recreate their social institutions (e.g. religion).

7. *Situational transcendence*: The ability of individuals and groups to frame their status and problems in terms that transcend the immediate situation and give it meaning (e.g. ethnic identity, cultural history) (pp. 333–334).

Empowering women is a process of supporting women and girls [10]:

- 'Analyse their situation from an age, gender and diversity perspective.

- Access information on their rights.

- Define their own priorities and

- Take action they consider appropriate to address inequalities and realise their full capacities and skills, so that they can attain a level of control over their own environment and livelihood' (pp. 13–14).

19.5 The impact of domestic violence on immigrant women's mental health

A review of literature by Rees and Pease [31] shows that while domestic and family violence is common in most societies, immigrant and refugee women are especially vulnerable. They found that domestic violence was not in fact higher in refugee communities, but 'it was specific experiences, including lack of host-language skills, unemployment, isolation from mainstream society and prior experiences of trauma related to oppressive political structures, fundamental religious beliefs and civil war that reinforced strategies by perpetrators and prevented women seeking assistance and early intervention' (p. 1). Moreover, structural inequalities (e.g. gender, class oppression and residency status) form the daily lives of refugee women and men. Intimate partner violence commonly reaches its highest level when culture communities are in transition, when women start to take in non-traditional roles or enter the labour force, or when men lose their ability to fulfil their culturally expected roles as providers and protectors. The impact can hardly be overestimated since 'violence erodes their self-esteem, and confidence to work at lifting themselves out of poverty' and 'fear of violence limits women's ability to perform their roles in many ways' [32, p. 5]. These impacts of violence exhaust the women's energy and capacity, and involve suffering and injustice.

Why do immigrant women sustain oppressive relationships?

Immigrant, stateless, returnee and refugee women experiencing domestic violence tend to face major structural obstacles that play a key role in sustaining oppressive relationships, including the state-level practise of immigration legislation as well as health and social service policy and provision. Therefore, 'explanations in terms of particular cultural practises and norms relating to gender relations can be seen to commit an equivalent error of cultural pathologisation that obscures more systematic state responsibilities and collusions with violence' [33, p. 72].

19.6 Access to mental healthcare services

A qualitative study [34] from the perspective of healthcare providers found that it is common that (i) immigrant women face many difficulties when accessing mental healthcare services due to cultural differences, social stigma and unfamiliarity with Western biomedicine, (ii) spiritual beliefs and practises influence immigrant women's mental healthcare practises and (iii) the healthcare provider-client relationship is a major influence on how immigrant women seek mental health service. The study also showed that cultural background exerts both positive and negative influences on how immigrant women seek mental healthcare. The conclusion was that even though cultural knowledge and practise influence immigrant women's coping choices and strategies, 'awareness of social and economic differences among diverse groups of immigrant women is necessary to improve the accessibility of mental healthcare for immigrant women' (p. 453).

Regardless of context, demographics and time factors, the field has several common themes and issues: (i) the prevalence of major depression and post-traumatic stress disorder (PTSD) across gender, age and ethnic groups; (ii) the interrelationships of not only the individual, but also the family and community; (iii) the interconnection of physical, psychiatric, psychological and social problems; (iv) the central role of culture and problems with equivalence (in concepts, language, metrics, norms) which interfere with the integration of immigrants into their host societies and (v) the persistent role of trauma and violence in precipitating long-lasting problems with mental illness and adjustment [35, p. 625]. While the prevalence and chronicity of PTSD may be higher among women, the construct is based on the experiences of male combat veterans, resulting in measurement problems that can influence both research and practise (for a review, see [36]). Further, memories of trauma need to be understood in a collective historical, political and human rights context [37].

At another level, communication of distress is universal but its meaning is not necessarily the same for everyone [38]. For instance, Nordanger [39] points to the limitations of PTSD as a Western measure of trauma and calls for a context-based conceptualisation of trauma. Informants' expressions of distress were found to be highly informed by the socio-cultural and socio-economic structures of Tigrayan society. The most reported complaints concerned (i) household erosion, (ii) social marginalisation and (iii) education abortion. Post-war psychosocial health problems were perceived as consequences of these aspects of impaired household economy, and were described in terms of their negative impacts on future income generation.

19.7 The ADAPT model (Adaptation and Development after Persecution and Trauma)

In general, the culture in which women are socialised helps to elucidate communication behaviours. Optimising efficient communication requires an understanding and knowledge of the cultural and social context in which communication takes place [40]. According to Hofstede [41], people in individualistic cultures tend to emphasise self-actualisation, individual initiatives and achievement, an 'I' identity, while people in collectivistic cultures stress fitting in, belonging to the in-group, and maintaining a 'we' identity.

Research on refugees and other immigrants' psychological wellbeing has focused up to now on deficiencies within the individual, such as feelings of distress and psychiatric symptoms. Intersectionality theory, introduced by African-American and Third World feminists, assumes that gender oppression is modified by intersections with other forms of inequality and oppression [31]. Ryan et al. [26] introduce a resource-based model which is understood in terms of the individual's needs and personal goals and the demands the person encounters during post-migration adaptation. These authors emphasise that each of these concepts must be examined in the context of the pre-migration, flight and post-migration phases. The additional concept of constraints on access to resources is particularly relevant to the post-migration phase.

An ecological model of psychosocial trauma by Harvey [42] noted that 'the efficiency of trauma-focused interventions depends upon the degree to which they enhance the person-community relationship and achieve 'ecological fit' within individually varied recovery contexts' (p. 3). Further, Moos [43] postulates that 'we need a fundamental paradigm shift in how to construe and examine the aftermath of life crises' (p. 79), that is, theories of posttraumatic development and maturation are not similar to theories of learned helplessness and PTSD.

A broad-based ecosocial model: ADAPT model [37, 44, 45] proposes five fundamental 'systems' of potentially threatened or disrupted health: (i) *safety and felt security* (PTSD); (ii) *attachment and bonds, networks and communities* (sense of belonging, grief); (iii) *justice* (feeling treated fairly and with dignity), (anger); (iv) *identity and roles* (being valued and useful, belonging) (marginalisation, liminality) and (v) *meaning and coherence* (social, political, cultural, religious, political): making sense (alienation). This model is applied below in the theory of change logic, using the clinical case as a tool to increase communication between clinicians and policy makers.

For individual survivors and their collectives to recover, it is necessary to repair damage to these systems and the institutions that support them. The ADAPT model understands trauma in a broader framework. Silove [37] postulates that reconstruction programmes need to reinforce broad ecosocial pillars that support general psychosocial recovery and, where necessary, provide relevant and useful interventions at the psychological level.

19.8 The case of Mrs Aba, her family and the community

Patient's demand

Mrs Aba screened positive for depression and PTSD in a primary psychiatric outpatient clinic in a suburb of Stockholm, the capital of Sweden.

Referral: Self-referred, willing to be evaluated after detection as checklist positive during a depression and PTSD screen before starting the language class at the community's introduction unit. During her flight from Iraq, the smugglers had raped her several times in the sight of her two children.

Brief anamnesis and previous history

1. *Family*: Mrs Aba is a 40-year-old Iraqi Christian woman who was resettled in Sweden at the beginning of 2007 due to violence and insecurity in Iraq after the fall of Saddam Hussein. Before her arrival, she had suffered multiple family losses, especially both her parents, her husband and their oldest son, all her three male siblings and several cousins. Her husband was a well-known manager in Baghdad. She also lost all material belongings, including their house, which she had to hand over to terrorists when they threatened to kidnap her (a common experience among asylum seekers from Iraq). These traumatic life events led to her flight.

2. *Professional*: Mrs Aba and her two remaining children (10-year-old son, 8-year-old daughter) came to her sister and family near Stockholm. After nearly one year seeking asylum, they were given permission to stay at the end of 2007. Mrs Aba is on the waiting list for a Swedish language course and her children have adjusted pretty well in school. Mrs Aba worries about her capacity to study. She has studied engineering and after her marriage worked part-time in an export company in Baghdad. She has nightmares and her depression is escalating.

3. *Medical*: Mrs Aba has had back pain for several years but does not know its cause. In Iraq she had some prescriptions that she cannot find in Sweden. She consumed Valium in Iraq on account of the violence and feeling unsafe. She wants such sedatives again when she feels depressed and has nightmares.

Immediate antecedents

She is anxious about her capacity to start the Swedish language course and feels worthless. She has some difficulties in bringing up her children and getting support from her sister and her family, who have been in Sweden for some years. Mrs Aba and her children live in a small apartment quite close to her sister.

Problematic behaviour

1. *Cognitive*: some of her thoughts are: 'Why should I survive', 'I have no future', 'I do not feel clean after rape' and hopeless; it is because I have lost my family.

2. *Emotional*: feels lonely, anxious, cries and has low mood, 'survivor's guilt', worthless, feels empty inside.

3. *Intellectual*: difficulties in concentrating, memory problems, thoughts of suicide.

4. *Behavioural*: feels tired, irritable, tries to hang on to her children, unable to do things she did in Iraq before the violence started about five years ago.

5. *Relational*: lack of trust, few social contacts.

6. *Spiritual*: Christian but has doubts that God helps.

7. *Physical/physiological*: cannot sleep at night due to nightmares, problems with food and appetite, stomach problems, vomiting, sweat, stress in muscles, pain in the back, heightened vulnerability to infection.

8. *Cause according to the patient*: the present situation.

Diagnosis according to diagnostic and statistical manual of mental disorder (DSM)-IV

Major depressive episode and PTSD.

Treatment strategies

Immediate:
- Improve her sleeping pattern.
- Manage stress and emotions with cognitive behavioural techniques; start a group of mental health promotion class for five weeks, two hour per week.

Long-term:
- Work on dysfunctional schema and coping skills due to her family loss and violence in her country before resettlement in Sweden.

- Build up social network.
- Individualise the language course, practical experience and job opportunities.

19.9 Theory of change logic: Mental health action planning

This section is based on the discussion in Lavelle and Wang [46] and questions raised from the policy planner's point of view. The case from Sweden presented above is used as an example. There is a need to overcome barriers to communication between scientists, service providers and policy makers by using a gender perspective. According to Ekblad [28], a basic prevention strategy for migrants includes:

- 'Recognition of human trafficking of women as an important social and health problem.
- Policy formulation and programme development to protect human rights.
- A psychosocial orientation to understand mental health behaviour and experience from a gender perspective in the context of society and culture.
- Partnerships and collaboration with a greater concern of newly arrived immigrants in host societies, resulting in greater emancipation and changing roles.
- Increasing efforts to match and access mental healthcare to the needs and expectations of immigrants.
- Training and preparation of all staff with responsibilities in the reception programme and health service of host countries to address the psychosocial needs of migrants' (p. 257).

Mental health policy and legislation

Mrs Aba's access to clinical care appears to play a significant role in the story of her health-seeking behaviour. 'How does access to and availability of primary health and mental health care in your country impact the individual and family seeking care? Do citizens have an equal right to health and mental health care? How does your government define mental health needs of a post-conflict society' [46, p. 49]. At present, asylum seeking adults in Sweden have access to emergency care only and the issue is being hotly debated since Sweden has one of the most restrictive policies in Europe. Adult asylum seekers (excluding hidden and undocumented who must pay all emergency care) have access only to emergency care by a new law from July 1, 2008 (Referens: Lagen om hälso- och sjukvård åt asylsökande m.fl. 2008:344). Mollica [1] came to believe that 'conventional psychiatric tools' would not be sufficient to help his Cambodian refugee patients. Further, fostering self-healing cannot be done until the traumatised woman understands her role in recovery. For Mrs Aba's health recovery, it is of significance to support her to be an active part of her self-healing process. The doctor or therapist should give her the question, 'What can we do together to make you healthy again', acknowledges that self-healing is a real process that needs to be consciously and actively supported.

During the asylum process, for women, one of the most potent stressful experiences is insecurity of legal status and their vulnerability for being dependent on others for living. Every effort should therefore be made to shorten the time during which asylum seekers have to live in this state of uncertainty, without compromising the quality of the appraisal. The negative effect of being denied access to legal employment should be taken into consideration. Exclusion from the labour force and forced dependence on social welfare result in disempowerment, stigmatisation, financial strain, boredom, social isolation and an insecure family situation. Women who work illegally are open to exploitation by employers.

Any policy and legislation have to be specifically grounded on the healing needs of female survivors of mass violence and traumatised populations. 'The mental health recovery needs are recommended to be accomplished by a culturally, linguistically and culturally competent service delivery system that general mental health legislation and policies would not be able to fully address' [46, p. 50]. The comprehensive recovery needs of female refugees are often not coordinated among providers and funding agencies.

Financing mental health recovery

The questions raised here are: What particular challenges does the current system pose for patients, families and communities? How does your government finance health, mental health and indigenous healing systems to provide the comprehensive care of trauma survivors? The comprehensive treatment, rehabilitation, support and coordination needs of a trauma survivor pose the financial question of what services are considered to be medical necessities.

Science-based mental health services

The connected questions are: 'How do we know that the care which Mrs Aba and her children will receive from the medical and mental health perspective is science-based best practise?' [46, p. 50]. When we measure clinical effectiveness should we also consider the impact on the patient of other social systems, such as alternative medicine, non-governmental organizations (NGOs), and so on? Which components of evidence-based practises for women's mental health recovery are evaluated and available for dissemination? Are there challenges for quantitative research in studying women's mental health treatment and outcomes?

According to Lavelle and Wang [46], the current literature on psychopharmacological intervention and cognitive behavioural treatment has demonstrated clinical efficacy in treatment of depression and PTSD. For instance, HPRT as a best-practise model focuses on the use of trauma story, mobilisation of individual resiliency and altruism, work and community re-engagement, social, familial and spiritual rediscovery, healthcare and nutrition and symptoms management and reduction are important factors for bio-psycho-social recovery of refugees.

Building on ongoing programmes of mental health education

Western countries generally have mandatory further education requirements for licensed professionals. Despite all the documentation on theoretical models for cultural competence training for clinical staff, there is no specific training requirement concerning refugees' mental health and staff are seldom asked for their views on such competency issues. HPRT's Master Class & Master's Certificate provides the only intensive multiple-disciplinary and cross-systems training on refugees' mental health. There is no infrastructure to focus on the needs and treatment outcomes of the survivors of mass violence.

The questions raised here are: 'Where ongoing education exists or where it is mandatory, are both short- and long-term training courses usually designed to provide state-of-the-art knowledge for health care practitioners? Is ongoing continuous 'mental health' education required or available in your country?' [46, p. 51]. What direct impact does training healthcare staff have on complicated, multiple problem cases like the story of Mrs Aba? Has your country established training across disciplines and systems to meet the training needs of all practitioners for this specialised population?

A study by Shahnavaz and Ekblad [47] using focus group interviews investigated whether the main concern of the participants (inter-professional teams in Swedish psychiatry) is to understand the culturally diverse in psychiatry rather than being culturally competent. Three major themes in the process of understanding emerged in the analyses: (i) diversity reflection, (ii) cultural knowledge and skill acquisition and (iii) communication. It was concluded that listening to clinical workers' competency needs may motivate greater sensitivity to the needs of their culturally diverse patients.

Coordination of international agencies, NGOs

The questions raised here are: 'Does the Mental Health Action Plan include specific actions and people responsible for the transition from humanitarian emergency aid to post-conflict recovery, including the role of all international, national and local agencies, donors and practitioners dealing with the mental health recovery of citizens affected by mass violence?' [46, p. 51].

One of the key challenges for both psychological services and NGOs is to facilitate access to social resources. Clinical staff need to work in conjunction with community and religious groups to maximise opportunities for social contact.

Mental health linkages to economic development

The questions raised here are: 'Research and its preliminary evidence suggest that significant economic costs are associated with mental illness among highly traumatised civilian populations in the following areas: Days of work lost (per week); Quality of job performance; Ability to plan for economic activities (e.g. farming); Increased domestic violence; Increased high-risk behaviour and its consequences (e.g. unsafe sex and HIV/AIDS); Increases in diabetes, cardiovascular disease and stroke; Premature death among the elderly; Negative impact on social capital, neighbourliness; Higher suicide rates and poor school performance by children and adolescents' [46, p. 52].

Mental health linkages to human rights

The UN Declaration of Human Rights, Article 25, Item 1, states:

> Everyone has the right to a standard of living adequate for the health and well-being of himself and his family, including food, clothing, housing, and medical care and necessary social services and the right to security in the event of unemployment, sickness, disability, widowhood, old age, or other lack of livelihood in circumstances beyond your control.

In your specific context, do you have a system that protects female patients' rights? Was Mrs Aba's 'right' to healthcare protected by this article of the UN Declaration of Human Rights? If yes, is it consistent during her new life in Sweden?

The natural linkage between mental health and human rights is often overlooked. While most people agree that recovery after a traumatic life event is a personal and public health issue, there tends to be less recognition that this is also a matter of social justice. UN and other agencies must facilitate studies in host countries, to understand their problems with the migrant and refugee populations, devise, improvise gold standards methods for intervention to help these countries.

Last but not at least, if the Mental Health Action Plan you adapt to a given female population emerging from mass violence and war fails to address this essential human right, you will most probably face a loss of credibility, hope and any possibility of fulfilling your mission.

References

1. Mollica, R.F. (2006) *Healing Invisible Wounds: Paths to Hope and Recovery in a Violent World*, Harcourt, New York.
2. Brody, E.B. (2007) Healing invisible wounds: paths to hope and recovery in a violent world: review. *The Journal of Nervous and Mental Diseases*, **195** (8), 709.

3. Annan, K. (2004) Review of the implementation of the Beijing Platform for Action and Women 2000: Gender, Equality, Development and Peace for the 21st Century. E/CN.6/2005/2, p. 22.

4. Ekblad, S., Kastrup, M.C., Eisenman, D.P. and Arcel, L.T. (2007) Interpersonal violence towards women section 7: mental health and illness in immigrants, in *Immigrant Medicine* (eds P.F. Walker, E.D. Barnett and J. Jaranson), WB Saunders, St. Louis, pp. 665–71.

5. World Health Organization. Mental health: a state of well-being. http://www.who.int/features/factfiles/mental_health/en.

6. Mollica, R. (2007) Global Mental Health: Trauma and Recovery. Introduction to the Course. Presented by The Harvard Program in Refugee Trauma, Massachussetts General Hospital and Instituto Superiore Di Sanita, Ministry of Health of Italy, 5 November 2007, Orvieto, Italy.

7. WHO (1998) Health Promotion Glossary, World Health Organization, Geneva.

8. Wilkinson, G.R. (2005) *The Impact of Inequality How to Make Sick Societies Healthier*, Routledge, London.

9. WHO (2001) Evaluation of Health Promotion: Principles and Perspectives (eds I. Roothman *et al.*), WHO regional publications. European Series No 92. Mental health: a state of well-being. http://www.who.int/features/factfiles/mental_health/en.

10. UNHCR (2008) Handbook for the Protection of Women and Girls. UNHCR, Geneva. Bird's Eye View of a Refugee's World. www.unhcr.org/events/47f48dc92.html.

11. Arcel, L.T. and Kastrup, C. (2004) War, women and health. *NORA*, **12** (1), 37–40.

12. Jaranson, J., Ekblad, S., Kroupin, V. and Eisenman, D.P. (2007) Epidemiology and risk factors. Section 7: mental health and illness in immigrants, in *Immigrant Medicine* (eds P.F. Walker, E.D. Barnett and J. Jaranson), Elsevier Saunders, St. Louis, pp. 627–32.

13. Silove, D., Ekblad, S. and Mollica, R. (2000) Health and human rights. The rights of the severely mentally ill in post-conflict societies. *Invited Lancet commentary*, **355** (9214), 1548–49.

14. Porter, M. and Haslam, N. (2001) Forced displacement in Yugoslavia: a meta-analysis of psychological consequences and their moderators. *Journal of Traumatic Stress*, **14**, 817–34.

15. Beiser, M. and Hou, F. (2001) Language acquisition, unemployment and depressive disorder among Southeast Asian refugees: a 10-year study. *Social Science and Medicine*, **53** (10), 1321–34.

16. Akhavan, S., Bildt, C.O., Franzen, E.C. and Wamala, S. (2004) Health in relation to unemployment and sick leave among immigrants in Sweden from a gender perspective. *Journal of Immigrant Health*, **6** (3), 102–18.

17. Akhavan, S., Bildt, C. and Wamala, S. (2007) Work-related health factors for female immigrants in Sweden. *Work*, **28** (2), 135–43.

18. Lindencrona, F., Ekblad, S. and Johanson Blight, K. (2005) *Integration Och Folkhälsa – en Kunskapsöversikt. Expertappendix i Integration 2005*, Integrationsverket, Norrköping, www.integrationsverket.se.

19. Inglehart, R. and Norris, P. (2003) *Rising Tide Gender Equality and Cultural Change Around the World*, Cambridge University Press, London.

20. Johansson Blight, K., Ekblad, S., Persson, J.-O. and Ekberg, J. (2006) Mental health, employment and gender. Cross-sectional evidence in a sample of refugees from Bosnia-Herzegovina living in two Swedish regions. *Social Science and Medicine*, **62** (7), 1565–830.

21. Johansson Blight, K., Persson, J.O., Ekblad, S. and Ekberg, J. (2008) Medical and licit drug use in an urban/rural study population of refugee background, 7–8 years into resettlement. *GMS Psycho-Social Medicine*, **5**, Doc04.

22. Rodriguez, E., Allen, J.A., Frongillo, E.A. Jr. and Chandra, P. (1999) Unemployment, depression, and health: a look at the African-American community. *Journal of Epidemiology and Community Health*, **53** (6), 335–42.

23. Tang, T.N., Oatley, K. and Toner, B.B. (2007) Impact of life events and difficulties on the mental health of chinese immigrant women. *Journal of Immigrant and Minority Health*. DOI: 10.1007/s10903-007-9042-1.

24. Gellis, Z.D. (2003) Kin and nonkin social supports in a community sample of Vietnamese immigrants. *Social Work*, **48**, 248–58.

25. Jaranson, J.M., Butcher, J., Halcon, L. *et al.* (2004) Somali and Oromo refugees, correlates of torture and trauma history. *American Journal of Public Health*, **94** (4), 591–98.

26. Ryan, D., Dooley, B. and Benson, C. (2008) Theoretical perspectives on post-migration adaptation and psychological well-being among refugees: towards a resource-based model. *Journal of Refugee Studies*, **21** (1). DOI: 10.1093/jrs/fem047.

27. Jaranson, J., Forbes Martin, S. and Ekblad, S. (2001) Refugee Mental Health, in Mental Health, United States, 2000 (eds R.W. Manderscheid and M.J. Henderson), US Department of Health and Human Services, Substance Abuse and Mental Health Services Administration (SAMHSA), Center for Mental Health Services, Rockville, pp. 120–33.

28. Ekblad, S. (2002) Gender and mental health in a multicultural society, in *Gender and Social Inequalities in Health* (eds S. Wamala and J. Lynch), Studentlitteratur, Lund, pp. 233–64.

29. Antonovsky, A. (1987) *Unraveling the Mystery of Health: How People Manage Stress and Stay Well*, Jossey-Bass, London.

30. Jablensky, A., Marsella, A.J. and Ekblad, S. (1994) Refugee mental health and well-being: conclusions and recommendations, in *Amidst Peril and Pain: The Mental Health and Wellbeing of World's Refugees* (eds A.J. Marsella, T. Bornemann, S. Ekblad and J. Orley), American Psychological Association, Washington, DC, pp. 327–39.

31. Rees, S. and Pease, B. (2007) Refugee Settlement, Safety and Wellbeing: Exploring Domestic and Family Violence in Refugee Communities. Paper Four of the Violence Against Women Community Attitudes Proejct. VicHealth, Immigrant Women's Domestic Violence Service Inc.

32. El-Bushra, J. and Lopez, E.P. (1993) Gender-related violence: its scope and relevance. *Focus on Gender*, **1** (2), 1–9.

33. Burman, E. and Chantler, K. (2005) Domestic violence and minoritisation: legal and policy barriers facing minoritzed women leaving violent relationships. *International Journal of Law and Psychiatry*, **28**, 59–74.

34. O'Mahony, J.M. and Donnelly, T.T. (2007) The influence of culture on immigrant women's mental health care experiences from the perspectives of health care providers. *Issues in Mental Health Nursing*, **28** (5), 453–71.

35. Jaranson, J. and Ekblad, S. (2007) Overview of the Mental Health Section. Section 7: Mental health and illness in immigrants, in: *Immigrant Medicine* (eds. P.F. Walker and E.D. Barnett, (Assoc Ed) J. Jaranson), Saunders, Elsevier, St. Louis, USA, pp. 625–626.

36. American Psychological Association (2007) Guidelines for psychological practice with girls and women. *The American Psychologist*, **62** (9), 949–79.

37. Silove, D. (2007) Mass Trauma, Survival and Adaptation. Presentation on the Course Global Mental Health: Trauma and Recovery. Presented by The Harvard Program in Refugee Trauma, Massachussetts General Hospital and Instituto Superiore Di Sanita, 7 November 2007, Ministy of Health of Italy, Orvieto, Italy.

38. Kleinman, A. (1988) *Rethinking Psychiatry: From Cultural Category to Personal Experience*, Free Press, New York.

39. Nordanger, D.O. (2007) Beyond PTSD: socio-economic bereavement in Tigray, Ethiopia. *Anthropology and Medicine*, **14** (1), 69–82.

40. Gao, G., Ting-Toomey, S. and Gudykunst, W.B. (1996) Chinese communication processes, in *The Handbook of Chinese Psychology* (ed. M. Harris Bond), Oxford University Press, Hong Kong, pp. 280–93.

41. Hofstede, G.H. (1980) *Culture's Consequences: International Differences in Work-related Values*, Sage Publications, Beverly Hills.

42. Harvey, M.R. (1996) An ecological view of psychological trauma and trauma recovery. *Journal of Traumatic Stress*, **9**, 3–23.

43. Moos, R.H. (2002) The mystery of human context and coping. An unravelling of clues. *American Journal of Community Psychology*, **30** (1), 67–68.

44. Silove, D. and Steel, Z. (2006) Understanding community psychosocial needs after disasters: implications for mental health services. *Journal of Postgraduate Medicine*, **52** (2), 121–25.

45. Ekblad, S. and Jaranson, J. (2004) Psychosocial rehabilitation, in *Broken Spirits. The Treatment of Traumatized Asylum Seekers, Refugees, War and Torture Victims* (eds J.P. Wilson and B. Drozdek), Brenner-Routledge Press, New York, pp. 609–36.

46. Lavelle, J. and Wang, E.D.S. (2007) Global Mental Health: Trauma and Recovery. Policy Case Study from Policy Planner's Point of View. Case Vignette & Discussion. In: Global Mental Health: Trauma and Recovery. On site training: November 6–17, 2006, Web-based training: December 4, 2006–May 13, 2007, pp. 47–52.

47. Shahnavaz, S. and Ekblad, S. (2007) Understanding the culturally diverse in psychiatry rather than being culturally competent – a preliminary report of swedish psychiatric teams' views on transcultural competence. *International Journal of Migration, Health and Social Care*, **3** (4), 14–30.

Further reading

Zur, J. (1996) From PTSD to voices in context: from an "experience-far" to an "experience-near" understanding of responses to war and atrocity across cultures. *International Journal of Social Psychiatry*, **42** (4), 305–17.

20

Work and women's mental health

Saida Douki

Faculty of Medicine of Tunis, Razi Hospital, Tunis, Tunisia

20.1 Introduction: A late but growing awareness

Over the past few decades there has been a number of research studies, in women's overall life circumstances and their relation to women's health status. Paid employment, in particular, has been considered an important part of women's living conditions as the number of women entering the labour market has grown constantly over the past decades. As a matter of fact, occupation ranks sixth amidst the 10 major risk factors for the global burden of disease 1990 that disproportionately affects women [1].

According to World Bank estimates, from 1960 to 1997, women have increased their numbers in the global labour force by 26% [2]. Today, women make up about 42% of the estimated global working population, making them indispensable as contributors to national and global economies [1]. This is true in developed and emerging countries. For example, in Sweden, today women constitute 48% of the total work force [3]. And in Tunisia, the percentage of women in the working population has increased sixfold between 1966 and 1999, from 5 to 30%.

However, gender differences in work-related health conditions have received little research attention. It's only over the past two decades that an extensive and relevant literature on women's work and mental health issues began to be brought out.

Women's work is generally associated with better health. Nevertheless, as women have become more assimilated into the workforce, they have realised

---

Contemporary Topics in Women's Mental Health   Edited by Chandra, Herrman, Fisher, Kastrup,
© 2009 John Wiley & Sons, Ltd   Niaz, Rondón and Okasha

considerable changes in their traditional roles which may contribute to health problems. In particular, the multiple roles that they fulfil in society render them at greater risk of experiencing mental problems than others in the community. Many studies seem to show that female workers may be exposed to some gender related stressors which could threaten their mental health and wellbeing.

20.2 The job burnout

The main work-related mental health problem is the so-called job burnout which was first identified in the 1970s by Bradley as a 'psychological condition which develops as a result of prolonged and unrelieved work stress'. Unlike acute stress reactions, which develop in response to specific critical incidents, burnout is a cumulative reaction to ongoing occupational stressors.

Definition

Burnout refers to a work-related syndrome of long-term exhaustion and diminished interest which is often construed as the result of a period of expending too much effort at work while having too little recovery.

The three key dimensions of this syndrome are an overwhelming exhaustion, feelings of cynicism and detachment from the job and a sense of ineffectiveness and lack of accomplishment [4]. The exhaustion component refers to feelings of being overextended and depleted of one's emotional and physical resources. The cynicism (or depersonalisation) component refers to a negative, callous or excessively detached response to various aspects of the job. The component of reduced efficacy or accomplishment refers to feelings of incompetence and a lack of achievement and productivity at work.

The well-studied measurement of burnout in the literature is the Maslach Burnout Inventory (MBI), a 22-item inventory, using the three components of the burnout syndrome. A high score on exhaustion and depersonalisation and a low score on personal accomplishment is an indication for burnout [5].

Self-evaluation

Burnout can occur when one feels overwhelmed and unable to meet constant demands (Table 20.1). As the stress continues, one begins to lose interest or motivation in the job. Burnout reduces productivity and saps energy, leading to increasing feelings of hopelessness, powerlessness, cynicism and resentment. Burnout expresses itself as irritability, may lead to snapping at people or making snide remarks about them. Other common manifestation of burn out are escapist behaviours such as drinking, drugs, sex, partying or shopping binges trying to escape from negative feelings. Relationships at work and personal life may begin to fall apart. Trust in people is lost, believing that people act out of selfishness and nothing can be done about it.

Table 20.1 Signs and symptoms of burnout

Fatigue, exhaustion, tiredness, a sense of being physically run down
Dysphoria
Irritability (anger at those making demands)
Crying jags
Anxiety attacks
Emotional outbursts
Anger attacks (exploding easily at seemingly inconsequential things)
Loss of appetite or weight gain
Overreacting
Teeth grinding
Increased drug, alcohol and tobacco use
Sleep disturbances, insomnia, sleeplessness, nightmares
Difficulties to concentrate, inability to concentrate, forgetfulness
Feelings of frustration
Feelings of powerlessness
Low productivity
Headaches, migraines
Neck or low back pain
Gastro-intestinal disturbances
Feelings of disillusion about one's job
Lost of the ability to experience joy
Feelings of dissatisfaction from one's achievements
Aversion for work, work 'phobia': to drag oneself into work and to
    have trouble getting started one arrived
To become less patient with co-workers, customers and clients
Feelings of having to face insurmountable barriers at work
Lack of energy to be consistently productive
To become more critical, cynical and sarcastic at work
A sense of being besieged, entrapped
Feelings of helplessness
Increased degree of risk taking

Diagnosis

There is no official diagnosis for burnout syndrome in the DSM-IV (American Psychiatric Association, 1994). Thus, in many countries, patients showing symptoms common to burnout syndrome are often classified by their primary symptom: fatigue, under undifferentiated somatoform disorder.

Burnout is by contrast listed in the ICD10 under the code Z73.0 to define a 'state of vital exhaustion'. However, some authors argue that the diagnosis 'neurasthenia' is more fit (Table 20.2). Most of these symptoms are indeed represented in the diagnosis for job-related neurasthenia given by the World Health Organization (WHO 1992), so recent research has been utilising this diagnosis as the psychiatric equivalent of burnout.

Table 20.2   ICD-10 diagnostic criteria for F48.0 neurasthenia

1. Persistent and distressing symptoms of exhaustion after minor mental or physical effort including general feeling of malaise, combined with a mixed state of excitement and depression.

2. Accompanied by two or more of these symptoms: muscular aches and pains, dizziness, tension headache, sleep disturbance, inability to relax and irritability.

3. Accompanied by two or more of these symptoms: increased cynicism or depersonalisation, diminished feelings of efficacy and emotional exhaustion.

4. Inability to recover through rest, relaxation or enjoyment.

5. Disturbed and restless, non-refreshing sleep, often troubled with dreams.

6. Duration of over one year.

7. Complaints are job-related.

8. Does not occur in the presence of organic mental disorders, affective disorder, panic or generalised anxiety disorder.

Table 20.3   Distribution of mental health problems

	Burnout syndrome (%)	Anxiety disorders (%)	Psychotic disorders (%)
Females	81	10.5	4.5
Males	68.5	3.5	19

Table 20.4   Percentage of workers who are low paid (1993–1995) UNDP

	Males	Females
Japan	20	37
Sweden	3	9
France	6	25
USA	13	33
UK	8	31

Burnout and depression

Is burnout a subtype of clinical depression? Good question. However, burnout is a problem that is specific to the work context, in contrast to depression, which tends to pervade every domain of a person's life.

Outcome of burnout

Burnout patients are known to avoid work, display a large amount of absenteeism, doing the bare minimum at work.

A common assumption has been that burnout precipitates negative effects in terms of mental health, such as depression, anxiety and drop in self-esteem. The implication of all this research is that burnout is an important risk factor for mental health and this can have a significant impact on both the family and the work life of the affected employee. Workers who experienced burnout are rated by their spouses in more negative ways and they themselves reported that their job had a negative impact on their family and that their marriage was unsatisfactory [4].

Risk factors

Six organisational risk factors were identified by Maslach *et al.* [4]: workload, control, reward, community, fairness and values. The first two areas are reflected in the demand-control model of job stress [6]. Reward refers to the power of reinforcements to shape behaviour. Community captures all of the work on social support and interpersonal conflict, while fairness emerges from the literature on equity and social justice. Finally, the area of values picks up the cognitive-emotional power of job goals and expectations. Too many responsibilities, too little control, too few rewards, too many conflicts, too much inequity, too much confusion about values and identity and no end in sight, all add up to burnout.

Burnout can affect workers of any kind, but high stress jobs are at higher risk. Generally, workers who have frequent intense or emotionally charged interactions with others are more susceptible to burnout. Thus, burnout research had its roots in care-giving and service occupations, in which the core of the job was the relationship between provider and recipient. Because of the nature of their work, professionals in healthcare and other fields such as teaching, policing and human services are thought to be at especially high risk for burnout [7].

A number of other factors were found to relate to high levels of burnout, these are:

- Traumatic events on the job. [8]
- Confusion, conflict and ambiguity to job role. [9]
- Risk and safety factors. [10]
- Being undermined by a superior, or the belief that one is undermined by a superior. [11]
- Low levels of social support. [12]
- Inadequate job resources. [13].

Burnout and women

Burnout was once thought to be a man's problem. Freudenberger [14] himself demonstrated in Women's Burnout that women are more and more exposed to this risk, explaining: 'In part, I think this is due to the expanded, multi-role lives they lead as mothers, wives and professionals'.

20.3 A higher risk for burnout

Actually, women are particularly exposed to the above defined organisational risk factors for burnout (Table 20.3).

Excessive workload: The multiple roles

According to Maslach [7], too many demands exhaust an individual's energy to the extent that recovery becomes impossible.

Actually, women's access to the labour market has resulted in multiple roles and an overload of responsibilities. Women play several simultaneous roles whereas men are allowed to have sequential roles. Women bear the burden of responsibility associated with being wives, mothers and carers of others.

Indeed, they hold today concurrently salaried jobs, domestic tasks and parenting roles. Women who have become more educated and free to move outside are today required to be in charge of tasks once performed by men, such as shopping or overseeing children's homework.

Women do more childcare, more care of elderly or disabled relatives and most of the housework and cooking while men have more leisure time.

In Tunisia, according to a recent community survey among 6000 families carried out by the Office National de la Population et de la Famille (ONFP) in 2002 [15], mothers are two to four times more involved than fathers in the education, schooling, health and punishment of their children. (Figure 20.1).

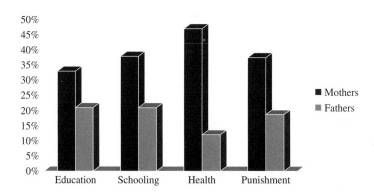

Figure 20.1 Parenting roles in Tunisia

In France, too, according to the INSEE [15], women dedicate twice as much time than men to domestic and parental tasks (33 hours a week).

This performance is not easy to achieve these days with the loss of extended family support and the limited options of childcare.

Lack of control: Lower status male-dominated occupations

Individuals who are overwhelmed by their level of responsibility may experience a crisis in control as well as in workload. Mismatch in control is reflected as one of responsibility exceeding one's authority. It is distressing for people to feel responsible for producing results, to which they are deeply committed while lacking the capacity to deliver on that mandate [7].

In Europe, women constitute the majority of clerical, service and sales workers. In France, 60% of female workers are concentrated in six jobs: private or public clerks, unskilled factory workers, teachers, health and social care (INSEE, 2002, *www.insee.fr/en*). In Sweden, where 67% of public sector workers are women, they still work primarily in municipal day-care, teaching, health services, clerical and retail work [3].

Lack of reward: Thirst for recognition

A third type of mismatch involves a lack of appropriate rewards for the work people do. Role strain may only occur when the demands of the roles outweigh the rewards and privileges [16]. The absence or presence of positive feedback can make all the difference between emotional wellbeing and burnout.

Insufficient financial rewards

It is well-known that in many countries, even the most developed, women are receiving lower wages for comparable levels of work and education and are more likely to work in low-paid employment. Gender segregation is a major factor in the gender pay gap, as women are disproportionately concentrated in lower paid jobs and the lower ranks of the better-paid managerial and professional occupations. Furthermore, women still earn less than men even when they have similar jobs, qualifications and experience, due to sex discrimination and unequal treatment [17].

According to the UNDP report (1993–1995), significantly more female workers receive low wages than their male counterparts (Table 20.4); moreover, relative income inequality penalising women and favouring men is structurally embedded as women typically earn around two thirds of the average male wage and this disparity has persisted over time.

A strong inverse relationship exists between social position and physical and mental health outcomes; adverse health outcomes are two to two and a half times higher amongst people in the most disadvantaged social position compared with those in the highest [1].

Social rewards

Recognition and appreciation of hard work values both the work and the workers. Lack of reward is closely associated with feelings of ineffectiveness. In addition, the lack of intrinsic rewards (such as pride in doing something of importance and doing it well) can also be a critical part of this mismatch.

Female workers in Tunisia [18] complain mostly about the lack of recognition of their efforts: at work, their family demands are ignored by a superior only concerned by their performance and efficiency; at home, their job needs are devalued by a husband only preoccupied by his personal comfort and household. They report feelings of failure and develop increasingly a loss of self-esteem, which opens the way to depression after exhaustion.

Lost of sense of community: Violence at work

People thrive in community and function best when they share praise, comfort, happiness and humour with people they like and respect. In addition to emotional exchange and instrumental assistance, this kind of social support reaffirms a person's membership in a group with a shared sense of values. Mutual respect between people is central to a shared sense of community.

Chronic and unresolved conflict with others on the job produces constant negative feelings of frustration and hostility, and reduces the likelihood of social support. Women are generally isolated and poorly integrated in the working world. Historically, the organisation and design of paid labour have tended to be sex-typed. Equipment, tools and spaces used for paid labour have tended to be designed for men [19, 20]. Work scheduling has presumed constant availability of the worker, with no constraints arising from responsibility for child care or elder care [21].

Therefore, women are considered uninvited and more likely to be exposed to experience disrespect, mobbing, bullying or harassment [22].Those who are increasingly choosing to enter traditionally male jobs such as engineering and technical jobs, are at special risk [23]. Such women may feel forced to take risks in order to prove that they are able to do the job and their mental health may be directly affected [24].

Sexual harassment is a major cause of stress for women workers and can produce significant and deleterious effects on work productivity of employees. Victims have reported decreases in work performance, development of stress-related complaints, for example, tension headaches, nervousness and development of physical illnesses. On a long term basis, other victims report switching jobs within their institutions, while others opt to resign from their positions so as to leave behind a hostile work environment. These abuses are rarely reported by women who run the risk of retaliation, ostracism, disbelief by coworkers or employers. On the other hand, legal remedies are uncertain, prolonged, financially and emotionally costly and may exacerbate psychological sequelae.

Unfairness: Gender discrimination, favouritism

Gender discrimination and unequal treatment raise multiple barriers to women's career opportunities and their health protection. A lack of fairness exacerbates burnout in at least two ways. First, the experience of unfair treatment is emotionally upsetting and exhausting. Second, unfairness fuels a deep sense of cynicism about the workplace.

For example, the following two classes of explanation can be given for the gender pay gap. One class of explanation is based on women being disproportionately employed in low-paid jobs – in other words, labour market gender segregation. The other class of explanation is based on discrimination against women – for instance, from employers, trade unions, the law or domestic norms – even when they have similar jobs and productivity levels, for example, in terms of education and experience, to men [17, 25].

An examination of data for 200 occupations (1970–1990) shows that one third of all workers in Finland, Norway and Sweden would have to change occupations to eliminate occupational segregation by sex [26] and a similar figure has been found in the United States of America [27].

Another Swedish study revealed that women and men are often offered different rehabilitation measures for similar work-related health problems. Men, more often than women, receive education in their rehabilitation programme, and women receive rehabilitation benefits for a shorter period of time than men [28].

Again, a similar study in Quebec showed that educational opportunities were more limited for injured women workers and compensation for inability to assume usual household responsibilities was more readily granted for household tasks usually done by men [29]. Even in countries where equality is guaranteed by law, application of occupational health and safety legislation may have discriminatory effects. Swedish and Canadian studies revealed that women and men are often offered different rehabilitation measures for similar work-related health problems. Men are more often offered training, access to a wider variety of new jobs and are offered more help in the home, while women receive rehabilitation benefits for a shorter time [30]. Women may have more difficulty in accessing compensation for their injuries because of discriminatory effects of seemingly neutral criteria [29, 30]. This means that systemic discrimination may be at work even if the legislation appears to be gender neutral. When prevention priorities are determined by compensation costs, women are then less likely to benefit from protective legislation [31].

With the increasing awareness and penalisation of gender discrimination, women suffer more from micro-inequities which are subtle forms of sexual harassment and gender discrimination that 'are not always illegal but negatively impact morale, job performance and opportunities for promotion and training' [32].

Another particular form of gender discrimination is tokenism. It refers to women who are less than 15% of the workforce and are viewed as 'tokens', with each woman standing as a representative of all members of her group. Token positions tend to be highly visible and often stressful [33].

Values: The role conflict

The sixth area of mismatch occurs when there is a conflict between values.

Besides overwork, women experience a role conflict which results from the '...psychological effects of being faced with two or more sets of incompatible (or contradictory) expectations and demands' [34]

It is still the case because most societies, even the most developed, continue to value in women their mothering role, delivering mixed messages to women who are confused about their life's goals, valued roles, priorities and identities.

In a traditional society like Tunisia, a survey among 4000 females aged between 19 and 45 years, revealed that 37% of the respondents considered that paid work does not contribute at all to their social promotion and 6% that paid work devalued their social status. By contrast, half of interviewed women (whatever their age) considered that the social status of a sterile woman is lower than that of a fertile mother. And moreover, one woman out of three considers a mother who did not give birth to a son to be inferior.

In France, too, the primacy of the mothering role is highly reaffirmed. Thus, 'Who is going to care for the children?' asked Laurent Fabius, former Prime Minister, commenting on the candidacy of Ségolène Royal (mother of four children) to the Presidency of the French Republic in 2006!

In Tunisia, similarly, a former Minister of Education declared in 1999: 'Neither at school, nor in offices, females are actually accepted; all happens as if the girl was prepared to get back definitively at home'.

Women feel internally burdened to prove themselves as workers, as wives and mothers. As explained by Freudenberger, another burnout-inducing extreme for a woman is the concept of all-around perfectionism, namely being 'The perfect wife, mother and professional'. He added that 'it's exactly the kind of impossible goal that leads to burnout'.

The risk of burnout is all the more heightened when the woman lacks spousal sympathy, is isolated from extended family members, when she lacks time to form other supportive relationships, to socialise or to enjoy private time and when she has difficulty in finding or keeping high-quality child care.

Gender traditional roles have bedevilled gender comparisons regarding health outcomes by the use of two different conceptual frameworks; in one, men are seen primarily in terms of their occupational role; in the other, women are primarily researched in terms of their family roles; the focus on the primacy of women's family roles has led to their paid work being regarded as an additional role rather than as a structural variable in its own right. The emphasis on women's reproductive health and women's roles as wives and mothers has been particularly evident in the health policies and health research conducted in developed countries. However, as Avotri and Walters [35] study of Ghanaian women showed, the main health concerns women identified were related to psychosocial health problems associated with heavy workloads.

Cultural-bound risk factors: Traditional ideologies, non traditional lives

Women's work is particularly distressing because it is a crucial threat to the male dominance in some traditional societies. Indeed, in Islamic countries, the superiority of males is strictly linked to their duty to maintain their family without any support from the spouse.

It is said in the Holy Book that 'Men are superior to women because Allah has made some of them to excel others and because they spend of their property; the good women are therefore obedient . . . ' (Quran, IV, 34)

The scholars explain that ' . . . Man is the person solely responsible for the complete maintenance of his wife, his family and any other needy relations. It is his duty by Law to assume all financial responsibilities and maintain his dependents adequately . . . woman has no financial responsibilities . . . If she is a wife, her husband is the provider; if she is a mother, it is the son; if she is a daughter, it is the father; if she is a sister; it is the brother, and so on. She is entitled to complete provision and total maintenance by the husband. She does not have to work or share with her husband the family expenses. She is free to retain, after marriage, whatever she possessed before it, and the husband has no right whatsoever to any of her belongings' [36].

With regard to the woman's right to seek employment it should be stated first that Islam regards her role in society as a mother and a wife as the most sacred and essential one [15]. However, there is no decree in Islam which forbids a woman from seeking employment whenever there is a necessity for it, especially in positions which fit her nature and in which society needs her most. Examples of these professions are nursing, teaching (especially for children) and medicine. Moreover, Islam grants women equal rights to contract, to enterprise, to earn and possess independently. Such rights apply to her properties before marriage as well as to whatever she acquires thereafter.

For all these reasons, an amendment to the Tunisian Labor Code came into force in July 1996 to establish the principle of non-discrimination between men and women in all aspects of employment, which assumes equality in respect not only of access to the labour market but also of security within this market in regards to work conditions, time schedules, promotion opportunities, salaries, and so on.

However, and despite the legal framework, work is not yet an established right whereas motherhood and obedience are still a duty!

So, Islamic female workers struggle with another crucial challenge: being independent without endangering their couple by weakening their husband's status. They are entrapped by the confusing messages both to be in the public area as autonomous and achieving and to be in the private sphere as submitted and dependent as in the previous generations of unemployed women!

20.4 Work and women's mental health issues

Research on the relationship between women's social roles and mental health has been equivocal.

The effect of multiple roles on women's psychological wellbeing remains controversial. Although it is well recognised that women's social roles affect their mental health, it is unclear whether the effects are beneficial or detrimental. Traditionally, this research has been conducted within two competing hypotheses: role strain theory proposes that because each person has limited time and energy, women with multiple roles often experience 'role conflict', which results in harmful effects on their mental and physical health. The job strain model as conceptualised by Karasek and Theorell [6] postulates that a combination of high psychological demands with low control at work leads to mental and physical illnesses. The opposing theory suggests that each additional role brings benefits, including increased social contacts and self-esteem, which contribute to better health and greater psychological wellbeing.

More recent research indicates that involvement in each role has both harmful and beneficial effects, and the balance between these varies depending on the characteristics of the role, the specific combination of roles and the socio-economic context of women's lives [37]. Socio-economic status creates different experiences and exposures in daily life and these, in turn, have consequences for women's psychological health. Of particular importance is the finding that as women's education and income levels rise, there is a decline in distress levels. In terms of combinations of roles, there is mixed evidence as to the effects of various combinations on women's psychological wellbeing. Although more roles often protect mental health, certain combinations can also lead to strain.

Studies, mainly from high-income industrialised countries show that women's increased participation in paid employment not only strengthens their social status and their individual and family's financial situations, but also is beneficial to their mental and physical health [38]. The same is true for men.

Although paid employment is generally beneficial for both women's and men's health, work also involves exposures to risks and hazards that can impair health.

These hazards are related to both physical (such as heavy lifting and carrying, repetitive working movements, night work, long hours, violence, noise, vibration, heat, cold, chemicals) and psychosocial exposures (e.g. stress related to high mental demand, speed, lack of control over the way work is done, lack of social support, lack of respect, discrimination, psychological and sexual harassment).

In general, women are more often than men exposed to some psychosocial risk factors at work, such as negative stress, psychological and sexual harassment and monotonous work [39]. Due to their low status in the work hierarchy, women exert less control over their work environment, a condition associated with cardiovascular, mental and musculoskeletal ill health [40]. The combination of paid and unpaid work affects women's health [41].

Consequently, work-related fatigue, repetitive strain injury, infections and mental health problems are more common among women than among men [42, 43].

When comparing men's and women's health, one of the most consistent findings is a higher rate of symptoms among women. The most commonly reported symptoms in women are depressive symptoms, symptoms of bodily tension and chronic pain from muscles and joints. As a matter of fact, in a study among a Swedish rural community with 13 200 inhabitants, Krantz and Ostergren [3] conclude that work related factors, such as non-employment and job strain, and circumstances within the private sphere, such as social network/support, seem equally important for middle aged women's health status.

Cheng *et al.* [44] showed that adverse psychosocial work conditions are important predictors of poor functional status and its decline over time, in a prospective study over four years among a cohort of 21 290 nurses in the USA. This survey revealed that, examined separately low job control, high job demands and low work related social support were associated with poor health status at baseline as well as greater functional declines over the four years follow up period. Examined in combination, women with low job control, high job demands and low work related social support had the greatest functional declines.

Chandola *et al.* [45] examined the effects of multiple roles on health to answer the question whether a combination of work and family roles may be either advantageous (role enhancement) or disadvantageous (role strain) for health. The study was conducted in three countries (UK, Finland and Japan) to compare the effect of work-to-family and family-to-work conflict on mental health within different welfare state arrangements and social norms. They found that both work-to-family and family-to-work conflict affect the mental health of men and women in the three countries, showing that the balance between work and family roles may be important for the mental health of both genders. As regards to the cultural context, Japanese women had the greatest conflict and poorest mental health while Helsinki women had the lowest conflict and best mental health. They explain that the family-friendly work policies in Finland may contribute to their lower levels of conflict and better mental health, especially for women. Correspondingly, the poorer mental health of working Japanese women could be attributable, in part, to their higher levels of work-to-family conflict. The gender stratification of the Japanese labour force, along with traditional gender attitudes to domestic labour, could result in higher levels of work-to-family conflict among Japanese women and consequently poorer mental health.

Tina Hallman *et al.* [46] carried out a study aimed at elucidating patterns concerning women's work, stress and living conditions that might affect their health and the progress of coronary heart disease (CHD). A questionnaire (The Stress Profile) was answered by 538 participants (97 women, 441 men), and a reference group (5308 women, 5177 men), aged 40–65 years. When comparing women's and men's results from the Stress Profile, women generally reported higher levels of stress than men did. Significant differences appeared concerning five areas: work content, workload and control, physical stress reactions, emotional stress reactions and burnout. When comparing women with CHD and healthy matched women, women with CHD reported a significantly higher level of burnout than the healthy matched group.

Soarez et al. [47] assessed the occurrence of low/high burnout among women and the demographic/socio-economic, work, lifestyle and health 'correlates' of high burnout. The sample consisted of 6000 randomly selected women from the general population, of which 3591 participated. The analyses showed that about 21% of the women had high burnout, and compared to those with low burnout, they were more often younger, divorced, blue-collar workers, lower educated, foreigners, on unemployment/retirement/sick-leave, financially strained, used more medication and cigarettes, reported higher work demands and lower control/social support at work, more somatic problems (e.g. pain) and depression. The regression analysis showed that only age, sick-leave, financial strain, medication, work demands, depression and somatic ailments were independently associated with high burnout.

In a review, Gjerdingen et al. [48] compared the distribution of women's work efforts in the areas of paid employment, household chores and childcare, in three countries (USA, Sweden and Netherlands) and addressed the impact of workload on their wellbeing and careers. They showed that heavy workloads may adversely affect women's health, especially in the presence of certain role characteristics (e.g. having a clerical, managerial, professional or executive position or caring for young children). Heavy work responsibilities may also undermine marital happiness, particularly if there is perceived inequity in the way partners share household work.

Artazcos et al. [49] addressed the issues of gender differences in health among married male and female workers and gender inequalities in the relation between family demands and health. They concluded that private changes such as sharing domestic responsibilities, as well as active public policies for facilitating family care are needed in order to reduce gender health inequalities attributable to the unequal distribution of family demands.

The same team [50] carried out similar research in Spain on a sample of 881 men and 400 women, aged 25–64 years, who were married or cohabiting. They found that family demands were not associated with men's health whereas married women who live in family units of more than three members had a higher risk of poor self-perceived health status and of psychosomatic symptoms. Among women, working more than 40 hours a week was also associated with both health indicators and, additionally, with a higher probability of medical visits. And the authors conclude once again that in order to fully understand social determinants of worker's health, besides social class, gender inequalities in the distribution of family responsibilities should be considered.

A Canadian team [37] explored the effects of different role combinations on women's mental health by examining associations with socioeconomic status and differences in women's distress (depressive symptoms, personal stress (role strain) and chronic stress (role strain plus environmental stressors). They showed that women with children, whether single or partnered, had a higher risk of personal stress. Distress, stress and chronic stress of mothers; regardless of employment or marital status, are staggeringly high. For partnered mothers, rates of personal stress and chronic stress were significantly lower among unemployed partnered mothers. Married and partnered mothers reported better mental health than their single counterparts. Lone, unemployed mothers were twice as likely to report a high level of distress compared with other groups. Lone mothers, regardless of employment status, were more likely to report high personal and chronic stress.

Hedman and Herner [51] compiled statistics from broad areas of health, work, reproduction and demography and analysed them for their impact on women's health and wellbeing in Sweden. In this country, women report more sick-leave. The authors concluded that, generally, women report less feeling of wellbeing than men in Sweden, probably because of the mean three extra hours of domestic work they do compared to men.

Developing countries

In Tunisia, Bouattour *et al.* [18] carried out a study among 1100 subjects on extended sick-leave (over one year) assessed for fitness-to-work. Seventy-three per cent were women and 13% of them had given up working for more than three years whereas men were only 6.5%.

They all were clerical, working in teaching and healthcare. They had a similar work experience, 15 years on average. The single significant difference was that women were far more likely to take care of dependent relatives (13.4% versus 4.1%). As regards the clinical characteristics, women have less personal history of mental disorders (30.8%) than men (42.8%).

The clinical picture in women was mainly featured by headaches, exhaustion, dysphoria, irritability with anger attacks, control impulse with violence and assaultive behaviour against children, difficulties in concentrating and forgetfulness, sleep disturbances and feelings of powerlessness and pessimism. They reported consistently a loss of sense of value and meaning ascribed to their existence and permanent feelings of guilt to never do anything properly, either at work or at home. In addition, marital conflicts were associated with depression in 57% of women. Concerning the triggering factors, 80% of women reported a family problem whilst 58% of men incriminated health or professional stressors.

During the assessment, most women declared a 'job phobia' arguing that they had burnt all their energy and become indefinitely incapable of working. They indeed have never recovered despite the many antidepressant treatments administered and each previous attempt to get back to work failed.

Ahmad-Nia [52] analysed the impact of work on mothers' health in Tehran (Iran) through a survey conducted among a representative sample of 1065 working (710) and non-working mothers (355) in 1998. Statistically significant differences between working and non-working women were not found in Tehran. It is argued that this is a result of the counter-balance of the positive and negative factors associated with paid work, such as increased stress on one hand and self-esteem on the other. Iranian society's particular socio-cultural climate has contributed to this finding, with its dominant gender-role ideology; the priority and extra weight placed on women's traditional roles as wives and mothers, and the remarkably influential impact of husbands' attitudes on women's health.

Sexual harassment

During the last decade an increasing number of studies have indicated adverse health consequences of sexual harassment at work [53–55]. Sexual harassment may result in guilt and shame, physical and mental health problems (anxiety, tension, irritability, depression, sleeplessness, fatigue and headaches, eczema, irritable bowel syndrome and other gastro-intestinal complaints, urinary tract infections, sexual dysfunctions, substance use and abuse and dependence) which in turn may lead to absenteeism, sick leave and reduced efficiency at work. Family, friendships and interpersonal work relationships are also often adversely affected [33, 56].

20.5 Management issues

Treatment issues

Treatment of women's work problems involves carefully evaluating the complex interplay, in each individual patient, among intrapsychic, developmental, family, sociocultural, workplace and other environmental factors; career life cycle issues should also be taken into account; career choice, career development, balancing between career and family or personal choices and midlife issues [33].

Group therapies in the workplace have been shown to be useful in providing feedback and support. Within these groups, people shared experiences with their peers, got a lot of gripes off their chests and received praise and understanding from the psychiatrists.

Preventive issues: Special treatment for women?

Recently, an increasing interest in quality of life issues and in better balancing personal and work lives for both genders has emerged. In order to enable workers to develop both sets of work and private skills, the work-family boundary will need to be relaxed and work redesigned so that all workers can better integrate work and personal life. That means changing the traditional image of an 'ideal' worker as someone with no outside responsibilities and with firm boundaries between work and personal life; it means regarding workers who blend public and private, work and family, rational and emotional, masculine and feminine; government policies need to support these changes.

Some employers have tried to help individual workers deal with workplace stress through stress management training programmes. Other employers have developed packages of 'family friendly' benefits, such as flexi-time, child care on site, paid parental and family leave, sabbaticals, part-time/shared-time positions and referrals for elderly care and child care.

Other employers and researchers seek ways to redesign the work setting more creatively so that all workers, not only women, can better integrate work and personal life. Redefining work-family boundaries, organisations have valued and rewarded skills associated with the traditional, usually Caucasian, male, public domains (task mastery, technical competence, autonomous action, competitiveness, linear reasoning) and have generally devalued skills associated with the private, traditionally female, domain (empathy, support, interdependence, contextual reasoning) [33].

Forensic issues

Psychiatrists and other mental health professionals may be misused by employers to retaliate against women who report sexual discrimination or harassment and regard them as mentally ill [33]. They have to be very cautious and systematically refer to their ethical framework. Occupational health policies and legislation should be advocated to promote and protect women's mental health in two key areas: the treatment of sex differences and gender segregation in the working world and the methods for handling discrimination, including sexual harassment.

20.6 Conclusion

Work plays an important part in determining women's and men's relative wealth, power and prestige. When differences in men's and women's working conditions and occupational positions are controlled in the analysis, the results revealed that women reported more work-related ill-health than men.

Women's work-related health cannot be understood without adding other frameworks related to gender roles and women's work in the domestic sphere. Workforce studies repeatedly document that paid employment is associated with better physical and mental health and less psychological distress for women. The fourth European Working Conditions Survey (EWCS, 53), reveal persistent gender inequalities. Such disparities include differences in working hours, occupation, economic sector and work-related health risks. Through their suffering, working women call for better integration of personal and professional lives for both genders.

Fostering a good work-life balance will improve the possibilities for women and men to enjoy both work and family, without being forced to choose between the two.

References

1. World Health Organization (2000) Women's Mental Health: An Evidence Based Review, Geneva.
2. World Bank (2001) *Engendering Development*, Oxford University Press, New York.
3. Krantz, G. and Östergren, P.O. (2000) Common symptoms in middle aged women: their relation to employment status, psychosocial work conditions and social support in a Swedish setting. *Journal of Epidemiology and Community Health*, **54**, 192–99.

4. Maslach, C., Schaufeli, W.B. and Leiter, M.P. (2001) Job burnout. *Annual Review of Psychology*, **52**, 397–422.

5. Maslach, C. and Jackson, S.E. (1986) *The Maslach Burnout Inventory*, Manual Edition, Consulting Psychologists Press, Palo Alto.

6. Karasek, R. and Theorell, T. (1990) *Healthy Work: Stress, Productivity, and the Reconstruction or Working Life*, Basic Books, New York.

7. Maslach C. (2006) Understanding job burnout, in *Stress and Quality of Working Life: Current Perspectives in Occupational Health* (eds A.M. Rossi, P.L. Perewwé and S.L. Sauter), Information Age Publishing, Greenwich, pp. 37–51.

8. Van der Ploeg, E., Dorresteijn, S. and Kleber, R. (2003) Critical incidents and chronic stressors at work: their impact on forensic doctors. *Journal of Occupational Health Psychology*, **8** (2), 157–66.

9. Posig, M. and Kickul, J. (2003) Extending our understanding of human burnout: test of an integrated model in no service occupations. *Journal of Occupational Health Psychology*, **8** (1), 3–19.

10. Leiter, M. and Robichaud, L. (1997) Relationships of occupational hazards with burnout: an assessment of measures and models. *Journal of Occupational Health Psychology*, **2** (1), 35–44.

11. Westman, M. and Eden, D. (1997) Effects of a respite from work on burnout: vacation relief and fade-out. *Journal of Applied Psychology*, **84** (4), 516–27.

12. Brown, C. and O'Brien, K. (1998) Understanding stress and burnout in shelter workers. *Professional Psychology: Research and Practice*, **29** (4), 383–85.

13. Lee, R. and Ashforth, B. (1996) A meta-analytic examination of the correlates of the three dimensions of job burnout. *Journal of Applied Psychology*, **81** (2), 123–33.

14. Freudenberger, H.J. and North, G. (1985) *Women's Burnout: How to Spot it, How to Reverse it and How to Prevent it*, R.R. Donnelley & Sons Company, Virginia.

15. Douki, S., Nacef, F., Benzineb, S. and Halbreich, U. (2007) Women's mental health in the Muslim world: cultural, religious and social issues. *Journal of Affective Disorders*, **102** (1–3), 177–89.

16. Reid, J. and Hardy, M. (1999) Multiple roles and well-being among midlife women: testing role strain and role enhancement theories. *Journals of Gerontology Series B: Psychological Sciences and Social Sciences*, **54** (6), S329–38.

17. Plantenga, J. and Remery, C. (2007) The Gender Pay Gap: Origins and Policy Responses. A Comparative Review of 30 European Countries, Office for Official Publications of the European Communities, Luxembourg.

18. Bouattour, M. (2001) Troubles Mentaux et Congés de Longue Durée, Faculté de Médecine de Tunis. Doctoral thesis in French.

19. Courville, J., Vézina, N. and Messing, K. (1992) Analyse des facteurs ergonomiques pouvant entraîner l'exclusion des femmes du tri des colis postaux. *Le Travail Humain*, **55**, 119–34.

20. Chatigny, C., Seifert, A.M. and Messing, K. (1995) Repetitive strain in non-repetitive work: a case study. *International Journal of Occupational Safety and Ergonomics*, **1** (1), 42–51.

21. Prévost, J. and Messing, K. (2001) Stratégies de conciliation d'un horaire de travail variable avec des responsabilités familiales. *Le Travail Humain*, **64**, 119–43.

22. Messing, K. and Östlin, P. (2006) Gender Equality, Work and Health. A Review of the Evidence, WHO, Geneva.

23. Asselin, S. (2003) Professions: convergence entre les sexes? Sociodemographic data at a glance (eng) Données sociodémographiques en bref. **7** (3), 6–8.

24. Messing, K. and Elabidi, D. (2003) Desegregation and occupational health: how male and female hospital attendants collaborate on work tasks requiring physical effort. *Policy and Practice in Health and Safety*, **1** (1), 83–103.

25. Grimshaw, D. and Rubery, J. (2007) Undervaluing Women's Work, Equal Opportunities Commission Working Paper, No. 53, Manchester.

26. Melkas, H. and Anker, R. (2001) Occupational Segregation by Sex in Nordic Countries: An Empirical Investigation, in Women, Gender and Work (ed. F.M. Loutfi), International Labour Office, Geneva.

27. Tomaskovic-Devey, D. (1993) *Gender and Racial Inequality at Work*, ILR Press, Ithaca.

28. Burell G. (2002). Gender Differences in Rehabilitation Programmes. A Case of Cardiovascular Rehabilitation, in Gender and Socioeconomic Inequalities in Health. (eds S Wamala and J Lynch), Studentlitteratur, Lund.

29. Lippel, K. (1999) Workers' compensation and stress: gender and access to compensation. *International Journal of Law and Psychiatry*, **22** (1), 79–89.

30. Lippel, K. (2003) Compensation for musculo-skeletal disorders in Quebec: systemic discrimination against women workers? *International Journal of Health Services*, **33** (2), 253–82.

31. Messing, K. and Boutin, S. (1997) La reconnaissance des conditions difficiles dans les emplois des femmes et les instances gouvernementales en santé et en sécurité du travail. *Relations Industrielles/ Industrial Relations*, **52** (2), 333–62.

32. Bernstein A.E. and Lenhart, S.A. (1993) *The psychodynamic treatment of women.* American Psychiatric Publishing.

33. Shrier, D.K. (2002) Career and workplace issues, in *Women's Mental Health, A Comprehensive Textbook*, Guilford Press, New York, pp. 527–41, 638.

34. Unger, R. and Crawford, M. (1996). *Women and gender: A feminist psychology.* New York: McGraw-Hill.

35. Avotri, J.Y. and Walters, V. (1999). "You just look at our work and see if you have any freedom on earth": Ghanaian women's accounts of their work and their health. *Social Science and Medicine*, **48** (9), 1123–33.

36. Badawi, J. (1971) The Status of Women in Islam (1971). Al Ittihad, vol. 8, N 2, september 1971, The American trust publication, PO box 38 Plainfield 46168.

37. Maclean, H., Glynn, K. and Ansara D. (2004) Multiple roles and women's mental health in Canada. *BMC Women's Health*, **4** (Suppl 1), S3. Published online 2004 August 25. doi: 10.1186/1472-6874-4-S1-S3.

38. Waldron, I., Weiss, C.C. and Hughes, M.E. (1998) Interacting effects of multiple roles on women's health. *Journal of Health and Social Behavior*, **39**, 216–36.

39. Arcand, R. and Labrèche, F. (2000) Environnement de Travail et Santé, in Enquête sociale et de santé 1998, Institut de la statistique du Québec, Québec, pp. 525–70.

40. Hall, E. (1989) Gender, work control and stress: a theoretical discussion and an empirical test. *International Journal of Health Services*, **19**, 725–45.

41. Brisson, C., Laflamme, N., Moisan, J. *et al.* (1999) Effect of family responsibilities and job strain on ambulatory blood pressure among white-collar women. *Psychosomatic Medicine*, **61**, 205–13.

42. Östlin, P. (2002) Gender Inequalities in Health: The Significance of Work, in Gender and Socioeconomic Inequalities in Health (eds S. Wamala and J. Lynch), Studentlitteratur, Lund.

43. Artazcoz, L. and Artieda, L. (2004) Combining job and family demands and being healthy: what are the differences between men and women? *European Journal of Public Health*, **14** (1), 43–48.

44. Cheng, Y., Kawachi, I., Coakley, E.H. *et al.* (2000) Association between psychosocial work characteristics and health functioning in American women: prospective study. *British Medical Journal*, **320** (7247), 1432–36.

45. Chandola, T., Martikainen, P., Bartley, M. and Lahelma, E. (2004) Does conflict between home and work explain the effect of multiple roles on mental health? A comparative study of Finland, Japan, and the UK? *International Journal of Epidemiology*, **33**, 884–93.

46. Hallman, T., Burell, G., Setterlind, S. *et al.* (2001) Psychosocial risk factors for coronary heart disease, their importance compared with other risk factors and gender differences in sensitivity. *Journal of Cardiovascular Risk*, **8** (1), 39–49.

47. Soares, J.J.F., Grossi, G. and Sundin, Ö. (2007) Burnout among women: associations with demographic/socio-economic, work, life-style and health factors. *Archives of Women's Mental Health*, **10** (2): 61–71.

48. Gjerdingen, D., McGovern, P., Bekker, M. *et al.* (2000) Women's work roles and their impact on health, well-being, and career: comparisons between the United States, Sweden, and The Netherlands. *Women Health*, **31** (4), 1–20.

49. Artazcoz, L. and Borrell, C. (2001) Gender inequalities in health among workers: the relation with family demands. *Journal of Epidemiology and Community Health*, **55** (9), 639–47.

50. Artazcoz, L., Artieda, L., Borrell, C., Cortès, I., Benach, J. and García, V. (2004) Combining job and family demands and being healthy: what are the differences between men and women? *European Journal of Public Health*, **14** (1), 43–48.

51. Hedman B., Herner E. (1988) Women's health and women's work in health services: what statistics tell us. *Women Health*, **13** (3–4), 9–34.

52. Ahmad-Nia, S. (2002) Women's work and health in Iran: a comparison of working and non-working mothers. *Social Science and Medicine*, **54** (5), 753–65.

53. Kauppinen, K. (1998) Sexual Harassment in the Workplace, in WHO. Women and Occupational Health, World Health Organization, Geneva.

54. Kisa, A. and Dziegielewski, S.F. (1996) Sexual harassment of female nurses in a hospital in Turkey. *Health Services Management Research*, **9** (4), 243–53.

55. Nicolson, P. (1996) *Gender, Power and Organisation: A Psychological Perspective*, Routledge, London.

56. Wilson, F.M. (1995) *Organisational Behaviour and Gender*, McGraw-Hill Book Company, London.

Further reading

Burchell, B., Fagan, C., O'Brien, C. and Smith, M. (2007) Working conditions in the European Union: The Gender Perspective, Office for Official Publications of the European Communities, Luxembourg.

21

Globalisation and women's mental health: Cutting edge information

Unaiza Niaz[1,2]

[1]*The Psychiatric Clinic & Stress Research Center, Karachi, Pakistan*
[2]*University of Health Sciences, Lahore, Pakistan*

According to the 1998 World Health Report: 'Women's health is inextricably linked to their status in society. It benefits from equality, and suffers from discrimination'. Today, the status and wellbeing of innumerable millions of women worldwide remain tragically low [1]. Women constitute more than 70% of the world's poor [2] and carry the triple burden of productive, reproductive and caring work. Even in developed countries, lone mothers with children are the largest groups of people living in poverty [3] and are at especially high risk for poor physical and mental health [4, 5]. Gender must be taken into account in looking at the way income disparities, inequalities and poverty in society, impacts on mental health.

21.1 Concept and process of globalisation

Globalisation is described as 'a new context, for a new connectivity among economic actors and activists throughout the world'. Globalisation has been made possible by progressive dismantling of barriers to trade and capital mobility, together with fundamental technological advances and steadily declining costs of transportation, communication and computing. Its integrative logic seems inexorable, its momentum irresistible [6].

Contemporary Topics in Women's Mental Health   Edited by Chandra, Herrman, Fisher, Kastrup,
© 2009 John Wiley & Sons, Ltd   Niaz, Rondón and Okasha

The process of globalisation is not homogeneous; it affects the economic systems and the social groups differently. Although this process has been spread throughout the world, it has a judgement that interferes with the limits; it has created and accentuated differences, deepening inequalities within and between nations.

It was understood that globalisation had the potential to increase prosperity in all countries; but it led to major challenges for the developing world. Existing inequalities between nations had made it difficult for this potential of prosperity to reach the poor women, poverty having a crippling effect on the advancement of women in particular. The vulnerable, high risk groups clearly are the worst sufferers of globalisations, with a negative impact on their mental health.

21.2 Gendered effects of globalisation

The gendered effects of global, national and local mal-governance must be seen in the context of overlapping domains of poverty and the widening gap between the rich and the poor in the context of escalating violence in developing and under developed countries. Mal-governance or poor governance, in the context of globalisation has gendered effects, with particular implications for women. Women's struggles for human rights generally, have been more pronounced with regard to violence against women than they have been concerned with economic rights.

Worldwide there are increasing intra-state conflicts than at any other time in human history, and the social fabric in many countries has been disintegrating, thus leading to increasing violence against women and girls. Undeniably, the use of gender-based violence, including rape and forced pregnancy, had been an increasingly appalling feature of ethnic conflicts.

As a result of different dimensions of global restructuring and the policies involved at the national, international and corporate levels, globalisation has led to an increase in the international movements of goods and services, capital and, increasingly, labour as people migrate for employment thus are induced to trafficking. The globalisation of criminal networks, the trafficking in women and children, drug trafficking and the arms trade have risen as problems without borders. Globalisation has also spread HIV/AIDS which has decimated entire communities and taken their productive members, leaving behind AIDS orphans in the care of the very old.

Globalisation produces new forms of commoditisation, to the extent of commoditising life itself. One of the consequences is human trafficking, the two groups most affected being women and children. Human trafficking involves 'moving men, women and children from one place to another and placing them in conditions of forced labour'. The practise includes various forms of forced labour, forced sex work, domestic servitude, unsafe agricultural labour, sweatshop labour and various forms of modern-day slavery.

A glaring example of the gendered implications for women, of the global and national governance agendas vis-à-vis the oil-producing areas of Nigeria, are worth mentioning. At the National Tribunal on Violence against Women (March 2001), women testified recounting their experiences of rape and degradation by soldiers and security agents, as happened in the town of Choba in 1999. *In the 1994 oil workers' strike, oil company employees 'refused to work in an impossible environment where murder, rape and looting were the order of the day'* [7–12].

In Nigeria, trafficking of children takes place within national borders as well as within the West African region. Nigerian women are most commonly trafficked across international borders for commercial sex work in Europe. Trafficking, as Orphant notes, has become 'big business', constituting the third-largest source of profits for organised crime, after drugs and guns, and generating billions of dollars each year. *As many as 20 000 Nigerian women are estimated to be engaged in commercial sex work in Italy. Most are from Edo state, but some come from other States in the South East and South-South zones* [7].

In South Asia [13] increase in women's employment is thought to modify the balance of power within the household. By bringing home income, women should attain a greater say in household expenditure decisions with respect to both utilisation and human capital investment. However practically, paid employment does not always mean empowerment for women in the health sector. Increasing female wages do not always result in positive benefits for women. They are excluded through traditional custom from deciding upon the use of their monetary contributions to the family budget, consequently the notion of family bargaining that states that an equal contribution to the household leads to equal power within the household does not hold for the working women at present.

21.3 The impact of globalisation and liberalisation on women's health

Social and cultural factors hinder women's economic equality

Social and economic inequality is detrimental to the health of any society. In South Asia, the society is diverse, multicultural, overpopulated and undergoing rapid but unequal economic growth. For instance, in India [14] there are obviously tensions within classes and communities. Gender inequalities permeate through the entire spectrum of society. The socio-cultural determinants of women's health have played a leading role in the perseverance and strengthening of health inequalities. Women's position in the family and society is partly based on matters like the birth of a son, restrictions on physical mobility, dowry, marriage, divorce, inheritance, literacy and education, work participation rates, dual burden. Working women still do not command equal power and rights in society.

Feminisation of labour

The effects of globalisation have been known to increase labour market flexibility, of employment and the proliferation of 'contingent' jobs which are typically temporary and unskilled. The feminisation of labour occurring as a part of the process of flexiblisation of labour has increasingly pushed women out of the core workforce and into a marginalised group of workers, consisting of part-time, temporary, casual and sub-contracted labour. In India, in the process of making the labour market informal; the labour force is affected broadly in two ways. Work is pushed out of the factories and formal work situations into small workshops (sweatshops), the homes and informal situations. Secondly, the workers who remain in the factories or in formal work situations are governed by looser contracts and have fewer social security benefits. New working conditions which include sub contract, flexible work, piece-rating, part timing and scheduling has marginalised them. As a consequence, they are not recognised as regular workers and their basic rights are not guaranteed.

According to [15] Vandana Shiva, an Indian eco-feminist and scholar,

> Globalization along with the support of organizations such as the WB & IMF has created slave wages. These wages are not necessarily the result of "unjust" societies, but of the fact that global trade devalues the worth of people's lives and work.

21.4 Education and empowerment in women

The most vital empowerment in women is intellectual, educational and skill development. Education of women, rather than emphasis entirely on economic activity, should be the long-term goal on women's empowerment.

This empowerment is enduring and economically viable and self-sustaining. These are crucial elements of women's empowerment which are bound to have long lasting effect and influence the cultural fabric of the society. Women's development is restricted due to lack of education, skills, training, thus further driving them towards the pressures of economics and society, where they get into exploitable positions; domestic servants and sex workers clearly prove this point.

Education enhances social and economic development of women

The potential benefits of education are always present, but female education often has a stronger and more significant impact than male education. In addition to the instrumental value of education, there are strong arguments for treating education as having an intrinsic value, following the perception of poverty as capability deprivation rather than income poverty.

Female education affects the way decisions are made in the household and have therefore great effects on subjects like, children's health, and children's (especially girls') school attendance and fertility. In gender-stratified cultures, even educated women expect to be excluded from making decisions, related to family finances [16].

The manifold benefits of female education are cumulative

1. In that it is reinforced over time, with the advantages transmitted across generations. Besides getting more productive and healthier, educated women are also more likely to educate their own children.

2. Education enables people to develop the skills for innovation leading to increase in productivity. In order to result in economic growth; the economy must be able to absorb the labour that will be the effect of the rising levels of productivity.

3. Regardless of region, culture and developmental level, well-educated women are observed to have fewer children than uneducated women. [17].

4. Fertility is affected by education, through influences on the supply and demand for children. Education influences supply by delaying the age of marriage, increasing the use of contraception, shortening the duration of breast-feeding and improving maternal and infant health and nutrition. Due to these effects, the final impact of education on the supply of children is ambiguous. The demand side includes value shifts towards a norm of fewer children and greater female autonomy, signifying less dependency on children.

21.5 The United Nations' and World Bank's approach to women's education

James D. Wolfensohn, President of the World Bank [18: ii] states that:

> All agree that the single most important key to development and poverty alleviation is education. This must start with universal primary education for girls and boys equally, as well as an open and competitive system of secondary and tertiary education. . . . Adult education, literacy, and lifelong learning must be combined with the fundamental recognition that education of women and girls is central to the process of development . . . pre-school education must be given its full weight . . . developments in science and technology and knowledge transfer offer a unique possibility to countries to catch up with more technologically advanced ones [18: i].

Kofi A. Annan, Secretary-General of the United Nations [19 : 4] believed that:

> Education is a human right with immense power to transform. On its foundation rest the cornerstone of freedom, democracy and sustainable human development [19].

The two quotations illustrate the difference between the World Bank and the UN in their approaches to education. The World Bank considers education an instrument in the surge for development and poverty alleviation. Therefore the World Bank finds it important to promote all levels of education. The education of girls is recognised as central *to the process of development*. Furthermore, considering the return on investment in education, the World Bank focuses on countries with an environment of good governance, political and macroeconomic stability, and broadly equitable access to social services [19:8].

In contrast, the UN considers education a human right. The UN also emphasises education's power to transform. But the basic approach is the perception of education as a human right, resulting in a plan more focused on achieving universal primary education for all, and reaching the targets of closing the gender gap in enrolment rates, agreed upon in the Dakar Framework for Action.

21.6 The global and local intersection of feminism in muslim societies

Review of the empirical studies of the Islamic Republic of Iran and the Republic of Azerbaijan [20], as well as on a review of studies of several other societies in Muslim societies in the South, is interesting. Through a brief review of Iran and a few references to post-Soviet Azerbaijan, one can see the interplay between local and global factors in shaping the course of women's movements and feminism. Attention apparently is paid primarily to the positive impact of two specific aspects of globalisation on women's movements and feminism in these two societies: the international human rights regime (comprised of the United Nations and international nongovernmental organisations such as Amnesty International and Human Rights Watch) and global feminism (comprised of feminist discourses, the international women's movement and transnational feminist networks).

Geo-political scenario's and globalisation

In colonial and postcolonial studies of Muslim societies, the gender- and class-based differential impacts of colonialism (in countries like Egypt, Syria, Iraq) or of Western hegemony (in countries that were never colonised, such as Iran, Turkey, Afghanistan) have been extensively studied. On women's rights movement and feminism also, colonialism or Western domination left contradictory impacts [21].

The external/global factor, due to the much more deeply penetrating and transformative processes of globalisation, is distinct from the colonial system of the past. Globalisation, is replete with contradictions, it is more like the Industrial Revolution in its impact on societies. Its interventions reach directly into daily life as well as economies, institutions of governance and world order [22, 23]. Because of increasing globalisation, no gender regime and therefore no women's movement in any locality (country or community) can be studied and understood without taking global influences into account. An obvious, recently illuminated case in point is the situation of women in Afghanistan. Women's status and rights in Afghanistan cannot be accounted for without understanding the interaction between the local (history, geography, geopolitics, political economy, culture and Afghan women's own agency and struggles) and the global or international factors, including the intervention of the superpowers (the Soviet Union and the United States), the regional powers (including Saudi Arabia, Pakistan and Iran) and the consequent interventions of international human/women's rights groups and feminist networks. Hence effects of globalisation, along with the local factors are irrelevant to these countries at present.

In the Muslim world, the geo-political scenarios along with the global influences have resulted in complex interactions and diverse results. For instance in the South, Iran, has been isolated globally by the monetary sanctions imposed on them. Therefore, effects of economic globalisation are not so significant as the local factors. In Iran women's movements escalated due to financial stressors and they entered the mainstream of economic activities and therefore they became significant and valuable contributors in society. Similarly in post Soviet Azerbaijan the interplay between local and global factors shaped the course of women's movements and feminist activities. Women in these two societies are evidently assertive, spirited and vocal in the expression and persistent in their struggles for their rights in society. Hence one can say that there is a positive impact on two aspects of globalisation on women's movements and feminism in these two societies. Undoubtedly the indigenous factors mentioned earlier played a significant major role in the positive impact on women's status in these societies rather than the effects of globalisation.

Globalisation and 'global feminism'

Globalisation processes, in particular since the 1970s, have affected feminist mobilisation for change in many different societies. Feminist interventions, in turn, have aimed to affect the parameters and course of globalisation processes [24]. The increasing globalisation and incorporation of the world through international trade, migration, faster and less expensive transportation, and new electronic communication and information technology, have led to a situation in which a growing number of women and men belong to more than one community. Communities and group identities are overlapping and de-territorialising, and a growing number of individuals who become multicultural and multilingual are adopting more fluid and multiple identities [25, 26] Globalisation is accompanied by an increase of consciousness of the world as a whole [27].

This and other effects of globalisation have important implications for gender relations and women's status in all societies. Giddens, for example, points to the indirect impact of global processes on social pressure for democratisation in the form of 'the expansion of social reflexivity and de-traditionalisation' [22]. As they become better informed about new and varied political alternatives in the world, populations become less likely to accept traditional models of political and gender regimes. Globalisation 'allows for the subversive possibility of women seeing beyond the local to the global' [28].

Even those who never physically leave their communities of origin are more likely now to evaluate their own lives by placing their rights, options and restrictions in a comparative and global perspective [29] Influences and issues framed in a global context can encourage the reflexive analysis of localised traditions and behaviour patterns and lead to the construction of new social relationships [30].

Gender differentially affects the power over these socioeconomic determinants, their access to resources, and their status, roles, options and treatment in society. Gender has significant explanatory power regarding differential susceptibility and exposure to mental health risks and differences in mental health outcomes. Gender differences in rates of overall mental disorder, including rare disorders such as schizophrenia and bipolar disorders, are negligible.

However, highly significant gender differences exist for depression, anxiety and somatic complaints that affect more than 20% of the population in established economies. Depression accounts for the largest portion of the burden associated with all the mental and neurological disorders. It is predicted to be the second leading cause of global burden of disease by 2020.

In many countries of the South-East Asia region, the mental and social wellbeing of women is at a low level mainly because of the socioeconomic factors. Women are second-rate citizens and are denied many basic rights. Access to healthcare is often denied to them. Due to a large family's poverty, illiteracy and the number of children problems multiply. Abuse of women, attitudes towards the female child, domestic violence and female infanticide are other aspects of the spectrum not auguring well for their wellbeing.

Women and common mental disorders

From the perspective of women and mental health, the key epidemiological finding is the much-replicated association of female gender and Common Mental Disorders (CMDs) such as depression and anxiety. Both community-based studies and studies of treatment seekers indicate that women are, on average, two to three times at greater risk of being affected by CMD [31, 32]. The obvious question thrown up by these findings is the reasons for this apparent vulnerability, and its significance. There are a number of potential factors, which may make women more vulnerable to depression. Davar has reviewed this issue in detail in a recent book on the mental health of women in India [33]. Some of the implications of the greater vulnerability of women to CMD are considered below.

There is considerable evidence demonstrating that stressful life events are closely associated with depression and such events are more common in the lives of women [34, 35]. Thus, women are far more likely to be victims of violence in their homes. The multiple roles played by women such as child-bearing and child-rearing, running the family home, caring for sick relatives and, in an increasing proportion of families, earning income, may lead to considerable stress. The reproductive roles of women, such as their expected role of bearing children, the consequences of infertility and the failure to produce a male child have been linked to wife-battering and female suicide [35, 36]. Women are far more likely to be denied educational and occupational opportunities and access to appropriate healthcare.

The impact of mental health problems also shows a gender differential. For example, whereas women were required to be the primary carers if their husbands were mentally ill, it was their own families that were responsible for their care if they were to become ill. Women with mental health problems are less likely to receive appropriate healthcare when sick and when they do seek help, a gender bias ensures that symptoms are taken less seriously than they are for men [35, 37].

Furthermore, the negative effects of globalisation and economic reform on public health are likely to hit women harder than men; for example, since the economic reforms and subsequent crisis in South-East Asia, there has been a rise in the incidence of reported domestic violence, rape and alcohol abuse [38] Indeed, 'it is not surprising that the health of so many women is compromised from time to time. Rather, what is more surprising is that stress-related health problems do not affect more women' [36].

21.7 Other impacts of globalisation

Healthcare: Accessibility and affordability

The economy is globally strained to the utmost under the challenges of globalisation, and most of the countries are finding it difficult to bear the burden of necessary healthcare expenses. The privatisation of healthcare has increased, with globalisation. For instance in countries like Great Britain, tremendous changes have been observed over the years; tourists from around the world have abused the National Health Service. Thus, these changes along with inflation, have forced healthcare in UK to be curtailed. Healthcare is now profit-driven. When there is a drive to derive a profit from healthcare, it ceases being a basic right and a basic social service. It becomes a privilege unreachable to the poorer segments of the population, enjoyed only by those who have resources. Also the spiralling costs of medicines are a growing barrier to healthcare. In developing countries if the country's economy has to fight an unequal battle with the developed countries in the international market, its society is doubly burdened by the inequities suffered by women, and then again by the effects of this unfavourable competition. The imposition of user charges and high costs of prescription drugs has denied access to many. The weaker sections, especially the women, are denied the physical care they deserve. Women themselves place their health needs last when cost is an issue, seeking medical care too late or not at all.

Social implications

Social development indicators include improved health and education such as declining infant mortality, rising literacy rates, reduced fertility. One most significant question is whether economic development leads to social development, particularly in ways that allow women to close the gap with men in measures such as health and education. There are large gender gaps in the education enrolment rates, indicating that cultural factors play an important role besides just economic development. Though in many Western countries women have higher access to higher education than men – even migrant women attain higher educational levels. The mixture of corporate capitalism and Western culture models is dissolving family and community social controls as witnessed by higher rates of family violence, rape, divorce and family breakdown.

Family is a strong social security mesh in most developing countries, particularly in South Asia. It has been a cultural norm to take care of the elderly. However, breaking up of the traditional joint family system and erosion of social values has made women more vulnerable in respect to their health status. They suffer from neglect, loneliness, alienation and poor nutrition status apart from physical ailments.

Grameeen Bank's experience of economic empowerment of women in Bangladesh has provided a strong evidence of economic independence leading to changes in social perceptions and roles [39, 40].

Globalisation has not ensured a good quality of life for the majority of South Asian women but has reinforced the existing gender inequalities. The Beijing platform while recognising the gender disparities in access to healthcare had noted 'women have different and unequal access to and use of basic health resources, including primary health services for prevention and treatment of childhood diseases, malnutrition, anaemia, and so on. Women's health is also affected by gender bias in the health system and by the provision of inadequate and inappropriate health services to women'. This access is further complicated due to gender differences at all levels. It is necessary to carefully filter cultural norms and biases, tackle poverty, improve literacy and increase consciousness for a girl child to be valued as highly as a boy.

Women's empowerment has to be seen in a 'relational context', for instance, obstacles to women's empowerment cannot be understood without a clear idea of the relationships, roles, responsibilities and inequalities between men and women. There are many dimensions to women's empowerment including personal, collective, global and national as well as social, economic and political. It is also imperative to position specific understandings of empowerment in day-to-day contexts realising that the concrete reality of women's lives differs in different regions of the world. The capability approach to a person's wellbeing would, therefore, entail assessing that person's ability to achieve various valuable functions and the ability to choose from a combination of alternatives as to how they lead their life.

There is a dire need for regulatory frameworks designed to protect women from the negative effects of globalisation with regards to health and safety, occupational standards, and so on. Governments should place restrictions to privatisation of public healthcare services and further ensure that adequate infrastructure is in place for women to reach these services. In regions where there is no adequate infrastructure, women should not be deprived of access to healthcare.

Urbanisation

The population distribution urbanisation, and internal migration and development, indicate that, strikingly, future population growth would be absorbed almost entirely by urban areas in developing countries [41]. From now until 2050, the urban population in developed countries would change little, remaining at about 1 billion, yet the urban population worldwide would continue rising, from 3.3 billion today, to well over 6 billion in 2050. Africa and Asia, currently the least urbanised regions, would have the most urban dwellers by 2030, with the urban population in those regions expected to double within a single generation. Urban growth would also continue in Latin America and the Caribbean, and in more developed regions, but at a slower pace. That wave of urbanisation was happening mostly in developing countries with very large increases occurring very rapidly.

Women's job opportunities and urbanisation

Renay Weiner (South Africa) [42] observed that the historical repression of the informal sector in South Africa, along with strict influx control policies, have shaped both the nature of activities as well as the development of the informal sector in the urban areas, thus tending to influence the concentration of women in certain activities: hawking; petty trade; commercial sex work and 'shebeening' (home-based trade in alcohol, entertainment, etc.). Fostering a more supportive environment in favour of women in the informal sector and a legal framework to facilitate women's entrepreneurship is vital to improve self-esteem and improve their mental health.

The rapidly changing cultural values and societal transformation, has a definite impact on the lifestyle of the working women in urban areas in Pakistan [43]. Women are entering the male job market, and holding senior managerial and executive positions. The women bankers, judges, scientists, politicians and business entrepreneurs are common in most of the large cities. The number of working women and industrial workers continues to rise, as they are needed in expanding textiles, garment, food processing and pharmaceutical industries.

Women' mental health issues in Pakistan like elsewhere in the world are depressive illnesses and anxiety disorders, sexual harassment, and so on. But the major social stressors are unique for Pakistan (and in some South Asian countries) are: (i) unreasonable pressure from parents and society to get married as soon as possible; (ii) and once they are married, the tremendous stress of producing a child, preferably a male child. The domestic violence, family conflict, pressures of joint family, in-laws demands and marital conflict have been repeatedly shown in clinical practise and research studies to trigger suicidal attempts and depressive illness, both in urban and rural women. Urban working women, often face hostility from in-laws and are blamed for neglecting their children and home. Several educated working women presented in the author's clinic with intense guilt, anxiety, depression and fatigue with suicidal preoccupations [43].

Urbanisation and suicide

Gender differences: In Western nations such as Greece, Mexico and the United States, male suicides outnumber female suicides three- to five [44]. Risk factors for suicide differ significantly by gender. Of the countries that provide suicide data, Hungary has the highest suicide rates for both elderly men and women: in 1991–1992, the suicide rate for men 75 years and older was as high as 177.5/100 000. A comparison of male and female suicide victims provides additional clues as to the gender differences for completed suicide [45].

In Pakistan most of the studies on suicide interestingly indicate most of the people who attempted suicide were less than 30 years of age, and more women than men were represented. An important difference from Western studies is that a larger number of married women compared to married men or single women were represented. The disturbing figures of married women points towards the marital and family conflicts and high incidence of domestic violence [46].

The Pakistani society is strongly patriarchal; women have few socially sanctioned ways of voicing their grievances. In most of the cases of deliberate self harm by ingesting insecticides in rural areas and ingesting psychotropic drugs in urban areas marriage appeared to be a significant source of stress in women [47].

Women's mental health/body image and the media

The image of 'sexy', of 'what's hot, what's not' that is portrayed by media is appalling. Media's depiction of 'ideal woman's body image' clearly affects women's mental health. Women must realise that beauty as represented in the media is an unhealthy depiction of reality. Girls often say 'I like being skinny' this idea comes from other girls at school, and girls often succumb to peer pressure.

Societal image of woman must be realistic. The way media depicts a woman or a man (but mainly women) is unrealistic and absurd. But this media created image will not change until the societal values and expectations from women change. Society must change its perception and attitude towards women's image and acquire respect for their individuality. Media is mostly cited to be to blame say young anorexic and bulimic girls, besides other factors. Anorexia Nervosa and Bulimia are known to occur in educated, urban young women.

The task of mental health promotion is daunting and will remain grossly underdeveloped in the face of such damaging media: to promote healthy body image and expand the definition of what makes people beautiful. The media has an important role to play in reducing the stigma of mental health problems, in general.

The role of the mass media in women's mental health is tremendous. The various forms of the mass media can be used to foster more positive community attitudes and behaviours towards women with mental health problems.

The media can only report correctly if Mental Health Professionals communicate and in a relevant and inspiring way with the media. Otherwise they will find other topics or stories to report, which may be detrimental to mental health.

Technological developments

The global village supposedly created by globalisation is not that global after all. It is obvious that power and resources do not seem to follow the majority/minority pattern of the world population, that is, globalisation has failed until now to democratically represent the world it has claimed to globalise. Critics point out that the Internet, for example, remains the realm of a privileged minority, as most of the world's population has never made a telephone call, let alone sent an email. Women recognised to be disadvantaged miss out in this area of scientific development. But in the last two decades, in some parts of the world women are higher users of certain parts of the Internet. It must be emphasised that the link between development and women's rights is vital. Societies with the greatest gender equality have grown the fastest, and it must be recognised that gender equality is critical to the development process.

21.8 Internet addiction

In the developed countries, in fact, technological developments have been shown to add to mental health problems [48]. Most of the empirical work has indicated that television watching reduces social involvement, physical activity, mental health and promotes boredom and unhappiness. Older persons and women are usually drawn to the socially interactive aspects of the Internet (conversation groups), while younger patients and men are more likely to access the interactive role playing games and pornography [49]. Bai et al., [50] found 67% of Internet addicts to be women. According to a person's age and education (average 15 years of education) certain behaviours emerge; this is called the Internet Behaviour Dependence, and interestingly gender or race are not reported to be significant. Students and housewives are particularly susceptible to this disorder [50].

After globalisation, the satellites, x-rated movies, horrible crimes videos, and so on have sensitised the population worldwide to violence which has serious consequences on mental health. Initial impressions of the excessive computer user, was of a young, computer savvy, introverted, object-oriented male [51–53]. This belief was challenged by Young [51], who found that 61% of her survey respondents were women.

Cyber-relationships or cyber-affairs, involve individuals married or unmarried who form on-line love relationships which may or may not develop into real-life affairs [54]. The user may lead as many of these affairs as desired in virtual safety and at the same time without leaving the house or office [51]. Often these innocent chat room affiliations can turn into a passionate cyber-affair, growing into intense mutual erotic dialogue (cyber-sex) with text-based fantasies.

Earlier research data on pathological Internet use shows that it is associated with significant psychosocial impairment such as increased depression, relationship friction, academic failure, financial debt and often job loss [51, 52, 55–59].

21.9 Mental health issues related to the use of internet and mobile phones in the developing countries

Negative effects

The mental health of women and men in developing countries is also falling prey to these addictions [60]. Increasing numbers of young and married working women have reported to psychiatric clinics in the last five years in Karachi, Pakistan. These women came in as emergency cases, in a state of acute distress, (anxiety, panic and depression, with suicidal preoccupations) following love affairs on the Internet or mobile phones (full blown physical and emotional involvement). They were all feeling lonely, bored or depressed at the time, and chatting on the Internet or mobiles to unknown people or acquaintances developed into sharing their lives, miseries and dissatisfaction in their relationships. Most of the participants in these 'relationships' were single, engaged and a few married, who professed undying love, but were not prepared for marriage.

The taboo of relations out of family, traditional and religious restrictions, seems to dwindle in the virtual world of the Internet, for these women. Boredom, loneliness and at times lack of emotional support in the family are the common causes for the development of love relationships in women. The strong religious values, expectations of family and their responsibility towards their marriage and children, all led to guilt and remorse, severe anxiety and depression. Interestingly none of the married women wanted to break up their marriages; they thought it was a harmless game/pasttime, or a means to get emotional support without obligations. Most of these women got immensely disturbed when they realised that they were emotionally involved. Intriguingly some of the women even met these men and got into physical relationships. Such behaviours until recently were extremely rare in Pakistan. These young women were devastated when they found out that they were used (as playmates). Men on the Internet usually chose women who were depressed, lonely, independent working married women. Because these women were 'safe', they made no financial demands nor did they put pressure on for commitment, being already married with the responsibility of their family.

Niaz [60] also reports increasing numbers of male patients referred in private by their wives, for addiction to Internet sex-sites. Briefly, their wives had brought them for treatment for their addiction as they sought sexual satisfaction on the Internet. All these men over a period of time had completely lost interest in their wives as sexual partners, and spent long hours on Internet/cyber sex. They had lost interest in work and their family. An Internet addict usually turns to the computer to find relief from moments of painful states of mental tension and agitation present in his or her life. In such instances, their use of the computer is less about using it as an information tool, and more about finding a psychological escape to cope with life's problems. Most of these men lost their jobs, as they were unable to work during the day; consequently adding to the financial stress, leading to further family conflict and in a few cases divorce/family breakup.

Positive effects

Internet use on the positive side is one option for the pursuit of additional educational credentials online and enhances career opportunities, for housewives. In the complex world today, women are recognising the need for further education. They can attend continuing education sessions such as conferences and seek additional degrees through formal academic institutions, with the Internet facility. For many women, the idea of finding time to attend classes on a campus or some other facility is extremely undesirable since busy schedules already make time and energy scarce resources. Taking a serious look at online opportunities is a creative way to expand desired learning options. This innovation in course delivery has opened the door for many women to pursue their educational goals. Even though it is a very popular option, not all individuals find online learning the best format for them, so discovering the most advantageous fit is extremely important. The Internet has enormous capacities for self-help groups, the use of depression net, and so on show how women may support each other; the positive sides are certainly not just educational.

For the first time in history, citizens around the globe are working with contemporaries from three other generations; possibly four. Because recruiting and retaining employees is more important than ever, learning strategies to understand each generational cohort is crucial. Happy, content workers are much more likely to remain employed, saving companies the orientation time and expense that comes from constant turnover. All four generations (the Silent Generation, the Baby Boomers, Generation X and Generation Y) in the workforce emphasise the commonalities of each group and the basic values they share. Different generations can maximise their similarities and turn their differences into strengths. Reaching harmony in the workplace is an achievable goal when all the generations discover and appreciate their underlying similarities and common goals. Each generation can see the value from the differences, working together becomes a great opportunity for discourse rather than a source of conflict.

21.10 Recommendations to counteract negative effects of globalisation

The United Nations Development Program (UNDP) has developed two measures of the disparity between men and women. The Gender Empowerment Measure (GEM) measures gender inequality in two key areas of economic and political participation and decision making. The other GDI (gender related development index) measures achievement in life expectancy, educational attainment and income. Based on all available data, UNDP [61] conclude that 'no society treats its women as well as its men'.

A concerted effect to change societal attitudes, elimination of all forms of biases, prejudices and discrimination, active participation of women in all spheres of life, incorporations of gender perspective in policies and plans, gender auditing and finally, making them 'visible' and being 'heard' at family, regional, national and international platforms. More emphasis should be placed on gender sensitive policies to address some of the gender inequalities associated with the new economic integration and expansion of markets resulting from globalisation.

There is a need to develop comprehensive international and national strategies and policies and devise and implement preventive programmes, develop and implement social welfare and health insurance systems to ensure sufficient funding for women's healthcare services. We also need to improve access and to evolve specialised women-friendly medical treatment and improve quality of life and health of menopausal and older women.

Identifying, women's health needs is crucial in this global world. Privatisation of healthcare commodifies and targets women's reproductive health needs. Similarly there is a great need to develop and implement a social welfare and health insurance system to make certain there is ample funding for women's healthcare economic integration and expansion of markets resulting from globalisation.

Globalisation is increasing inequalities between men and women. Globalisation has both positive and negative definite effects on mental health. The vulnerable, high risk groups clearly are the worst victims of globalisation's negative impact on their mental health. Globalisation of justice is what women need.

References

1. WHO (1998) The World Health Report. Executive summary, World Health Organization, Geneva.
2. UNDP (1995) Gender and Human Development. Human Development Report, published for UNDP by Oxford University Press, New York.
3. Organista, P.B., Chun, K.M. and Marin, G. (Eds.). (1998). *Readings in Ethnic Psychology*. Routledge, New York.
4. Macran, S., Joshi, H. and Dex, S. (1996) Employment after childbearing: a survival analysis. *Work Employment and Society*, **10** (2), 273–96, DOI: 10.1177/0950017096102004 © 1996 BSA Publications Ltd.

5. Lipman, E.L., Offord, D.R. and Boyle, M.H. (1997) Socio-demographic, physical and mental health characteristics of single mothers in Ontario. *Canadian Medical Association Journal*, **156** (5), 639–45.

6. Annan, K. (2005) Secretary General Kofi Annan's UN Reform Proposals Report the Second UN Millennium Summit.

7. Orphant, M. (2001) Trafficking in Persons: Myths, Methods, and Human Rights, Population. Reference. Bureau, 2 December.

8. Pereira, C. (2003) Configuring "global," "national," and "local" in governance agendas in Nigeria. *Social Research*, **69** (3), 781–804.

9. Pereira, C. (2001) Innovative Human Rights Work in Nigeria. Report for the Heinrich Boll Foundation, July 2001. pp. 14–41.

10. Ekine, S. (2001) *Blood and Oil*, Center for Democracy and Development, London; Human Rights Watch (1999) *The Price of Oil*, Human Rights Watch, New York.

11. Turner, T. (1980) Nigeria: imperialism, oil technology and the comprador state, in *Oil and Class Struggle* (eds P. Nore and T. Turner), Zed Press, London, pp. 199–223.

12. Turner, T. (1997) Oil workers and oil communities: counterplanning from the commons in Nigeria, in *Feminism, Women's Struggles and the State in Post-colonial Nigeria* (eds C. Pereira and K. Shettima), Pluto Press, London. Forthcoming.

13. Niaz, U. (1997) *Contemporary Issues of Pakistan Women: A Psycho-Social Profile*, Pakistan Association for Women's Studies, University of Karachi, Pakistan, isbn 9698400-1.

14. Gupta, K.S. (2004) Impact of Globalization & Liberalization on Women's Health in India. Presentation at Hawaii International Conference on Social Sciences Honolulu, Hawaii.

15. Shiva, V. (2008) On Globalization/Vandana Shiva Slave Wages, http://www.physicsforums.com/showthread.php?t=206839 as retrieved on 31 January 05:31:40 GMT.

16. Jejeebhoy, S.J. (1995) *Women's Education, Autonomy, and Reproductive Behaviour: Experience from Developing Countries*, Oxford University Press, Oxford, pp. 16, 43f.

17. O'Gara, C. and Robey, B. (1998) Fertility trends and factors affecting fertility, in *Women in the Third World–An Encyclopedia of Contemporary Issues* (ed. N.P. Stromquist), Garland Publishing, Inc., New York and London, pp. 176–84.

18. Wolfensohn, J.D. (2001) President of the World Bank, World Bank, p. 3.

19. Annan, K.A. and Bellamy, C. Secretary-General of the United Nations (1999) *The State of the World's Children 1999: Education*, UNICEF, New York.

20. Tohidi, N. (2002) Global-Local Intersection of Feminism in Muslim Societies: The Cases of Iran and Azerbaijan–Social Research, Fall.

21. Abu-Lughod, J. (1991) Going beyond global babble, in *Culture, Globalization and the World-System* (ed. A.D. King), Macmillan, Basingstoke.

22. Giddens, A. (1994) *Beyond Left and Right: The Future of Radical Politics*, Polity Press, Cambridge, pp. 5–7, 111.

23. Held, D., McGrew, A., Goldblatt, D. and Perraton, J. (1999) *Global Transformations: Politics, Economic, and Culture*, Stanford University Press, Stanford.

24. Eschle, C. (2001) *Global Democracy, Social Movements, and Feminism*, Westview Press, Boulder, p. 192.

25. Jaggar, A.M. (1998) Globalizing feminist ethics. *Hypatia*, **13** (2), (Spring), 7–31.

26. Appadurai, A. (1995) Modernity at large: cultural dimensions of globalization, Minneapolis, in *The Challenge of Local Feminism: Women's Movements in Global Perspective* (ed. A. Basu), Westview Press, Boulder.

27. Robertson, R. (1996) *Globalization: Social Theory and Global Culture*, Sage Publications, London.

28. Eisenstein, Z. (1997) Women's publics and the search for new democracies. *Feminist Review*, **57** (17), 140–67.

29. Jaggar, J. and Alison, M. (1998) Globalizing feminist ethics. *Hypatia*, **13** (2), (Spring), 7.

30. Eschle, C. (2001) *Global Democracy, Social Movements, and Feminism*, Westview Press, Boulder, p. 147.

31. Patel, V., Araya, R., Lima, M.S. *et al.* (1999) Women, poverty and common mental disorders in four restructuring societies. *Social Science and Medicine*, **49**, 1461–71.

32. Mumford, D.B., Saeed, K., Ahmad, I. *et al.* (1997) Stress and psychiatric disorder in rural Punjab. A community survey. *The British Journal of Psychiatry*, **170**, 473–8.

33. Davar, B. (1999) *The Mental Health of Indian Women: A Feminist Agenda*, Sage Publications, New Delhi.

34. Hussain, N., Creed, F. and Tomenson, B. (2000) Depression and social stress in Pakistan. *Psychological Medicine*, **30**, 395–402.

35. Gittelsohn, J., Bentley, M.E. and Pelto, P.J (1994) Listening to Women Talk about their Health: Issues and Evidence from India, Ford Foundation, New Delhi.

36. Dennerstein, L., Astbury, J. and Morse, C. (1993) Psychosocial and Mental Health Aspects of Women's Health, WHO/FHE/MNH/93.1, World Health Organization.

37. Malik, S. (1993) Women and mental health. *Indian Journal of Psychiatry*, **35**, 3–10.

38. Subramaniam, V. (1999) The impact of globalization on women's reproductive health and rights: a regional perspective. *Development*, **42**, 145–49.

39. Rahman, A. (2001) *Women and Microcredit in Rural Bangladesh: Anthropological Study of Grameen Bank Lending*, Westview Press, Boulder, p. 4. isbn 0-8133-3930-8.

40. Yunus, M. (2005) Grameen Bank's Struggling (Beggar) Members Programme (English), Grameen Communications, July Retrieved on 2008-01-31.

41. Department of Public Information (2008) News and Media Division New York Commission on Population and Development. Forty-first Session.

42. UNESCO (1995) Meeting of Experts on Women in the Informal Sector United Nations Centre, Gigiri, near Nairobi, 25–27 September 1995.

43. Niaz, U. (1997) *Contemporary Issues of Pakistani Women: A Psych-Social Profile*, Pakistan Association of Women's Studies, University of Karachi, Pakistan, isbn 969-8400-00-1.

44. Murthy, R.S. (2001). The World Health Report 2001: Mental Health: New Understanding, New Hope. Published by World Health Organization, 2001.

45. Brent, D.A., Baugher, M., Bridge, J. *et al.* (1999) Age- and sex-related risk factors for adolescent suicide. *Journal of the American Academy of Child and Adolescent Psychiatry*, **38** (12), 1497–505.

46. Khan, M.M. and Reza, H. (2000) The pattern of suicide in Pakistan. *Crisis*, **21** (1), 31–35.

47. Khan, M.M. (1998) *Crisis: The Journal of Crisis Intervention and Suicide Prevention*, **19** (4), 172–6.

48. Kraut, R., Lundmark, V., Patterson, M., Kiesler, S., Mukopadhyay, T., and Scherlis, W. (1998). Internet paradox: A social technology that reduces social involvement and psychological well-being? *American Psychologist* **53** (9), 1017–31. Online document: http://www.apa.org/journals/amp/amp5391017.html.

49. Mitchell, P. (2000). Internet addiction: Genuine diagnosis or not? *The Lancet*, **355**, 632.

50. Bai, Y.M., Lin, C.C. and Chen, J.Y. (2001) Internet addiction disorder among clients of a virtual clinic. *Psychiatric Services*, **25**, 1397.

51. Young, K.S. (1998a) Internet addiction: the emergence of a new clinical disorder. *CyberPsychology and Behavior*, **1** (3), 237–44.

52. Young, K.S. (1998b) *Caught in the Net: How to Recognize the Signs of Internet Addiction and a Winning Strategy for Recovery*, John Wiley & Sons, Inc., New York.

53. Griffiths, M. (1997) Does Internet and Computer Addiction Exist? Some Case Study Evidence. Paper presented at the 105th Annual Meeting of the American Psychological Association August 15, 1997, Chicago.

54. Brent, D.A., Baugher, M., Bridge, J. *et al.* (1999) Age- and sex-related risk factors for adolescent suicide. *Journal of the American Academy of Child and Adolescent Psychiatry*, **38** (12), 1497–505.

55. Young, K.S. (1997) What Makes the Internet Addictive: Potential Explanations for Pathological Internet Use, Online document, http://www.netaddiction.com/articles/habitforming.htm. Retrieved October 4, 2002, from source.

56. Griffiths, M. (2001) Sex on the internet: Observations and implications for internet sex addiction. *Journal of Sex Research*, **38** (4), 333–42.

57. Krant, R., Patterson, M., Lundmark, V. *et al.* (1998) Internet Paradox: a social technology that reduces social involvement and psychological well-being? *The American Psychologist*, **53**, 1017–31.

58. Morahan-Martin, J. (2001) Incidence and correlates of pathological Internet use. *The Journal of Communication*, **51** (2), 366.

59. Scherer, K. (1997) College life online: healthy and unhealthy internet use. *Journal of College Student Development*, **38**, 655–65.

60. Niaz, U. (2008) Addiction with Internet and mobile phones: an interview, *JPPS*, July–Dec., **5** (2), 72–5.

61. Pillarisetti, J. and McGillivray, M. UNDP (1998) Human development and gender empowerment: methodological and measurement issues. *Development Policy Review*, **16** (2), 197.

22

The impact of culture on women's mental health

Marianne Kastrup[1] and Unaiza Niaz[2]

[1]*Transcultural Psychiatry, Psychiatric Department, Rigshospitalet, Copenhagen, Denmark*
[2]*The Psychiatric Clinic & Stress Research Center Karachi, Pakistan; and University of Health Sciences, Lahore, Pakistan*

22.1 Introduction

Women and men differ in biology and life circumstances, so it is not surprising that their psychiatric morbidity and disease manifestations differ. When studying female morbidity we have to take into consideration the biological set up, gender roles, the socio-political circumstances, the norms of society, as well as the cultural context [1] Gender factors may influence help-seeking behaviour, treatment outcome and impact of mental illness [2].

Until recently we have however seen an emphasis on the biological and reproductive aspects of women's mental health, whereas the cultural dimension and the impact of culture on mental health have received less attention. Yet we know that the cultural dimension may play a different role in the two sexes.

Culture contributes to female psychopathology in various ways depending on the nature of psychopathology but also on the individual with the disorder [3].

On a global level about 25% of all get a psychiatric or behavioural disorder at a certain moment in their life [4]. Thus mental health problems are one of the major health problems facing women across the world.

Psychiatric disorders like depression, and anxiety, as well as psychological distress, sexual or domestic violence affect women to a greater extent than men across countries and across different cultural settings. Factors like poverty, hunger,

Contemporary Topics in Women's Mental Health   Edited by Chandra, Herrman, Fisher, Kastrup,
© 2009 John Wiley & Sons, Ltd   Niaz, Rondón and Okasha

malnutrition, overwork, domestic violence and sexual abuse, all contribute to women's poor mental health irrespective of cultural background and we find that the frequency and severity of such factors are positively related to the mental health problems in women [5].

Pressures created by the multiple roles women fulfill; the discrimination against them; their life conditions; and the societal stressors all contribute to this. Furthermore, gender inequalities and their consequences that are linked to the cultural context may have a negative impact on women's mental health [1].

Virtually all societies up until recently have relegated women to a subordinate rank and justified their behaviour as a consequence of women's 'natural' inferiority. Throughout history, philosophers, scientists and the clergy have underlined women's 'natural' inferiority, thus sanctioning and perpetuating their restricted and debased status. Hence growing up in almost any patriarchal culture with its associated belief systems has a significant effect on women's mental health. Cultural and religious traditions have been used as an excuse to justify discriminatory and abusive treatment of women including wife-battering for defiant behaviour or even killing wives or daughters for 'dishonouring' the family. Many cultures treat women as second-class citizens, under control of their fathers, brothers or husbands. Such gender-role stereotyping is highly correlated with domestic violence [6].

Culture is only one of many important factors influencing health-related beliefs along with individual factors, educational factors, socio-economic factors and environmental factors [7]. All these factors may have an impact on women's mental health. Depending on the context, women may in some situations be very influenced by their cultural background whereas their personality in other situations may have a decisive influence on their mental health.

Furthermore, women's ethnic identity plays a core role in how women experience their own self-value and thereby influencing the causes and courses of mental distress [8].

In the present chapter we shall discuss issues like: What role do social expectations and gender roles play in women's mental illnesses? What do their illnesses and 'psychological problems' indicate? What is the impact of violence and subordination on women's health?

An overview will be presented of the impact of culture on women's mental health. Particular emphasis will be given to the gender-based violence in the light of which this topic has received insufficient attention hitherto despite its huge public mental health dimension and related costs for society.

22.2 Definitions

Culture

Although many different definitions of culture exist, it is generally agreed that culture is a dynamic concept. Culture may be defined as the learned, shared beliefs, values, attitudes and behaviours characteristic of a society or population

[9]. One of the most widespread definitions of culture, namely that of Tylor, state that culture is the complex whole which includes knowledge, belief, art, morals, law, custom and any other capabilities and habits acquired by man as a member of society [7]. Cultures are described as constructs that are ever changing and emerge from interactions between individuals, communities and institutional practises [10].

From a health perspective, culture has an impact on, for example, the causes, symptoms and manifestations of mental disorders; the explanatory models; the coping mechanisms; the help seeking behaviour; and the social response [10].

Mental health

Mental health is in the chapter defined using the definition of World Health Organization (WHO) [11]. Here mental health is not just the absence of mental disorder. It is defined as a state of wellbeing in which every individual realises his or her own potential, can cope with the normal stresses of life, can work productively and fruitfully, and is able to make a contribution to her or his community.

Sex/Gender

The chapter comprises both the 'sex' aspects, that is, the biological characteristics as well as the 'gender' aspects, that is, the socially constructed distinguishing features, but with an emphasis on the gender aspects in recognition of the social determinants of mental health.

Gender based violence

A commonly used definition of violence is the WHO definition stating that violence is 'the intentional use of physical force or power, threatened or actual, against oneself, another person or against a group or community, that either results in or has a high likelihood of resulting in injury, death, psychological harm, mal-development or deprivation' [12].

Using the UN Declaration on the Elimination of Violence Against Women [13] violence may be defined as: 'any act of gender-based violence that results in, or is likely to result in, physical, sexual or psychological harm or suffering to women'.

Within the last 10–15 years, we have experienced an increasing awareness of violence as a serious public mental health problem, particularly in women. One should however keep in mind that defining outcomes in terms of injury or death as the WHO definition does may not pay sufficient attention to the fact that many forms of violence against women do not necessarily lead to injury or death [14]. Many countries have carried out surveys on the extent; the characteristics; and the consequences of violence against women, but surveys of the possible gender differences in the relationship between physical violence, sexual violations and mental health problems are scarce [15].

22.3 Epidemiological perspectives

Up until recently it has been a belief by many that psychiatric disorders were occurring less frequently in developing countries than in industrialised nations, but today it is common knowledge that regardless of the level of industrial development, stressors occur in all cultures and mental disorders are commonly found among women in all cultures [16].

In the WHO World Health Report [4], the leading causes of disability-adjusted life years (DALYs) are listed for women in all ages. From this it appears that unipolar depression on a global level ranks 4 of all disorders, and that among females aged 15–44 we find mental disorders in 4 out of the 10 most common causes of disability (Unipolar depression, schizophrenia, bipolar affective disorders and self-inflicted injuries).

Furthermore, results from the international investigations carried out by the World Health Organization on schizophrenia; on determinants of serious mental disorders; and on depression [17–19] indicate similarities in the incidences of mental disorders among women globally, in particular the most severe ones.

What differs are the socio-cultural factors that have a significant impact on the incidence of minor mental disorders [20] which is in line with previous findings that gender differences in psychiatric morbidity cannot be explained by biomedical models but are related also to marital status, social roles and expectations [21].

22.4 Cultural aspects of stress

Gender is one way of defining a hierarchy that assigns entitlement and superiority to one group over another [22], and the female gender is on a global level and in all cultural settings disproportionately highly represented among the poor, the illiterate and otherwise disadvantaged groups of the world. There is no indication that the lifetime prevalence in males and females differ regarding exposure to traumatic life events even though the kinds of events may differ. Yet, a higher prevalence of post traumatic stress disorders (PTSDs) is reported consistently in women. In fact, women in general have an almost twice as high risk of developing PTSD at some time during their lifetime than men; the condition is more likely to run a chronic course; it is prevailing in all cultures, and it is neither the type of event nor its perception that may explain these gender differences [23].

Irrespective of culture, women fulfil the role of nurturers and providers of emotional support, and they have usually the main responsibility for care giving in the family. In a number of occasions, like disaster, or forced migration this may overload women's capacity to cope, as preoccupation with the needs of the family may lead to the situation where they are not able to consider their own needs especially if they become widows [22].

On the other hand, the care giving role may have a protective function as women contrary to their partners have a natural role and identity in the new environment.

It is well established that gender role conflicts and adverse life events may precipitate anxious and depressive disorders in women with young children.

Women's health status is directly linked to their culture and the position they occupy within it [24] We must recognise that norms, values and behaviour are socially defined for each gender, which determines the roles of men and women in society. Many stress factors; biological, psychological and societal, may contribute to stress.

From a cultural perspective certain aspects are of particular concern as they greatly interfere with the mental health of women. To link all these factors into a coherent theoretical model explaining the prevalence of psychological and psychiatric distress in women is a major challenge [25]. Among such factors are poverty, migration, refugee status, violence and consequences of globalisation.

Poverty

There is ample documentation that among those living in poverty mental disorders are more common. As a consequence the burden of mental disorders is heavier in the impoverished part of the population [26]. As women comprise an overwhelming majority among the impoverished layers of society – and that is related to the cultural context – it is impossible to discuss the interaction of poverty, mental health and culture without referring to gender. Poverty and hunger places a heavy burden on women and the multiple risk factors may be predictive of psychiatric morbidity [25]. Further that women, due to their disproportionately higher burden of poverty, are more vulnerable to getting a depressive episode [2].

We also see an interaction of risk factors as women who live under deprived socioeconomic circumstances are more at risk of experiencing partner violence, or having a partner with problems of substance abuse, thus seeing that the multiple risk factors may be predictive of psychiatric morbidity [2].

Migration

Migration is a process which is particularly prone to causing psychosocial stress factors. Distinctions must be made between the individual woman migrating; the motives for and circumstances surrounding her migration; the relationship to her home country; the differences between the new and the original culture; as well as the degree of acceptance the woman has achieved in the host country.

It is well documented that migration can be a key trigger in the development of stress-related illnesses. Thus, migration does not only relate to the development of post traumatic disorders but also to depressive disorders, anxiety disorders as well as psychosomatic reactions [18, 27, 28]. In order to get a comprehensive picture of the complex interaction between culture, mental health and migrant women, one has to take into consideration a number of factors including the women's current living conditions, for example, family structure, poverty, pre-migratory stressful events, post-migratory stressors, other health problems as well as their personality structure and subjective sense of control and self-efficacy [29].

Refugee status

Among the world's refugees, women make up approximately half the population, but as pointed out by Kastrup and Arcel [22] many refugee reports make reference to the proportion of women and implicitly suggest that all refugee women are vulnerable which may be difficult to reconcile with today's notion of gender equity and the empowerment of women [30]. Furthermore, gender profiles are more readily available for refugee populations in developing countries than in the industrialised world.

Yet, we find only a few studies with a focus on gender particularities, and findings are inconsistent. Some report a relatively higher level of psychological distress in females and relate this finding to the accumulation of live stressors that refugee women face in exile. As an example, studies of Cambodian refugees and Tamil refugees report that women are at greater risk of a war-related PTSD (e.g. [31, 32]).

Others report of sex differences, for example, Thulesius and Håkansson [33] among Bosnian refugees in Sweden and among Cambodian refugees in the US [34].

Until now, the role of marital status for the adjustment in the new society and the emergence of posttraumatic stress has received limited attention. The different social roles and expectations of the two sexes are reflected in a study among Bosnian refugee couples in USA [35] in which women's marital satisfaction was predicted by their husband's PTSD, but not vice versa, which seems to indicate that women are more orientated towards others.

Among refugee women – irrespective of culture – those with young children need particular attention as they have an increased vulnerability to stress and a heightened risk of mental disorders [36]. Cambodian mothers living as refugees in Australia report that the number of trauma events prior to birth was related to psychological morbidity following childbirth and that the number of support people did not predict the level of symptoms.

Globalisation

From a gender and mental health perspective globalisation has a number of consequences. The rapid transformations we are witnessing particularly in developing countries imply [37] that the generations of women growing up today face a future that is so entirely different from that of the former generations that few of the skills of these generations of women are useful today.

Because of this globalisation, the experience of stress in vulnerable women can increase and cultures can lose their psychologically protective function, as individual and collective identities are questioned [38]. The particular problems of women are discussed elsewhere (see chapter on globalisation).

Resilience

Not all women exposed to psychosocial stressors develop mental health problems.

Among the protective factors we find, for example, political involvement, spirituality, the existence of an inner locus of control and self-reliance, emotional disclosure to others [39].

The study of resilience factors and its association with the prevailing culture is important, but there is still a lack of research in order to understand the positive aspects, and protective function of a given cultural background and so it is important not to only focus on the negative impact of circumstantial stressors on different female populations.

Mental health professionals tend to focus on the negative and pathological impact of existing traumatic and societal factors and less on the resources these women possess; the defence mechanism employed; coping styles; social involvement; and cognitive styles that women may utilise to adapt to changed life circumstances or a new cultural context.

As Dennerstein *et al.* [21] pointed out; it is surprising – not that many women have compromised mental health – but rather that not more suffer from stress-related mental health problems.

22.5 Diagnostic considerations

Culture specific aspects in western classification systems

The aim of classification is to be universally applicable and culture free, if cultural factors are allowed to influence diagnosis we run the risk of politisation [40]. From a gender perspective we should keep in mind that the delineation of illnesses are a product of social and political as well as cultural factors reflecting normality and abnormality [40].

Knowledge of the cultural background including socio-cultural factors, religious beliefs, cultural norms, values and standards of behaviour, as well as experiences – all contribute to a more reliable assessment of women's mental health [31]. There is an increasing recognition of the need for a diagnostic classificatory system that takes a cross-cultural approach and includes culturally-typical standard forms of behaviour or with due recognition of gender specific issues.

Furthermore, in order to assess properly the mental status of women there is a need for a particularly careful, biographical history that can provide information on the ethnic and cultural reference group and identity of the women.

It should be kept in mind that misinterpretation of symptoms has been brought forward as an explanatory factor for the high prevalence of certain mental disorders in women.

Suicide/Attempted suicide

Suicide is the 13th most common cause of death on a global level today. About 813 000 die annually as a result of suicide, out of which only 305 000 are women. It is well known that suicide rates are highly related to country and cultural background. Cultural factors including religious beliefs, and socio-economic factors like partner violence and poverty are, together with mental illness, key factors determining the risk of suicide.

As pointed out by WHO [41], women show in some countries higher suicide rates than men, for example, in China where there is evidence that the large and rapid social transitions are a risk factor and may contribute to the rise in suicide in particular among rural women.

Suicide is the second-leading cause of death for Asian-American women aged 15–24. It is not surprising that young Asian-American women have the highest suicide rate among women of any race, ethnicity between the age of 15 and 24. Probably, the Asian-American women suffer from higher suicide rates because the mental health community has not caught up with the demands of a multicultural society. Depression and thoughts of suicide are prevalent amongst women of all races, but psychological treatment is largely founded upon Western ideals. The high rates of depression amongst Asian-American women are a consequence of poor outreach to the Asian-American community, to combat stigmas of mental disease, and of poor resources specifically addressing concerns unique to Asian-American women [42].

In Pakistan males have a higher suicide rate, but when controlling for marital status it is noteworthy that married women have a much higher rate compared to married men and single women. This suggests that the limited autonomy that married women may experience is a cultural stress factor and may be a contributory factor to their higher risk of suicidal behaviour [43].

There is clear evidence that attempted suicide is more common in certain cultural groups, a fact that has been linked to culture conflict producing cognitive dissonance between the women and their surroundings, and feelings of powerlessness, hostility and hopelessness may contribute [44]. Several countries – as different as Singapore and Trinidad – all report high rates of suicide attempts among young Indian women [44]. Troubles with in-laws and interpersonal relationships are given as frequent reasons for attempted suicides among young Indian women.

It is also noteworthy that the two sexes react differently to the ongoing transition of the Eastern European countries, as males in times of unemployment due to their role as primary provider may be at greater risk of suicidal acts [2].

Women are at less risk and we still need to elucidate what are the protective factors for women in this culture.

Cultural aspects of gender based violence

According to the former UN Secretary General Kofi Annan [45] violence against women may be seen as the most pervasive, yet least recognised, human rights abuse.

Interpersonal violence permeates the lives of a large group of women in all cultures. It is often an integrated part of gender inequality and has a heavy impact on the mental health of the women involved as well as their surroundings.

Violence has many forms and leads to further discrimination against women as it adds to women's exclusion from the public domain. It takes place frequently in the private domain, hidden and inescapable. It may be part of war and strife in the form of rape and sexual assaults.

That women frequently are emotionally or financially dependent upon their violators intensifies the problem and has implications for how the problem should be dealt with [46].

Historically, culture, customs, traditions and beliefs have fostered in their own way various forms of violence against women, all of which need not take the form of atrocious assaults. Society in many cultures demands that widows, however young they are, lead a rigidly austere life, and social isolation and total lack of access to men have all been considered as necessary measures to keep them from temptation and sin.

Women, living in situations of power and control often experience domestic and/or sexual violence. The gender-based violence may include intimidation, threats, economic deprivation, sexual and psychological abuse apart from physical violence [47]. For instance in Puerto Rico nearly 64% of all abused women were also suffering from some form of mental illness. According to some studies 50% of all women referred to psychiatric services in Puerto Rico had been physically abused, and about one third of women victims of domestic violence had attempted suicide.

Abused women are known to develop alcoholism, drug dependence or eating disorders. Nevertheless, a large number of these women's mental health problems are erroneously diagnosed as psychoses, neuroses or personality disorders when they are really reactions to frequent and prolonged violence and emotional torment [48].

Unfortunately, many professionals do not recognise the effect that violent partners have on women's lives. Women on the contrary are frequently blamed for the abuse they receive. Stigma or 'labels' given to abused women have a crucial impact on whether or not a woman is permitted to maintain custody of her children or whether she is retained in her job.

The treatment of women's mental health problems must start from theoretical or practical approaches grounded in women's own experiences. Clinical care must provide an environment of security and protection in which their empowerment is encouraged and the real causes of their illnesses are tackled, like the physical, psychological and social factors that condition their lives. Simultaneously women must demand and explore new models of mental health, where women can express their 'female' malaise [49].

There is increasing recognition of the particular risks that displaced and refugee women are subjected to in refugee settings or areas of war, as they are disproportionately affected by violence [46].

Honour killings

Honour crimes are acts of violence, usually murder, committed by male family members against female family members, who are perceived to have brought dishonour upon the family. A woman can be targeted by (individuals within) her family for many reasons. The mere perception that a woman has behaved in a specific way to 'dishonour' her family, is sufficient to trigger an attack [50]. The phenomenon of honour-related crimes against women is global. Honour killings are prevalent in various countries, such as Albania, Brazil, Canada, Denmark, Ecuador, Egypt, Germany, Iran, Iraq, Israel, Italy, Jordan, Morocco, Palestinian territories, Sweden, Turkey, Uganda, the United Kingdom and the United States [51–55].

In the United States, until recent times, wife-killings by husbands (especially against adulterous wives whether or not they were premeditated) were not considered a crime in some jurisdictions. Such practises, to a large extent, have ceased to be endemic in North America although some immigrants from North Africa and the Near East have brought the practise with them in recent decades [56, 57].

In Europe, honour killings have mostly been reported within some Muslim and Sikh communities [58].

Many cases of honour killings have been reported in Pakistan [59]. The rise of religious/extremist fundamentalism in this patriarchal society has made women the prime victims, helpless under the law and under social mores. Honour killing is often regarded as a private matter for the affected family alone. The practise is condemned by human rights supporters for being a double standard and sexist, since males will not be killed for such an 'offence'; that is, if a man rapes a woman, it is the woman who 'brings dishonour' to her family and not the rapist.

Women's equal participation is fully supported by Islamic teachings and by Pakistan's legislation. Islamic teachings exemplify justice and equality for women, while in the Constitution of Pakistan the full participation of women next to men is endorsed. But practically none of these are implemented [60].

The concept of women as property and honour are deeply entrenched in the socio-cultural fabric of Pakistan. As a result, many individuals, including women, support this ritual.

22.6 Cultural and social practices and their impact on mental health

Examples from different regions

Impact of culture in South Asia

South Asia is the most heavily populated and amongst the poorest regions in the world. It faces enormous social, economic and health challenges, including pervasive inequality, violence, political instability and high burden of diseases. When women's health has been addressed in this region, issues associated with reproduction, such as family planning and childbearing, and women's mental health has been relatively neglected.

Women's socialisation is influenced by economic and cultural pressures. In traditional societies, like South Asia, the role of mother, wife and daughter are projected to the extent that a woman's identity as an individual is not recognised. Women exist only in the context of some relationship with a male family member, and in general women are inferior partners. Women are themselves socially conditioned to accept this as their proper status and thus help to uphold and perpetuate this attitude [61].

Even in the new millennium, women in South Asia are deprived of their socio-economic and legal rights. They live in a system where religious injunctions, tribal codes, feudal traditions and discriminatory laws are prevalent. They are beset by a lifetime social and psychological disadvantage, coupled with long years of child bearing. They often end up experiencing poverty, isolation and psychological disability. In some urban regions of South-Asian countries, women's social roles have changed to some extent [62]. They have now comparatively more opportunities for education, employment and enjoyment of civil rights within society. However, the de-stereotyping of the gender roles which have been traditionally assigned by our society is still far away.

In this region, some ancient traditions and customs are still followed, promoting various forms of violence against women. These include honour killings, exchange marriages, marriage to the Quran, Karo-kari, bride price, dowry, female circumcision, questioning women's ability to testify, confinement to home, denying their right to choose their partner. In some rural areas of Sindh, Pakistan and Punjab, India, girls are deprived of their marriage rights only to keep the property in the family. A cruel custom asking the girl to swear on the Quran that she will leave her share of property to brothers adds misery to the already miserable lives of these incarcerated women [63].

The cultural norms prevailing in South-East Asia perpetuate the subordinate position of women socially and economically. In this region, very often young unmarried girls and women suffer tremendous physical and psychological stress due to the violent behaviour of men. The nature of violence includes wife-beating, murder of wife, kidnapping, rape, physical assault and acid throwing. The most frequent causes for acts of violence are domestic quarrels due to the inability of a woman's family to make dowry payments at the time of marriage [64].

In some regions of South East Asia, violence has reached staggering levels; in a recent population-based study from India, nearly half of women reported physical violence [65]. Annually an estimated one million pregnant Pakistani women are physically abused at least once during pregnancy [66]. Besides that, many women and young children from South-East regions are trafficked and forced into prostitution, undesired marriages and bonded labour [67].

Sri Lankan women, whether they are Sinhala, Tamil or Muslim, continue to be viewed as the reproducers, nurturers and disseminators of 'tradition', 'culture', 'community' and 'nation'. With the exception of the Mothers' Fronts in the north, east and the south, which received unprecedented popular sympathy and support and were consistently valorised by the media [68], the other groups of women working as garment-factory workers, housemaids, as well as the war widows frequently suffer at the hands of their families, communities and the nation as a whole [69].

The changing role of women in Sri Lanka countering the societal pressures has been a tremendous uphill struggle. Debates on the 'woman question' in Sri Lanka, which were centrally concerned with questioning and transforming such strictures and pressures on women, have also been over determined by ethno nationalism and the civil war in the north and east from the late 1970s onward. Thus, while there still remains a small but vibrant feminist movement in the country, it is frequently pushed into a reactive rather than a proactive role. Many organisations that agitated against the cultural oppression of women or their exploitation in the labour market are now primarily involved in the fields of development and human rights – setting up micro credit schemes for displaced women, offering skills training in refugee camps and monitoring human rights violations. In the same way that the left deferred the liberation of women until after the socialist revolution, feminists in Sri Lanka seem to be pushed to defer the transformation of societal strictures on women until the civil war in the island has ended [70].

In China the Communist government came to power in 1949 with one of the major policy initiatives of the Communist government to do away with unequal treatment of women. However, it is very easy to demonstrate that significant discrimination against women still exists. This discrimination may be due to 'remnants of feudal thinking'. There are aspects of current Chinese society that encourage the continuation of this cultural tradition [71].

Impact of culture in the Arab World

In the Arab World, women experience what Deniz Kandiyoti (2000: xiv) [72] has called a 'double jeopardy'. They are not only subject to the widespread restrictions on civic and political participation affecting both sexes, but are further denied autonomy by discriminatory 'personal status laws'. Under variants of these laws, it is not women but their male guardians who have the authority to decide issues such as whether they may work or travel, or whom they may marry. Historically structures of patriarchy were not uniform across the region before colonialism.

Nevertheless the Western model of the nation-state, complete with its gendered concepts of citizenship, became the compulsory model for Middle Eastern states emerging from colonialism, where it was imposed on already gendered systems of social stratification. The resulting 'intersection' of patriarchies created a historically specific momentum of increasing control exercised over women by men, families, communities and the state [73].

Several traditional cultural practises – such as honour crimes, the stoning of women accused of adultery, virginity tests or female genital cutting in Muslim societies, including the Middle East, have increasingly drawn the attention of the Western media and public in recent years as human rights abuses [74]. The lack of information on Islam and on the wide diversity of Muslim societies; the parallel rise of the Islamic religious right, which claims such customary practises to be Islamic; and the tendency to 'essentialise' Islam are some of the factors that have led to the incorrect portrayal in the West of such practises as Islamic. This depiction is not only misleading, but also stands in sharp contrast to the efforts of women's movements in Muslim societies, which, in their fight against such practises, are campaigning to raise public consciousness that these practises are against Islam [75].

The sexual oppression of women in the Middle East and elsewhere in the Muslim world is not the result of an oppressive vision of sexuality based on Islam, but a combination of historical, sociopolitical and economic factors. Although an analysis of the Quran and the literature traditionally accepted as establishing the normative practises of Islam, leads to contradictory conclusions about the construction of women's sexuality in early Islam, several customary practises that allow violations of women's human rights in the region: honour crimes, stoning, female genital cutting or virginity tests – have no Koranic basis, as women researchers and activists in the region point out. Moreover, the prevalence of these practises varies greatly among the countries in the region.

The last decade of the twentieth century saw considerable innovation at the organisational level in the Arab world. The burgeoning of women's groups in the region can be described in numerical terms and with reference to United Nations conferences on women and women's rights guarantees contained in international law. An account based on numbers would note the rise of NGOs focusing on women's status, the creation by governments of national commissions for women, and the increase in the number of women entering the workforce in countries where women's participation in paid labour was previously very low [76].

There has been mounting public rejection of any policy perceived to foster a 'Western agenda', the distance has still to go before all governments in the region outlaw discrimination against women, and the high levels of female illiteracy. Moreover, female employees of deregulated privatised business are often working today under worse terms and conditions than applied when those businesses were state owned. As indicated by the Palestinian example, homegrown activism concerning women and the media in Arab countries has been buttressed in recent years by international financial or logistical help.

Example: For instance, the Western Asia Regional Office of the United Nations Development Fund for Women (UNIFEM-WARO) backed a 16-day campaign in 1998 to encourage the Egyptian, Jordanian, Lebanese, Palestinian and Yemeni media to break long-standing taboos on reporting about violence against women. The campaign built on breakthroughs already achieved by Jordanian crime reporter Rana Husseini in exposing the phenomenon of so-called honour crimes, which involve the murder or attempted murder of women alleged to have besmirched their family's reputation by being found in the company of an unrelated male. Husseini's coverage of this form of family violence provided evidence for a petition aimed at changing the Jordanian law that promises leniency for male perpetrators of such crimes. Parliament rejected the change in November 1999 but the issue of honour killing had been brought into public view [77]. This was the climate in which a veteran woman journalist, Mahassen Imam, founded the Arab Women's Media Center (AWMC) in the Jordanian capital, Amman, in December 1999. Endorsed by the Jordanian royal family, the centre trains, supports and celebrates media women working in Jordan and other parts of the Arab world. Also in 1999, North African activists, working under the umbrella of the group Collectif 95 Maghreb Egalite, compiled a groundbreaking report in which they drew a direct link between physical and symbolic violence against women. Analysing in detail the negative stereotyping of women on Moroccan television, and the media's failure to provide a voice for thousands of women subjected to organised rape during the Algerian civil strife that erupted in 1992, the report's authors pointed out that the boundary between physical and symbolic violence is highly porous. Since each type of violence feeds on the other, they wrote, neither should be trivialised or downplayed (Collectif 95, 1999: 9) [78] Municipal elections took place in Qatar in March 1999, women were allowed to vote and stand for public office, in stark contrast to norms of political participation in other Arab Gulf states at that time. Literacy among women in Arab states has remained exceptionally low. Although the start of the twenty-first century found higher literacy among adult women than men in the Gulf emirates of Qatar and the UAE, elsewhere in the region this ratio was reversed, with female illiteracy reaching 76% in Yemen, 65% in Morocco, 57% in Egypt, 44% in Algeria and 34% in Saudi Arabia (UNDP, 2001: 210–12) [79].

Impact of culture in Latin America

Latin America is one of the most unequal regions in the world with 220 million people, most of them women, living in poverty, while the economic indicators show a steady upward trend. Access to healthcare has diminished in the region in the last two decades, due to inadequate reforms in health, the lack of appropriate insurance and social protection. In Brazil, as in most Latin American countries, crime and punishment have been defined in relation to the dominant figure of the white, high-income male. It has been so because throughout time, this is the group that has the resources and the influence to determine what is order and disorder, deviant and legitimate in Brazilian society, which largely accounts for the impunity with which domestic violence, including the murder of a wife has been treated. There are major paradigmatic shifts when this violence is recognised as a crime and this crime as a human rights violation [80].

Patriarchal ideology gives privileges to the male, which are reinforced by law until recently, and has shaped male identity as dependent on power, economic independence and hence control over women. Lack of upward social mobility and the persistence of ethnic and class divisions and exclusions have been accentuated by internal migration and the increase in the use of alcohol and other substances to increase violence in all its forms. Exclusion and poverty are threats to the traditional male identity that can be solved by exerting power in the house in the form of sexual and physical violence against the woman.

The Brazilian position at the 1993 Vienna human rights conference was once again continued by the country's normative frame. The 1988 constitution (as a result of feminist advocacy) states that it is the duty of the state to create mechanisms to avoid violence in the family. This makes family violence a state responsibility; the government can be rendered accountable for failing to attend victims and for failing to provide mechanisms to prevent family violence [81, 82].

22.7 Therapeutic issues

Access to services and treatment gap

Cultural/Social barriers to help seeking

Gender is one of the important factors determining help-seeking. It determines the type and quality of care you are offered. and in most cultures women are the primary consumers of medication, psychotherapy and other treatments related to mental health [83].

In some cultures however we find that women in need of psychiatric care are more likely to experience stigma against getting access to health, and mental health programmes specifically targeting women are rare [2].

Women in certain cultures are facing deprivation and denial of opportunities, thereby having fewer options also regarding health and consequently having a greater likelihood of being denied adequate access to mental healthcare. Further, mentally ill women are more likely in some cultures to be stigmatised compared to mentally ill men as women's mental illness has a greater impact on the function of the family life [2]. Studies from, for example, India show that if a married woman develops mental illness the husband may want a divorce and the negative attitude by the husband and his family further adds to the burden of the mentally ill woman [84].

In the WHO report [85] from the European Ministerial Conference it is noteworthy that the chapter on treatment gap lists several vulnerable groups but does not report on gender differences, and the question is whether this is due to lack of a gender focus or whether it is a reflection of that gender treatment gap in the European region is not a pertinent issue.

Therapeutic concerns

Therapists and patients may come from different social and cultural backgrounds and here it is important to be aware of the cultural attunement, that is, the process when a therapist and a patient from different cultural contexts try to establish a common ground in understanding, and defining the problems presented and to find an agreement concerning goals for treatment [22]. Establishing a therapeutic alliance demands greater effort from both parts than when client and therapist are from the same culture. To achieve a sustainable relationship it is important that the therapist is able to avoid any negative stereotypes about women from other cultural and educational backgrounds in particular from non-Western countries.

Cultural attunement aims to reduce the power balance between therapist and female patient, to respect diversity and avoid over-generalisations, and to overcome oppression in the client's life without suppressing the woman's own values [22].

It requires maturity, and cognitive flexibility of the therapist to stay true to one's own professionalism and yet meet the woman in her cultural context.

Working therapeutically with women from other cultures has several challenges. One needs to keep in mind that verbalising problems may not be usual in some cultures and women may look for a fast biological cure and not be ready for an interactive therapy or revealing very private matters. We also frequently see a discrepancy between how the woman herself perceives her problems and how the therapist does [22].

The role of the family needs consideration as women in some cultural settings are under social control and it may create obstacles to engage in a therapeutic intervention that may result in an empowerment of the woman. Family members may openly oppose such interventions thereby preventing the woman from changing her situation.

Further many women have been subjected to several very traumatic life events, violence, and so on acting cumulatively and all adding to their mental health problems. All these problems need consideration and the women may only trust the therapist if their current stressors are also being taken care of [22].

22.8 Perspectives

Global mental health is closely related to political and economic welfare. But to what degree is mental health a fundamental human right for women? Access to psychiatric help is a close function of economic differences inter as well as intra nationally [86], and access to adequate mental health service is still inaccessible to many women in diverse cultural settings.

Globally, it is evident from research data that women are generally aware of their fundamental human rights in society. Despite awareness of gender discrimination at home and work, and basic human rights, women continue to suffer differential treatment. In developing countries poverty and undoubtedly the long lasting effects of traditions and culture are the primary causes for women's insubordination, for violence against them, all issues that may have an impact on their mental health problems.

With increasing migration, new directions for action are needed [46]. The particular problems of migrant women receive increasing attention from international organisations. Such women are at risk of being victims of violence, and this is particularly so among refugee women, and many of them are faced with a life situation with new and unfamiliar responsibilities placed on them [22].

The commitment of civil society and governments must focus on changing community and societal norms and on raising the status of women [46].

Investing in the education and health of women should have high priority if we want to improve the mental health of the populations in low- and middle-income countries [25] and women's mental health should be of primary concern for policymakers [25]. Many ways may be taken, but a global awareness of the complex interaction of women's life situation, socio-cultural stressors and mental health is a necessary prerequisite to move forward.

References

1. Petersson, B. and Kastrup, M. (1995) Gender and mental health, in *Clinical Psychiatry. Epidemiological Psychiatry* (ed. A. Jablensky), Bailliere, London.
2. Patel, V. (2005) Gender in Mental Health Research, WHO, Geneva.
3. Tseng, W.-S., Bhugra, D. and Bhui, K. (2007) Culture and psychopathology: general view, in *Textbook of Cultural Psychiatry*, Cambridge University Press, Cambridge.
4. WHO (2001) World Health Report, WHO, Geneva.
5. Kastrup, M. (2008) Global burden of mental health, in *Handbook of Disease Burden*, Springer Verlag, Berlin, in press.
6. Niaz, U. (2004) Women's mental health in Pakistan. *World Psychiatry*, **3**, 60–61.
7. Helman, C.G. (2001) *Culture, Health and Illness*, Arnold, London.
8. Bibeau, G. (1997) Cultural psychiatry in a creolizing world: questions for a new research agenda. *Transcultural Psychiatry*, **34**, 9–41.
9. Bhugra, D. and Mastrogianni, A. (2004) Globalisation and mental disorders. Overview with relation to depression. *The British Journal of Psychiatry*, **184**, 10–20.
10. Kirmayer, L.J. (2001) Cultural variations in the clinical presentation of depression and anxiety: implications for diagnosis and treatment. *The Journal of Clinical Psychiatry*, **62** (Suppl 13), 22–28.
11. WHO (2008) http://www.who.int/features/qa/62/en/index.html.
12. WHO (1996) Global Consultation on Violence and Health, Violence: A Public Health Priority (document WHO/EHA/SPI.POA.2), WHO, Geneva.
13. United Nations (1993) Declaration on the Elimination of Violence against Women, United Nations General Assembly, New York, 5 pages. http://www.un.org.
14. WHO (2002) World Report on Violence and Health, WHO, Geneva.
15. Helweg-Larsen, K. and Kastrup, M. (2007) Consequences of collective violence with particular focus on the gender perspective. – Secondary publication. *Danish Medical Bulletin*, **54**, 155–56.

16. Sartorius, N. (2000) Psychiatrie in Entwicklungsländern, in *Psychiatrie der Gegenwart. Band 3: Psychiatrie spezieller Lebenssituationen. 4. Auflage* (eds H. Helmchen *et al.*), Springer, Berlin Heidelberg New York, pp. 425–46.

17. WHO (1973) The International Pilot Study of Schizophrenia, WHO, Geneva.

18. Jablensky, A., Sartorius, N., Ehrenberg, G. *et al.* (1992) *Schizophrenia: Manifestations, Incidence and Course in Different Cultures: A World Health Organization Ten Countries Study*, Psychological Medicine, Monograph Supplement, vol. 20, Cambridge University Press, Cambridge.

19. Sartorius, N., Davidian, H., Ehrenberg, G. *et al.* (1983) Depressive Disorders in Different Cultures: Report on the WHO-Collaborative-Study on Standardized Assessment of Depressive Disorders, WHO, Geneva.

20. Jilek, W.G. and Jilek-Aall, L. (2000) Kulturspezifische psychische Störungen, in *Psychiatrie der Gegenwart. Band 3: Psychiatrie spezieller Lebenssituationen. 4. Auflage* (eds H. Helmchen *et al.*), Springer, Berlin Heidelberg New York.

21. Dennerstein, L., Astbury, J. and Morse, C. (1993) Psychosocial and Mental Health Aspects of Women's Health, WHO, Geneva.

22. Kastrup, M. and Arcel, L. (2004) Gender specific treatment. Gender specific treatment of refugees with PTSD, in *Broken spirits The Treatment of Traumatized Asylum Seekers, Refugees, War and Torture Victims* (eds J. Wilson and B. Drozdek), Brunner and Routledge, New York.

23. ISTSS (International Society Traumatic Stress Studies) (2000) Guidelines for treatment of PTSD. *Journal of Traumatic Stress Studies*, **13**, 539–88.

24. Londono, L. (1993) Mujer y Salud en el Contexto Politico. Diosas, Musas y Mujeres. (Violence, subordination and women's mental health.) (Consequences . . . Caracas: Monte Avila, pp. 161–70.

25. Desjarlais, R., Eisenberg, L., Good, B. and Kleinman, A. (eds) World Mental Health (1995) *Problems and Priorities in Low-income Countries*, Oxford University Press, Oxford.

26. Patel, V. and Kleinmann, A. (2003) Poverty and mental health in developing countries. *Bulletin of the World Health Organization*, **81**, 601–5.

27. Pfeiffer, W. (1994) *Transkulturelle Psychiatrie*, Thieme Verlag, Stuttgart, New York.

28. Tseng, W.S. (2003) *Clinician's Guide to Cultural Psychiatry*, Academic Press, San Diego.

29. Kastrup, M., Calliess, I., Behrendt, K. and Machleidt, W. (2008) Cultural Aspects of Depression. WPA Educational Program on Depression, in press.

30. UNHCR (2001) UNHCR Statistical Yearbook, UNHCR, Geneva.

31. Mollica, R., Wyshak, G. and Lavelle, J. (1987) The psychosocial impact of war trauma and torture on SouthEast Asian refugees. *The American Journal of Psychiatry*, **144**, 1567–72.

32. Reppesgaard, H. (1997) Studies on psychosocial problems among displaced people in Sri Lanka. *European Journal of Psychiatry*, **11**, 223–34.

33. Thulesius, H. and Håkansson, A. (1999) Screening for posttraumatic stress disorder symptoms among Bosnian refugees. *Journal of Traumatic Stress*, **12**, 167–74.

34. Cheung, P. (1994) Posttraumatic stress disorder among Cambodian refugees in New Zealand. *International Journal of Social Psychiatry*, **40**, 17–26.

35. Spasojevic, J., Heffer, R.W. and Snyder, D.K. (2000) Effects of posttraumatic stress and acculturation on marital functioning in Bosnian refugee couples. *Journal of Traumatic Stress*, **13**, 205–17.

36. Matthey, S., Silove, D.M., Barnett, B. *et al.* (1999) Correlates of depression and PTSD in Cambodian women with young children: a pilot study. *Stress Medicine*, **15**, 103–7.

37. Brundtland, G.H. (1999) International Consultation on the Health of Indigenous Peoples, Speech at Sweet Briar College 23.11.1999.

38. Kirmayer, L.J. and Minas, I.H. (2000) The future of cultural psychiatry: an international perspective. *Canadian Journal of Psychiatry*, **45**, 438–46.

39. Arcel, L.T., Folnegovic-Smalc, V., Tocilj-Simunkovic, G. (1998) Ethnic cleansing and post-traumatic coping, in *War Violence, Trauma and the Coping Process* (ed. L.T. Arcel), IRCT, Copenhagen.

40. Fabrega, H. and Mezzich, J. (1996) Cultural and historical foundations of psychiatric diagnosis, in *Culture and Psychiatric Diagnosis* (eds J. Mezzich *et al.*), APA Press, Washington.

41. WHO (2004) Gender in Mental Health Research, WHO, Geneva.

42. Cohen, E. (2007) Push to achieve tied to suicide in Asian-American women Posted: 8:45 p.m. EDT, May 16, 2007 CNN.

43. Khan, M.M. and Prince, M. (2003) Beyond rates: the tragedy of suicide in Pakistan. *Tropical Doctor*, **33**, 63–69.

44. Bhugra, D., Desai, M. and Baldwin, D. (1999) Suicide and attempted suicide across cultures, in *Ethnicity: An agenda for Mental Health* (eds D. Bhugra and V. Bahl), Gaskell, London.

45. Annan, K. (2004) Review of the implementation of the Beijing Platform for Action and Women 2000: Gender, Equality, Development and Peace for the 21st Century, E/CN.6/2005/2, p. 22, December 2004.

46. Ekblad, S., Kastrup, M., Eisenman, D. and Arcel, L. (2007) Interpersonal violence towards women: an overview and clinical directions, in *Immigrant Medicine* (eds P. Walker and E. Barnett), Saunders, Philadelphia.

47. Rios, T. and Caceres, V. (1999) *Violence, Subordination and Women's Mental Health. Consequences... La violencia domestica desde la perspectiva sindical*, El Exento, Rio Piedras, pp. 6–7.

48. Mullender, A. (2000) *La Violencia Domestica Una Nueva Vision de un Viejo Problema*, Paidos, Barcelona.

49. Burin, M. (1991) *El Malestar de las Mujeres: La Tranquilidad Recetada*, Paidos, Buenos Aires.

50. Cohn, M.R. (1999) They kill their own in the name of honor, in *The Toronto Star*, 8/01/1999.

51. Brand, A.L. (1998) *Women, the State and Political Liberalization, Middle Eastern and North African Experiences*, Columbia University Press, New York, pp. 132–39.

52. Antoun, R.T. (1977) *Arab Village: A Social Structural Study of a Trans-Jordanian Peasant Community*, Indiana University Press.

53. B'tselem (1994) The Israeli Information Center for Human Rights 'Morality, Family Honour and Collaboration', In: Collaborators in the Occupied Territories: Human Rights Abuses and Violations, The Israeli Information Center for Human Rights in the Occupied Territories. January 1994, 89–99, B'Tselem Report – Collaborators in the Occupied Territories.

54. Hamzeh-Muhaisen, M. (1997) Violence Against Women: Who Will Stop the Men? Palestine Report, October 10, 1997; 8–10.

55. l-Khayyat, S. (1993) *Honour and Shame: Women in Modern Iraq*, Saqi Books, London.

56. Stillwell, C. (2008) *Honor Killings: When the Ancient and the Modern Collide*, Wednesday, January 23, 2008. SF Gate online service Hearst Communications Inc., www.sfgate.com.

57. Spatz, M. (1991) Lesser' crime: a comparative study of legal defences for men who kill their wives. *Columbia Journal of Law and Social Problems*, **24**, 597–638.

58. Anwar, M. (1998) *The Family and Marriage In: Between Cultures, Continuity and Change in the Lives of Young Asians*, Routledge, London.

59. Constable, P. (2000) Women Pay The Price of 'Honor'. Washington Post, Monday, May 8, 2000.

60. Sharon, O. (2005) Islam: Governing Under Sharia, Copyright 2008 by the Council on Foreign Relations (*associate director*,cfr.org).

61. Niaz, U. and Hasan, S. (2006) Culture and mental health in women in South Asia. *World Psychiatry*, **5** (2), 57–65.

62. O'Hare, U. (1999) Realizing human rights for women. *Human Rights Quarterly*, **21**, 368–69.

63. Niaz, U. (2003) Violence against women in South Asian countries. *Archives of Women's Mental Health*, **6**, 173–84.

64. Leslie, J. (1996) Dowry, 'Dowry Deaths', and violence against women. *Journal of South Asia Women Studies*, **2** (4), 4.

65. Jejeebhoy, S. (1999) Wife battering in rural India; husband's right? Evidence from Survey Data. *Economic and Political Weekly*, **33**, 855–6212.

66. Fikree, F.F., Jafarey, S.N., Korejo, R. *et al.* (2006) Intimate partner violence before and during pregnancy: experiences of postpartum women in Karachi, Pakistan *Journal of the Pakistan Medical Association*, **56**, 252–57.

67. UNICEF (2000) Domestic Violence against Women and Girls, May 2000.

68. Abeyesekera, S. (1990) Women in Struggle: Sri Lanka 1980–1986. Paper presented at the Second National Convention on Women's Studies, CENWOR, Colombo.

69. Hensman, R. (1992) Feminism and ethnic nationalism in Sri Lanka. *Journal of Gender Studies*, **1**, 501–6.

70. Hoole, R., Somasundaram, D., Sritharan, K. and Thiranagama, R. (1990) *The Broken Palmyrah*, Sri Lanka Studies Institute, Claremont.

71. Pearson, V. (1995) Aspects of the Medical Care System in the People's of China. *Social Science and Medicine*, **41**, 1159–73.

72. Kandiyoti, D. (1995) Reflections on the politics of gender in Muslim societies: from Nairobi to Beijing, in *Faith and Freedom: Women's Human Rights in the Muslim World* (ed. M. Afkhami), I.B. Tauris, London, pp. 19–32.

73. Joseph, S. and Slyomovics, S. (2001) Introduction, in *Women and Power in the Middle East* (eds S. Joseph and S. Slyomovics), University of Pennsylvania Press, Philadelphia.

74. Sakr, N. (2000) Optical illusions: television and censorship in the Arab world. *Transnational Broadcasting Studies*, Fall/Winter.

75. Ikkaracan, U.P.; Women for Women's Human Rights (WWHR)-New Ways (2000) Muslim Societies (2000) and The Myth of a Warm Home: Violence in the Family.

Women and Sexuality in Muslim Societies (in Turkish), NGOs, Women for Women's Human Rights (WWHR) and New Ways, Turkey, pp. 417–26.

76. al-Afifi Abdel-Wahab, N. and Abdel-Hadi, A (1996) (eds). *The Feminist. Movement in the Arab World*. Cairo: Dar Al-Mostaqbal Al-Arabi/New. Woman Research and Study Center.

77. ADFM (Association Democratique des Femmes du Maroc) (2001) Convention CEDAW: Rapport Parallele, ADFM, Rabat.

78. Suad, J. and Najmabadi, A. (2003) Encyclopedia of Women & Islamic Cultures -Women, 682 pages. Collectif 95 Maghreb Egalite. Les Maghrebines entre violences symboliques et violences physiques. Collectif 95 Maghreb Egalite, Rabat, 1999.

79. UNDP (United Nations Development Program) (2001) *Human Development Report 2000*, Oxford University Press, Oxford.

80. Estrada, D. (2002) Latin America: Women Victims of Violence Face Hurdles to Justice, Santiago, September 13 (IPS).

81. Lykes, B., Brabeck, M., Ferns, T. and Radan, A. (1993) A human rights and mental health among Latin American women in situations of state-sponsored violence. *Psychology of the Women Quarterly*, **17**, 525–44.

82. Alvarez, S. (1990) *Engendering Democracy in Brazil: Women's Movements in Transition Politics*, Princeton University Press, Princeton.

83. Bleichmar, D. and Prefacio, E. (1991) Hacia una feminizacion de la norma, in *El Malestar de las Mujeres: La Tranquilidad Recetada* (ed. G. Burin), Paidos, Buenos Aires.

84. SCARF (1998) A Study of Mentally Disabled Women, Schizophreniz Research Foundation, Chennai.

85. WHO (2005) Mental Health: Facing the Challenges, Building Solutions. Report WHO European Ministerial Conference WHO.

86. Saraceno, B. and Saxena, S. (2004) Bridging the mental health research gap in low- and middle-income countries. *Acta Psychiatria Scandinavica*, **110**, 1–3.

23
Female mutilation

Amira Seif Eldin

Department of Community Medicine, Faculty of Medicine, Alexandria University, Alexandria, Egypt

23.1 Definition

Female genital mutilation (FGM) or female circumcision (FC) as it is alternatively known constitutes all procedures which involve partial or total removal of the external female genitalia or other injury to female genital organs whether for cultural or any other non-therapeutic reasons [1].

23.2 Introduction

Every year, 3 million girls and women are subjected to genital mutilation/cutting, a dangerous and potentially life-threatening procedure that causes unspeakable pain and suffering. This practise violates girls' and women's basic human rights, denying them of their physical and mental integrity, their right to freedom from violence and discrimination, and in the most extreme case, of their life [2].

Female genital mutilation/cutting (FGM/C) is a global concern. Not only is it practised among communities in Africa and the Middle East, but also in immigrant communities throughout the world. Moreover, recent data reveal that it occurs on a much larger scale than previously thought. It continues to be one of the most persistent, pervasive and silently endured human rights violations [3].

More than 2 million girls each year – or approximately 5500 girls every day – undergo FGM, the partial or total removal of the female external genitalia. It is estimated that some 100–140 million girls, the great majority of whom live

Contemporary Topics in Women's Mental Health   Edited by Chandra, Herrman, Fisher, Kastrup,
© 2009 John Wiley & Sons, Ltd   Niaz, Rondón and Okasha

in Africa, have been subjected to this traditional practise, which is associated with serious health consequences [4].

Short-term complications include haemorrhage, wound infection, urine retention, shock and sepsis.

Long-term complications include formation of keloids (scarring) and cysts; obstructed labour, which can lead to perineal lacerations, bleeding, infection and brain damage to infants; fistula formation and sexual and psychological problems. Some women die from the procedure. In the Central Africa Republic, Egypt and Eritrea alone, reliable survey data indicate that 1 million women have suffered the adverse health effects of genital cutting [5]. In recent years, there has been increasing recognition among many African governments, women's organisations and the international community that FGM violates women's bodily integrity, health and human rights. In cultures where FGM is practised, however, it is viewed as having important social, cultural, hygienic and even economic functions. The most common reasons given by communities that practise FGM are that it prevents female promiscuity, preserves virginity and promotes cleanliness.

Parents of girls in these communities believe that circumcision is necessary to avoid social rejection and increase the chances that their daughters will marry, thereby improving their wellbeing and the family's financial position. They fear that uncircumcised girls will become 'loose' women whose genitalia are abhorrent and frightening to men and even dangerous to newborns and health workers during childbirth [6].

23.3 Historical background

It is uncertain when FGM was first practised, but it certainly preceded the founding of both Christianity and Islam. There is no basis for the belief that the procedure was advocated or approved by Mohammed nor is it in any way part of the Islamic faith. Though the operation is largely confined to Muslims, it is also performed in certain Christian communities in Africa. FGM is practised in various forms in over 28 African countries and also in Oman, the Yemen and the United Arab Emirates and by some Muslims in Malaysia and Indonesia, while it is not practised in Iran, Iraq, Jordan, Libya or Saudi Arabia [7].

There is no religious justification for this practise. All three major monotheistic world religions define man as a perfect creation of the Almighty, and condemn doing any harm to God's creation. In Sura 95, Verse 4, the Koran states: 'We have created man in our most perfect image'. Besides, in Islam men and women are meant to experience sexual fulfillment, and it is considered the husband's matrimonial duty to satisfy his wife, a nearly impossible task when a woman is circumcised.

FGM is not prescribed by any religion. This is not, however, the general perception, especially regarding Islam. Although there is a theological branch of Islam that supports FGM of the *sunna* type, the Koran contains no text that requires the cutting of the female external genitalia, and it is widely accepted that the practise was current in Sudanese or Nubian populations before Islam. Moreover, the majority of Muslims around the world do not practise FGM. There is no evidence of the practise in Saudi Arabia and it is not found in several North African Muslim countries, including Algeria, Libya, Morocco and Tunisia [8].

23.4 Classification

Where FGM takes place, it is often performed during infancy, childhood or adolescence. FGM has traditionally been called 'female circumcision'. Recognition of its harmful physical, psychological and human rights consequences, however, has led to use of the term 'female genital mutilation', a term that more accurately describes the consequences of the procedure and distinguishes it from the much milder male circumcision.

There are several types of FGM. The following is based on the World Health Organization typology [1].

1. *Type I (commonly referred to as clitoridectomy)*: Excision (removal) of the clitoral hood with or without removal of all or part of the clitoris.

2. *Type II (commonly referred to as excision)*: Excision (removal) of the clitoris together with part or all of the labia minora (the inner vaginal lips). This is the most widely practised form.

3. *Type III (commonly referred to as infibulation)*: Excision (removal) of part or all of the external genitalia (clitoris, labia minora and labia majora) and stitching or narrowing of the vaginal opening, leaving a very small opening, about the size of a matchstick, to allow for the flow of urine and menstrual blood.

4. *Type IV (Unclassified)*:
   a. Pricking, piercing or incision of the clitoris and/or labia.
   b. Stretching the clitoris and/or labia.
   c. Cauterisation by burning of the clitoris and surrounding tissues.
   d. Scraping (angurya cuts) of the vaginal orifice or cutting (gishiri cuts) of the vagina.
   e. Introduction of corrosive substances into the vagina to cause bleeding, or introduction of herbs into the vagina to tighten or narrow the vagina.
   f. Any other procedure that falls under the definition of FGM.

In Type III, the girl or woman's legs are generally bound together from the hip to the ankle so she remains immobile for approximately 40 days to allow for the formation of scar tissue. In some communities where no stitching is used, adhesive substances including sugar, eggs, and in rare cases, even animal excreta are sometimes placed on the wound to allow it to heal. Overall, approximately 15% of women who have experienced FGM undergo this form. However, where it is practised, it sometimes affects 90–100% of the women.

23.5 Epidemiology of FGM

It is estimated that over 130 million girls and women have undergone female genital utilation. It is also estimated that 2 million girls are at risk of undergoing some form of the procedure every year. Most of the women and girls affected live in more than 28 countries in Africa mainly in northeast Africa and in a belt reaching from east to west north of the equator [11]. About 90% of women in northern Sudan have undergone FGM, although some live in the Middle East and Asia [10, 12]. Affected women and girls are also increasingly found in Europe, Australia, New Zealand, Canada and the USA, primarily among immigrant communities from Africa and southwestern Asia [13]. The practise is also seen in the Middle East (parts of Oman, the United Arab Emirates and Yemen) and in other countries such as Indonesia and Malaysia [14]. Even though many people re-evaluate and abandon the practise when they emigrate [15]. There is evidence that it continues in Europe [16]. Many Somali girls living in London have been subjected to genital mutilation after moving from their home country [17]. In the United Kingdom, though data on prevalence are scarce, there are thought to be 3000−4000 new cases every year [18].

FGM will continue indefinitely unless effective interventions are found to convince communities to abandon the practise. Many campaigners, development and health workers from the communities where FGM is a traditional practise recognise the need for change, but do not know how to achieve such an extensive social transformation [19].

Recent analysis reveals that some 3 million girls and women are cut each year on the African continent (Sub-Saharan Africa, Egypt and Sudan). Of these, nearly half are from two countries: Egypt and Ethiopia. Although this figure is significantly higher than the previous estimate of 2 million, this new figure does not reflect increased incidence, but is a more accurate estimate drawn from a greater availability of data [3].

The Egypt demographic health survey published in 2001, revealed a nationwide prevalence rate of FGM of 97% among ever-married women. Besides, the survey indicated widespread support for the practise, claiming that 81% of Egyptian women support its continuation. It is practised at all levels of Egyptian society, without respect to social class, educational background or religious affiliation. Both Muslims and Coptic Christians practise FGM throughout the country [20].

The age at which large proportions of girls are cut varies greatly from one country to another. About 90% of girls in Egypt are cut between the ages of 5 and 14 years, while in Ethiopia, Mali and Mauritania, 60% or more of girls surveyed underwent the procedure before their fifth birthday [12]. In Yemen, the Demographic and Health Survey carried out in 1997 found that as many as 76% of girls underwent FGM/C in their first two weeks of life. In-country variations are also apparent, often reflecting the distribution of ethnic groups. In Sudan, a cohort study in 2004 found that at least 75% of girls had undergone FGM/C by the age of 9−10 in South Darfur, a State which has a predominantly Fur and Arab population, while in Kassala, which has a predominantly Beja population,

75% of girls had already been cut by the age of 4–5 [10]. Despite many decades of campaigns and legislation, FGM is still highly traditionally been practised and is still practised in girls from these areas now living in Europe.

23.6 Physical complications of FGM

FGM causes extreme damage to a woman or a girl, sometimes resulting in death. In cases where the procedure is carried out in unsanitary conditions and unsterile equipment is used, the dangers of infection are great. When it is performed in the sanitary conditions of a hospital by qualified personnel risk of infection may be reduced, but the long-term consequences remain.

Examples of short-term consequences include: bleeding (often haemorrhaging from rupture of the blood vessels of the clitoris); post-operative shock; damage to other organs resulting from lack of surgical expertise of the person performing the procedure and the violence of the resistance of the patient when anaesthesia is not used; infections, including tetanus and septicemia, because of the use of unsterilised or poorly disinfected equipment; urine retention caused by swelling and inflammation; severe bleeding sometimes leading to death.

Examples of long-term consequences include: chronic infections of the bladder and vagina. In Type III, the urine and menstrual blood can only leave the body drop by drop; the build up inside the abdomen and fluid retention often cause infections and inflammation that can lead to infertility; dysmenorrhoea or extremely painful menstruation; excessive scar tissue at the site of the operation; formation of cysts on the stitch line; child birth obstruction, which can result in the development of fistulas; tearing in the vaginal and/or bladder wall and chronic incontinence; risk of HIV infection. (There is a growing speculation of a potential risk of HIV/AIDS associated with the procedure, especially when the same unsterile instruments are used on multiple girls.) Reinfibulation must be performed each time a child is born. When infibulation (Type III) is performed, the small opening left in the genital area is too small for the head of a baby to pass through. Failure to reopen this area can lead to death or brain damage of the baby and death of the mother. The excisor must reopen the mother and restitch her again after the birth. In most ethnic groups the woman is restitched as before with the same tiny opening. In other ethnic groups the opening is left only slightly larger to reduce painful intercourse. (In most cases, not only must the woman be reopened for each childbirth, but also on her wedding night when the excisor may have to be called in to open her so she can consummate the marriage.) For a woman who has been infibulated, first coitus is invariably a difficult process. Even later intercourse may be painful (dyspareunia). Couples may complain of infertility, though the real problem is the inability of the husband to achieve penetration.

Problems at pregnancy and delivery: at time of delivery, fear or obstruction (if the scar fails to dilate) may cause delay and prolonged second stage of labour. Obstructed labour may be dangerous to the mother and the child: the mother may suffer lacerations or tears, keloid formation and implantation dermoids.

Fayyad gives a horrifying account of the death of a woman in Egypt after the operation was done by force. The baby may suffer brain damage as a result of an insufficiency of oxygen (anoxia) [21]. In Africa, prolonged or obstructed labour may occur if there is inadequate obstetric care. Dirie and Lindmark in Somalia found that even in otherwise normal deliveries anterior and mediolateral episiotomies were required [22].

In Britain, with proper obstetric care there is rarely any difficulty in the second stage of labour, though an incision of the web of tissue across the vagina is often necessary. In hospitals unused to looking after women with genital mutilation there may be hostility and incomprehension, particularly if the woman requests resuturing [23].

23.7 Psychological complications

Scientific studies are needed on the precise psychological effects of FGM on a girl or woman. However, changes have been observed in some girls who have been subjected to the procedure. Nightmares, depression, shock, passivity, feelings of betrayal are not uncommon among these girls.

The study done in Kenya [24] reported that for many girls and women, FGM is an acutely traumatic experience that leaves a lasting psychological mark and may adversely affect their full emotional development. Here too, scientific research is limited, but the anecdotal evidence from girls and women who have undergone the practise is testament to the impact it has had on their lives. Girls are generally conscious when the operation is performed, and for many, it is a shocking experience marked not only by acute pain, but also by fear and confusion. In cases where there has been some preparation for the operation, girls are often expected to suppress such feelings and collaborate in the proceedings. The experience of FGM/C (female genital mutilation/cutting) has also been related to a range of psychological and psychosomatic disorders such as disturbances in eating and sleeping habits, moods and cognition. Symptoms of these include sleeplessness, recurring nightmares, loss of appetite, weight loss or excessive weight gain, as well as panic attacks, difficulties in concentrating and learning, and other symptoms of post-traumatic stress [24].

To appreciate why this operation is performed some understanding is required of the cultural background associated with FGM. In the least destructive operation, when only the prepuce of the clitoris is removed, the object is to reduce the woman's sexual desire and hence to ensure her virginity until she is married. The more extensive operations, involving stitching of the vagina, have the same aim of ensuring chastity until marriage. The reduction in the size of the vaginal orifice is supposed to increase the husband's enjoyment of the sexual act; there is no good evidence for this and initially penetration may be difficult and painful for both partners. From the family's point of view the operation ensures a satisfactory bride price; an eligible man would not consider marrying a girl who had not had the operation. The procedure is arranged by the mother or grandmother and in Africa is usually performed by a traditional birth attendant, a midwife making a little extra money or by a professional exciser. FGM is supported and encouraged by men; indeed the operation can be regarded as an exercise in male supremacy and the oppression of women.

FGM, representing a violation of someone's physical intactness, can be classified as a psychological trauma according to DSM-IV and a potential cause of posttraumatic stress disorder (PTSD).

The results of the study done by Behrendt and Moritz [18] indicated that FGM is likely to cause various emotional disturbances, forging the way to psychiatric disorders, especially PTSD. The high rate of PTSD of more than 30% in this group is comparable to the rate of PTSD of early childhood abuse, which, on average, ranges between 30 and 50%. Despite the fact that FGM presents a part of the participants' ethnic background, the results imply that cultural embedment does not protect against the development of PTSD and other psychiatric disorders. In agreement with other studies, PTSD rather than trauma was associated with declarative memory dysfunction [18].

There are no figures for the incidence of emotional or psychological effects, but it is probable that this would be small in communities where social pressures are strongly in favour of the operation. Conversely, in such circumstances, the uncircumcised girl may be the object of disapproval and derision.

One of the early psychological changes for girls after FC, was reported by teachers in Sudan who said that after FC their students acted differently, avoiding boys, no longer teasing them, sitting shyly apart. Such modesty on the part of girls is more common at the start of puberty; it can be observed in societies where FC is not performed [25].

23.8 Posttraumatic stress disorder and memory problems after FGM

In many cases, girls and women who have been traumatised by FGM/C remain silent about their experience. In some cultures they have no socially acceptable means of expressing their feelings of psychological unease or distress. In cases where they cannot or will not speak openly about a psychosocial difficulty, individual women or girls may present it in terms of a physical complaint. Some evidence of the psychological effects of FGM is also emerging among immigrant communities in Europe, America, Australia and New Zealand. Migrant women who have undergone FGM/C often face an additional psychological burden, since both the values associated with FGM/C and its physical and psychological impact are poorly understood in their host country [3].

23.9 Obstacles facing changing harmful social convention: Female genital mutilation/cutting

Most societies that practise FGM view it as an important part of their cultural identity. In addition to the fear that their daughters will not be marriageable, both parents and daughters fear being ostracised by their community and peers if they were to stop the practise. Maintaining social cohesion and group membership is a powerful motivating force that drives the continuation of the practise. However, there are some signs of change that indicate the potential for eventual abandonment of the practise. Although any cutting of a healthy female organ is a threat to the girl's health and a violation of her rights to bodily integrity, in some countries a move away from the practise of infibulation (Type III), the most severe form of FGM, towards less radical forms of cutting (Types I and II) is being observed [26].

In Sudan the type of FC called the 'Sunna' is frequently used to refer to circumcision in the Sudan. Men generally use the word without any understanding of different types of FC. ' Sunna' literally means (according to the tradition of the Prophet Mohammed) and, in reference to circumcision, perpetuates and reflects misunderstanding of Islamic injunctions. There is a great debate on the support of female circumcision. There are no verses in the Holy Koran that support FGM, however, there were associated practises with the hadith or sayings in which Prophet Mohamed instructed the circumciser to 'Cut off the foreskin (the prepuce or outer fold of skin of clitoris), and do not cut off deeply (not cutting the clitoris itself), for this is brighter for the face and more favourable with the husband'. This hadith is quoted by many Islamic scholars such as Al-Hakim, Al-Baihaqi. The purpose and importance of FGM varies from community to community and, very often, from family to family. Proponents contend that FGM is justified as part of socialisation into womanhood or because it has religious significance (especially among Muslims), curbs female sexual desires, or has aesthetic, purifying or hygienic benefits [7]. FGM does reward its practitioners if they charge for services or receive social recognition and status. One of the main factors behind the persistence of FGM is its social significance for females. In most regions where it is practised, a woman achieves recognition only through marriage and childbearing, and many men refuse to marry a woman who has not undergone FGM. Therefore to be uncircumcised is to have no access to status or a voice in these communities [27].

Usually female circumcision is considered an important occasion in the life of a girl in such communities. She is for once the centre of attention. She receives presents. There is a celebration. Girls learn circumcision is necessary to be accepted in society and to marry. It is not surprised that even though girls fear the operation itself, they look forward to the event. Although different types of circumcision did not appear to affect sexual satisfaction significantly, but here certainly social and psychological factors, as well as physical ones, are likely to affect women's response. Survey data on sexual problems were not especially reliable. The importance of the ceremonial aspects associated with FGM is declining in many communities. This trend may also be related, in part, to the existence of legislation to prohibit FGM that discourages public manifestations of the practise [28].

The physical dangers of FC, the harm it can do, is indisputable medically. Yet large parts of the population fail to perceive FC as hazardous to the health. Males especially seem ignorant, content to dismiss damage arising from FC as part of the natural, inevitable consequences of being born a woman. Many women share this predisposition. This is one of the reasons why FC persists, sustain the practise and survive. Certain ideas about sex and marriage are practically ubiquitous among African cultures that infibulation is necessary as a safeguard of virginity, and to insure a husband's pleasure. Boys and girls acquire such notions as part of their socialisation and education. Men will not marry an uncircumcised woman; she is unclean, immoral [14].

Of the five countries that demonstrate the highest rates of prevalence (Egypt, Guinea, Mali, Somalia and Sudan) – none have shown any evidence of change in prevalence over time [3].

At the community and at the family level, strong pressure is brought to bear on women and girls to ensure continuation of the practise of FGM. Women who are not excised face immediate divorce (Somalia) or forcible excision (most communities). As initiates, girls are sworn into secrecy so that the pain and ordeals associated with the procedure of FGM will not be discussed, especially with unexcised women (Kenya and Sierra Leone). Songs and poems are used to deride unexcised girls (most communities). The fear of the unknown through punishment by God, ancestral curses and other supernatural powers is instilled in them [29].

Prior to the 1995 and 2000, Egyptian Demographic and Health Surveys, the belief that FGM was on the decline and the ideas that this attitude prevails mainly among illiterate populations, the lower and lower middle class was a false one and on the other hand, despite the battle over FGM that followed the 1994 International Conference on Population and Development (ICPD) held in Cairo. Several national surveys and community-based studies have revealed that FGM remains a highly challenging public health problem in Egypt [20, 30]. The Demographic and Health Survey in Egypt published in 2001 revealed a nationwide prevalence of 97% among ever-married women. In addition, the survey indicated widespread support for the practise and claimed 81% of women supported its continuation. It is practised at all levels of Egyptian social class, educational background or religious affiliation.

The 'medicalisation' of FGM, whereby girls are cut by trained personnel rather than by traditional practitioners, is on the rise. This trend may reflect the impact of campaigns that emphasise the health risks associated with the practise, but fail to address the underlying motivations for its perpetuation. Analysing survey data by age group reveals that in Egypt, Guinea and Mali, the medicalisation of FGM/C has increased dramatically in recent years [11].

In a study done by Mostafa *et al.* to explore the knowledge, beliefs and attitudes of medical students (future physicians) about FGM; 52% of them support the continuation of the practise and 73.2% are encouraging its medicalisation as a risk reduction strategy [31].

Taking note of the Government's 1996 decision to prohibit FGM and the 1997 ministerial decree banning this practise in Ministry of Health service outlets, as well as various efforts to educate the public about the harm caused by this practise, including campaigns in the media and in the curricula, the Committee is concerned that the practise is still widespread [3].

23.10 The basic concept for FGM elimination (The mental map for FGM)

The three overlapping reasons for the practise of FGM are the myth of: Religion (spiritual cleanliness), Hygiene and Aesthetics (fear about ugly look and bad odour), and Society (to be accepted).

Spiritual and religious reasons, sociological reasons, hygienic and aesthetic reasons – seem to indoctrinate society into the practise without explicitly address-ing women's sexuality. According to these reasons, the clitoris and external genitalia are believed to be ugly and dirty, and if not excised can grow to unsightly proportions. In addition, they are purported to make women spiritually unclean. Their removal is thus required by religion. The clitoris is also believed to prevent women from reaching maturity and having the right to identify with a person's age group, the ancestors and the human race. According to the numerous myths associated with this set of beliefs, the external genitalia have the power to make a birth attendant blind; cause infants to become abnormal, insane or die or cause husbands and fathers to die [32, 33].

While the overall 'mental map' is similar in most of the countries which practise FGM, some reasons are more prominent in certain countries than others. For example, Muslim countries tend to associate the practise with tradition as well as with Islam; some communities emphasise the rite of passage from childhood to adulthood (Burkina Faso, Ethiopia, Kenya and Sierra Leone) or to humanity (some Eritreans) and others emphasis the mythological aspects (e.g. in Nigeria some people believe that if the head of the baby touches the clitoris, the baby will die). Understanding the different components of 'the mental map' and their relative strength is crucial for any intervention strategy.

Like other social behaviours, the practise of FGM derives from varied and complex belief systems (Box 23.1). It is tempting to simplify matters by isolating a piece of the behaviour and explaining it as a separate item, for example, 'FGM has negative health consequences'. Yet it is crucial to see the big picture – the connections among all aspects of the behaviour. The challenge of taking the whole picture into consideration may seem daunting, but social behaviour involves a vast range of influences – defined by culture. Culture acts as a lens or filter through which people view, understand and interpret the world. Each culture is selective in what is filtered out and what reaches the human consciousness. Some things may pass unchanged (basic human needs) while others may undergo subtle shifts in emphasis. The filter effect of culture has great importance for health communication programmes (Box 23.2). Because culture is not static and changes constantly and because of the inherent functions of culture, it is important for healthcare providers and community workers to strive towards gaining cultural competency by assessing their own values and biases – their own 'filters' and 'mental maps' – and by respecting the values, culture and biases of others [28, 34].

23.11 Recommendations in countries where FGM is commonly practised

1. The wrong concept that FGM tends to be considered mainly from the woman's point of view and has become identified as a feminist issue should be corrected.

2. It seems a mistaken policy as FGM would die out if men ceased to insist on it. It is therefore important that men should be included and involved in educational programmes.

3. The cooperation of local press and radio stations should be sought, and help should be requested from local newspapers and news sheets in the relevant languages.

Box 23.1 Statements from Islamic and Coptic Church Leaders

Islamic Shari'a protects children and safeguards their rights. Those who fail to give rights to their children commit a major sin. [. . .] FGM is a medical issue, what doctors say we heed and obey. There is no text in Shari'a, in the Koran, in the prophetic Sunna addressing FGM. The Grand Imam, Sheikh Mohammed Sayed Tantawi, Sheikh of Al-Azhar. Cairo Conference (2003 [9]).

It has been proven to us with authenticated religious evidence that there is no rightful Shariat evidence on which to base the legitimacy of any form of FGM/C. Moreover any type has associated harm, as stated by trusted doctors. Signed statement by 30 Sheikhs from the eight largest Sufist groups in Sudan, 2004 [10].

From the Christian perspective – this practise has no religious grounds whatsoever. Further, it is medically, morally and practically groundless. When God created the human being, he made everything in him/her good: each organ has its function and role. So, why do we allow the disfiguring of God's good creation? There is not a single verse in the Bible or the Old or New Testaments, nor is there anything in Judaism or Christianity – not one single verse speaks of female circumcision. Bishop Moussa, Bishop for Youth of the Coptic Orthodox Church and Representative of Pope Shenouda III. Cairo Conference (2003) [9].

Box 23.2 A Mother's Story: Challenges Faced by Those Who Begin the Process of Change

Khadija is a devout Ansar Sunna Muslim from the Beni Amer tribal group in Eastern Sudan. She lives with her extended family. When she leaves the house, she covers herself in a black abaya (garment) and face veil to be properly modest. As a girl, she underwent infibulation, known in Sudan as 'pharaonic' cutting, according to Beni Amer tradition. Now she has a six-year-old daughter who has not yet been cut. Khadija attended a programme about harmful traditional practises, where she learned about the health complications associated with FGM/C. Along with other women, she registered her daughter with the group of uncircumcised girls. Yet Khadija is troubled. Although she doesn't want her daughter to suffer from the health complications she heard about, she knows that men favour the practise for religious reasons. She also expects that her mother-in-law will have something to say about it. 'If I don't cut her, there won't be anyone to marry her,' says Khadija. 'I wish I didn't have daughters, because I am so worried about them' [7].

---

4. Provide all healthcare providers (doctors, nurses, midwife) with knowledge and life skills education related to FGM in their undergraduate curricula and part of their in services training.

References

1. WHO (1999) Female Genital Mutilation Program to Date: What Works and What Doesn't Work, WHO/CHS/WMH/99.5, Geneva.
2. Mackie, G. (2000) in *Female Genital Cutting: the Beginning of the End* (eds B. Shell-Duncan and Y. Hernlund) Female Circumcision in Africa: Culture, Controversy and Change. Lynne Rienner, Boulder, pp. 253–282.
3. UNICEF (2004) UNICEF Global Consultation on Indicators, NYHQ, Child Protection, November 11–13, 2004.
4. Elmusharaf, S., Elhadi, N. and Almroth, L. (2006) Reliability of self reported form of female genital mutilation and WHO classification cross sectional study. *British Medical Journal*, **333** (7559), 124.
5. Carr, D. (1997) *Female Genital Cutting, Findings from the Demographic and Health Surveys Program*, Macro International Inc., Calverton.
6. Redwan, A., Salentine, S. and Hassett, P. (2004) *Female Genital Cutting in Ethiopia: a Rapid Appraisal of Knowledge, Beliefs and Practice of Men, Women and Community Leaders in Harar and Jijiga Cities, Awomer and Burqa Farmers Associations, Manna Woreda in Jimma Zone*, The PRIME II Project, IntraHealth International, Inc., Addis Ababa, Chapel Hill.

7. Toubia, N. (1993) *Female Genital Mutilation: a Call for Global Action*, Women, Inc., New York, p. 9.
8. Bayoumi, A. (2003) Baseline Survey on FGM Prevalence and Cohort Group Assembly.
9. Population Council (2003) Female Circumcision in Indonesia: Extent, Implications and Possible Interventions to Uphold Women's Health Rights, Population Council, Jakarta.
10. Maiga, C.O. (1997) Femmes Musulmanes: une Identite Reaffirmee, Le Soudanais, No 141, December 1997, p. 3.
11. Shell-Duncan, B. (2001) The Medicalization of Female Circumcision; Harm Reduction or Promotion of Female.
12. Family Health Department (1996) Safe Motherhood Needs Assessment, Ethiopia Ministry of Health, Addis Abbaba.
13. Dorkenoo, E. and Elworthy, S. (1992) Female Genital Mutilation: Proposals for Change, Minority, London.
14. WHO (2000) Female Genital Mutilation, Fact sheet no. 241, World Health Organization, Geneva.
15. Johnsdotter, S. and Essen, B. (2004) The Conflictual Feelings Experienced by Migrant Women are Described.
16. Sami, I.R. (1986) Female circumcision with special reference to the Sudan. *Annals of Tropical Paediatrics*, **6**, 99–115.
17. El Dareer, A. (1983) Complications of female circumcision in the Sudan. *Tropical Doctor*, **13**, 131–33.
18. Behrendt, A. and Moritz, S. (2005) Post traumatic stress disorder and memory problems after female genital mutilation. *The American Journal of Psychiatry*, **162**, 1000–2.
19. World Health Organization (WHO) (2001) Female Genital Mutilation: Policy Guidelines for Nurses and Health Workers.
20. El-Zanaty, F. and Way, A. (2001) Egypt Demographic and health survey 2000, Ministry, Calverton.
21. Fayyad, S. (1993) *Voices*, Marion Boyars Publishers, London, pp. 102–7.
22. Dirie, M.A. and Lindmark, G. (1991) A hospital study of the complications of female circumcision. *Tropical Doctor*, **21**, 146–48.
23. Dorkenoo, E. and Elworthy, S. (1992) Female Genital Mutilation: Proposals for Change, Minority Rights Group, London.
24. Kagondu, G. (2002) Female Genital Mutilation Eradication Project: Pilot Project in Four Districts of Kenya, Mid-term Evaluation Report, Maendeleo Ya Wanake Organization (MYWO) and Program for Appropriate Technology in Health (PATH).
25. Rushwan, H., Slot, C., El Dareer, A. and Bushra, N. (1983) Female Circumcision in the Sudan. Prevalence, Complications, Attitudes and Changes, Faculty of Medicine, University of Khartoum, Khartoum.
26. Mohamud, A., Radney, S. and Ringheim, K. (2002) Protecting and empowering girls: confronting the underlying roots of female genital mutilation, in *Responding to Cairo: Case Studies* (eds N. Haberland and D. Measham).
27. Mohamud, A., Ali, N. and Yinger, N. (1998) Review of Female Genital Mutilation Programs in Africa.

28. UNICEF (2005) Innocenti Digest. Changing A Harmful Social Convention: Female Genital Mutilation/Cutting.

29. WHO (1996) Female Genital Mutilation and Obstetric Outcome.

30. Egypt Report of Female Genital Mutilation (FGM) or Female Genital Cutting (2001) http://www.state.gov/g/wi/rls/rep/crfgm/10096pf.htm, US Department of State. Released by the Office of the Senior Coordinator for International Women's Issues, Washington, DC.

31. Mostafa, S., Zeiny, N., Tayel, S. and Moubarak, E. (2006) What Do Medical Students in Alexandria Know About Female Circumcision.

32. Mohammud, A. (1992) FGM a Continuing Violation of Young Women's Rights, Passages (Field Notes Section), Advocates for Youth, March 1992.

33. Mohammud, A. (1997) The Role of Youth and Youth Serving Organizations. Paper Presented at the African Adolescent Forum, Program for Appropriate Technology in Health (PATH), Addid Ababa, January 20, 1997.

34. WHO (2006) Collaborative prospective study in six African countries. *Lancet*, **367**, 1835–41.

SECTION 5

Gender, social policy and implications for promoting women's mental health

Jane Fisher[1] and Helen Herrman[2]

[1]Key Centre for Women's Health in Society, WHO Collaborating Centre in Women's Health, University of Melbourne, Melbourne, Australia

[2]Orygen Youth Health Research Centre, The University of Melbourne; WHO Collaborating Centre in Mental Health, Melbourne, Australia

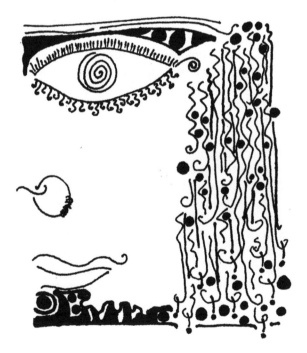

Contemporary Topics in Women's Mental Health   Edited by Chandra, Herrman, Fisher, Kastrup,
© 2009 John Wiley & Sons, Ltd   Niaz, Rondón and Okasha

Commentary

Social and political context and the promotion of women's mental health

There is debate about the causes of mental health problems in women and this has implications for mental health promotion, primary prevention, early intervention and treatment. Although exact estimation is limited by methodological constraints, the overall prevalence of severe mental illnesses in adult populations appears similar in women and men. Between 0.2–2.0% of adults develop schizophrenia and 0.4–1.6% a bipolar mood disorder across the lifespan [1]. However, in the countries in which large comprehensive community prevalence studies of mental illness have been undertaken, women are consistently more likely than men to experience some of the common mental disorders. Women aged 18–64 are for example, between 1.6 and 2.6 times more likely to experience Major Depression in their lifetimes than men are. This difference is most apparent during the life phase of reproduction and caring for dependent children. Panic Disorder occurs two to three times more commonly in women than men. Somatisation or the tendency to experience clinically significant symptoms, which cannot be explained by a known medical condition, is diagnosed 10 times more frequently in women than in men. Borderline, Histrionic and Dependent Personality disorders are diagnosed more frequently in women than in men. Co-morbidity or the co-occurrence of more than one diagnosable condition, in particular the common mental disorders, is associated with higher disability and is more common in women than in men [2].

A number of hypotheses are proposed to explain this phenomenon of higher rates of common mental disorders in women. Many investigators have presumed that differences in rates of mental disorders between sexes are biologically determined. The hormonal differences between females and males, especially those associated with the menstrual cycle and reproduction, are assumed to be responsible and to render women intrinsically vulnerable to poor mental health. While biological differences may contribute, as yet the notion that these underpin different rates of psychological disturbance between women and men is unproven [2, 3].

The second group of theories ascribes women's greater vulnerability to individual psychological functioning. In particular the presumption that women worry excessively and are 'neurotic', with less adaptive and more 'emotion-focused' coping styles in the face of adverse life events [4, 5]. These theories are predicated on the presumption that the events are not ones that should arouse anxiety and that disproportionate anxiety renders women vulnerable to more sustained mental health problems.

It is also proposed that clinicians and researchers, who are socialised and shaped within cultures, form stereotypes about what constitutes normality in females and males and therefore what divergence from these should be regarded as abnormal. Broverman *et al.*'s classic study [6] demonstrated that 79 currently active mental health professionals' clinical judgements about what constituted healthy adult functioning were governed significantly by gender stereotypes. Similar characteristics were assigned by both male and female clinicians to a notionally healthy man and a healthy adult whose sex was not specified. However, a healthy female was characterised by being more submissive, suggestible, non-aggressive, non-competitive, concerned about appearance, emotional, excitable and disinterested in mathematics and science than a healthy man or adult of non-specified sex. Diagnostic decisions are significantly influenced by the gender of the patient, with women being more likely than men to be diagnosed as depressed and prescribed antidepressants than men presenting with the same symptoms [7].

The last general explanation covers social causation hypotheses, that it is aspects of women's and men's lives which make them more or less vulnerable to different patterns of ill health, including mental health. In these, the contribution of the different social position occupied by women is integral to both the higher level of risk factors for poor mental health that they face and the lower levels of protective factors to which they have access. Chen *et al.* [8] undertook a multilevel analysis of self-reported depression symptoms collected from more than 7700 women and publicly available data from the 50 American states in which they lived. These data included: political participation (number of female elected officers, availability of a legislative body for the status of women and number of females registered to vote); reproductive rights (state-supported access to legal abortion, modern contraception and fertility treatment); economic autonomy (legislated right to equal employment, number of female owned businesses and proportion of women with incomes below the poverty line) and employment and earning (median female income and rates of female labour force participation). Women who lived in states in which female political participation was high, reproductive rights recognised and employment and economic autonomy assured had significantly lower average levels of depressive symptoms than others. It was concluded that as there is no basis to presume that women in general are biologically or psychologically different between states, that social determinants outweigh both intrinsic biological and individual psychological factors in explaining gender differences in rates of depression.

Mental health is related inextricably to an individual's life circumstances and personal experiences. However, wider contextual factors, including a society's concern for gender, ethnicity and the human rights to education, equal social and economic participation, safety, individual autonomy and freedom from discrimination are also closely related to mental health [9]. A social model of health takes all these factors into account and presumes that an individual's state of health or experience of illness is determined by personal experiences, social circumstances, culture and political environment in addition to inherited or biological factors [2].

Reflecting this social model of health the World Health Organization (WHO) defines mental health in broad terms as:

> ... the capacity of the individual, the group and the environment to interact
> with one another in ways that promote subjective well-being, the optimal

development and use of mental abilities (cognitive, affective and relational), the achievement of individual and collective goals consistent with
justice and the attainment and preservation of conditions of fundamental
equality . . . [10].

This definition makes it clear that daily experiences regarding opportunities
to use individual abilities and skills; to experience personal achievement and a
sense of effectiveness are fundamental to experiencing an inner, subjective sense
of wellbeing. The definition also emphasises the importance of development over
the whole course of life, that early experiences and opportunities influence later
capacities for participation. Further, there is acknowledgement of the central
importance to the individual of relationships with other people, including of
trust, intimacy and the giving and receiving of affection, support and care;
collaboration and the opportunity to work together to achieve common goals
and to have shared experiences. The social, cultural, economic and political living
environment is crucial and mental health cannot be realised without justice and
equality of human rights; inclusion of all and fairness of opportunity and access
to adequate resources on which to live [9]. These are intrinsically gendered. Even
in the contemporary world women's rights to equality of access to education,
personal safety, reproductive choice and freedom from discrimination are not
recognised universally.

Following the establishment of WHO, the United Nations oversaw the formation of formal covenants enshrining health as a human right. The International
Covenant on Economic, Social and Cultural Rights (ICESCR) (1966) [10] states
the right of every person to the enjoyment of the highest attainable standard of
physical and mental health and that this includes the right to skilled healthcare
and accessible, affordable health services.

Thirty years after the establishment of the WHO, the International Conference
on Primary Health Care, held at Alma-Ata, USSR, in September 1978 wrote the
Alma-Ata Declaration (1978). It reaffirmed the definition of health as being more
than the absence of illness; identified again the gross inequalities in the health
status of people living in developing compared to those from developed countries
and stated that this disparity was of common concern to all countries. It did not
however, make specific reference to mental health or to differences in the health
status of women and men. In 1981 the WHO published a paper on the social
aspects of mental health, but it did not highlight the particular social risks faced
disproportionately by girls and women [11].

In 1995, 30 years after the ICESCR was signed, these disparities were addressed
specifically in the United Nations sponsored Fourth World Conference on
Women in Beijing, China. The principal themes of the Conference were: the
advancement and empowerment of women in relation to women's human rights;
women and poverty; women and decision-making; the girl child and violence
against women as pervasive areas of concern in women's lives including to their
health. The Beijing Declaration and Platform for Action (1995) states explicitly
that women's health involves their mental as well as their physical and social
wellbeing and is determined by the interpersonal, social, cultural, political and

economic contexts of their lives, as well as by biology. It identifies distinctly the adverse effects of social exclusion and powerlessness; excessive work and sexual and gender-based violence to women's health, including their mental health. Astbury and Cabral de Mello [2] in their influential evidence based review on women's mental health for the WHO in 2000 argued persuasively that the notion of a social model of mental health, while of intrinsic value, had to be a revised to become a gendered social model of health.

It was clear by 2000 that the aspirations of the Alma Ata declaration were still to be met and that further whole of government and international agency approaches were needed to address development disparities including their impact on health. In September 2000, 189 member states ratified the United Nations Millennium Declaration that every woman man and child has the right to development and freedom from want and that progress was to be measurable and demonstrable. In order to ensure this aim, it defines goals, targets and indicators for combating poverty, hunger, disease, illiteracy, environmental degradation and, most crucially, discrimination against women as central to development. The Millennium Development Goals (MDGs) are the central reference against which global development is assessed. While MDG 3 to: promote gender equality and empower women refers directly to girls and women, addressing pejorative stereotypes and inequalities is of importance to every MDG. The WHO Department of Gender and Women's Health, acknowledging that development impacts differentially on the lives of women and men has identified the particular gender-related risks faced by the poorest groups and targets and indicators of the health-related MDGs in which gender might influence achievement of the goal. For example, the eradication of extreme poverty and hunger (MDG 1) can only be realised if malnutrition eradication programmes disaggregate monitoring data by sex to ensure that in settings where sons are preferred, girl children are equally likely to receive adequate nutrition or nutritional supplements. Reducing mortality in children under the age of five (MDG 4) requires women's work to be addressed, in particular increasing the resources available to support the work of mothering. Reducing maternal mortality (MDG 5) requires change in the social norms in some countries which require women to obtain the consent of a male family member before seeking health care which can prevent them participating in health promotion programmes and receiving essential treatment [12].

In 2005 the WHO established the Commission on the Social Determinants of Health (CSDH) [13] to 'marshal the evidence on effective strategies to promote health equity'. It reported in 2008 that in all contexts there are social gradients in health, with the poorest having much worse health than those who are socioeconomically advantaged. These disparities reflect diverse factors, not just health services and systems, but are indicators of social injustice. The report of the CSDH states clearly that addressing inequalities in social organisation including those between women and men is central to addressing health inequities. The Commission calls for a 'new global agenda for health equity' emphasising in its recommendations the importance of early childhood development and complete education for girls as well as boys. Improving the circumstances in which children are born will improve the wellbeing of all girls and women. The CSDH suggests that a stronger focus on social determinants, of which gender is a key exemplar, is required in order to understand persistent health inequalities and that these should be monitored routinely by national governments and international organisations. Health practitioners as well as researchers and policy makers require a comprehensive understanding of the social determinants of health and incorporation of these in practise.

Poor mental health is of serious public health concern and it is expected that by the year 2020 the common mental disorder of Major Depression will be the second most important contributing factor to disability as a burden of disease in the world [14]. It will be the leading cause of disability for females and not only the most frequently encountered women's mental health problem but the leading women's health problem globally [15].

Overall, in all countries, women carry a disproportionate share of the unpaid workload of care for children or other dependent relations and household tasks. They are more likely to be poor and less able to influence personal or household financial decision-making. They are more likely to experience violence and coercion from an intimate partner or other family member than are men. Women are also less likely to have access to the protective factors of full participation in education, paid employment and political decision-making. Brown and Harris's [16] influential social theory derived from research with socially disadvantaged women concluded that it was the coincidental experiences of entrapment and humiliation that led to despair, hopelessness, worry and depression. Entrapment and humiliation are intrinsic to poverty, violence and gender discrimination.

> Women's [mental] health is inextricably linked to their status in society. It benefits from equality and suffers from discrimination. Today the status and well-being of countless millions of women worldwide remains tragically low. As a result, human well-being suffers, and the prospects for future generations are dimmer . . . .
>
> The World Health Report (WHO) 1998 [17]

Mental health promotion requires comprehensive knowledge of the factors that contribute to mental health problems and identification of those that are modifiable so that they can be targeted directly. These can be grouped into three elements: the individual, her society and the cultural and political environment [9, 18]. Environmental factors include: adequate housing; domestic and public safety; access to good education for all; fair working conditions and legal recognition of rights to freedom from discrimination. Social factors include: the benefits of strong early emotional attachments; access to secure relationships characterised by affection and trust; abilities to communicate, negotiate and participate and attainment of autonomy. Individual determinants are: capacities to regulate emotions and thoughts; to learn from experience; to manage conflict; to tolerate life's unpredictability and grow in resilience [9, 18].

In Section 5 some of the specific gendered risk factors for mental health problems, the social policies that relate to these and their implications for the promotion of women's mental health are addressed. Takashi Izutsu's chapter provides a comprehensive review of the international covenants and related social policies that apply to all member countries of the United Nations. He demonstrates through analysis of these that women's mental health reflects the recognition of human rights and that the status of women's mental health is a powerful indicator of socio-political differences between countries. Toshiko Kamo's chapter provides the evidence from both psychological and neurobiological research about the profound adverse effects on women's general health of experiencing violence from an intimate partner. She outlines how mental health improves dramatically when violence ceases because a woman leaves her dangerous domestic setting. The improvements are sustained after being in a safe place where women are treated with respect and assisted to recognise that there are other ways of living to which they have a right. This exemplifies the importance of cross-sectoral interventions, including legislation making domestic violence a crime, and the provision of safe houses for victim survivors of intimate partner violence in addition to interventions provided within the health system.

Wenhong Chen identifies how families act as agents of gender socialisation and can determine self-regard, personal confidence and capacity to participate in girl children and women. This is especially salient in countries and cultures with a strong preference for male children and in which the rights of girls can be overlooked, ignored or actively transgressed. While socio-political recognition of the rights of women is crucial, it is also important that stereotypes within families about the needs, capacities and rights to participate of girls are emphasised and that public education about the equal rights of girl children are still required.

Linda Richter and Tamsen Rochat review the profound contribution that women make to the world in their work as mothers. All communities, societies and countries benefit from women's unpaid work in nurturing newborns, infants, young children, older children and adolescents. Women's skills in responding contingently, knowledgeably and sensitively to their children's needs promote optimal development, which in turn permits adults to function well and promotes social cohesion. Yet this immeasurable workload is unwaged, undervalued and poorly defined. It is not dignified with the language and descriptors of work. Policy makers, public commentators and clinicians generally use the stereotypes that mothering is not work and that only women who are employed are entitled to be called 'working mothers'. Jane Fisher's chapter identifies common gender stereotypes that govern conceptualisations of the work of mothering and proposes a new model, including the ways that the language used to describe the work of mothering in research, health practise; social policy and public discourse require modification.

Gender and social policy have clear implications for treatment, but also for local, national and international strategies to reduce mental health problems, through reducing risk factors and through gender-informed strategies to promote women's mental health [9, 18].

References

1. American Psychiatric Association (1994) *Diagnostic and Statistical Manual of Mental Disorders*, 4th edn, American Psychiatric Association, Washington, DC.
2. Astbury, J. and Cabral de Mello, M. (2000) Women's Mental Health: An Evidence Based Review, World Health Organization, Geneva.
3. Piccinelli, M. and Wilkinson, G. (2000) Gender differences in depression: critical review. *The British Journal of Psychiatry*, **177**, 486–92.
4. Astbury, J. (1996) *Crazy for You. The Making of Women's Madness*, Oxford University Press Australia, Melbourne.
5. Ussher, J. (1991) *Women's Madness: Misogyny or Mental Illness?* Harvester Wheatsheaf, Exeter.
6. Broverman, I., Broverman, D., Clarkson, F. *et al.* (1970) Sex-role stereotypes and clinical judgments of mental health. *Journal of Consulting and Clinical Psychology*, **34** (1), 1–7.
7. Dowrick, C. (2004) *Beyond Depression: A New Approach to Understanding and Management*, Oxford Medical Publications, Oxford University Press, Oxford.
8. Chen, Y-Y., Subramanian, S.V., Acevedo-Garcia, D. and Kawachi, I. (2005) Women's status and depressive symptoms: a multilevel analysis. *Social Science and Medicine*, **60**, 49–60.
9. Herrman, H. and Jane-Llopis, E. (2005). Mental health promotion in public health. *Promotion and Education*, **12** (Suppl 2), 42–47.
10. International Covenant on Economic, Social and Cultural Rights (ICESCR). Office of the Unitied Nations High Commissioner for Human Rights, Geneva. http://www. unhchr.ch/html/menu3/b/a_cescr.htm. Retrieved on 12-07-2008.
11. World Health Organization (1981) Social Dimensions of Mental Health, World Health Organization, Geneva.
12. World Health Organization (2003) 'En-gendering' the Millennium Development Goals (MDGs) on Health, World Health Organization, Geneva.
13. CSDH (2008) Closing the Gap in a Generation: Health Equity through Action on the Social Determinants of Health. Final Report of the Commission on Social Determinants of Health, World Health Organization, Geneva.
14. World Health Organization (2001) World Health Report 2001. Mental Health: New Understanding, New Hope, World Health Organization, Geneva.
15. Murray, C.J.L. and Lopez, A.D. (1996) *The Global Burden of Disease: A Comprehensive Assessment of Mortality and Disability from Diseases, Injuries and Risk Factors in 1990 and Projected to 2020*, Harvard School of Public Health.
16. Brown, G.W. and Harris, T. (1978) *The Social Origins of Depression. A Study of Psychiatric Disorder in Women*, Tavistock Publications, London.
17. World Health Organization (1998) The World Health Report 1998 – Life in the 21st Century: A Vision for All, World Health Organization, Geneva.
18. Herrman, H., Saxena, S. and Moodie, R. (2005) Promoting Mental Health: Concepts, Emerging Evidence, Practice, World Health Organization, Geneva.

24

Women's mental health in the context of broad global policies

Takashi Izutsu

United Nations Population Fund, New York, USA

24.1 Introduction

Disparity in mental health in women is observed internationally. In particular, women in developing countries tend to be more susceptible to mental health problems, have fewer mental health services available and face more barriers to access these limited services. For example, one in three to one in five women in developing countries have a significant mental health problem during pregnancy and after childbirth, in many cases without any access to mental health services while 1 in 10 have these difficulties with some access to health services in developed countries [1]. Women, especially those living in developing countries, are more exposed to risk factors which increase their susceptibility to mental health problems. Some of these include less valued social roles, poorer socioeconomic status, gender-based violence and less access to mental health services. The right to mental health is for all. However, in reality, women in developing countries suffer disproportionally with more risks, more needs, higher burden and less access to services.

To realise mental health on the ground, especially in developing countries, awareness raising and advocacy, pointing out the high prevalence and burden of mental health problems and the development of quality mental health policies are critical. However, in addition to these important activities, it is also necessary to integrate mental health into the priorities of the international community

Contemporary Topics in Women's Mental Health Edited by Chandra, Herrman, Fisher, Kastrup,
© 2009 John Wiley & Sons, Ltd   Niaz, Rondón and Okasha

as identified in the Millennium Development Goals (MDGs), particularly the health MDGs; for example, MDG 4: To Reduce Child Death; MDG 5: To Promote Maternal Health and MDG 6: To Combat HIV/AIDS, Malaria and Other Diseases.

In order to address women's mental health in the context of the global priorities of the development and political community, it is necessary to understand and strategically utilise legal and political instruments such as conventions, and other internationally agreed consensuses to justify and mobilise commitment from stakeholders and secure funding. There have been several international instruments which highlight the importance of the mental health of women and utilising these can serve as a key bridge between the mental health community and the global development and political community.

In addition, to address the development of mental health services, it is crucial to understand and address the financial reality in the country, especially budget allocations in the health sector, so that budgets for mental health programmes can be mobilised. In so doing, understanding and preparing for the 'new aid environment' which includes Sector-Wide Approaches (SWAps) and the Poverty Reduction Strategy Paper (PRSP) which is expanding rapidly, is critical.

Thus, this chapter describes the useful international instruments for advocating and integrating mental health into international development and political priorities, and the new aid environment to mobilise necessary funding.

24.2 Definitions of health and the right to health made by the United Nations

Mental health is already an important and major component of health and the right to health as defined by the United Nations system.

First, the definition of 'health' outlined in the *Constitution of the World Health Organization* (WHO) (1946) [2] is 'a state of complete physical, *mental* and social *well-being* and not merely the absence of disease or infirmity' (Preamble).

'The right to health' stated in the *International Covenant on Economic, Social and Cultural Rights* (ICESCR) (1966) [3] is 'the right of everyone to the enjoyment of the highest attainable standard of physical and *mental health*' (Article 12) (for substantive issues arising in the implementation of the ICESCR, see The Right to the Highest Attainable Standard of Health, General Comments [4] Paragraph 17 (The right to health facilities, goods and services), 18 (Non-discrimination and equal treatment), 22 (Children and adolescents), 26 (Persons with disabilities), 27 (Indigenous peoples), 34 and 36 (Specific legal obligations)). The ICESCR is a component of the International Bill of Human Rights which also includes the Universal Declaration of Human Rights (UDHR) (1948) [5] and the International Covenant on Civil and Political Rights (ICCPR) (1966) [6] and its two Optional Protocols [7, 8]. These are the most fundamental principles of the United Nations and broader global community's activities.

24.3 The Fourth World Conference on Women: Platform for Action (1995)

The United Nations facilitated the Fourth World Conference on Women in 1995 in Beijing, China. The principal themes were the advancement and empowerment of women in relation to women's human rights, women and poverty, women and decision-making, the girl child, violence against women and other areas of concern. The Beijing Declaration and Platform for Action was developed as the outcome document of the Conference. The Platform for Action is still one of the guiding principles for activities on gender issues in the global community [9].

The Platform for Action reaffirmed that women have the right to enjoy the highest attainable standard of physical and *mental health*, and that the enjoyment of this right is vital to their life and wellbeing as well as their ability to participate in all areas of public and private life. In addition, it states that women's health involves their *emotional*, social and physical wellbeing and is determined by the social, political and economic context of their lives, as well as by biology (Para. 89). It pays special attention to sexual and gender-based violence, including physical and *psychological* abuse, trafficking in women and girls, sexual exploitation and states women are at high risk of physical and *mental trauma* due to these types of abuse (Para. 99). It clearly mentions '*mental disorders* related to marginalisation, powerlessness and poverty, along with overwork and stress and the growing incidence of domestic violence as well as substance abuse, are among other health issues of growing concern to women' (Para. 100).

Concerning the girl child, the Platform for Action states that they have less access to *mental health care* (Para. 39), and the existing discrimination in their access endangers current and future health (Para. 266). Therefore, it states that all barriers must be eliminated to enable girls to develop their full potential and skills through equal access to physical and *mental health* care and related information (Para. 272).

The Platform for Action calls for action by governments and relevant stakeholders to 'reaffirm the right to the enjoyment of the highest attainable standards of physical and *mental health*, protect and promote the attainment of this right for women and girls and incorporate it in national legislation' (Para. 106. b.) and 'integrate *mental health services* into primary healthcare systems or other appropriate levels, develop supportive programmes and train primary health workers to recognise and care for girls and women of all ages who have experienced any form of violence such as domestic violence, sexual abuse or other abuse in armed and non-armed conflict' (Para. 106. q.). Furthermore, governments are urged to take steps to ensure that full assistance is provided to the victims of systematic rape and other forms of inhuman and degrading treatment of women as a deliberate instrument of war and ethnic cleansing for their physical and *mental rehabilitation* (Para. 144. c.). In particular, there is a call for governments to protect the girl child from economic exploitation and from performing any work that is likely to be hazardous or interferes with the child's education, or is harmful to the child's health or physical, *mental*, spiritual, moral or social *development* (Para. 282. a.). In addition, it calls for action by governments and partners to 'take appropriate legislative, administrative, social and educational measures to protect the girl child, in the household and in society, from all forms of physical or *mental violence*, injury or abuse, neglect or negligent treatment, maltreatment or exploitation, including sexual abuse' (283. b).

The Platform for Action also calls for action by governments, the United Nations system, health professions, research institutions, non-governmental organisations, donors, pharmaceutical industries and the mass media, as appropriate, to conduct research to understand and better address the determinants and consequences of unsafe abortion, including its effects on health conditions including *mental health* (Para. 109. i.).

Finally, it calls for action by governments and relevant stakeholders to place special focus on programmes to educate women and men, especially parents, on the importance of girls' physical and *mental health and well-being* (Para. 277) and to strengthen and reorient health education and health services, particularly primary healthcare programmes that meet the physical and *mental needs* of girls and women (Para. 281. c.).

24.4 Conventions

Conventions are legally binding tools for governments which have ratified them. After ratification governments need to change their laws and policies in compliance with the Conventions.

Convention on the Rights of Persons with Disabilities (CRPD) (2006)

In 2006, the United Nations General Assembly adopted, the Convention on the Rights of Persons with Disabilities (CRPD) by consensus. Article 1 of the Convention states that: 'Persons with disabilities include those who have long-term physical, *mental, intellectual* or sensory impairments which in interaction with various barriers may hinder their full and effective participation in society on an equal basis with others'. Article 25 on Health mentions that countries must take all appropriate measures to ensure that persons with disabilities have access to health services that are gender-sensitive, with the same range, quality and standard of free or affordable healthcare and programmes as provided to other persons. In particular, women and girls with disabilities are subject to multiple discrimination, and the Convention calls for State Parties to take all appropriate measures to ensure the full development, advancement and empowerment of women, for the purpose of guaranteeing them the exercise and enjoyment of the human rights and fundamental freedoms set out in this Convention (Article 6) [10].

Convention on the Rights of the Child (CRC) (1989)

The Convention on the Rights of the Child (CRC) recognises the rights of children including girls with regard to mental health [11].

The Convention states that every child must have a standard of living adequate for the child's physical, *mental*, spiritual, moral and social development (Article 27). It also mentions that children need to be directed to ensure the development of the child's personality, talents and *mental* and physical *abilities* to their fullest potential (Article 29). In addition, the Convention recognises the importance of the mass media and shall ensure that the child has access to information and material which aims to promote his or her social, spiritual and moral wellbeing as well as physical and *mental health* (Article 17).

The Convention states that children need to be protected from economic exploitation and from any work that is likely to be hazardous or interfere with the child's education, or is harmful to the child's health or physical, *mental*, spiritual, moral or social development (Article 32). In addition to economic exploitation, the Convention calls for all appropriate legislative, administrative, social and educational measures to protect the child from all forms of physical or *mental violence* (Article 19). Additionally, States Parties need to take all appropriate measures, including legislative, administrative, social and educational measures, to protect children from the illicit use of *narcotic drugs and psychotropic substances* (Article 33).

In Article 23, the rights of children *with mental or physical disabilities* are recognised and promotion of the international exchange of appropriate information in the field of preventive healthcare and of medical, *psychological* and functional treatment of children with disabilities is encouraged. Also, States Parties have to recognise the right to periodic review of treatment provided to children who are placed in institutions for care, protection or treatment of his or her physical or *mental health* (Article 25).

Finally, Article 39 says all appropriate measures must be taken to promote the physical and *psychological* recovery and social reintegration of child victims of any form of neglect, exploitation, abuse or torture among other cruel, inhuman or degrading treatments or punishments including armed conflicts.

Convention against torture and other cruel, inhuman or degrading treatment or punishment (CAT) (1984)

This Convention is also relevant to the mental health of women. Article 1 defines torture as 'any act by which severe pain or suffering, whether physical or *mental*, is intentionally inflicted on a person for such purposes as obtaining from him or a third person information or a confession, punishing him for an act he or a third person has committed or is suspected of having committed or intimidating or coercing him or a third person, or for any reason based on discrimination of any kind, when such pain or suffering is inflicted by or at the instigation of or with the consent or acquiescence of a public official or other person acting in an official capacity' [12].

24.5 Other international tools

Declaration on the elimination of violence against women (1993)

The Declaration defined violence against women as 'any act of gender-based violence that results in physical, sexual or *psychological harm or suffering* to women', and emphasised the importance of *psychological aspects* (Article 1) [13].

The Declaration declares States should take appropriate measures to promote their safety and physical and *psychological rehabilitation* (Article 4.g).

International Conference on Population and Development (ICPD) programme of action (1994)

The International Conference on Population and Development (ICPD) in 1994 in Cairo defined reproductive health as 'a state of complete physical, *mental and social well-being*' (Para. 7.2). Therefore, family planning, maternal health, gender-based violence and other areas mentioned as part of reproductive health include mental health in its definition [14].

United Nations Population Fund (UNFPA) strategic plan 2008–2011

Based on these international tools, United Nations Population Fund (UNFPA) has started to integrate mental health concerns into its mandate on universal access to reproductive health, particularly as it relates to the achievement of MDG 5 as one of the leaders in this area among United Nations agencies. In addition to holding an expert meeting and issuing publications on integrating mental health into reproductive maternal, newborn and child health in collaboration with WHO, UNFPA also included mental health in its principle policy 'Strategic Plan 2008–2011' as part of a set of goals and outcomes. Although this constitutes a big step towards change, much needs to be realised in the area of systematically integrating mental health into larger development efforts. UNFPA and WHO have jointly initiated a programme to integrate mental health needs into existing maternal and child health policies and programmes based on this [15].

The Inter-Agency Standing Committee (IASC) guidelines on mental health and psychosocial support in emergency settings

The Inter-agency Standing Committee (IASC) was established in 1992 as the primary mechanism for facilitating inter-agency decision making in response to complex emergencies and natural disaster, in response to the United Nations General Assembly Resolution 46/182. The IASC is formed by a broader range of United Nations and non-United Nations humanitarian organisation. The IASC Guidelines provide essential advice on how to facilitate an integrated approach to address the most urgent mental health and psychosocial issues in emergency situations. The Guidelines pay special attention to women's needs in mental health and psychosocial support [16].

24.6 New aid environment: Sector wide approaches and the poverty reduction strategy paper

Globally, health expenditure is 8.7% of the gross domestic product and annual government expenditure on health is USD 382 per capita [17]. When we look at Africa and South East Asia, these figures are 6% and USD 22, respectively in Africa and 4% and USD 8, respectively in South East Asia [17]. It is extremely difficult to compete with other pressing health agendas, such as HIV/AIDS, to try to obtain money for mental health from the small amount of money allocated for health. Rather, it is better to place mental health into priority agendas such as reproductive maternal, newborn and child health and HIV programmes so that these large scale programmes can at the same time deliver mental health services.

In order to do so, it is critical to understand financial flow in countries, especially budgeting in the health sector. Understanding and preparing for the new aid environment is necessary in this regard.

Building on the international consensus on what is needed to be done as expressed by world leaders at the Millennium Summit in 2000 (including the Millennium Declaration and MDGs) [17], and following international agreement on required resources at Monterrey in 2002, the Paris Declaration on Harmonization and Alignment [18] in 2005 proposed new aid modalities which were subsequently endorsed at the World Summit in 2005.

SWAps is a new modality of development activities. Rather than each donor running projects by themselves outside of the government, in these new modalities, donors provide resources to partner governments. The partner government then takes leadership and an ownership role for planning and implementation and coordinates external partners including donors. External partners are expected to focus on providing financial and/or technical support to government based on the governmental plan, so that government itself can lead and manage its own development and develop national capacity with result-oriented activities. This can reduce duplication of work by many entities, governmental administrative load and transaction fees.

The PRSP began as a tool for debt relief, but is increasingly being considered as a common vehicle through which (i) countries develop and express their nationally owned poverty-reduction strategies and policies, (ii) the Bretton Woods Institutions such as the World Bank identify lending requirements and appropriate policy environments and (iii) the donor community and the United

Nations system align and coordinate assistance strategies and budgets for poverty reduction at the national level.

These measures have brought about a new way of working in health in developing countries. In SWAps and PRSP, countries usually develop their own national plan for the health sector, based on their situation and priorities, in collaboration with donors and the United Nations system. Following analysis, health budgets are then allocated based on the health sector plan. The health sector plan usually consists of actions for HIV and AIDS, malaria, immunisation for infectious diseases and child health. It is becoming increasingly difficult to create an independent plan for mental health. Therefore, it is crucial to integrate priorities such as child health, maternal health and HIV and AIDS. If we can integrate the mental health module into these areas of work, health workers might be able to provide mental health services as part of their own work.

24.7 Conclusion

One of the missing links in mental health was the association of mental health with broader non-mental health communities. In addition to our endeavours to develop mental health policies, psychiatrists and other specialised mental health professionals, it is also critical to try to integrate mental health into other priority areas, particularly health priorities such as reproductive maternal, newborn and child health and HIV and AIDS. For example, if mental health can be part of maternal health intervention protocol, mental health service will be widely provided by maternal health community in collaboration with mental health community.

In order to realise this, it is important to understand the surrounding broader legal and political issues. The utilisation of international Conventions and other instruments with an understanding of the financial flow, particularly paying attention to the new aid environment would promote networking with other priority areas and the broader development and political community as a whole.

In addition to these political level endeavours, it is essential to have closer collaboration of mental health professionals with professionals in the other health areas at clinical level. It is important to build stronger partnership with maternal, newborn and child health and HIV and AIDS professionals so that they can integrate mental health smoothly with active knowledge sharing and referral support from mental health professionals.

It is now necessary to work with development, political and health communities outside the mental health sector to make mental health a reality for all, including those living in the world's resource constrained countries.

References

1. World Health Organization United Nations Population Fund (2008) Maternal Mental Health and Child Health and Development in Low and Middle Income Countries. Report of the WHO-UNFPA Meeting, WHO, Geneva.

2. United Nations (1946) Constitution of the World Health Organization (WHO), United Nations, New York.

3. United Nations (1966) International Covenant on Economic, Social and Cultural Rights, United Nations, New York.

4. United Nations (2000) The Right to the Highest Attainable Standard of Health: E/C.12/2000/4: General Comments, United Nations, New York.

5. United Nations (1948) Universal Declaration of Human Rights, United Nations, New York.

6. United Nations (1966) International Covenant on Civil and Political Rights, United Nations, New York.

7. United Nations (1966) Optional Protocol to the International Covenant on Civil and Political Rights, United Nations, New York.

8. United Nations (1989) Second Optional Protocol to the International Covenant on Civil and Political Rights, Aiming at the Abolition of the Death Penalty, United Nations, New York.

9. United Nations (1995) United Nations 4th World Conference on Platform for Action: Women Platform for Action, Beijing.

10. United Nations (2006) Convention on the Rights of Persons with Disabilities, United Nations, New York.

11. United Nations (1989) Convention on the Rights of the Child, United Nations, New York.

12. United Nations (1984) Convention against Torture and Other Cruel, Inhuman or Degrading Treatment or Punishment, United Nations, New York.

13. United Nations (1993) Declaration on the Elimination of Violence against Women, United Nations, New York.

14. United Nations (1994) United Nations International Conference on Population and Development (ICPD): Programme of Action, Cairo.

15. United Nations (2007) United Nations Population Fund (UNFPA) Strategic Plan 2008–2011, United Nations, New York.

16. IASC (2007) IASC Guidelines on Mental Health and Psychosocial Support in Emergency Settings, Geneva.

17. United Nations (2000) United Nations Millennium Declaration, New York.

18. OECD (2005) Paris Declaration on Aid Effectiveness: Ownership, Harmonisation, Alignment, Results and Mutual Accountability, Paris.

Further reading

United Nations Population Fund (2008) UNFPA Emerging Issues: Mental, Sexual & Reproductive Health, United Nations Population Fund, New York.

World Health Organization, United Nations Population Fund (2008) Improving Maternal Mental Health, World Health Organization, Geneva.

World Health Organization, United Nations Population Fund (2009) Mental Health Aspects of Women's Reproductive Health: A Global Review of the Literature, World Health Organization, Geneva.

25

Families of origin as agents determining women's mental health

Wenhong Cheng

Department of Child and Adolescent Psychiatry, Shanghai Mental Health Center, Medical School, Shanghai Jiaotong University, Shanghai, China

25.1 Introduction

Families of origin have a lifetime impact on many aspects of the developing child. They affect not only physical and personality development during childhood, but also interpersonal relationships as realised in marriage, parenthood and occupation and mental health during adulthood. Each parent's sex, personality, mental and physical health, capacity for intimacy and attitudes towards and valuing of the child's sex will produce different effects on the growth, mental health and future of their sons and daughters. While biological differences might contribute to differences in ways of thinking and emotional reactions between boys and girls, parental behaviours interact with these to shape development. There is consistent evidence about the fundamental importance of the family's role in children's development. Abdelgalil *et al.* [1] interviewed the families of 58 street adolescents in Brazil. Most of the families shared characteristics including being headed by a female single-parent and depending on their children for income. The parents were mostly poor, and had low levels of education. Many reported drug abuse, unemployment and immigration, and themselves had a history of living on the streets, childhood work and premature pregnancy. Parents thought that it was more dangerous for girls than boys to live outside the home,

Contemporary Topics in Women's Mental Health Edited by Chandra, Herrman, Fisher, Kastrup,
© 2009 John Wiley & Sons, Ltd   Niaz, Rondón and Okasha

and these gendered views influenced the engagement of boys and girls in income generation. While the boys worked on the streets, most of the girls worked as maids or waitresses. From this example we can see that even in extreme circumstances children are affected by family gender stereotypes.

25.2 The impact of the family of origin's perspectives about females on the growth of women

When a female newborn comes into their lives, the parents' attitudes towards her will affect her development as a woman and her self-acceptance. Expectations of parents about the sex of the newborn vary across cultures, with some having a strong preference for sons. If the parents expect a boy, but a girl is born, parents may feel disappointed and resist relinquishing the illusion of having a boy. In this circumstance a girl may feel denied and discriminated against emotionally and unconsciously, and this is likely to affect her emotional development as a female. As an adolescent, she may doubt her role as a woman, or feel inferior and a low sense of entitlement. After puberty she may refuse to adopt a female identity and physical form, and rather perform the masculine role or present with psychological symptoms that suggest as a refusal to grow up. A number of studies confirm the role of parents' views about infant sex as being very important. Girls tend to develop character traits reflecting the parents' perception of girls, and such an effect is quite stable in life [2, 3].

Parents' attitudes towards the baby's emotional reactions will also affect the baby. Parents are more likely to be demonstrative with girls than boys, as in being together and sharing feelings. They tend to have protective attitudes towards girls, and encourage girls to express their negative feelings, to accept help from others, express more love such as hugging and want girls to avoid harm [4, 5]. While community awareness of gender stereotypes typically moulds the behavioural characteristics of girls in this way, this varies with different times, ethnic groups, social class and levels of education, with different effects on the female adult psychological adaptation.

Appropriate protection and emotional support together with parents' positive perspective towards females is conducive to the healthy growth of women, and assists them to deal with interpersonal relationships and express love and emotion. This then is conducive to helping them to understand others easily, and desire to reproduce and be well-equipped to mother in turn. On the other hand, when parents or society treat the female newborn or girl child as 'weaker', and as needing more special care than a boy, women will be less likely to develop appropriate self-confidence, courage, independence and ambition towards various goals from childhood. Such types of stigma and gender stereotype from parents will limit the woman's development in many aspects of life, and is likely to increase her vulnerability to emotional problems.

Among the major schools of gender identity development theory, only psychoanalysis proposes that gender-related psychological characteristics arise from biological origins. Other theories propose that the interactions within families, communities and societies determine gender identity. Whether the former or the latter, the formation of gender identity is related to the parents' care at an early stage and the relationship between the parents and children. According to the theory of psychoanalysis [6], a three-year-old girl in the Oedipus phase will begin to discover differences between male and female sexual anatomy, and respond to her father with heterosexual love. She will tend to identify with her mother to resolve the conflict in the triangular relationship with her father and mother. This process of female identification with her mother will affect her female identification and mental health in the future, and the process is affected by her parents. For example, if a father is narcissistic, he may need a feeling of superiority in front of his wife and daughter, and this may make it more likely that his daughter will feel inferior as a female, and later be vulnerable to mental disorders such as depression and anxiety. If a mother is depressed, it might be difficult for her to help her daughter complete female identification. Social learning theory emphasises that a girl becomes a female through identifying with and imitating her mother [7]. The relationship between mother and daughter, and the mother's ability to mother will affect the quality of female identification in her daughter. An intimate relationship between mother and daughter, and a mother's good health will help her daughter grow up as a healthy, competent woman.

25.3 Impact of parenthood on women's mental health

In addition, parents' own emotions will affect parenthood and girls' development and mental health. For example, when parents' own anxiety and insecurity is serious, it is likely that they will control their girl-child through over-protection. Their daughter will lack the chance to have a sense of self-control. When she grows up, she is vulnerable to being over-dependent, and to lack of self-confidence. She may lack the necessary assertiveness and sense of competition, and be withdrawn and shy in the workplace. This in turn can lead to an anxious personality, a sense of incompetence and depression. This mechanism underpins inter-generational transmission of traits and disorders, and continues to affect the next generation. As Chambless *et al.* [8] report in their review of the literature that when a mother over-protects a daughter, the girl is likely to develop anxiety disorders earlier in childhood. Parents' over-protection can contribute to children adapting poorly to society. On the other hand, if a mother does not have enough time to take care of her daughter, the girl may also lack a sense of security and develop avoidant and dependent behaviours.

Bowlby [9] suggested that the mother and infant relationship was the base on which the infant was able to develop self-control and independence, and was a prototype of attachment with others in her or his adulthood. Further research provides inconsistent evidence on this point [10, 11]. Attachment depends on inner characteristics as well as the environment. A number of environment factors are very important [12]. These include the parents' mental health and their experience of stress events. However the infant's temperament is another important influence on the attachment type [13]. Most researchers agree that the early attachment type developing from the parent-child relationship is among the factors important to the later psychosocial function of the child. The psychosocial function of the child is influenced by multiple interacting developmental factors. A pilot study [14] investigated the attachment styles of 18 women with anxiety disorders, of whom 14 met the diagnostic criteria for panic disorder. The study found that all 18 women patients had abnormal attachment. These women had a total of 20 preschool children. Sixteen of the children had unusual attachment, and 13 had the same attachment methods as their mothers. This suggests that parents' behaviour towards their children may affect the attachment development.

If the parents' care is poor, it will affect the normal emotional development of girls. When girls grow to puberty, they may have difficulty establishing a good relationship with their parents. As adults, their relationships with other people may not mature. If a girl does not develop secure attachment during early life, she may have poor self-control and poor capacity for independence, and develop chronic anxiety or other mental illness in adulthood. Lipsedge studied the family characteristics of 87 adult patients with agoraphobia, a disorder more common in women than men [15]. The families of origin for 58% of the patients had a history of bickering, violence or alcohol abuse, or family breakdown related to death, chronic disease or violent behaviour in at least one of the parents.

In recent years, the relationship between trauma in early life and mental health in adulthood has had more and more attention. The Adverse Childhood Experiences (ACEs) Study has revealed a powerful relationship between adverse experiences in childhood and mental disorders as well as physical disorders in adulthood [16]. The adverse experiences include physical, emotional or sexual abuse; emotional or physical neglect; having one or no parents; alcohol or drug abuse in the home; family member incarcerated; severe or chronic mental illness and seeing the mother treated violently. This work suggests that the more types of childhood trauma to which the child is exposed, the greater is the likelihood of adult health risk behaviours and diseases.

Many studies have found that women are vulnerable to sexual abuse or sexual assault, at several times the rate reported in men [17] (see also p). Most sexual abuse begins early in life. Over 90% of children experiencing sexual abuse also suffer other kinds of abuse such as physical violence. Usually the abusers are males, and in some cases the father is the perpetrator [18]. These girls experience significant adverse effects. There is consistent evidence that adults with a history of childhood sexual abuse have a higher probability than others of mental disorders including depression, post-traumatic stress disorder, anxiety disorder, conduct disorder and substance abuse and of suicide [19, 20].

Physical and emotional abuse such as that related to domestic violence is increasingly recognised as important for women's mental health. Researchers estimated 20 years ago that over 3.3 million American children aged 3–17 years were at least once a year at risk of parents' violence towards them or at risk of observing inter-parental violence [21]. They speculated that the children witnessing violence far outnumbered those suffering from physical abuse directly [22]. While people living long-term in such families might not recognise a problem, many will suffer and gradually develop inappropriate ways to adapt. In the violent family, the man is most often the attacker and the woman a victim. Suh *et al.* [23] estimated that 40–60% of children who were victims of physical violence once or more saw their mother suffer abuse from father or her male partner. A young daughter may learn and agree with the mother's victim role, and may not protect herself well with a violent man in her own adult life. She is at risk of distorted adult relationships with men, and more vulnerable to mental health problems. A woman is also more likely than a man to be seriously injured [24]. The children exposed to these various harms may have developmental, social and behavioural problems, and also more severe mental and physical diseases. Garnefski *et al.* surveyed 7638 school girls aged 12–19 years, among whom 594 girls had a self-reported history of sexual abuse. The girls reporting sexual abuse also reported considerably more problems than the other girls in four categories: emotional problems, aggressive and criminal behaviours, addiction and risk behaviours and suicidality. Twenty-five per cent of those with a sexual abuse history had aggressive or criminal behaviour, and 41% had emotional problems. Logistic regression analyses showed a strong association between a history of sexual abuse and these problems, especially suicidality [25].

There is a gender difference in the long-term response to domestic violence. Men with this exposure tend to show destructive and aggressive behaviour towards people and objects [26, 27]. Women tend to have increased rates of physical discomfort, and more passive and dependent behaviours [28]. In adolescence, girls may show extreme distrust of men and have a negative attitude towards marriage. When the girls start dating, they are more likely than other girls to suffer physical violence from a male friend, but to perceive it as inevitable or even as an expression of love. While the men and women adapt in different ways, the difference is not static or extreme. It reflects a difference in coping and protection mechanisms [22, 29].

25.4 Families, social change and women's mental health

Social changes have been dramatic in recent decades, and the male and female roles in life are being challenged. In both the East and West, women are no longer necessarily in charge of domestic life and child-rearing. An increasing number of married women in many countries retain their professional identities, or resume employment after a few months to several years of raising a baby at home. Now society is more likely to respect women working outside the home, encourage women to keep a career and encourage equal competition with men. The traditional relationship between parents and daughter has also been challenged, and pubertal and growing women experience friction between traditional parents and modern society. This kind of conflict will affect female identity, particularly in the rapidly developing countries in recent decades. In China, for example, parents still tend to control girls more than boys with respect to moral and gentle values. On the other hand, society's role in differentiating between the sexes is becoming weaker, giving more and more space for females to overthrow tradition. This can cause worry for parents and conflict between parents and pubertal girls. Family conflict and associated confusion in the identification of young women can cause more and more psychological problems for girls.

This may be reflected in increasing mental health problems among females during recent decades. For example, the rate of smoking has increased more among female than male adolescents over the past 20 years [30, 31]. Health Canada [32] statistics show that the rate of increase in the numbers of women who smoke is twice than that of young men [32]. This is being reflected in increasing rates of smoking-related female psychological problems. Other women's problems are also increasing, such as the rate of women committing violence and crime and involved in substance abuse globally.

25.5 Conclusion

Families of origin have an important role in the development of women and their mental health throughout life. Family factors such as the parents' expectations and perspectives on women's roles, and the parents' own mental health and experience of being parented can affect women's emotional relationships within and beyond families of origin, and their independence, intimacy and mental health. With the global changes in societies, women are likely to meet more challenge and conflict from families, and mental health problems are increasing. We need to know more about how women may be protected from early life in their families of origin, especially as societies change rapidly. We also need to understand what policymakers and professionals can do to influence the social, family and personal factors that may improve women's mental health or decrease the problems related to women's mental disorders or problems.

References

1. Abdelgalil, S., Gurgel, R.G., Theobald, S. and Cuevas, L. (2004) Household and family characteristics of street children in Aracaju, Brazil. *Archives of Disease in Childhood*, **89**, 817–20.
2. Rubin, J.Z., Provenzano, R. and Luria, Z. (1974) The eye of the beholder: parents views on sex of new-borns. *The American Journal of Orthopsychiatry*, **44**, 512–19.
3. Karraker, K.H., Vogel, D.A. and Lake, M.A. (1995) Parents' gender-stereotyped perceptions of new-borns: the eye of the beholder revisited. *Sex Roles*, **33**, 687–701.
4. Leaper, C., Hauser, S.T., Kremen, A. *et al.* (1989) Adolescent-parent interactions in relation to adolescents' gender and ego development pathway: a longitudinal study. *The Journal of Early Adolescence*, **9**, 335–61.

5. Fitzpatrick, M.A. and Marshall, L.J. (1996) The effect of family communication environments on children's social behavior during middle childhood. *Communication Research*, **23**, 379–407.

6. Frued, S. (1965) Femininity, in *New Introductory Lectures on Psychoanalysis* (ed. J. Strachey), Norton, New York, pp. 112–35.

7. Bandura, A. (1969) Social-learning theory of identificatory processes, in *Handbook of Socialization Theory and Research* (ed. D.A. Goslin), Rand McNally, Chicago, pp. 213–62.

8. Chambless, D.L., Gillis, M.M., Tran, G.Q. *et al.* (1996) Parental bonding reports of clients with obsessive compulsive disorder and agoraphobia. *Clinical Psychology and Psychotherapy*, **3**, 77–85.

9. Bowlby, J. (1969) *Attachment and Loss*. Attachment, vol. 1, Basic Books, New York.

10. Thompson, R.A. (2000) The legacy of early attachments. *Child Development*, **71**, 145–52.

11. Teti, D.M., Sakin, J., Kucera, E. *et al.* (1996) And baby makes four: predictors of attachment security among preschool-aged firstborns during the transition to siblinghood. *Child Development*, **67**, 579–96.

12. Holden, G.W. and Miller, P.C. (1999) Enduring and different: a meta-analysis of the similarity in parents' child rearing. *Psychological Bulletin*, **125**, 223–54.

13. Belsky, J. (1997) Theory testing, effect-size evaluation, and differential susceptibility to rearing influence. The case of mothering and attachment. *Child Development*, **64**, 598–600.

14. Manassis, K., Bradley, S., Goldberg, S. *et al.* (1994) Attachment in mothers with anxiety disorders and their children. *Journal of the American Academy of Child and Adolescent Psychiatry*, **33**, 1106–13.

15. Bowlby, J. (1973) *Attachment and Loss*, Separation: Anxiety and Anger, vol. II, Basic Books, New York, p. 300.

16. Felitti, V.J., Anda, R.F., Nordenberg, D. *et al.* (1998) Relationship of childhood abuse and household dysfunction to many of the leading causes of death in adults. *American Journal of Preventive Medicine*, **14**, 245–58.

17. Fegert, J.M. (2007) Sexueller Missbrauch an Kindern und Jugendlichen. Bundesgesundheitsballt, Gesundheitsforschung. *Gesundheits Schutz*, **50**, 78–98.

18. Niederberger, J.M. (2002) The perpetrator's strategy as a crucial variable: a representative study of sexual abuse of girls and its sequelae in Switzerland. *Child Abuse and Neglect*, **26**, 55–71.

19. Copeland, W.E., Keeler, G., Angold, A. *et al.* (2007) Traumatic events and posttraumatic stress in childhood. *Archives of General Psychiatry*, **64**, 577–84.

20. Dube, S.R., Anda, R.F., Whitfield, C.L. *et al.* (2005) Long-term consequences of childhood sexual abuse by gender of victim. *American Journal of Preventive Medicine*, **28**, 430–38.

21. Carlson, B.E. (1984) Children's, in *Battered Women and Their Families* (ed. A.R. Roberts), Springer, New York.

22. Holden, G.W. and Ritchie, K.L. (1991) Linking extreme marital discord, child rearing, and child behavior problems: evidence from battered women. *Child Development*, **62**, 311–27.

23. Suh, E.K. and Abel, E.M. (1990) The impact of spousal violence on the children of the abused. *Journal of Independent Social Work*, **4**, 27–34.

24. Halpern, C.T., Oslak, S.G., Young, M.L. *et al.* (2001) Partner violence among adolescents in opposite-sex romantic relationships: findings from the national longitudinal study of adolescent health. *American Journal of Public Health*, **91**, 1679–85.

25. Garnefski, N. and Diekstra R.F. (1997) Child sexual abuse and emotional and behavioral problems in adolescence: gender differences. *Journal of the American Academy of Child and Adolescent Psychiatry*, **36**, 323–29.

26. Rosenbaum, A. and O'Leary, K.D. (1981) Children: the unintended victims of marital violence. *The American Journal of Orthopsychiatry*, **51** (15), 692–99.

27. Wolfe, D.A., Jaffe, P., Wilson, S. *et al.* (1985) Children of battered women: the relation of child behavior to family violence and maternal stress. *Journal of Consulting and Clinical Psychology*, **53**, 657–65.

28. Hughes, H.M. (1986) Research with children in shelters: implications for clinical services. *Children Today*, **8**, 21–25.

29. Sternberg, K.J., Lamb, M.E., Greenbaum, C. *et al.* (1993) Effects of domestic violence on children's behavior problems and depression. *Child Development*, **29**, 44–52.

30. Waldron, I., Lyle, D. and Brandon, A. (1991) Gender differences in teenage smoking. *Women and Health*, **17**, 65–90.

31. French, S. and Perry, C. (1996) Smoking among adolescent girls: prevalence and etiology. *Journal of the American Medical Women's Association*, **51**, 25–28.

32. Health Canada (1999) National Population Health Survey Highlights, Minister of National Health and Welfare, Ottawa.

26

The unpaid workload: Gender discrimination in conceptualisation and its impact on maternal wellbeing

Jane Fisher

Key Centre for Women's Health in Society, WHO Collaborating Center in Women's Health, University of Melbourne, Melbourne, Australia

26.1 Introduction

Women in all nations carry a disproportionate share of the unpaid workload of household tasks and the care of dependent children. This workload is neither readily nor usually quantified, and is unnamed, poorly defined and never complete. It is most strikingly apparent to mothers of newborns, particularly those who are making the transition from childlessness to parenthood. There is growing consciousness of the mental health problems women can experience at this life phase, but the contribution of the unpaid workload to postpartum psychological distress is rarely considered. Demographic analyses and investigations of time use, labour force participation, leisure hours and discretionary time rarely describe the personal experiences of women as they adapt to the unpaid workload of motherhood. There are very few investigations of the mental health of the poorest mothers in resource-constrained contexts and none about the impact of the unpaid agricultural labour or other subsistence work which they frequently combine with infant care. The mental health of women in resource constrained countries is of great importance, but as there is as yet so little evidence available

Contemporary Topics in Women's Mental Health   Edited by Chandra, Herrman, Fisher, Kastrup,
© 2009 John Wiley & Sons, Ltd   Niaz, Rondón and Okasha

about their needs, the focus of this chapter is on the situation of women in industrialised countries.

26.2 Maternal desire

Maternal desire can transcend language and is a much-debated construct 'at once obvious and invisible', defined as the 'longing felt by a woman to nurture her children and to participate in their mutual relationship' [1]. This intrinsic desire is sometimes dismissed as a reflection of traditional patterns of socialisation that constrain women to become providers of care. However, dismissing maternal desire in this way as merely a dated social construction can actually create a taboo and inhibit women from expressing a desire to care for children [1]. In contemporary industrialised democracies women face the unavoidable dilemmas of balancing the maternal desire to care well for children against income generation, self-realisation through professional ambition and social and political participation [2]. Personal agency in making decisions about the number and timing of children can be more readily realised in settings in which women have reproductive choice, access to effective contraception including for those who are single, well developed perinatal health services and paid and unpaid maternity leave. Maternal desire is more complex in the context of an unintended or unwelcome pregnancy. Women in this circumstance nonetheless face comparable dilemmas when a pregnancy is continued to birth.

Equality of access to education and employment, defined here as paid work, might moderate but does not remove maternal desire. In settings where autonomous reproductive choice is sanctioned, surveys of women of reproductive age consistently find that more than 95% want to have children and few have an absolutely clear and sustained wish not to have children [3]. If a woman desires to care for children, her interaction with the workplace and the nature of her work are inevitably changed.

Clinical considerations of maternal desire and the work of motherhood reflect social conceptualisations and gender stereotypes that are not described in formal public policies. Presumptions that it is pathological for women to protest and feel distress in the face of adjustment to these dilemmas might reflect limited awareness of gender stereotypes and the social processes in which they are embedded.

26.3 Disenfranchised grief and motherhood

There is never a perfect time in a woman's life to have a baby. One of the inevitable but least anticipated experiences of motherhood is how much is lost when an infant is born. When a woman has a first baby she experiences overnight the quite dramatic loss of almost all that has formed her identity until that point. In giving birth, women lose, at least temporarily, professional identity, capacity to generate an income, social and leisure activities, bodily integrity, autonomy and liberty, but these are disenfranchised or unrecognised losses. There is little public recognition of these losses, no ritual to acknowledge them and often an insensitive and envious response which suggests that mothering a baby is easier and more gratifying than paid employment. Stereotypically, there is a marked gender difference in the losses arising from the birth of an infant. While men can experience a loss of primacy within their intimate partnerships, they can otherwise lose very little and might, in fact, participate less in domestic life after the birth of the baby than before. This brings about a gendered divide in daily experience that was unanticipated and proves difficult, at least initially, for most couples to negotiate fairly.

In parenthood we are powerfully reconnected not only with our own infancy and early experiences but also with our notions of what constitutes a mother's and a father's work [4]. There is potential for inaccuracy of memory and idealisation, reflected in the not uncommon masculine fantasy that his own mother was highly competent, available and uncomplaining and that managing the needs of children and household tasks was unproblematic to her [5]. Sometimes women's mothers-in-law collude with these idealised memories and criticise their daughters-in-law for seeking a different distribution of domestic responsibilities than they themselves experienced. Contemporary women more often seek not to duplicate the restrictions that confined their mothers to the domestic sphere, economic dependence and limited external engagement, preferring to explore ways in which taking good care of their children can be combined with economic participation. However, they might lack the language to name these needs and the ambivalence aroused by departure from the traditional model of mothering [5].

26.4 Fantasies of motherhood

Women have usually imagined having a baby for decades, adolescent girls have already thought quite actively about whether or not to have a baby, and little girls' play often involves baby caretaking with dolls and prams [4]. Commonly, though what is imagined, perhaps romantically, is that life will be enhanced and that, in some way, a baby will bring joy, completion, a sense of connection, affection and mutuality, and that maternal desire will be gratified.

The usual language to connote this life transition from the childless state to having a first baby promotes the notion that it is to be anticipated with delight. It is described as 'giving up work' to become a 'lady of leisure'. The common question to pregnant women in both clinical and social settings is, 'When are you stopping work?'

26.5 Fantasies about the workload

These descriptions imply that mothering a newborn is an entirely pleasurable activity, the fantasy being that it will bring discretionary time, increased relaxation and flexibility, and that it will be intrinsically satisfying. Unlike most other major life transitions, this one is permanent and irreversible; a baby cannot be divorced or traded in for an alternative life. This transition is rarely conceptualised as being from one workplace to another workplace which is extraordinarily demanding and constant. In reality, infant care requires the equivalent of working a double shift and remaining on call for the third shift each day, but this workplace is not dignified with the language or descriptors of work. Mothers who undertake the major obligation of primary caretaking are described consistently in public discourse as 'not working'.

One of the first hallmarks of a workplace is that there is some definition of the tasks or expectations of a worker, most commonly in the form of a position description or a statement of duties. In their absence, the workload is diffuse and usually profoundly undervalued, especially by those who have never done it. Nulliparous women in advanced pregnancy underestimate two fundamental realities: first, the time and active endeavour required each day to keep a baby alive and manage a household in which a baby lives; and second, the power of attachment and that an infant is not a mechanical object whose care can be managed unemotionally.

26.6 Workload of motherhood

The actual unpaid workload of infant care and coincidental household tasks has proved difficult to define and to measure. Time-use surveys require informants to complete detailed descriptions of their activities at repeated time increments over 48 hours [6]. The completion of detailed paper surveys is itself time-consuming and there is less evidence from informants at this life stage than others. Smith and Ellwood [7] have recently attempted to quantify the unpaid 'caring workload' in the Australian National University Time Use Survey of New Mothers in a non-clinical sample of 188 mothers of infants recruited from the community [7]. Data were collected by a portable electronic recording device in which each of more than 25 defined activities were programmed to individual buttons which could be pressed as the activity was initiated and again when it was completed. The device produces a data file in which the date and duration of each activity is recorded. Data were collected by each mother for 24 hours a day over seven consecutive days. As the device is only able to capture one task, the authors acknowledge that multi-tasking is not captured and that actual work is underestimated.

Infant care activities alone are very frequent and cannot be anticipated or planned. At infant age three months there were on average 49 breast or bottle feeds a week which lasted a mean of 20 minutes but up to 75 minutes. On average there were 70 other occasions a week when mothers were carrying, holding or soothing their infants for around 13–18 minutes each time. Smith and Ellwood [7] conclude that active and passive infant care occupy about 23 hours of each day in the first year after birth and found that, in total, mothers were responsible for or with their infants for an average of 165.4 of the 168 hours of the week.

While it is far more time consuming than can be imagined to care well for a baby, all other household activities are slower and much more difficult to complete when caring simultaneously for an infant. Smith and Ellwood conclude that it is not accurate to define the times when an infant is asleep as leisure, not only because there are always other household tasks to complete but also because there is no true freedom either to rest or to pursue leisure activities at this time because of the essential primary responsibility for the infant. The tasks do not remit on weekends and, in general, women have much less leisure than had been imagined. Together, the repetitive work of managing a household and caring for an infant cannot be completed by one person. Nevertheless, the prevailing stereotype is that paid employment is defined as work and mothering responsibilities as 'not work'. Many women seek, therefore, to assume this workload single handed and to spare their partners who 'are working'.

The notion that procreation, quintessentially female because it requires ovulation, gestation and lactation, had as its inevitable consequence the arrest of other aspects of development was widespread until the early to mid-twentieth century in Western countries. Women who used abstract thinking were 'masculinised exceptions' [8]. Education was thought to be wasted on women and participation in non-maternal occupations socially proscribed. Healthy motherhood was thought to be all-consuming and to require self-sacrifice [8]. Although challenged powerfully by feminist scholars and activists, these stereotypes still prevail in modified forms. Many women seek to undertake the tasks of household management and infant care single handed, believing that this is the role of a mother. In incorporating this stereotype, the fact that the work can never be completed, especially not perfectly, leads to a sense of incompetence and shame [5].

26.7 Occupational fatigue as a determinant of maternal mood?

One of the hallmarks of a recognised workplace, especially those in which shift work is required, is an occupational health and safety policy on the serious consequences of occupational fatigue. Work-related fatigue is the subject of substantial scholarly research, most focused on the military, manufacturing, transport, media and communications and health sectors. Severe occupational fatigue is associated with prolonged or irregular working hours, particularly with early starting times and overnight work. Any work taking place between 1 a.m. and 6 a.m. is more likely to incur risk because of the disruptions to the circadian rhythm. It is especially problematic in highly mentally and emotionally demanding work in which there are inadequate rest breaks. Insufficient sleep and circadian disruption are associated with 'shift work sleep disorder' or 'nightshift lag' [9]. Occupational fatigue is known to affect both health and performance. It has adverse effects on emotional, cognitive and physical domains and is accompanied by poor judgement, slower reactions to events, decreased skills, increased clumsiness, reduced concentration and vigilance and impaired memory. Severe fatigue leads to increased irritability, agitation, reduced empathy and sociability, low mood and a general loss of insight and capacity to recognise these changes in the self [9].

The domestic setting is not, however, conceptualised or named as a workplace. In consequence, the domestic workplace does not benefit from the attention to occupational safety that is formally considered in workplace assessments of environmental hazards. Occupational fatigue is rarely considered as an explanatory factor for poor maternal functioning after childbirth.

Australia's residential early parenting centres are unique in the world and provide brief structured psycho-educational programmes to assist mothers with mild to moderate mood disturbance who are caring for infants with unsettled behaviour, particularly crying, resistance to soothing and frequent overnight waking. Some services are freestanding in either purpose-built facilities or buildings adapted from historical use as institutions for the care of children relinquished for adoption. More recently, others have been developed within maternity services. There are similarities in the therapeutic approach and most services offer a programme requiring joint admission of mother and baby for four or five nights.

The health and social circumstances of women admitted to one residential early parenting service were investigated in a survey of a consecutive cohort of women attending Masada Private Hospital Mother Baby Unit in Melbourne, Australia. Among other study-specific and psychometric measures, the 109 participants completed the Profile of Mood States (POMS) [10 #3741] and the Edinburgh Postnatal Depression Scale (EPDS) [10] to assess dimensions of self-reported mood, including anxiety, depression, irritability, functional efficiency, cognitive clarity and fatigue [11].

Participants were aged on average 33.3 ($\pm$4) years and their babies 22 weeks; 36% were primiparous. Most (71%) were working full-time as mothers, a few (5%) were also in full-time employment and the remainder were in part-time employment. Their partners, almost all of whom were employed full-time, spent longer than average hours away from home in their workplaces. Women undertook all or most of the domestic and infant care work in 62% of households; it was shared evenly in only 10% [11]. Leisure hours were defined as time without direct responsibility for the baby or other tasks, and these participants spent on average 3.8 hours (less than an hour per day) in leisure; their partners spent almost double that time in leisure (7.9 hours per week, $p < 0.01$). It was found that 90% of women were having fewer than 6 hours sleep in 24 and these were usually interrupted by infant waking. In most households, women defining themselves as 'not working' undertook all the overnight infant care. More than 90% were clinically fatigued (POMS Fatigue-Inertia subscale score $\geq$13); functional efficiency (POMS Vigour-Activity subscale score $\leq$11) was severely compromised in 69%; and cognitive clarity (POMS Confusion-Bewilderment subscale score $\geq$14) diminished in 59%. However, fewer (48%) scored in the clinical range of $\geq$13 on the EPDS.

Cluster analyses of the POMS and EPDS scores revealed three groups. The smallest group (28% of participants) was probably depressed with scores in the clinical range on all measures; a second group (35%) were clinically exhausted and had elevated anxiety, but on average depression scores lower than the clinical cut-off; and the third group (37%) only had elevated fatigue scores. The groups are not obviously clinically distinct at admission and these data suggest that severe occupational fatigue had compromised mood and functioning in most of these mothers of newborns, but that less than a third were accurately regarded as depressed.

In Smith and Ellwood's [7] study, mothers' sleep hours were obtained in 18 different episodes in the tracking week, with each stretch of sleep averaging just over 3 hours (188 minutes). Mothers were kept awake on average six nights a week, for around three-quarters of an hour on each occasion.

The Australian Occupational Health and Safety Act [12] outlines principles relating to the management and prevention of occupational fatigue in workplaces in which there are long and irregular hours, including air traffic controllers, pilots, flight crew, long distance and heavy vehicle drivers, nurses, junior doctors, miners, military personnel and journalists. There is to be a maximum of 12 standard safe working hours in 24 hours; at least four nights of consecutive rest in order to recover in each 14-day period of shift work; night shifts are not to be undertaken on more than two to three consecutive days; and no worker can be rostered to have less than 6 hours available for uninterrupted sleep between shifts for more than three consecutive days. Fatigued workers are known to place themselves and others at risk, with effects similar to those of an elevated blood alcohol level.

However, there are no workplace safety requirements, especially about occupational fatigue, for the work of mothering an infant. In a later follow-up study of mothers admitted to the same residential early parenting programme, in which mothers are taught, among other skills, sustainable infant settling strategies and how to reduce frequency of overnight waking, it was demonstrated that, one month after the intervention, maternal sleep had increased, numbers of overnight wakings had decreased and maternal mood was improved dramatically [13].

26.8 Recognition and valuing of work and occupational satisfaction

Unlike employment, in which completed tasks are noted in some way and remunerated, the tasks of infant care and household work are unremunerated and visible only when not done.

Occupational satisfaction is essential in order to maintain engagement with work and the desire to undertake tasks as well as possible. In 2006 a major national survey required employees from all levels of occupation in the United Kingdom to identify and then rank sources of occupational satisfaction [14]. The first was salary: the work of mothering and household tasks is unremunerated, and most countries lack social protection schemes in which universal maternity benefits are paid. Second was the social environment, especially interactions with colleagues: most women in developed countries do not live in multi-generational households and the domestic setting is often socially isolated. Third, were creative and intellectual challenges: mothering is frequently described as challenging, but usually emotionally rather than intellectually, and many tasks are repetitive and do not stimulate imagination. Fourth was feeling valued and respected: in the workplace of motherhood, these depend on the infant. If the baby is responsive and rewards the mother by quieting to her soothing, smiling, interacting, suckling easily and developing at least along an average trajectory, the baby provides gratification. In contrast, an infant who resists soothing, cries inconsolably or is difficult to breastfeed can be experienced as critical and unappreciative. Fifth was external recognition of contribution, including constructive feedback: after the birth of a baby, women have greatly increased dependence on their partners, including the need for recognition of their endeavours. However, this need can be unfamiliar, unexpected and difficult to name. Women can feel ashamed about appearing excessively needy in asking their partners to recognise and praise the day's endeavours. As is usual when attempting to learn new skills, vulnerability to criticism is increased; one of the most prominent predictors of depression after childbirth in women is to feel criticised by her partner for infant care and household management that are perceived to be inadequate.

Gratification in a workplace is also associated with experiences of success and mastery in the completion of tasks. The least satisfaction is found in work that is experienced as onerous, repetitive, monotonous and poorly waged. Completion, success and mastery are much less achievable in the workplace of motherhood, where the outcome is arguably the long-term one of a well-adjusted young adult. The need for gratification in completion of tasks is legitimate and, if the domestic sphere is recognised as a workplace, then opportunities to experience gratification can be identified and provided. To do so, however, requires a conceptual shift.

26.9 Training and education for mothering

In any occupation requiring specialist knowledge and technical proficiency, education and continuing training are provided. Caring well for an infant is sophisticated and technically skilled, requiring in addition to knowledge of a newborn's developmental capacities, maturities of emotional responsiveness and sensitivity. In any other context, there would be training and frequent professional education to develop and maintain these skills. However, the usual advice mothers are given is just to trust their intuition, although the nature and formation of maternal intuition is generally unquestioned by healthcare providers or consumers.

I sometimes ask mothers of newborns in my clinical care to imagine being a recent school leaver given responsibility to keep alive a patient in an intensive care unit just by trusting their intuition. This notion, recognised as exaggerated, is nevertheless readily identified as illustrating the situation of infant care and why it is intrinsically anxiety arousing. Most of them struggle to define intuition. Intuition is defined technically as understanding that is achieved without effort, ready insight independent of previous experiences or empirical knowledge and a sensing beyond conscious understanding. The formation of intuition about infant care is more speculative, but many popular guides to baby care suggest that it grows spontaneously and rapidly.

It is suggested to be an amalgam of memories, observations, information and values formed through experience of care in earlier life. It is related, perhaps, to the construct of attachment style, founded in John Bowlby's and Mary Ainsworth's theories about the ways in which parental responsiveness shapes an infant's later capacities to trust and form sustained, affectionate interpersonal relationships [15, 16]. The 70% of people who have a secure attachment style are able to trust others and form mutually interdependent relationships relatively easily and predictably. However, for the 30% with anxious and insecure attachment styles, this is not a steady or reliable state and they face the task of trying not to duplicate insensitive or abusive caretaking from their own early experiences or are preoccupied with anxiety about the baby's intrinsic vulnerability, mothering in ways that are more driven by their own needs than infant cues.

The formation of a confident maternal identity is usually a slow developmental process, captured by Daniel Stern and colleagues in the wonderful phrase that 'the birth of a baby is the birth of a mother' [4]. They describe how a new identity of the self as a mother gradually emerges from the repeated experiences that mothering an infant involves, but that it requires a 'fundamentally different mindset' and a 're-organisation of mental life'.

When we are uncertain we are especially vulnerable to unsolicited advice. This is often provided by others with conviction, but is usually derived from personal experience and rarely from what would be regarded as an evidence base. Fashions of infant care change with knowledge; practises from previous generations are not always congruent with current best practise. The example of neonatal sleeping position is a powerful illustration. Until the late 1980s it was believed that newborns slept most soundly and were least likely to choke on regurgitated milk if put to sleep prone, in a bassinet with a soft mattress and a padded lining. In 1991 it was found that this sleeping position was associated with an increased risk of unexplained infant death [17]. There were rapid revisions in infant care advice to ensure that infants were placed in a supine sleeping position in a well-aired cot with a firm mattress; unfortunately, implications for infant settling and alterations to maternal skills were not developed at the same time.

The widespread directive to mothers as they initiate breastfeeding is to 'feed on demand', but this guidance is rarely operationalised in practical terms. The usual interpretation by mothers of newborns is that every infant cry indicates hunger and that the only appropriate response is to offer the breast or the bottle. It is rare for mothers to be taught comprehensive management of infant crying, including that much crying is difficult to explain and that a range of interpretations and comfort responses is needed. Comfort strategies are often contested and hard to implement as parents negotiate between the imagined ideal of having a constantly happy infant who is never distressed and the reality of an infant with a range of emotional expressions but no language to describe the underlying need. Prolonged infant crying and resistance to soothing, especially when coupled with a partner who is experienced as critical and disengaged from infant care, is associated with diminished maternal confidence and depression. Teaching mothers to recognise infant tiredness, establish sustainable routines of daily care in which the infant's needs for feeding, playing and sleeping are well met, and to manage frequent waking leads to marked and rapid improvements in maternal mood and infant manageability [13, 18].

26.10 Presumptions about the contributions of others to the workload

Another pregnancy fantasy, especially among nulliparous women, is that other people will be as passionately absorbed by the baby as they and their partners are and that their baby will be loved as much by others as by them. Their own parents and siblings, childless friends and colleagues from the workplace are imagined to want to share this work. Reality rarely matches this fantasy. After the initial celebration of the baby's birth, regular voluntary sharing of the unpaid work by a wider circle is not common. A slow reality has to grow that the work and its associated adjustments and compromises are primarily undertaken by parents.

This process is sometimes precipitated when a mother first takes her new baby to visit her workplace, imagining it to be unchanged, that her original place remains, and that colleagues will make time to talk and make the baby welcome. Instead she finds that their attention remains with the workplace and the baby is, at best, of passing interest. The predicament demands recognition of and adjustment to losses: what will never be experienced again and is lost permanently; what can be restored, perhaps in a modified form; and, of great importance, what can be experienced in this developmental phase that could not have been known without motherhood.

26.11 Collegial relationships

Perhaps it is not surprising that the only solution to the predicament is thought to be a flight to the familiar, including to rapid resumption of employment and relinquishment of the newborn to non-maternal care [2]. However, in advanced pregnancy, the ease of resumption of external activities is often underestimated. Pregnant nulliparous women can imagine that it will be straightforward to leave a young infant with someone else and resume adult activities. The power of emotional attachment to the baby cannot be readily imagined and the difficulty of being separated from the baby, even if liberty is yearned for, is often underestimated until it is a real rather than a theoretical possibility. In reality, mothers can find the power of protective attachment and separation from an infant surprisingly intense and preoccupying. An infant is not a mechanical object; it is not straightforward to leave the infant in another person's care and be able to concentrate on other activities. Stern *et al.* [4] describe mothering as an 'intimate responsibility' in which the 'the baby should be held by me and not by others' and that there can be vivid fantasies of the baby coming to harm if in the care of others [4].

Stern *et al.* [4] also confirm the need for mothers to turn towards other women and join the quintessentially feminine world of mothers and infants [4]. Extending the analogy of the workplace, a mother needs to build new collegial relationships in the workplace of motherhood; coffee mornings and mothers' groups are staff meetings in this new workplace, providing an excellent forum for the exchange of experiences and mutual consultation which are helpful to adjustment and the growth of confidence. However, all too often these gatherings, too, are trivialised or envied: 'all you do is have coffee with your friends and play with the baby all day'.

Women then encounter the reality that, in whatever way they seek to combine the work of motherhood with external activities, including employment, it will arouse differences of opinion. Susan Chira [19], in her book *A Mother's Place: Taking the Debate About Working Mothers Beyond Guilt and Blame* [19], articulates this is in her summary of how mothers are blamed for whatever they do: work (if they are middle class), not work (if they are on welfare), work too much (if they are ambitious) or work too little (if they are not ambitious enough). She argues that middle-class women are occupied with the adverse effects on professional progression of time away from the workforce, and simultaneously with the dilemmas of deciding whether guilt about being separated from the infant is appropriate or excessive, necessary or socialised. Many provide personal anecdotes that babies love childcare. However, others are acutely conscious that the systematic investigations, difficult both to complete and to interpret suggest that prolonged non-maternal care for very young children has some adverse effects on development and attachment theory argues powerfully that experiences of caretaking in the early years govern later adjustment.

Mothers have to grow in the realisation that there is a need to become politicised and assertive as advocates for their infants' human rights, and to balance these with the rights of parents. Inevitably this process arouses ambivalence and the particular loneliness that accompanies individual decision-making about contentious social dilemmas. It also arouses ambivalence in caretakers, many of whom will already have faced this dilemma, and might be asked to disclose it. However, their obligation is not to impose their individual resolution on the woman seeking advice, rather to assist her to make her own decision.

26.12 Honouring the work of motherhood in practice and policy

It is common for mothers of first newborns to ask, 'Why didn't anyone tell me...?' or even to suggest that there has been a conspiracy of silence about these realities. Perhaps the permanence and constancy of this task and the adjustment to loss, change, extraordinary responsibility and the new emotional sequelae cannot be described. Even with this knowledge, the power of maternal desire appears to outweigh other considerations. The beliefs and stereotypes of healthcare providers, including mental health clinicians, govern the language they use. Interactions in routine practise provide a unique opportunity to honour the work of mothering and promote adaptive ways of conceptualising these changes.

Asking a pregnant woman when she is giving up work or the mother of a newborn when she is going back to work carries the clear stereotyped message that infant care is not work. Rephrasing the questions as, 'When are you starting work as a mother?' or, 'When are you adding employment to your workload?' suggest a more respectful understanding and carry different implications which challenge the notion that work is being 'given up'. Similarly, guidance to encourage partners to 'help' implies that it is *her* work with which he is assisting, rather than *his* work to share. Reframing this question, ideally to them both, as 'How is household work and infant care shared between you?' with the follow-up question 'Does this feel fair?' conveys quite different assumptions. Gender stereotypes are usually not revealed until this phase of life and are demonstrated in presumptions about who does what after the baby's birth. Women can be helped to recognise when these gender stereotypes are apparent. For example, his statement that, 'I'll do the washing-up for you' or 'I'll get up to the baby for you' reveals his (perhaps unconscious) beliefs about mothers' responsibilities. She can be coached to draw this to his attention and to discuss in non-confrontational ways whether these are acceptable or appropriate to their circumstances.

Ussher [5] describes how mothers who protest about the realities of motherhood are regarded as bad or unfeminine, and that they face the impossible paradox of seeking to be a good mother while balancing, in silence, the costs that it imposes on their lives. Mothers frequently describe themselves as being 'good' or 'bad', perhaps reflecting this highly socialised construction. It entails their belief that this work should be accepted without protest and, if it is done imperfectly, that it reveals their intrinsic incompetence or unsuitability for motherhood. The language of 'coping' and 'not coping' is in the same paradigm. It is an exceptional achievement, deserving congratulation, for any woman to keep an infant alive. However, she might legitimately want to experience greater confidence, pleasure and sense of effectiveness as she does so. Clinicians can emphasise the predicament rather than the person and acknowledge that confidence is eroded by miscarriage; infertility and assisted conception; pregnancy illness and operative birth. Clinicians can also convey their understanding that this predicament is much more difficult for women who live a long way from or have a poor relationship with their family of origin, have worries in addition to caring for the baby, or are caring for a baby who will not settle and cries inconsolably.

Such recognition and sensitivity are also essential in public policy and discourse in which mothers who are in paid employment are referred to as 'working mothers', while those providing exclusive primary care for an infant, an extraordinary and unrelenting workload, are referred to as 'stay-at-home' mothers with the clear implication that they are not working. Neither descriptor is just. All mothers of infants and young children work; some are also in employment. There are interesting parallels with the process of dignifying prostitution; it is argued that naming it as 'sex work' was an essential first step in the establishment of a safe and legitimised working environment and sector-specific health and social services.

26.13 Conclusion

In conclusion, mothering is work of immense but unrecognised value to societies. In failing to name and honour this work, inaccurate and gendered stereotypes are confirmed. The dominant stereotype is that mothering is a leisure activity to which women are intrinsically suited and that it enhances rather than complicates their lives. By careful consideration of their assumptions and how these are reflected in their language and recommendations, clinicians and policy makers are ideally positioned to promote the formation of a confident maternal identity in women who are working as mothers of infants.

References

1. de Marneffe, D. (2004) *Maternal Desire. On Children, Love and Inner Life*, Little, Brown and Company, Time Warner Book Group, New York.
2. Manne, A. (2005) *Motherhood: How Should We Care for Our Children?* Allen and Unwin, Crows Nest.
3. Weston, R., Qu, L., Parker, R. and Alexander, M. (2004) "It's not for Lack of Wanting Kids". A report on the fertility decision making project. Report No. 11, Australian Institute of Family Studies, Melbourne.
4. Stern, D., Bruschweiler-Stern, N. and Freeland, A. (1998) *The Birth of a Mother*, Basic Books, New York.
5. Ussher, J. (1991) *Women's Madness: Misogyny or Mental Illness?* Harvester Wheatsheaf, Exeter.
6. Australian Bureau of Statistics (1999) *Time Use Survey, Australia: Information Paper*, Australian Bureau of Statistics, Canberra.
7. Smith, J. and Baxter, J. (2007) Breastfeeding, Infants' and Mothers' Time Use: A Comparison of the Longitudinal Study of Australian Children and Time Use Survey of New Mothers, Australian Institute of Family Studies presentation Melbourne.
8. Hrdy, S.B. (1999) *Mother Nature: A History of Mothers, Infants and Natural Selection*, Pantheon, New York.
9. Rogers, N. and Grunstein, R. (2005) Working and sleeping around the clock. Sleep loss symposium report. *The Medical Journal of Australia*, **182**, 444–45.
10. McNair, D.M., Lorr, M. and Droppleman, L.F. (1981) *Profile of Mood States: EdITS Manual*, Educational and Industrial Testing Service, San Diego.
11. Fisher, J.R.W., Feekery, C.J. and Rowe-Murray, H.J. (2002) Nature, severity and correlates of psychological distress in women admitted to a private mother-baby unit. *Journal of Paediatrics and Child Health*, **38** (2), 140–45.

12. Commonwealth of Australia (1991) Occupational Health and Safety Act, Department of the Attorney General, Canberra.

13. Fisher, J., Feekery, C. and Rowe, H. (2003) Treatment of maternal mood disorder and infant behaviour disturbance in an Australian private mothercraft unit: a follow-up study. *Archives of Women's Mental Health*, **7** (S1), s1–s5.

14. Jobsite (2008) Work-satisfaction guaranteed? www.jobsite.co.uk (accessed 30 March 2008).

15. Bowlby, J. (1969) *Attachment and Loss*. Attachment, vol. 1, Institute of Psychoanalysis, The Hogarth Press, London.

16. Ainsworth, M. and Bowlby, J. (1965) *Child Care and the Growth of Love*, Penguin Books, London.

17. Dwyer, T., Ponsonby, A., Gibbons, L. and Newman, N. (1991) Prone sleeping position and SIDS: evidence from recent case-control and cohort studies in Tasmania. *Journal of Paediatrics and Child Health*, **27** (6), 340–43.

18. Fisher, J., Rowe, H. and Feekery, C. (2004) Temperament and behaviour of infants aged four to twelve months on admission to a private mother-baby unit and at one and six months follow up. *The Clinical Psychologist*, **8** (1), 15–21.

19. Chira, S. (1998) *A Mother's Place: Taking the Debate About Working Mothers Beyond Guilt and Blame*, HarperCollins, New York.

27

Foundations of human development: Maternal care in the early years

Linda M. Richter and Tamsen Rochat

Child, Youth, Family and Social Development Programme, Human Sciences Research Council, Durban, South Africa

27.1 Child development and human culture

The science of child development has advanced rapidly since the 1970s, particularly with the introduction of new assessment technologies and theoretical cross-fertilisation from other disciplines. The most important advances occurred as a result of: (i) observational technology such as film and videotape which made it possible to observe infants and young children in real time in everyday situations, especially whilst interacting with their intimate caregivers [1]; (ii) the influence of psycho-linguistics and speech act theory which sensitised researchers to the importance of studying communication, and the development of communication and language in context [2] and (iii) very rapid developments in the neurological sciences that enabled the neurophysiological and behavioural antecedents and consequences of variations in the care of offspring to be studied in animal models and amongst humans [3].

What these advances in technology, knowledge and theory demonstrate is that the intense emotional and communicative interaction that occurs between parents and young children during caregiving is universal, whether the children and caregivers are biologically related or not [4]. The early emotional sharing

---

Contemporary Topics in Women's Mental Health   Edited by Chandra, Herrman, Fisher, Kastrup,
© 2009 John Wiley & Sons, Ltd   Niaz, Rondón and Okasha

and engagement with one or more adults, very often the mother, is essential to children's development of language, empathy and cooperation. To a considerable degree, caregiver-infant interactions seem to be driven by biological predispositions on the part of both the adult and the child [5]. Despite variations in form and intensity, prolonged eye contact, imitative facial expressions and mouth movements, synchronised conversation-like vocalisations and emotional attunement between intimate caregivers and infants have been noted in all observed cultures [4].

Baby talk or *motherese*, which refers to the characteristically high pitch, intonation and simplified speech adopted when talking to babies, is used not only by mothers, but also by older children, men and older people when addressing infants and attempting to establish responsive interaction with them [5]. This form of interaction between infants and more mature individuals is theorised to be essential for the development of human characteristics such as language, interpersonal and emotional understanding, empathic reasoning and morality, self-regulation and self-identity [6–8]. Babies are uniquely dependent on particular forms of early experience with other people. The incomplete development of children deprived – for a variety of reasons, including cruel neglect and isolation – of warm, responsive, interpersonal care, demonstrates the importance of these types of interaction in the phenotypic expression of unique human capacities [9]. It is through these interactions that young children are inculcated into shared human culture, as well as into their own specific linguistic and ethnic way of life.

The infant is prepared to enter into communication with other human beings through predisposed *pro forma* sensory, motor, linguistic and cognitive capacities, as well as by what has been called experience-expectant and experience-dependent brain development [1, 2, 5]. Amongst other things, newborn babies preferentially focus on the human face, turn to the human voice and imitate basic mouth movements. Their brains anticipate certain types of experience, especially with other human beings [10]. These predispositions create a curriculum of anticipated and required stimulation, contingency and responsiveness towards the child, to which emotionally involved parents respond.

On their side, parents and other intimate caregivers also enter relationships with young children with seemingly predetermined feelings and behaviours. For example, motherese is unconsciously responsive to babies. *Intuitive parenting* refers to parental counterparts to the infant's dependency and expectancy [11]. Sensitive caregivers observe and respond to the cues of infants and young children, enable the child's perceived intentions (for example by pulling a desired object to within reach), imitate infant behaviour and attempt to elicit communication signals. These behaviours are not learned and they don't proceed from rational analysis and decision. Instead, they are prompted and reinforced by the adult's affection for and strong motivation to care for the child and engage with them. In this sense, motivation for parenting primes the adult and opens the way for intuitive responsiveness [12].

27.2 Interactions and relationships

In the early weeks and months of life, parenting is directed primarily to establishing emotional contact with the child, and caring for their physical needs. This includes learning how to 'read' the child so as to know how best to comfort them, draw and hold their attention, make them smile, and so on. It also refers to meeting needs for feeding, hygiene, sleep and healthcare. The predilection of both adult and child to engage with one another, their success at doing so, and their shared pleasure are repeated in bursts or 'packages' of maternal stimulation [13]. Initially, the infant's responses are not person-specific. Over time, as interactions become familiar, their intimacy and predictability begin to constitute relationship templates that can be understood in terms of attachment theory [14].

Attachment is described as a bio-ecological system to ensure the caregiver and child's proximity to one another, to safeguard the infant's survival and protection. Infants have innate signalling capacities, such as crying, that bring and keep the caregiver close. In turn, caregivers respond to these signals with varying warmth, urgency and predictability. The attachment relationship to the primary caregiver develops over the first six to nine months, at which time an attachment type, along a dimension of security, is discernible.

The importance of security for the young child is twofold. Firstly, security and exploration for the child exist in balance [15]. Secure infants venture beyond the mother to explore objects and learn about the world. But they look back and return frequently to the caregiver, especially when they encounter unknown conditions. Through social referencing, they look to the caregiver for cues on how to interpret new experiences [16]. The caregiver's confidence and encouragement enable the young child to explore and acquire competences unimpeded by anxiety and insecurity.

Secondly, the first attachment creates a mental representation, or an internal working model, of people who will be encountered in the future. This mental model influences children's expectations of future relationships and, consequently, their behaviour in relation to new people. There is a great deal of evidence to support the connection between attachment security, a young child's cognitive and language development, and later peer relations and social adjustment [17].

A number of factors influence the establishment, maintenance and quality of parent-child relationships. These include the wider social environment, such as resource constraints and social support, as well as influences at the level of the child and the caregiver. Together these constitute an integrated, multilevel, ecology of human development [18]. Belsky [19] for example, posits three categories of determinants of the quality of parenting:

- Contextual sources of stress and support, such as socioeconomic status and the quality of the parental partnership.

- Characteristics of the child, such as temperament, disability and gender.
- Psychological resources of the caregiver, importantly including low morale and depression.

Care for young children is driven by parental motivations, such as the desire to be a good mother, preventing one's child from coming to harm and the like. It is also affected by mental and emotional states [12]. Preoccupation with worries, in particular, interfere with the capacity to be sensitive and responsive to young children. Stress, including the ongoing hardship and insecurity associated with poverty, can disrupt parenting and fragment the attention a caregiver gives a young child.

27.3 Maternal mental health and children's development

Factors commonly associated with depression include severe negative life events, early childhood adversity, low perceived and actual social support and lack of social capital [20]. Depression among women with young children has long been known to be high in resource-rich countries, with rates of up to 40% reported among non-working poor mothers of preschool children [21]. Recently, growing evidence also points to high rates of depression among women in resource-poor countries [22]. For example, in South Africa an estimated prevalence of depression of 34.7% has been reported [23]; in India, 23% [24] and in eastern Turkey, 27% [25].

Depressed mood during pregnancy is associated with inadequate antenatal care, low birth weight and preterm delivery, thus increasing the risks of poor maternal and child health outcomes [24]. Recent research indicates that low socioeconomic status, poverty and single motherhood are associated with increased antenatal depression and, importantly, that depression during pregnancy is the strongest predictor of post-partum depression (PPD) [26].

Depression is characterised by self-preoccupation, irritability, diminished emotional involvement, increased hostility and resentment, fatigue and helplessness [27]. A very large number of studies demonstrate that depressed mothers are withdrawn and/or insensitively intrusive in their interactions with their infants and young children, and that children show disturbed reactions to this maternal behaviour [23]. Follow-up studies indicate that the adverse effects of maternal depression on children may persist well into childhood and early adolescence in the form of behaviour disorders, anxiety, depression and attentional problems [28]. The effects of maternal depression are exacerbated by other risks, such as low socio-economic status and extended duration of the depressive episode [29].

Apart from its indirect effects on children's adjustment and attention, caregiver depression may threaten the survival, growth and health of children more directly through lack of adequate care, and decreased concern with the child's safety [29], For example, Rahman *et al.* [30, 31] have suggested that maternal depression plays a role in the risk of infant illness and growth impairment in developing countries through decreased child surveillance and lack of attention to simple health promotion activities.

Postnatal depression is an important issue for public health in developing countries; it has been shown to be of high prevalence and to have serious consequences for both maternal and child health [32]. In these settings, gender inequality and poverty exacerbate other challenges to the wellbeing of women and children.

27.4 Maternal care

As described earlier, the interactive nature of caregiving, and its role in facilitating early child development, is well established. It is generally accepted that early learning by young children is enabled by a warm, consistent and responsive caregiver. Activities and processes which facilitate children's learning require intense emotional investment, and psychological availability on the part of the primary caregiver, most often a mother. Together, these constitute what has been called the *holding environment*, a physical and psychological space in which a baby is protected. Donald Winnicott referred to caregiver devotion to these caring activities as a state of *maternal preoccupation*, or the ability of a mother to identify closely and intuitively with her infant [33].

Available evidence points to the importance of social support networks for safeguarding and maintaining maternal mental health. Thus, enabling responsive caregiving is not limited to the maternal caregiving figure alone. Rather there is a shared, contextual environment, optimally a supportive familial framework, which provides for the economic, social and psychological security and protection of both the child and the mother. Attention to the contextual nature of the early developmental relationship leads us to better understand how negative life events, social adversity, marital or relationship conflict and a lack of social support not only affect maternal mental health and morale, but also directly and indirectly challenge a young child's development. Poverty and adversity often compound these contextual influences, exposing women and children to a multitude of physical and social risks.

The extent of these risks and threats to early child development are significant [34], and there is an increasing urgency to recognise the important role of parenting factors in determining child outcomes. Key risk factors include cognitive stimulation and child learning opportunities, caregiver sensitivity and responsivity, maternal depression and exposure to violence [35]. These key areas offer a guiding framework for reflecting on the importance of mental health interventions for caregivers, to ensure that their children can grow towards their full human potential in adverse conditions.

27.5 Implications for mental healthcare

PPD is a significant problem among women with young children, with important implications for the mental health of mothers, and the health and wellbeing of their children. Recent evidence has also begun to indicate similar risks to children whose fathers suffer from depression [36]. For this reason, the development of effective systems for the screening, early detection and appropriate treatment of depression are crucial to improving child and adult mental health outcomes.

A number of factors predict postnatal depression. A recent meta-analysis including over 14 000 subjects, and subsequent studies of nearly 10 000 additional cases, found that the strongest predictors of PPD were depression before pregnancy, anxiety, experiencing stressful life events during pregnancy or during the early post-partum period, low levels of social support and a previous history of depression [26]. Since all of these risk factors can be assessed during routine pregnancy care, it is important that antenatal healthcare providers, as well as women more generally, are educated about risk factors in order to increase early detection and health service use.

Several simple and effective PPD screening tools are available, the one in most widespread use is the Edinburgh Postnatal Depression Scale (EPDS), a 10-item screening questionnaire which has been found to be user-friendly and acceptable in most cultures internationally [37, 38]. In addition, several useful assessment schedules have been developed for use by nurse-practitioners, such as the Earthquake Assessment Model for Mental Health [39], which is helpful in recognising early signs of depression and developing a response.

Several treatment approaches have been found to be effective, acceptable and safe for women with PPD. Optimal treatment is prompt, includes an interdisciplinary team, and uses a family-centred approach, all of which tend to improve longer term outcomes [40]. Treatments which have been shown to be effective include cognitive behavioural therapy (CBT) and interpersonal therapy (IPT), using individual and group approaches, supportive counselling, psycho education and, in more severe cases, treatment with antidepressant medications [41–44]. Group IPT interventions have also been validated and have shown promising results in clinical trials in resource-poor settings such as Uganda [45].

27.6 Increased choices for women

Given the potential tensions between women's paid work and child care, and the impact of these on child outcomes, it is important to reflect on the implications of access to quality child care services available to parents in contemporary societies. Quality of care includes not only structural issues, such as staff-child ratio, group sizes, staff training and physical environmental factors, but also processes of care, such as warmth, responsiveness and emotional tone.

Often the most at-risk dyads are those struggling under crippling socio-economic factors, which introduce a cumulative set of practical and social challenges which would, in part, be alleviated by increased access to household income and resources. However, evidence suggests that the cost of high quality care often negates any increase in household income for low income woman [46]. Likewise, longitudinal studies indicate that low-income women who return to work, and are forced to access alternative child care in order to do so, are often disadvantaged by the poor quality of child care [47]. Findings also suggest that the children of these women have poorer outcomes as a result of the low quality of the out-of-home care they can afford. For women around the world, the choice between caring for their children at home and paid work outside the home is only meaningful when quality child care is available outside of the home at a reasonable cost.

27.7 Conclusion

Children's development depends critically on a caring environment for the full expression of their human capacities. Mothers, by virtue of pregnancy, birthing and breastfeeding, are frequently at the heart of a child's proximal environment, although other intimate adults also contribute to it, and can and do function as parents. Biological predispositions on the part of both the newborn and young infant, as well as other parenting adults, create conditions for the formation of strong socio-emotional caregiver-child attachment. This attachment forms the basis for children's emotional and social functioning. However, broader contextual factors exert a strong influence on the quality of attachment, including characteristics of the infant, such as low birth weight; psychological resources of caregivers such as emotional state, and ongoing stresses and supports, including the involvement of marital partners and other family. Because care for young children is driven by parental motivation, low morale and depression can interfere with the capacity for sensitive and responsive child care. In turn, lack of appropriate care can endanger the survival of young children, threaten growth and health, and lead to adjustment and other problems. For this reason, care of women's health and mental health is integral to children's development, including the need to address the undue burden of poverty borne by women and the difficult choices women face in finding good quality care for children while they work to provide for their family.

References

1. Schaffer, H. (1977) *Studies in Mother-Infant Interaction*, Academic Press, London.
2. Bullowa, M. (1979) *Before Speech: The Beginning of Interpersonal Communication*, Cambridge University Press, London.
3. Schore, A. (1994) *Affect Regulation and the Origin of the Self: The Neurobiology of Emotional Development*, Lawrence Erlbaum, Hillsdale.
4. Richter, L. (1995) Are early adult-infant interactions universal: a South African view. *South African Journal of Child and Adolescent Psychiatry*, **7**, 2–18.

5. Trevarthen, C. (1983) Interpersonal abilities of infants as generators for transmission of language and culture, in *The Behaviour of Human Infants* (eds A. Oliviero and M. Zappella), Plenum Press, London, pp. 145–76.

6. Kaye, K. (1982) *The Mental and Social life of Babies*, Harvester Press, Sussex.

7. Pinker, S. (2002) *The Blank Slate: The Modern Denial of Human Nature*, Viking-Penguin, New York.

8. Stern, D. (1985) *The Interpersonal World of the Infant: A View from Psychoanalysis and Developmental Psychology*, Basic Books, New York.

9. Curtiss, S. (1977) *Genie: A Psycholinguistic Study of a Modern-Day "Wild Child"*, Academic Press, New York.

10. Cozolino, L. (2006) *The Neuroscience of Human Relationships: Attachments and the Developing Social Brain*, WW Norton, New York.

11. Papousek, H. and Papousek, M. (1987) Intuitive parenting: a dialectic counterpart to the infant's precocity in integrative capacities, in *Handbook of Infant Development*, 2nd edn (ed. J. Osofsky), John Wiley & Sons, Inc., New York, pp. 669–720.

12. Dix, T. (1991) The affective organization of parenting: adaptive and maladaptive processes. *Psychological Bulletin*, **110**, 3–25.

13. Beebe, B. and Gerstman, L. (1984) A method of defining "packages" of maternal stimulation and their functional significance for the infant with mother and strangers. *International Journal of Behaviour and Development*, **7**, 423–40.

14. Bowlby, J. (1969) *Attachment and Loss: Attachment*, Vol. **1**, Basic Books, New York.

15. Ainsworth, M.D. and Bell, S.M. (1970) Attachment, exploration, and separation: Illustrated by the behaviour of 1-year-olds in a strange situation. *Child Development*, **41**, 49–67.

16. Blackford, J. and Walden, T. (1998) Individual differences in social referencing. *Infant Behaviour and Development*, **21**, 89–102.

17. Weinfeld, N., Sroufe, L. and Egeland, B. (2000) Attachment from infancy to early adult hood in a high-risk sample: continuity, discontinuity and their correlates. *Child Development*, **71**, 695–702.

18. Bronfenbrenner, U. (ed.) (2005) *Making Human Beings Human: Bioecological Perspectives on Human Development*, Sage Publications, Thousand Oaks.

19. Belsky, J. (1984) The determinants of parenting: a process model. *Child Development*, **55**, 83–96.

20. Harris, T. (2001) Recent development in understanding the psychosocial aspects of depression. *British Medical Bulletin*, **57**, 17–32.

21. Puckering, C. (1989) Annotation: maternal depression. *Journal of Child Psychology and Psychiatry*, **30**, 807–17.

22. Husain, N., Creed, F. and Tomenson, B. (2000) Depression and social stress in Pakistan. *Psychological Medicine*, **30**, 395–402.

23. Cooper, P.J., Tomlinson, M. and Swartz, L. *et al.* (1999) Post-partum depression and the mother-infant relationship in a South African peri-urban settlement. *British Journal of Psychiatry*, **175**, 554–58.

24. Patel, V., Rodriges, M. and DeSouza, N. (2002) Gender, poverty, and postnatal depression: a study of mothers in Goa, India. *American Journal of Psychiatry*, **159**, 43–47.

25. Inandi, T., Elci, O., Ozturk, A. *et al.* (2002) Risk factors for depression in postnatal first year, in eastern Turkey. *International Journal of Epidemiology*, **31**, 1201–7.

26. Robertson, E., Grace, S., Wallington, T. and Stewart D. (2004) Antenatal risk factors for postpartum depression: a synthesis of recent literature. *General Hospital Psychiatry*, **26**, 289–95.

27. Weissman, M., Paykel, E. and Klerman G. (1972) The depressed woman as a mother. *Social Psychiatry*, **7**, 98–108.

28. Galler, J.R., Harrison, R.H., Ramsey, F. *et al.* (2000) Maternal depressive symptoms affect infant cognitive development in Barbados. *Journal of Child Psychology and Psychiatry*, **41**, 747–57.

29. McLennan, J. and Kotelchuck, M. (2000) Parental prevention practices for young children in the context of maternal depression. *Pediatrics*, **105**, 1090–95.

30. Rahman, A., Bunn, J. and Creed, F. (2007) Maternal depression increases infant risk of diarrhoeal illness: a cohort study. *Archives of the Diseases of Childhood*, **92**, 24–28.

31. Zeitlin, M., Ghassemi, H. and Mansour, M. (1990) *Positive Deviance in Child Nutrition*, United Nations University Press, Tokyo.

32. Tomlinson, M., Cooper, P. and Stein, A. *et al.* (2006) Post-partum depression and infant growth in a South African peri-urban settlement. *Child Care Health and Development*, **32**, 81–86.

33. Winnicott, D. (1960) The theory of the parent-child relationship. *International Journal of Psychoanalysis*, **41**, 585–95.

34. Grantham-McGregor, S., Bun Cheung, Y. and Cueto, S. (2007) Developmental potential in the first 5 years for children in developing countries. *Lancet*, **369**, 60–70.

35. Walker, S.P., Wachs, T.D. and Meeks Gardner, J. International Child Development Steering Group (2007) Child development: risk factors for adverse outcomes in developing countries. *Lancet*, **369**, 145–57.

36. Ramchandani, P., Stein, A., Evans, J. and O'Conner, T. ALSPAC Study Team (2005) Paternal depression in the postnatal period and child development: a prospective population study. *Lancet*, **365**, 2201–5.

37. Cox, J.L., Holden, J.M. and Sagovsky, R. (1987) Detection of postnatal depression: development of the 10-item Edinburgh Postnatal Depression Scale. *British Journal of Psychiatry*, **150**, 782–86.

38. Eberhard-Gran, M., Eskild, A., Tambs, K. *et al.* (2001) Review of validation studies of the Edinburgh Postnatal Depression Scale. *Acta Psychiatrica Scandinavica*, **104**, 243–49.

39. Watson Driscoll, J. (2005) Recognizing women's common mental health problems: the earthquake assessment model. *Journal of Obstetric Gynecological and Neonatal Nursing*, **34** (2), 246–54.

40. Andrews Horowitz, J. and Goodman, J.H. (2005) Identifying and treating postpartum depression. *Journal of Obstetric Gynecological and Neonatal Nursing*, **34** (2), 264–73.

41. Charbol, H., Teissedre, F., Saint-Jean, M. *et al.* (2002) Prevention and treatment of postpartum depression: a controlled randomised study of women at risk. *Psychological Medicine*, **32**, 1039–47.

42. Cooper, P.J., Murray, L., Wilson, A. and Romaniuk, H. (2003) Controlled trial of the short and long term effect of psychological treatment for postpartum depression. *British Journal of Psychiatry*, **182**, 412–19.

43. O'Hara, M.W., Stuart, S., Gorman, L.L. and Wenzel, A. (2000) Efficacy of inter-personal therapy for postpartum depression. *Archives of General Psychiatry*, **57**, 1039–110.

44. Misri, S., Kostaras, X., Fox, D. and Kostaras, D. (2000) The impact of partner support in the treatment of postnatal depression. *Canadian Journal of Psychiatry*, **45**, 554–58.

45. Bolton, P., Bass, J., Neugebauer, R. *et al.* (2003) Group interpersonal psychotherapy for depression in rural Uganda: a randomized controlled trial. *Journal of the American Medical Association*, **289**, 3117–24.

46. Toroyan, T., Roberts, I., Oakley, A. *et al.* (2003) Effectiveness of out-of-home day care for disadvantaged families: randomised controlled trial. *The British Medical Journal*, **327**, 906.

47. Leach, P., Stein, A. and Sylva, K. (2005) A Prospective Study of the Effects of Different Kinds of Care on Children's Development in the First Five Years, Families Children and Child Care Project.

28

The adverse impact of psychological aggression, coercion and violence in the intimate partner relationship on women's mental health

Toshiko Kamo

Tokyo Women's Medical University, Institute of Women's Health, Tokyo, Japan

28.1 Introduction

There is ample research evidence demonstrating that intimate partner violence (IPV) occurs in all countries, and is apparent in all social, economic, religious and cultural groups. IPV is recognised as a serious human rights violation, and increasingly as an important public health problem with significant consequences for women's physical, mental, sexual and reproductive health, and their economic circumstances which have been overlooked for a long time.

28.2 Prevalence and nature of intimate partner violence

The World Health Organisation's World Report on Violence [1] drew on evidence from population-based surveys undertaken between 1984 and 1999 in 48

Contemporary Topics in Women's Mental Health   Edited by Chandra, Herrman, Fisher, Kastrup,
© 2009 John Wiley & Sons, Ltd   Niaz, Rondón and Okasha

countries. It found that between 10 and 69% of women reported being physically assaulted by an intimate male partner at some point in their lives [1]. Further data were generated in a recent World Health Organization (WHO)-led multi-country study which used standardised population-based household surveys in 15 selected sites in 10 countries: Bangladesh, Brazil, Ethiopia, Japan, Namibia, Peru, Samoa, Serbia and Montenegro, Thailand and United Republic of Tanzania [2]. This study found that the lifetime prevalence of either physical or sexual partner violence, or both, varied from 15 to 71%, and the prevalence in the past year was estimated as being between 4 and 54%.

Psychological aggression including intimidation, constant belittling and humiliation and various controlling behaviours are forms of abuse and although measurement of them is not yet fully standardised, they are important for a comprehensive understanding of IPV. A recent government study undertaken in 1283 married or previously-married women in Japan for instance, found that 26.7% of the informants had experienced physical violence by an intimate partner in their lifetime, 15.2% sexual coercion and 16.1% psychological aggression [3].

There is substantial overlap between physical violence, sexual coercion and psychological aggression, which can occur simultaneously or separately. In most sites in the WHO Multi-Country Study between 30 and 56% of women who had ever experienced any violence reported both physical and sexual violence. In a study in Leo'n, Nicaragua (2000), 28.1% of women who had experienced IPV reported physical, sexual and psychological abuse and 41.1% of them reported both physical and sexual abuse [4]. In a Japanese nationwide survey of victims of violence using public or private refuges in 2006, 801 women volunteered to participate and then completed questionnaires. It was found in the survey that experiencing multiple types of abuse simultaneously or alternately was six times more common in these abused women than experiencing a single type of violence [5].

It is also known that IPV lasts usually for an extended period of time. Even though there are major obstacles to leaving abusive relationships, many abused women eventually seek refuge from violent partners, sometimes after many years of abuse; usually once the children have grown up or once they have been almost killed. In the study in Leo'n, for example, the median time that women spent in a violent relationship was around six years, although younger women were more likely than older women to leave sooner [6].

In summary IPV is characterised as multi-dimensional violence consisting mainly of physical assault, sexual coercion and/or psychological aggression, which carries serious consequences including damage to social life and both physical and mental health for abused women. From the viewpoint of traumatic stress studies IPV can be regarded as long-lasting repetitious stress or trauma, and the impact on health is comparable to child abuse and neglect by parents and other caregivers.

28.3 Impact of intimate partner violence on general health

Violence has been associated with a host of adverse health outcomes, both immediate and long-term. Although violence can have direct health problems, including injuries, being a victim of violence also increases a woman's risk of future ill health and violence is a demonstrated risk factor for a variety of diseases and conditions. These include chronic functional disorders such as irritable bowel syndrome, fibromyalgia, gastrointestinal disorders and various chronic pain syndromes [7], which are estimated to be more common than direct injuries. Reproductive health is also affected, including unwanted pregnancy and/or sexually transmitted infection through sexual coercion. Repeated pregnancies and a large number of children are thought both to contribute to risk of IPV because of the increased stress of caring for a large number of children, but also might reflect abuse, through lack of reproductive choice. Ellsberg *et al.* and the WHO Multi-country Study on Women's Health and Domestic Violence against Women Study Team [8] reported very recently, newly analysed data about 24 097 women aged 15–49 years from the WHO Multi Country population-based survey. There were significant associations between lifetime experiences of IPV and self-reported poor health (odds ratio, OR 1.6). In this study, between 19 and 55% of women who had ever been physically abused by their partner were injured. Although the interval since experiencing violence varied, specific physical health problems in the previous four weeks were more prevalent in women reporting IPV than in non-abused women. These included difficulty walking (OR 1.6), difficulty with daily activities (OR 1.6), pain (OR 1.6), memory loss (OR 1.8), dizziness (OR 1.7) and vaginal discharge (OR 1.8).

28.4 Mental health problems among women affected by intimate partner violence

In the last two decades of the twentieth century, the relationship between IPV and mental health problems has become more apparent and there is now much greater recognition of the links between them. Mental health problems are likely to be observed even more commonly than physical health problems after IPV. In the WHO study significantly more women who had experienced partner violence at least once in their lifetime reported serious emotional distress, including suicidal thoughts (OR 2.9) and suicidal attempts (OR 3.8) than non-abused women. Although the available research has not yet addressed many criteria for causal inferences, the existing research is consistent with the hypothesis that IPV increases risk for mental health problems.

Golding [9] reviewed the then available literature on the prevalence of mental health problems among women with a history of physical IPV [9]. In this review, data from an earlier review of violence against women by Koss *et al.* in 1994 were used and 33 further English-language studies were identified through systematic searches and included. The studies were reviewed for associations of IPV with depression, suicidality, posttraumatic stress disorder (PTSD) and substance abuse. Golding [9] found that the weighted mean prevalence of mental health problems among battered women was 47.6% (95% CI 15–83%) in 18 studies which had assessed depression; 17.9% in 13 studies which examined suicidality; 63.8% (95% CI 31–84.4%) in 11 studies of (PTSD); 18.5% in 10 studies of alcohol abuse and 8.9% in 4 studies of drug abuse. Additionally dose-response relationships of violence to depression and PTSD were observed, namely, severity and duration of violence was associated with prevalence and severity of depression and of PTSD. Most studies on both depression and PTSD in the general population have found higher lifetime prevalence of depression and PTSD in women than in men. However, the rates of depression and PTSD among women with a history of IPV are even higher than those in the general population of women. The lifetime risk of developing depression is 10–20% in females in developed countries and slightly less in males, and it is well known that women are twice as likely as men to develop PTSD during their lifetimes (10.4% versus 5.0%) [8]. Olff *et al.* [10] reviewed the empirical evidence for a range of explanations of this difference, including gender differences in trauma exposure, in acute stress reactions and in psychological and biological stress response mechanisms. They concluded that women's higher PTSD risk may be due to the type of trauma they experience. These included: younger age at the time of trauma exposure; stronger perceptions of threat and loss of control; higher levels of peritraumatic dissociation; insufficient social support resources and greater use of alcohol to manage trauma-related symptoms like intrusive memories and dissociation. In addition there are gender-specific acute psychobiological reactions to trauma.

There is also a high rate of comorbidity between depression and PTSD, which is apparent in women abused by IPV at the same or even higher levels than in studies of other traumatic exposures. Stein and Kennedy [11] reported that major depressive disorder (MDD) and IPV-related PTSD were more frequently comorbid than would be expected by chance. In an investigation of 44 women who were victims of IPV, 43% of those with current IPV-related PTSD also had (MDD) [11]. In addition severity of depressive and PTSD symptoms were highly correlated in this study. Nixon *et al.* [12] recruited 142 women from domestic violence assistance agencies and shelters. They found using structured clinical interviews, high levels of PTSD (75%), MDD (54%) and comorbid PTSD/MDD (49%) in women who had experienced an incident of physical abuse in the six months prior to assessment. The PTSD/MDD group were significantly more likely to have suffered an adult rape (outside of the abusive relationship) than the PTSD/No MDD group, and reported greater psychological aggression than either the No PTSD/No MDD or PTSD/No MDD groups. The PTSD/MDD group also endorsed more maladaptive beliefs than the other two groups so that the authors estimated cognitions and schemas in meaning of cognitive theory may play an important role in understanding why depression develops in the context of PTSD.

Follow-up studies [13] of women abused by intimate partners conclude that rates of depression in those who entered a battered women's shelter declined significantly across time. Surtees [14] found prevalence rates of depression in 32 women were lower six months after entering a Women's Aid refuge than they had been when first seeking assistance. Similarly, Campbell *et al.* [13] observed depressive symptoms across time in 141 women who had used a domestic violence shelter three times: immediately after shelter exit, 10 weeks thereafter and six months later. There were substantial decreases in symptoms between the immediate period after seeking refuge from IPV and six or more months later. Whereas 83% of the women reported at least mild depression on the Center for Epidemiological Studies Depression (CES-D) scale upon shelter exit, only 58% were depressed 10 weeks later. This change was sustained and had not reverted at the six month follow-up. The authors suggested that, after controlling for previous levels of depression, the women's feelings of powerlessness, experience of abuse and decreased social support contributed to their depression symptoms. Mood improved when abuse ceased, social support was provided and a sense of personal agency fostered. Yanagita *et al.* [15] administrated the General Health Questionnaire 28 (GHQ-28) and the Impact of Event Scale Revised (IES-R) to 87 IPV women victims in a Japanese public emergency shelter to investigate short time outcome of their mental health state after they entered the shelter and when leaving it. They found that the severely disturbed mental states including traumatic stress symptoms observed on admission to the shelter (mean total scores of GHQ-28 : 17.8 and IES-R: 41.6) recovered significantly by discharge to GHQ-28 : 10.1 and IES-R: 33.7 respectively. This was achieved despite the mean duration of stay by women in the shelter being only 22 days [15]. It is very important that the results indicate mental disorders represented by depression in abused women remit quite rapidly in a safe environment where they can be confident that IPV will not occur. There is not nearly enough evidence to know, however, their long-term outcome of depression and whether this also improved their general quality of life.

Although there are as yet no follow-up studies of IPV-related PTSD, biological findings from investigations of women abused by their intimate partners are gradually accruing especially from the research field of traumatic stress. Alterations of the hypothalamic–pituitary–adrenal (HPA) axis function and sympathetic-adrenal activity have been proposed as key elements in biological models of PTSD, and research related to the HPA axis is especially advanced in this area. There is positive evidence that the HPA axis is dysregulated in women who are experiencing IPV, however, it is still not clear whether women's basic cortisol level is likely to be low [16, 17] or high [18]. Seedat *et al.* [16] examined morning plasma samples collected for cortisol determination in 22 women with histories of IPV (10 with current PTSD, 12 without current or lifetime PTSD) and 16 non-abused controls. In this study it was recognised that mean cortisol levels were significantly lower in IPV subjects compared with controls, but did not distinguish IPV subjects with and without PTSD. Griffin *et al.* [17] assessed 70 female domestic violence victim-survivors and 14 non traumatised women who were matched for age and ethnicity. They found that IPV survivors with PTSD, regardless of whether or not they had comorbid depression, had significantly lower baseline cortisol levels at 9:00 a.m. than healthy women and trauma survivors with no diagnosis. In contrast, Inslichta *et al.* [18] found that female survivors of IPV with lifetime (current or remitted) PTSD (n = 29) had significantly higher salivary cortisol levels across the day compared to women who were exposed to IPV but never developed PTSD (n = 20).

There is also an emergent body of research about brain morphometry. Fennema-Notestine *et al.* [19] using quantitative magnetic resonance imaging estimated that there were smaller supratentorial cranial vaults and smaller frontal and occipital grey matter volumes in women with IPV (n = 22) compared to non-victimised women (n = 17). This might reflect the influence of early trauma on neurodevelopmental processes or denote brain morphometric characteristics of persons experiencing serious psychosocial adversity regardless of life stage. A further study by Seedat *et al.* [20] using single voxel proton magnetic resonance spectroscopy reported that IPV exposed women with PTSD (n = 7) had significantly higher anterior cingulate choline/creatine than IPV women without PTSD (n = 9). These findings suggest the existence of metabolite alterations in general in PTSD caused by additional stressors to the IPV. However, the authors also found that the participants with PTSD had experienced more severe IPV as measured by the Conflict Tactics Scale-Revised than the non-PTSD group, suggesting a possible dose related effect.

It has been suggested that women are rendered vulnerable to abusive relationships because of deficits in cognitive capacity and a number of explanatory models are proposed. The battered woman syndrome proposes that sufferers have low self regard and distorted cognitions, believing that the abuse is their fault. The diagnostic category of Masochistic (or Self-Defeating) Personality Disorder was proposed to describe a person who avoided pleasure, was attracted to relationships or social circumstances in which suffering would be experienced and resisted assistance from others. However, it was strongly criticised as blaming victims for their predicaments and was not included in the Diagnostic and Statistical Manual of Mental Disorders-III's operational diagnostic criteria for psychiatric disorders by the American Psychiatric Association [21]. There is a small body of neuropsychological research about the cognitive functioning of women abused by intimate partners. Stein *et al.* [22] investigated neuropsychological function in female victims of IPV. They found that cognitive deficits in IPV subjects were confined to measures of working memory, visuo-construction and executive function; were subtle; and were not uniformly worse among those with current PTSD. The tendency to having low self-esteem, self-criticism, guilty conscience and re-entering to a violent relationship is explained often by learned helplessness due to IPV itself. It might also reflect the experience of child abuse including watching violence between their parents or reflect psychiatric disorders which may be caused also mostly by IPV. Ehrensaft *et al.* [23] used a prospective longitudinal birth cohort design, with repeated measures of mental disorder before and after the experience of an abusive relationship in New Zealand. In a comparison between 38 people who had experienced abuse and 411 who had not, they found that males and females who had psychiatric disorders in adolescence were at greatest risk of becoming involved in abusive adult relationships. After the authors controlled for earlier psychiatric history, women who were involved in abusive relationships, but not men, had an increased risk of adult psychiatric morbidity including depression, marijuana dependence and especially PTSD. They concluded that the result lends support to clinical theories proposing that women who are abused by a partner develop mental health problems.

28.5 Intimate partner violence, children and intergenerational patterns of abuse

IPV also has a profound impact on the mental health of children. Children who witness marital violence, in particular those whose mothers are abused by an intimate partner, are themselves at higher risk for a whole range of emotional and behavioural problems, including anxiety, depression, poor school performance, low self-esteem, disobedience, nightmares and physical health complaints [24]. There is a shortage of comparison studies in this research area, but Kernic *et al.* [25] observed that 2- to 17-year-old children exposed to maternal IPV (n = 167) were more likely to have borderline to clinical level scores on externalising (aggressive and delinquent) behaviours (relative risk (RR) = 1.6, 95% confidence interval (CI): 1.2–2.1) and total behavioural problems (RR = 1.4, 95% CI: 1.1–1.9) compared to the Child Behaviour Checklist (CBCL) normative sample (n = 2736) after adjusting for age and sex. The answer to the question about whether childhood exposure to family violence is associated with an increased risk of IPV, will become an important watershed in establishing the seriousness of the problems associated with IPV. There is as yet only a small body of research concerning the intergenerational chain reaction of IPV. Bensley *et al.* [26] conducted a population-based telephone survey asking a representative sample of 3527 English-speaking, non-institutionalised adult women about whether they had been physically or sexually assaulted or witnessed interparental violence in childhood, and whether they had experienced physical assault or emotional abuse from an intimate partner in the past year. They found that women reporting childhood physical abuse or witnessing interparental violence were at a four- to sixfold increase in risk of physical IPV, and women reporting any of the experiences measured in the study were at three- to fourfold increase in risk of partner emotional abuse. Very recently McKinney *et al.* [27] analysed data about the relationship between childhood exposure to family violence and adult perpetration or victimisation of IPV in 1615 couples from an American national population-based study. According to the research, men who experienced moderate (adjusted odds ratio (AOR) 3.9, 95% CI, 1.3–11.8) or severe (AOR 4.5, 95% CI: 1.1–19.3) child physical abuse were at increased risk of nonreciprocal male-to-female partner violence; a male history of severe childhood physical abuse or witnessing interparental violence was associated with a twofold increased risk of reciprocal IPV. Women who witnessed interparental threats of violence (AOR 1.9, 95% CI, 0.8–4.6) or interparental physical violence in childhood (AOR 3.4, 95% CI, 1.5–7.9) were at increased risk of nonreciprocal female-to-male partner violence. Women exposed to any type of childhood family violence were more than 1.5 times as likely to engage in reciprocal IPV [27]. These data have clear implications that in order to prevent IPV, interventions are required for children who are victimised by family violence.

28.6 Conclusion

Overall therefore there is copious evidence about the severe adverse impact of psychological aggression, coercion and physical violence in intimate relationships on women's mental health. It is still underestimated by governments and public policy makers, but it is at this level that action is required to reduce this modifiable risk factor for poor mental health in women. From the clinical standpoint while large scale, longitudinal, prospective studies are required to know about the mental health outcomes of the victims, the most urgent need is for interventions to reduce IPV to be developed and trialled. Even in the absence of this it is essential for clinicians caring for women with mental health problems to assess exposure to IPV as a matter of routine and to ensure that treatment recommendations are well informed about strategies to protect women's safety and improve psychological functioning through violence reduction. The public provision of places of safety for women leaving situations of domestic violence is an essential strategy to reducing mental health problems. IPV is a crime, but is not recognised as illegal in many jurisdictions. The promotion of women's mental health requires appropriate public and private recognition of the destructive impact of IPV.

References

1. World Health Organization (2002) World Report on Violence and Health, World Health Organization, Geneva.
2. Garcia-Moreno, C., Jansen, H., Ellsberg, M. *et al.* (2006) Prevalence of intimate partner violence: findings from the WHO multi-country study on women's health and domestic violence. *Lancet*, **368**, 1260–69.
3. Gender Equality Bureau (2005) *Survey on Violence between Men and Women*, Japanese Cabinet Office, Tokyo.
4. Ellsberg, M.C., Peña, R., Herrera, A. *et al.* (2000) Candies in hell: women's experience of violence in Nicaragua. *Social Science and Medicine*, **51**, 1595–610.
5. Gender Equality Bureau (2007) (Survey on Support for Independence of Victims of Violence between Spouses, Translated by Kamo), Japanese Cabinet Office, Tokyo.

6. Ellsberg, M., Winkvist, A., Peña, R. and Stenlund, H. (2001) Women's strategic responses to violence in Nicaragua. *Journal of Epidemiology and Community Health*, **55**, 547–55.

7. Campbell, J.C. (2002) Health consequences of intimate partner violence. *Lancet*, **359**, 1331–35.

8. Ellsberg, M., Jansen, H., Heise, L. *et al.* WHO Multi-country Study on Women's Health and Domestic Violence against Women Study Team (2008) Intimate partner violence and women's physical and mental health in the WHO multi-country study on women's health and domestic violence: an observational study. *Lancet*, **371**, 1165–72.

9. Golding, J.M. (1999) Intimate partner violence as a risk factor for mental disorders: a meta-analysis. *Journal of Family Violence*, **14** (2), 99–132.

10. Olff, M., Langeland, W., Draijer, N. and Gersons, B.P. (2007) Gender differences in posttraumatic stress disorder. *Psychological Bulletin*, **133** (2), 183–204.

11. Stein, M. and Kennedy, C. (2001) Major depressive and post-traumatic stress disorder comorbidity in female victims of intimate partner violence. *Journal of Affective Disorders*, **66**, 133–38.

12. Nixon, R., Resick, P. and Nishith, P. (2004) An exploration of comorbid depression among female victims of intimate partner violence with posttraumatic stress disorder. *Journal of Affective Disorders*, **82**, 315–20.

13. Campbell, R., Sullivan, C.M. and Davidson, W.S. (1999) Women who use domestic violence shelters: changes in depression over time. *Psychology of Women Quarterly*, **19**, 237–55.

14. Surtees, P.G. (1995) In the shadow of adversity: the evolution and resolution of anxiety and depressive disorder. *British Journal of Psychiatry*, **166**, 583–94.

15. Yanagita, T., Yoneda, Y., Hamada, T. *et al.* (2004) Acute trauma reaction and recovery in victims of domestic violence, during a brief stay in a public shelter. *Journal of Japanese Clinical Psychology*, **22** (2), 152–62.

16. Seedat, S., Stein, M., Kennedy, C. and Hauger, R. (2003) Plasma cortisol and neuropeptide Y in female victims of intimate partner violence. *Psychoneuroendocrinology*, **28**, 796–808.

17. Griffin, M., Resick, P. and Yehuda, R. (2005) Enhanced cortisol suppression following dexamethasone administration in domestic violence survivors. *The American Journal of Psychiatry*, **162**, 1192–99.

18. Inslichta, S., Marmar, C., Neylan, T. *et al.* (2006) Increased cortisol in women with intimate partner violence-related posttraumatic stress disorder. *Psychoneuroendocrinology*, **31**, 825–38.

19. Fennema-Notestine, C., Stein, M.B., Kennedy, C.M. *et al.* (2002) Brain morphometry in female victims of intimate partner violence with and without Posttraumatic Stress Disorder. *Biological Psychiatry*, **51**, 1089–101.

20. Seedat, S., Videen, J., Kennedy, C. and Stein, M.B. (2005) Single voxel proton magnetic resonance spectroscopy in women with and without intimate partner violence-related posttraumatic stress disorder. *Psychiatry Research-Neuroimaging*, **139**, 249–58.

21. Hutchins, H. and Kirk, S.A. (1997) *Making us Crazy DSM - The Psychiatric Bible and the Creation of Mental Disorders*, The Free Press, New York.

22. Stein, M., Kennedy, C. and Twamley, E. (2002) Neuropsychological function in female victims of intimate partner violence with and without posttraumatic stress disorder. *Biological Psychiatry*, **52**, 1079–88.

23. Ehrensaft, M., Moffitt, T. and Caspi, A. (2006) Is domestic violence followed by an increased risk of psychiatric disorders among women but not among men? A Longitudinal Cohort Study. *American Journal of Psychiatry*, **163**, 885–92.

24. Krug, E.G., Dahlberg, L.L., Mercy, J.A. *et al.* (2002) World Report on Violence and Health, World Health Organization, Geneva.

25. Kernic, M.A., Wolf, M.E., Holt, V.L. *et al.* (2003) Behavioral problems among children whose mothers are abused by an intimate partner. *Child Abuse and Neglect*, **27**, 1231–46.

26. Bensley, L., Van Eenwyk, J. and Wynkoop Simmons, K. (2003) Childhood family violence history and women's risk for intimate partner violence and poor health. *American Journal of Preventive Medicine*, **25** (1), 38–44.

27. McKinney, C.M., Caetano, R., Ramisetty-Mikter, S. and Nelson, S. (2009) Childhood family violence and perpetration and victimization of intimate partner violence: findings from a national population-based study of couples. *Annual of Epidemiology*, **19** (1), 25–32.

28. Koss, M.P. (1993) Detecting the scope of rape: a review of prevalence research methods. *Journal of Interpersonal Violence*. **8**, 198–222.

Index

Abbas, Sarvath 6, 97–116
abortions 195, 202–3
ACBT *see* affective cognitive behavioural
    therapy
accidents, trauma types 150–1, 159–64
ACE *see* Adverse Childhood Experiences
acute and transient psychoses, concepts 26
ADAPT model, migration 412–13
adolescents 99, 191, 264, 283, 317–20,
    397–8, 518–22, 555–6
Adverse Childhood Experiences (ACE)
    520–1
advocacy interventions, intimate partner
    violence 390–1, 398
affective cognitive behavioural therapy
    (ACBT) 81
Afghanistan 160, 363, 372–3, 448–9
Africa 41–2, 49–50, 76–8, 141–4, 169–77,
    200–2, 228–9, 237–8, 259, 261, 263,
    291, 320, 362, 363–4, 371–7, 390,
    453, 485–96
age at onset 12, 17, 259–60, 267
ageing women, schizophrenia 16
agents of gender socialisation, parents 505,
    517–22
agoraphobia
    see also anxiety disorders
    concepts 4, 38–55, 520
Alami, Khadija Mchichi 4, 37–64
alcohol dependence, concepts 139–47
alcohol and substance abuse 7, 12, 19, 20,
    41, 85–6, 122–3, 126–9, 131,
    139–47, 158, 162–4, 169–72, 187,
    199, 201–2, 262, 293–4, 318–20,
    329–33, 424–5, 451, 471–2, 477,
    511–14, 522, 552–6

BPD 19, 20
burden and stigma 140–1, 169–72, 187
causes 140–1, 162–4, 451, 471–2
concepts 7, 126–9, 131, 139–47, 158,
    169–72, 187, 199, 201–2,
    318–20, 329–33, 451, 471–2,
    477, 511–14, 552–6
consumer voices 169–72, 187
definitions 139–40
depression 19, 20, 41, 552–6
epidemiology 140–3, 162–3, 329,
    471–2, 522, 552–6
genetics 140
HIV 7, 141–3, 145–6
interventions 144–7, 169–72
patterns of drinking 140–1
pregnancy 144–5, 199, 201–2, 293–4
price increases 126, 131
PTSD 141, 145, 158, 162–4, 201–2,
    552–6
recommendations 145–6
research needs 145
risky health behaviours 141–3, 262
schizophrenia 12
sexual interest/functioning 141–3,
    162–3
social/economic consequences 143–4
stigma 143, 145
suicides 122–3, 126, 127–9, 131, 199
terminology 139–40
types of substance 139–40, 169–72
violence 7, 131, 139–40, 144, 146,
    162–4, 262, 471–2, 552–6
alcohol use disorder (AUD) 139–47
alexithymia 75–6
Algeria 160, 373–4, 476, 487

Alma-Ata Declaration (1978) 502
AMEND intervention programme,
    intimate partner violence 393,
    394–5
amenorrhoea 13
American Psychiatric Association
    110
Amnesty International 361, 448
AN *see* anorexia nervosa
Angola 375
angry/hostility personality trait 127
Annan, Kofi A. 361, 447–8, 471
anorexia nervosa (AN) 6, 97–111, 128,
    454–5
    see also eating disorders
anticonvulsants 22–3, 24, 295, 349–50
antidepressants 25, 42–4, 80–1, 109, 130,
    311–12, 338–54, 501
    see also psychotropic drugs
antipsychotic agents 12–13, 24–5, 27,
    292–6, 338–54
    see also psychotropic drugs
antisocial personality disorder 41, 329
anxiety disorders
    see also agoraphobia; generalised. . .;
        obsessive-compulsive. . .;
        panic. . .; phobias;
        post-traumatic stress. . .; social. . .
    biological factors 44–5, 505, 553–4
    children and adolescents 283, 318–20,
        519–22, 555–6
    comorbidities 39–41, 65–6, 81, 127–9,
        156, 159–64, 238–46, 552–3
    concepts 4, 37–55, 65–6, 127–9, 156,
        159–64, 180–6, 201–2, 230,
        238–46, 266–76, 287–96,
        304–12, 318–20, 323–33,
        369–83, 388–99, 426, 450–8,
        463–79, 500–1, 519–22, 530–7
    depression 39–41
    disasters 362–3, 369–83
    epidemiology 37–41, 161–2, 201–2,
        287–96, 318–20, 323, 329, 426,
        450–8, 500–1, 520–1, 552–6
    gynaecological cancers 242–6
    gynaecological infections 238–9
    hysterectomies 236–8
    infertility 230–5
    lifespan changes 50–5, 264–76, 292–6,
        318–20, 324–33
    medications 42–4

menopause 41, 45, 51, 54–5, 194,
    235–8, 259–76, 294–6
motherhood 53–5, 201–2, 351–4,
    530–7
PCOD 241, 346–7
PMS/PMDD 41, 50–1, 294–5, 325–6
pregnancy 45, 52–5, 201–2, 287–8,
    292–6, 307–12, 542–5
prenatal genetic screening 202
prevalence 38–9
social factors 46–50, 414–18
suicides 127–9, 318–20, 470–1, 551–2
treatments 42–4, 181–6, 389–99
violence impacts 47–50, 160–4, 272–3,
    388–99, 450–8, 463–79,
    519–22, 543–5, 549–56
Arab women 48–50, 54, 79, 150–64,
    169–72, 209, 361, 371–7, 433,
    448–58, 472–6, 485–96
ART *see* assisted reproductive technology
assisted reproductive technology (ART)
    230–2, 234–5, 536–7
Astbury, Jill 194, 259–80, 503
asylum-seekers 406–18
    see also migration; refugees
attachment to the infant 541–2, 545
attention deficit hyperactivity disorder
    318–20
auditory startle 157
Australia 11, 120, 125–6, 141, 151–2,
    180–6, 259, 261, 264–7, 269–70,
    396, 488, 491, 530–1
autonomic dysfunction, somatisation and
    dissociation 73, 74
Ayurveda 3, 76–8
Azerbaijan 448–9

baby talk 540
Baingana, Florence 7, 139–48
Bangladesh 229, 375, 550
BasicNeeds 169–72
batterer interventions, intimate partner
    violence 366, 388, 391–9
Beck Depression Inventory 212
BED *see* binge eating disorder
behavioural therapy 80, 84–5, 88, 105–6,
    130
Belmont Report 289–90, 291–2, 340
Benjet, Corina 283, 317–22
benzodiazepines 350
beyondblue 180–6

Bhugra, Dinesh 15
binge drinking 140–7
binge eating disorder (BED) 99–111, 241
biological factors 3, 41, 44–5, 70–4,
      126–7, 155–6, 505, 539–45, 553–4
bipolar affective disorder (BPD)
   age at onset 17
   alcohol and substance abuse 19, 20
   anticonvulsants 22–3, 24, 295
   burden and stigma 15, 173–7
   cognitive dysfunction 19
   comorbidities 18–19, 20
   concepts 6–7, 9, 13, 17–28, 38, 52, 158,
         173–7, 187, 204–5, 284–5,
         287–96, 301–12, 352–4, 466,
         500–1
   consumer voices 173–7, 187
   course 17–18
   definitions 17, 18
   epidemiology 17–18, 38, 287–96, 466,
         500–1
   marriage 13
   medications 21–5
   menopause 20
   mixed mania 17, 18
   mortality 18–19
   outcomes 17–18
   phenomenology 19
   postpartum period 20, 204–5, 352–4
   pregnancy 20, 21–5, 52, 174–7
   rapid cycling findings 18, 25
   suicides 18–19
   treatments 21–5, 173–7, 294–5
   types 17–25
birth defects 21–3, 53
blood vengeance 153
blueVoices 182
BMI 110
BN see bulimia nervosa
body image 454–5
borderline disorders 75–6, 85–6, 88, 500
Bosnia 363, 371–2, 375, 408
BPD see bipolar affective disorder
Brahmanda 179
Brazil 201, 231–2, 472, 476–7, 517–18, 550
BRCA1/BRCA2 gene mutations 244–5
breast cancer 263
breastfeeding 194, 208, 282–3, 345–54,
      528–9, 533–4
Bretton Woods Institutions 513–14
brothels 371–2

bulimia nervosa (BN) 6, 97–111, 128,
      454–5
   see also eating disorders
bupropion 339, 344, 350, 353
burden and stigma 7, 14, 15, 16, 140–1,
      143, 145, 169–87, 432, 518–22
busiprone 350

Cambodia 371, 375, 376, 415–16, 468
Canada 141, 151–2, 264–8, 272, 396, 431,
      436–7, 472, 488, 522
cancers 162, 228, 238, 240–6, 263
candidiasis 239
carbamazepine 22–4, 344, 349, 350
cardiovascular diseases 240, 263, 347, 418,
      435–6
caregivers, schizophrenia 15, 16
Carnegie, Dale 176
CAT *see* Convention Against Torture and
      Other Cruel, Inhuman or Degrading
      Treatment or Punishment
CBT *see* cognitive-behavioural therapy
cervical cancer, concepts 242–4
Chandra, Prabha S. 1–8, 189–96,
      227–57
Chaturvedi, Santosh K. 65–95
Cheng, Wenhong 505, 517–24
child abuse 194, 240, 320, 363–4, 511–14,
      520–31, 550, 554–6
child care 544–5
childbirth 190–6, 197–214
   see also motherhood; postpartum...
childhood experiences
   menopause 268–70
   mental disorders 519–22, 544–5,
      555–6
children 194, 208, 210–14, 268–70, 283,
      317–20, 362, 376, 397–8, 443–7,
      505, 509–14, 517–22, 525–37,
      539–45, 555–6
Chile 284–5, 301–12
China 10, 11, 12, 76, 118–22, 124–5, 130,
      143, 201–3, 212, 230, 236, 261, 361,
      377, 408, 474, 502–3, 522
Chira, Susan 535
chlorpromazine 24–5, 338–54
cholinesterase inhibitors 344
choriocarcinoma 242
Christians 413–18, 486–7, 488, 495
chronic fatigue syndrome (CFS) 68–9, 79
   see also somatisation

chronic pelvic pain syndrome (CPPS) 69,
79–80, 191, 239–40
see also somatisation
citalopram 344, 345
classification systems, cultures 469–70
clinical depression *see* major depressive
disorder
clinical practice, definition 338–40
clinical research 287–96, 338–54
clomipramine 345–6
clozapine 12–13, 25, 338–54
cocaine 139–40, 169–72
cognitive dysfunction 19, 72–3, 263, 554–5
cognitive therapy 43–4, 81–5, 88, 130–1,
212–13, 273–6, 544–5
cognitive-analytic therapy 88
cognitive-behavioural therapy (CBT)
concepts 43–4, 81–5, 88, 106–8, 130,
212–13, 232–3, 273–6, 353, 393,
394–5, 414–18, 544–5
critique 273–6, 395
collective violence, trauma types 151, 153,
159–64, 191–2
collectivistic cultures 412–13
collegial relationships, motherhood
534–5
Columbia 374
combat experiences, trauma types 150–3,
159–64, 191–2, 295–6, 362–3,
369–83, 406–18, 444–58
'comfort women' 371–2
Commission on the Social Determinants of
Health (CSDH) 324, 503–4
commoditisation 362, 444–58
communications, child development
539–45
comorbidities 18–19, 20, 39–41, 65–6, 81,
127–9, 155–64, 239–46, 287–96,
552–3
Composite International Diagnostic
Interview (CIDI) 150–1
conduct disorder 318–20, 520–2, 555–6
Congo 195
consumer voices 7–8, 169–87
contributions of others, motherhood 504,
534–7, 545
control benefits, menopause 267–70
Convention Against Torture and Other
Cruel, Inhuman or Degrading
Treatment or Punishment (CAT)
(1984) 511–12

Convention on the Rights of the Child
(CRC) (1989) 511
Convention on the Rights of Persons with
Disabilities (CRPD) (2006) 510
conversion disorder
see also somatisation
concepts 68–9, 71–2, 74–88
epidemiology 81–2
symptoms 68–9, 82
treatments 82–3
coping 274–6, 409–10, 414–18, 469,
500–1, 536–7
see also resilience
Coptic Christians 488, 495
corpus callosum 72
cortisol levels 73–4, 155–6, 553–4
couple-focused interventions, intimate
partner violence 396–7
CPPS *see* chronic pelvic pain syndrome
crack 140
CRC *see* Convention on the Rights of the
Child
criminal justice interventions, intimate
partner violence 391–5, 396, 505,
556
criminal networks, globalisation 444–58
CRPD *see* Convention on the Rights of
Persons with Disabilities
crying infants 208, 530, 533–4
crystal methamphetamine 140
CSDH *see* Commission on the Social
Determinants of Health
cultures 4, 41–2, 67–8, 76–9, 87–9,
117–31, 150, 158–9, 194, 202–3,
208–10, 228–9, 237–8, 259–76,
361, 377–83, 399, 407–18, 432–3,
445–6, 463–79, 485–96, 505,
507–14, 517–22, 549–56
classification systems 469–70
concepts 361, 463–79, 505, 517–22
definition 464–5
diagnostic considerations 469–72
epidemiological perspectives 466
FGM 48–50, 361, 363–4, 475, 485–96
'honour killings' 150, 361, 464–5, 472,
475–6
intimate partner violence 361, 399,
410–18, 463–79, 549–56
Muslim women 48–50, 79, 150–64,
169–72, 361, 371–7, 433,
448–58, 472–6, 485–96

parents as agents of gender socialisation 505, 517–22
preferences for sons 202–3, 208–14, 505, 517–22
stereotypes 202–3, 208–14, 500–1, 505, 517–22, 535–7
suicides 117, 125–6, 470–1
therapeutic issues 477–9
current themes in psychiatric disorders 1–8
cyber-sex 456–8
cynicism, job burnout 424–6

Dare, Christopher 108–9
daughters, cultural preferences for sons 202–3, 208–14, 505, 517–22
DBT see dialectical behaviour therapy
de Mello, Meena Cabral 197–225, 503
Declaration on the Elimination of Violence Against Women (1993) 512
Declaration of Madrid 331
delusional disorder 26, 204–5, 352–4
see also schizophrenia
Denmark 119, 129, 360, 472
dependent personality disorder 500
depersonalisation/derealisation syndrome 68–9, 86–7, 424–5
see also dissociation
depression 4, 6–9, 13, 17–18, 37–55, 65–88, 122–9, 154–64, 180–6, 198–202, 203–10, 229–46, 284–5, 287–96, 301–12, 318–33, 337–54, 369–99, 411–18, 426–8, 436–9, 450–8, 463–79, 490–4, 500–5, 519–22, 530–2, 542–5
see also bipolar affective disorder; dysthymia
alcohol and substance abuse 19, 20, 41, 552–6
anxiety disorders 39–41
biological factors 41, 44–5, 505, 553–4
children and adolescents 283, 318–20, 519–22, 542–5, 555–6
Chile 284–5, 302–12
comorbidities 39–41, 65–6, 81, 127–9, 156, 159–64, 229–36, 239–46, 552–3
consumer voices 180–6, 187
cultural variations 41–2, 208–14, 463–79
disasters 362–3, 369–83
divorce/separation 47

epidemiology 17–18, 37–41, 161–2, 200–2, 205–10, 265–7, 287–96, 318–20, 323, 329, 450–8, 463–4, 466, 490–4, 520–1, 542–5, 552–6
FGM 363–4, 490–4
future prospects 504
gender paradox 122–3
gynaecological cancers 242–6
gynaecological infections 238–9
hysterectomies 236–8
infertility 229–35
job burnout 426–8, 436–9
lifespan changes 50–5, 264–76, 292–6, 318–20, 324–33
marriage 13, 46–7
medications 25, 42–4, 80–1, 109, 130, 311–12, 337–54, 414–18, 511–14, 544–5
menopause 41, 45, 51, 54–5, 194, 235–8, 259–76, 294–6
migration 399, 411–18, 466–8
motherhood 53–5, 198–200, 203–10, 352–4, 530–7, 542–5
oestrogens 41, 45, 51
PCOD 241, 346–7
PMS/PMDD 41, 50–1, 294–5, 325–6
postpartum depression 54, 203–10, 294–5, 307–12, 351–4, 530–7, 542–5
pregnancy 20, 21–5, 45, 52–5, 198–202, 287–8, 292–6, 307–12, 542–5
schizophrenia 11, 13, 20
serotonin system 45, 51, 127
social factors 46–50, 414–18
stigma 180–6, 325, 329–33
sub-Saharan Africa 41–2, 50–1
suicides 18–19, 122–3, 127–9, 182, 198–200, 318–20, 451, 454, 470–1, 551–2, 553
treatments 25, 42–4, 80–1, 109, 130, 180–6, 200–2, 212–14, 232–5, 294–5, 306–12, 329–33, 337–54, 389–99, 414–18, 501, 543–5
violence impacts 47–50, 160–4, 272–3, 388–99, 411–18, 450–8, 463–79, 519–22, 543–5, 549–56
Desai, Geetha 227–57

Descartian mind–body dualistic
    approach 3
DHEA 156, 347
diabetes 418
dialectical behaviour therapy (DBT) 106
diazepam 339, 414–18
disabilities in women, NHIS data 15–16
disasters 2, 150–3, 159–64, 191–2, 295–6,
    362–3, 369–83, 406–18, 444–58,
    466–8
discrimination 407–18, 430–3, 445, 464,
    502, 504, 525–37
disenfranchised grief, motherhood 526–7
dissociation
    biological factors 3, 70–4
    causes 66–8, 70–81, 85
    classification systems 68–9
    clinical features 66–9, 76–7, 78–9,
        85–7
    comorbidities 65–6, 81
    concepts 2–3, 65–88, 156, 332–3
    cultural variations 67–8, 76–7, 78–9,
        87–8
    definitions 66–8
    diagnosis 68–9
    epidemiology 77–8, 85–6
    lifespan changes 77
    psychosocial factors 74–81
    subtypes 86–7
    symptoms 66–8, 76–7, 78–9, 85–7
    trauma responses in women 74–8, 332
    treatments 69, 79–81, 87–8
dissociative identity disorder 86
divalproex 21
divorce/separation, depression 47
'domino' hypothesis, menopause 264–6
Douki, Saida 360–1, 423–42
dowry payments 473–4
drugs see alcohol and substance abuse;
    medications
DSM III-R 161–2, 271, 302–3, 554
DSM IV 26, 68–9, 83, 85, 102–3, 140,
    154–5, 159, 160, 206, 330, 414–15,
    425–6, 491
dysphoria 3, 41, 50–1, 294–5, 325–6, 425
dysthymia 37–55
    see also depression

Earthquake Assessment Model for Mental
    Health 544
earthquakes 363, 377–83

eating disorders (EDs)
    assessments 100, 101–2
    body image 454–5
    causes 98–100, 241, 454–5, 471–2
    concepts 6, 97–111, 128, 241, 287–96,
        329–33, 454–5, 471–2, 490–4
    diagnosis 100–4
    distribution 100, 111
    engagement 101, 104
    in-patient management needs 109–10
    legal compulsion 110–11
    management 104–5, 109–11
    media pressures 454–5
    medications 109
    presentation 100–1
    psychological treatments 105–9
    puberty 99
    risk factors 98–100
    suicides 111, 128
    symptoms 100–2, 103
    treatments 104–11
eating disorders not otherwise specified
    (EDNOS) 6, 102–11
Ebstein's anomaly 21–2
ecological fallacy, suicides 6, 123–4
economic costs to society, mental disorders
    418
ecstasy 140
ECT see electro convulsive therapy
Edinburgh Postnatal Depression Scale
    (EPDS) 530–1, 544
EDNOS see eating disorders not otherwise
    specified
education 45–50, 269–70, 284–5, 302–12,
    323–4, 329–33, 380–3, 397–8, 417,
    446–9, 457–8, 479, 494–6, 505,
    517–22, 530–1, 532–4, 544–5
    see also socio-economic status
    Arab women 48–50
    benefits 446–9
    disaster recovery 380–3
    FGM 494–6
    globalisation 45–7, 446–8, 479
    health care professionals 417, 496
    Internet benefits 457
    intimate partner violence interventions
        397–8
    motherhood 530–1, 532–4, 544–5
Egypt 448–9, 472, 476, 486, 488–9, 493
Ekblad, Solvig 364–5, 405–21
El-Sabbagh, Salim 149–68

Eldin, Amira Seif 363–4, 485–98
electro convulsive therapy (ECT) 182, 337–8
EMERGE intervention programme, intimate partner violence 393, 394–5
emotional sharing, child development 539–45
employment status 269–70, 302–12, 323–4, 329–33, 360–1, 364–5, 407–18, 423–39, 445, 446–58, 470–1, 501–2, 504
  see also job burnout; socio-economic. . .; working women
empowerment 329–30, 410, 446–58
endometriosis 240, 243–4, 294–5, 346–7
EPDS *see* Edinburgh Postnatal Depression Scale
epidemiology 10–11, 17–18, 37–41, 77–8, 81–2, 84, 85–6, 118–24, 198–214, 228–32, 235–8, 259–76, 287–96, 302–12, 317–20, 323, 338–40, 387–8, 423–39, 455–8, 463–79, 488–9, 500–1, 520–2, 542–5
epilepsy 22–4, 82
equality principle, gender-sensitive psychiatric care 327–8
Eritrea 486
estazolam 350
ethics 285, 287–96, 338–40
Ethiopia 488, 494, 550
European Working Conditions Survey (EWCS) 439
evidence-based medicine 340–1, 416–17
existential concerns, menopause 272–5
experience-dependent/expectant brain development 540
experiential reports 233–5, 237–8
exploiting gender inequalities, definition 325–6
extended families, migration 409–10
eye movement desensitisation and reprocessing (EMDR) 88

fainting 157
Fairburn, Christopher 107
families of origin
  see also parents
  agents of gender socialisation 505, 517–22
family-friendly work policies 435, 438–9

fantasies of motherhood 527–8, 534
FDA *see* Food and Drug Administration
female circumcision (FC) 48–50, 361, 363–4, 475, 485–96
female genital mutilation (FGM) 48–50, 361, 363–4, 475, 485–96
  church leaders 495
  classification 487, 489, 490–2
  concepts 48–50, 361, 363–4, 485–96
  definition 485, 487
  education programmes 494–6
  elimination concepts 494–6
  epidemiology 488–9
  historical background 486–7
  memory lapses 490–1
  obstacles to change 491–4
  physical complications 363–4, 485–6, 487, 489–90, 492–6
  practising countries 49, 486–7, 488, 493–4
  psychological complications 363–4, 490–4
  reasons 361, 486, 492–5
feminists 9, 377, 393, 446–58, 529
'fight or flight' responses, trauma 156
financing issues, services 416–17, 513–14
Finland 120–1, 129, 141, 195, 209, 231, 431, 435
Fisher, Jane 193–4, 197–225, 499–506, 525–38
fluid retention 343
fluoxetine 109, 232–3, 339, 344, 353
flurazepam 350
fluvoxamine 339, 344, 346, 353
Food and Drug Administration (FDA) 293, 340–2, 349–50
foster parents 27
Fourth World Conference on Women 1995 502–3, 509–10
France 209, 235, 259, 373–4, 426, 429
Freud, Sigmund 81, 150

GABA 45
gabapentin 350
GAD *see* generalised anxiety disorder
galactorrhoea 13
Gambia 229–30, 239
Gender Empowerment Measure (GEM) 458
gender equality issues 325–6, 380–1, 445–6, 458, 465–79

gender integration strategies, definition 326
gender paradox, suicides 6, 121–2
gender-sensitive psychiatric care
    basic strategies 325–8
    characteristics 328–33
    concepts 283, 317–20, 323–33,
        338–42, 458
    equality principle 327–8
    knowledge and commitment principle
        327–8
    knowledgeable staff 332–3
    principles 327–8
    relationships principle 327–8, 333
    respectful relationships 333
    restraint/seclusion uses 329, 331–2
    safety issues 330–3
    sexual safety issues 330–3
    voices of women 326
gender-specific issues, therapy 3
generalised anxiety disorder (GAD) 37–55,
    159–64, 230, 304–12
    see also anxiety. . .
genocide 371–7
geo-political scenarios, globalisation 448–9
Germany 106–8, 119, 141, 151–2, 472
Ghana 169–72, 432
global policies 435, 438–9, 502–5, 507–14
    see also United Nations. . .
globalisation 2, 362, 443–58, 468–9
    concepts 362, 443–58, 468–9
    definition 443–4
    education 446–8, 457–8, 479
    gendered effects 444–5, 468–9
    geo-political scenarios 448–9
    healthcare impacts 451–5, 458
    inequalities 445–6, 458, 468–9
    Internet addictions 455–8
    job opportunities 453–4
    mal-governance 444–5
    mental disorders 450–8, 468–9
    mental health impacts 362, 445–6,
        468–9
    mobile phones 456–8
    Muslim societies 448–58
    positive aspects 448–9
    process 443–4
    recommendations 458
    social implications 451–3
    suicides 451, 454
    urbanisation 453–4
Google Earth 406

Grameen Bank 452
group therapy 233–5, 274–6, 381, 414–18,
    438, 544–5
Guinea 371, 374, 493
Gulf Wars 372–3
gynaecological cancers 228, 238, 240–6
gynaecological conditions/procedures 192,
    227–46, 346–7
gynaecological infections 192, 228, 238–42

Hadlaczky, Gergö 6, 117–37
hallucinations 88, 204–5, 352–4
    see also schizophrenia
haloperidol 344
headaches, menopausal symptoms 261–4
health, definitions 405–6, 465, 502, 508–9
health visitors 212–13
health-related quality of life (HRQL) 241,
    243–4, 274, 438–9
heavy episodic drinking 140–7
hepatitis B/C 143
heroin 139–40
Herrman, Helen 499–506
Herzegovina 375
Hindu women 177–80
histrionic personality disorder 500
HIV/AIDS 7, 27, 141–3, 145–6, 163, 191,
    195, 263, 390, 406–7, 418, 444, 489,
    508, 513–14
holding environment, definition 543
holistic approaches 329–33
homelessness, schizophrenia 14–15, 27,
    178–9
Hong Kong 17, 119, 201, 203, 207
'honour killings' 150, 361, 464–5, 472,
    475–6
hormone replacement therapies (HRTs)
    194, 262–5
Horton, Richard 370
hot flushes, menopausal symptoms 260–7,
    274
HPA *see* hypothalamic–pituitary adrenal
    axis
HPRT 416–17
HRTs *see* hormone replacement therapies
human development 194, 208, 210–14,
    369–70, 505, 517–22, 529–37,
    539–45
    baby talk 540
    experience-dependent/expectant brain
        development 540

foundations 505, 539–45
Oedipus phase 519
parents as agents of gender socialisation
        505, 517–22
scientific advances 539–40
secure infants 541–2
human papilloma virus (HPV) 242–4
    see also cervical cancer
human rights 361, 362–5, 383, 406–18,
        443–58, 463–79, 485–96, 501–5,
        508–14, 535, 549–56
Human Rights Watch 448
human trafficking 362, 444–58, 509–14
Hungary 17, 120, 121, 454
Hurricane Katrina 381
Hussein, Alhaji 170–2
Husseini, Rana 476
hyperprolactinaemia 347
hypochondriacal worry 66, 78, 83–5,
        155–6
    see also somatisation
hypothalamic–pituitary adrenal axis
        (HPA) 44–5, 73–4, 127, 155–8,
        346–7, 553–4
hysterectomies 227–8, 235–8, 264
    see also infertility
hysteria 66, 81–8, 373–83
    see also conversion disorder

IASC see Inter-Agency Standing
        Committee
ICCPR see International Covenant on Civil
        and Political Rights
ICD-10 68–9, 87, 102, 205, 302–4, 425–6
Iceland 141, 209
ICESCR see International Covenant on
        Economic, Social and Cultural
        Rights
ICPD see International Conference on
        Population and Development
IDPs see internally displaced persons
illicit drugs, definition 140
imipramine 339, 346
immunological mechanisms, somatisation
        and dissociation 70–1
in vitro fertilization (IVF) 192, 230–2,
        234–5
in-patient management needs, EDs 109–10
'inability to forget' problems, trauma 157
India 4, 13, 15–16, 26–7, 76–8, 119–22,
        124–6, 177–80, 198–9, 201–3, 207,

210–11, 228–9, 239, 361, 445–6,
        450–1, 470–1, 477–8, 542
individualistic cultures 412–13
Indonesia 486, 488
inequalities, globalisation 445–6, 458,
        468–9
infants
    attachment to the infant 541–2, 545
    breastfeeding 194, 208, 282–3, 345–54,
        528–9, 533–4
    crying 208, 530, 533–4
    mother-infant relationships 194, 208,
        210–14, 369–70, 505, 517–22,
        529–37, 539–45, 555–6
    postpartum depression 208–10, 542–5
    SIDS 533–4
infertility
    anxiety disorders 230–5
    concepts 192, 227–46, 432, 451, 489,
        536–7
    definition 228
    depression 229–35
    epidemiology 228–32
    experiential reports 233–5
    FGM 489–90
    IVF 192, 230–2, 234–5
    psychological factors 229–35
    psychological interventions 232–5
    psychosocial factors 192, 228–35
    social mobility factors 233–4
    socio-cultural factors 228–9
    stigma 192, 228–9, 432
    suicides 192
information technology 443–4, 455–8
informed consent 283, 290–1, 317–20,
        340
injection drug use (IDU) 139–40
insight focused therapy 273–6
intensive residential therapy 43–4
Inter-Agency Standing Committee (IASC),
        Guidelines on Mental Health and
        Psychosocial Support in Emergency
        Settings 512–13
internally displaced persons (IDPs) 406–18
International Bill of Human Rights 508–14
International Conference on Population
        and Development (ICPD) 512
International Consensus on Women's
        Mental Health 324–5, 331
International Covenant on Civil and
        Political Rights (ICCPR) 508

International Covenant on Economic,
    Social and Cultural Rights
    (ICESCR) 502, 508
Internet 328, 455–8
interpersonal psychotherapy (IPT),
    concepts 106–8, 130–1, 233, 544–5
interpersonal violence 150–64, 191–2, 193,
    203, 207–8, 213, 262, 283–4,
    317–20, 329–33, 361, 364–6,
    387–99, 405–18, 444–58, 463–79,
    520–2, 549–56
intimate partner violence (IPV) 163, 193,
    203, 207–8, 213, 262, 283, 361,
    364–6, 387–99, 405–18, 450–8,
    463–79, 504, 505, 520–2, 549–56
  advocacy interventions 390–1, 398
  AMEND intervention programme 393,
    394–5
  batterer interventions 366, 388, 391–9
  biological consequences 505, 553–4
  CBT 393, 394–5
  children 283, 397–8, 555–6
  concepts 361, 365–6, 387–99, 410–18,
    450–8, 463–79, 504, 505, 520–2,
    549–56
  couple-focused interventions 396–7
  criminal justice interventions 391–5,
    396, 505, 556
  cultural factors 361, 399, 410–18,
    463–79, 549–56
  Duluth intervention model 393–4
  education 397–8
  EMERGE intervention programme 393,
    394–5
  general health consequences 551, 553–6
  interventions 365–6, 387–99, 553–6
  mental health consequences 365–6,
    387–9, 549–56
  migration 364–5, 399, 405–18
  nature 549–50
  prevalence 549–50
  prosecutions 391, 393, 399, 556
  protection orders 391, 392
  psychological aggression 505, 549–56
  public awareness programmes 365–6,
    397, 556
  school programmes 398
  sexual coercion 504, 549–56
  shelter stays 389–90, 398, 505, 553–6
  social support enhancements 389–90
  victim-focused interventions 388–91

intuition 532–3, 540
involuntary childlessness 192, 227–46
    see also infertility
IPT see interpersonal psychotherapy
IPV see intimate partner violence
IQs 23
Iran 231, 377, 437–8, 448–51, 472, 486
Iraq 160, 363, 371–3, 413–18, 448–9, 472,
    486
irritable bowel syndrom, see also
    somatisation
irritable bowel syndrome 68–9, 78–9,
    239–40
Islam 48–50, 79, 150–64, 169–72, 371–7,
    433, 448–58, 472–6, 485–96
Israel 374, 472
Italy 19, 209, 377, 472
Izutsu, Takashi 197–225, 505, 507–15

Jadresic, Enrique 284–5, 301–15
Janet, Pierre 85
Japan 26, 119, 209, 230, 261, 310, 377, 380,
    426, 435, 550
job burnout
  concepts 424–39
  cultural issues 432–3
  definition 424
  depression 426–8, 436–9
  diagnosis 425–6
  outcomes 427
  rewards 426, 429–31
  risk factors 424, 427–33
  role conflicts 432–3, 435–6
  sense of community 430
  sexual harassment 430, 438–9
  symptoms 424–5, 435
  treatments 438–9
  values 432
  women 426, 428–33
job strain model 434–5
Jordan 476, 486
Judaism 495

Kadri, Nadia 4, 37–64
kaleidoscopic views 2–3
Kamo, Toshiko 505, 549–58
Kanaiya, Lillian 174–7
Karam, Elie G. 5, 149–68
Karpinski, Janis 372
Kashmir 373, 378–80
Kastrup, Marianne 359–68, 463–83

Kennerly, Kerri-Anne 183
Kenya 173–7, 493–4
knowledge and commitment principle,
      gender-sensitive psychiatric care
      327–8
knowledgeable staff, gender-sensitive
      psychiatric care 332–3
Kobe earthquake of 1995 377
Korea 79, 202, 261, 372
Kosovo 375
Kurds 371
Kuwait 229

lamotrigine 339, 344, 350
landmines 376
Lasegue, Charles 101
Latin America
      see also individual countries
      cultural impacts 476–7
Lebanon 160–3, 374, 476
legal compulsion, EDs 110–11
legislation issues, migration 415–16
lesbians 192–3
Liberia 191–2, 371–2, 374–5
Libya 486–7
life course perspectives, menopause
      267–70
life expectancies 259
lifespan changes 50–5, 77, 190–6, 264–76,
      292–6, 318–20, 324–33
      see also menopause; pregnancy
lithium 21–2, 339, 344, 346, 347, 350
locus of control 267–70, 409–10, 412–13,
      427–8, 429, 469, 519–20
loss and separation, migration 409

major depressive disorder (MDD) 37–55,
      127–9, 154, 159–64, 180–6, 200–2,
      205–14, 271–6, 287–96, 302–12,
      352–4, 373–83, 411–18, 426–8,
      500–4, 552–6
      see also depression
mal-governance, globalisation 444–5
Malach Burnout Inventory (MBI) 424
malaria 508, 514
Malaysia 486, 488
Mali 488, 493
man-made disasters 362–3, 369–83
management
      concepts 104–5, 109–11
      treatment contrasts 105

working women 438–9
manic depression see bipolar affective
      disorder
MAOIs see monoamine oxidase inhibitors
maprotiline 350
marijuana 140, 169–72, 555
marriage 13–14, 27–8, 46–7, 48–50
maternal care in the early years 505,
      518–22, 525–37, 539–45
maternal desire, concepts 526–7
maternal mood, occupational fatigue
      529–31
maternal preoccupation, definition 543
maternal wellbeing 505, 525–37, 539–45
      see also motherhood
Maudsley Method, concepts 108–9
Mauritania 488
MDD see major depressive disorder
MDGs see Millennium Development Goals
media pressures
      body image 454–5
      FGM elimination 361, 495
Medical Women's International
      Association 328
medically unexplained physical symptoms
      (MUPS) 66–88
see also somatisation
medications 12–13, 21–5, 27, 42–4, 80–1,
      83, 84–5, 88, 109–10, 292–6,
      337–54, 414–18, 511–14, 544–5
      see also psychotropic drugs; treatments
meditation 233
memory lapses 261–4, 266–7, 491, 551
menarche 41, 50
menopause 20, 41, 45, 51, 54–5, 190–6,
      235–8, 259–76, 294–6, 343
      age at onset 259–60, 267
      BPD 20
      breast cancer 263
      CBT 273–6
      childhood experiences 268–70
      concepts 194, 259–76, 294–6, 343,
            346–54
      control benefits 267–70
      cultural issues 194, 260–4
      definition 259–60
      depression and anxiety disorders 41, 45,
            51, 54–5, 194, 235–8, 259–76,
            294–6
      'domino' hypothesis 264–6
      epidemiology 259–76

menopause (*continued*)
  existential concerns 272–5
  HRTs 194, 262–5
  life course perspectives 267–70
  methodological research difficulties
      270–1
  midlife depression 264–7
  multidimensional models 270–1
  partners 262, 266–76
  perceptions 260, 272–5
  psychosocial factors 194, 259–76
  reductions in onset age 259–60
  religious attendance benefits 267–8
  research evidence 262–4, 294–6
  risk assessment 264
  schizophrenia 287–96
  shame issues 267–8
  socio-economic status 259–60, 265–70
  somatisation and dissociation 71–2
  stressors 264–76
  symptoms 260–7, 271–6
  therapeutic approaches 271–6
  violence 262, 272–3, 275
  woman-centred counselling 272–6
menstrual cycle 41, 50–1, 54–5, 71–2, 241,
    294–5, 325–6, 343, 346–54
mental disorders 46, 156–64, 302–12,
    318–20, 323–33, 371–2, 374, 375,
    399, 406–18, 450–8, 466–9, 470–1,
    479, 509–14, 519–22, 544–5,
    549–56
  see also individual disorders; psychiatric
      disorders
mental health
  see also wellbeing
  Alma-Ata Declaration (1978) 502
  Chile 284–5, 301–12
  concepts 405–6, 465–79, 500–5,
      507–14, 519–22, 549–56
  cultures 4, 41–2, 67–8, 76–7, 78–9,
      87–9, 117–31, 150, 158–9, 194,
      202–3, 208–10, 228–9, 237–8,
      259–76, 361, 377–83, 399,
      407–18, 432–3, 445–6, 463–79,
      485–96, 505, 507–14, 517–22
  definitions 405–6, 465, 501–2, 508–9
  FGM 363–4, 490–4
  Fourth World Conference on Women
      1995 502–3, 509–10
  global policies 502–5, 507–14
  globalisation 2, 362, 445–58, 468–9
  Internet 455–8
  intimate partner violence 365–6,
      387–9, 410–18, 549–56
  marriage 46–7
  menopause 20, 41, 45, 51, 54–5, 190–6,
      235–8, 259–76, 294–6
  migration 364–5, 399, 405–18, 466–8,
      479
  parents as agents of gender socialisation
      505, 517–22
  pregnancy 20, 21–5, 45, 52–5, 125,
      128–9, 144–5, 174–7, 189–96,
      197–214, 287–8, 292–6,
      307–12, 345–54, 542–5
  promotion issues 500–5
  science-based services 416–17
  socio-political differences between
      countries 505, 507–14
  working women 360–1, 423–39,
      544–5
mental health facilities, constraints 9–10,
    65–6
mental health professionals 190–6,
    213–14, 245–6, 284–5, 301–12,
    323–33, 383, 388–99, 407–18,
    477–9, 496, 500–1, 535–7, 544–5
mental rehabilitation 16, 25, 83, 129–31,
    509–14
mentalhealth@Work 180–6
Messaoudi, Khalida 373–4
meta-analysis, concepts 338–41
Middle East wars 374
migration 364–5, 371–2, 375, 399,
    405–18, 466–8, 479
  see also refugees
  ADAPT model 412–13
  intimate partner violence 364–5, 399,
      405–18
  legislation issues 415–16
  loss and separation 409
  mental disorders 371–2, 375, 399,
      411–18, 466–8, 479
  mental health 364–5, 399, 405–18,
      466–8, 479
  the Mrs Aba case 413–18
  policy needs 415–18
  resilience and coping factors 409–10,
      414–18
  risk factors 408–9
  services 407–18
milk substitutes 194, 208, 528–9

Millennium Development Goals (MDGs) 508, 512–14
milnacipran 346
mirtazapine 344, 350
miscarriages 151, 153, 199–200, 202, 536–7
mixed mania 17, 18
see also bipolar affective disorder
mobile phones 456–8
moclobemide 339, 344, 345–6
modernisation effects, suicides 125–6
Mollica, Richard F. 405
Monari, Mary 173–7
monoamine oxidase inhibitors (MAOIs) 338–54
Montenegro 550
Montia, Sayibu 170–2
mood stabilisers
see also psychotropic drugs
list 344
Morocco 48, 51, 54–5, 77, 472, 476, 487
mortality 10–11, 13, 16, 18–19, 117–31, 198–200, 485–96
mother-infant relationships 194, 208, 210–14, 369–70, 505, 517–22, 529–37, 539–45, 555–6
motherhood 13–14, 20, 27–8, 53–5, 189–96, 198–214, 292–6, 307–12, 351–4, 518–22, 525–37, 539–45
see also parents; postpartum. . .; pregnancy
attachment to the infant 541–2, 545
baby talk 540
collegial relationships 534–5
contributions of others 504, 534–7, 545
depression 53–5, 198–200, 203–10, 352–4, 530–7, 542–5
disenfranchised grief 526–7
education 530–1, 532–4, 544–5
fantasies 527–8, 534
human development 194, 208, 210–14, 369–70, 505, 517–22, 529–37, 539–45
intuition concepts 532–3, 540
maternal care in the early years 505, 518–22, 525–37, 539–45
occupational fatigue 529–31
occupational satisfaction 531–2
politicisation needs 535
recognition factors 531–7

unpaid workload 504, 505, 525–37, 539–45
workload measures 528–37
Mozambique 375–6
multiple roles of women 46–7, 149–50, 264, 360–1, 428–39, 443, 450–8, 464–79, 521–2, 527
MUPS *see* medically unexplained physical symptoms
Muslim women 48–50, 79, 150–64, 169–72, 361, 371–7, 433, 448–58, 472–6, 485–96

Namibia 550
National Health Service (NHS) 105
National Institute for Clinical Excellence (NICE) 105, 108
National Institutes of Health (NIH) 288–9
natural disasters 362–3, 369, 377–83
nazis 371
neonatal toxicity, valproic acid 23–4
Nepal 195, 375
Netherlands 111, 119, 229, 231–2, 266, 436
neural circuitry, somatisation and dissociation 72
neural tube defects 24
neurasthenia
see also job burnout
concepts 425–6
neurobehavioural teratogenicity, antiepileptic drugs 23
neurobiological factors 3, 70–4, 155–6, 505, 539–45, 553–4
neuroendocrine dysregulation, somatisation and dissociation 73–4
neuropsychology, somatisation and dissociation 72–3
neurosis 105–6, 269, 500–1
neurotransmitter dysfunction, somatisation and dissociation 73, 74
New Zealand 108, 488, 491, 555
NHIS data, disabilities in women 15–16
Niaz, Unaiza 359–68, 369–86, 443–61, 463–83
Nicaragua 550
Nigeria 141, 143–4, 193–4, 197–214, 229, 445, 494
night sweats, menopausal symptoms 260–5
NIH *see* National Institutes of Health
non-epileptic seizures 69, 82–3, 159–64
see also conversion disorder

non-governmental organizations (NGOs)
416–18, 475
non-specific supportive clinical
management 108
norepinephrine 45
Norris, Fran H. 377
Norway 141, 144–5, 431

obesity 13, 98, 268–9, 271
see also eating disorders
obsessive-compulsive disorder 19, 38,
52–5
see also anxiety. . .
occupational fatigue, maternal mood
529–31
occupational satisfaction, motherhood
531–2
Oedipus phase 519
oestrogens 12, 41, 45, 51, 71–2, 156,
262–3, 266, 294–5, 345–54
Okasha, Ahmed 1–8
olanzapine 12–13, 25, 109, 339, 344
Oman 486, 488
oral contraceptives 51, 265, 347
Oromo refugees 364–5, 408–9
osteoporosis 346–7
ovarian cancer, concepts 242, 244–6
ovaries 235–8, 294–5
oxcarbazepine 23–4, 350
Oxfam 378
oxytocin 45, 156

'packages' of maternal stimulation 541
Padmavati, R. 9–35
Pakistan 26–7, 145, 194, 201, 207, 234, 261,
361, 363, 373, 377, 378–80, 449,
453–4, 456–7, 470–1, 472, 474
Palestine 160–2, 374, 472, 476
paliperidona 344
Palmer, Robert L. 6, 97–116
panic disorder (PD) 19, 37–55, 159–64,
287–96, 500–1, 520–2
see also anxiety. . .
parents 13–14, 27–8, 177–80, 194, 200–3,
208–14, 268–70, 369–70, 428–9,
470–1, 505, 517–22, 525–37,
539–45
see also motherhood
quality determinants 541–2
schizophrenia 13–14, 27–8, 177–80
skills 28

unpaid workload of motherhood 504,
505, 525–37, 539–45
paroxetine 339, 344, 345–6, 350, 353
partners 163, 193, 203, 206–8, 211, 213,
232–5, 262, 266–76, 283, 361,
364–6, 387–99, 405–18, 432–3,
450–8, 463–79, 504, 505, 520–2,
534–7, 545, 549–56
see also intimate partner violence
PCOD *see* polycystic ovarian disease
PD *see* panic disorder
perimenopause 194, 259–76, 287–96
see also menopause
personal experiences, trauma types
150–64, 191–2
personality disorders 41, 75–6, 127–9, 329,
500–1
Peru 377, 550
pesticides 124, 130
pharmacodynamics, concepts 342–3
pharmacokinetics, concepts 342–3
pharmacotherapy 13, 80–1, 83–5, 87–8,
130–1, 306–12, 337–54
Phencyclidine (PCP) 140
phenomenology, BPD 19
philosophies of medicine 3
phobias 37–55, 287–96, 304–12
see also anxiety. . .
physiological factors, trauma 157
physiotherapy 83
placebo trials 290–6, 340–1, 345–6
PMDD *see* premenstrual dysphoric
disorder
PMS *see* premenstrual syndrome
Pol Pot regime 371
police 366, 391–9
policy needs
global policies 502–5, 507–14
migration and mental health 415–18
postpartum period 213–14, 535–7,
544–5
unpaid workload of motherhood 504,
535–7, 544–5
polycystic ovarian disease (PCOD),
concepts 240–1, 294–5, 346–7
polygamy 48–50, 230
POMS *see* Profile of Mood States
possessions 4, 66, 68–9, 76–8, 86
post-traumatic stress disorder (PTSD) 5,
37–55, 65–6, 85, 88, 141, 145–6,
150–64, 193–214, 240, 273–6,

287–8, 295–6, 330–3, 365–6,
371–83, 388–99, 407–18, 466–79,
490–4, 520–2, 552–6
see also anxiety. . .
alcohol and substance abuse 141, 145,
158, 162–4, 201–2, 552–6
causes 159–64, 240, 371–83, 388–99,
411–18, 466–79, 490–4, 520–31
comorbidities 159–64, 240, 552–3
concepts 5, 150–64, 240, 273–6, 287–8,
295–6, 330–3, 365–6, 371–83,
388–99, 411–18, 466–79,
490–4, 520–1, 552–6
FGM 364, 491–4
migration 399, 411–18, 466–8
postpartum period 193–4, 197–214
research needs 295–6
treatments 88, 212–13, 273–6, 295–6,
375, 379–83, 389–99, 414–18
postpartum blues, concepts 203–4,
351–4
postpartum depression
Chile 284–5, 307–12
concepts 54, 203–10, 294–5, 307–12,
351–4, 530–7, 542–5
cultural specificity 208–14
infant factors 208–10, 542–5
partners 206–8, 211, 213
psychosocial factors 206–8, 307–12
single mothers 310–12
socio-economic status 310–12
treatments 212–13, 351–4, 544–5
postpartum morbidity 193, 203
postpartum period 20, 53–4, 129, 190–6,
197–214, 294–5, 307–12, 347–54,
526–37, 542–5
see also motherhood
policy needs 213–14, 535–7, 544–5
research needs 213–14
service needs 214, 544–5
suicides 198–200
postpartum psychosis, concepts 26–7,
198–200, 203, 204–5, 351–4
poverty 38, 210–11, 376–7, 380–3,
408–18, 443–58, 463–4, 467–79,
502–5, 508–14, 517–22, 541–5
Poverty Reduction Strategy Paper (PRSP)
508–14
PPD *see* postpartum depression
preferences for sons 202–3, 208–14, 505,
517–22

pregnancy 20, 21–5, 45, 52–5, 71–2, 125,
128–9, 144–5, 174–7, 189–96,
197–214, 228–9, 285, 287–8,
292–6, 307–12, 345–54, 489–90,
526–37, 542–5
see also infertility; motherhood;
postpartum. . .
alcohol and substance abuse 144–5,
199, 201–2, 293–4
anxiety disorders 45, 52–5, 201–2,
287–8, 292–6, 307–12,
542–5
cultural preferences 202–3, 208–14,
505, 517–22
depression 20, 21–5, 45, 52–5,
198–202, 287–8, 292–6,
307–12, 542–5
FGM 489–90
mental health aspects 20, 21–5, 45,
52–5, 125, 128–9, 144–5,
174–7, 189–96, 197–214,
287–8, 292–6, 307–12, 345–54,
542–5
policy needs 213–14
psychotropic drugs 347–51
research needs 213–14, 285, 292–6
self-harm 198–200
service needs 214, 544–5
suicides 125, 128–9, 198–200
violence 193, 203
premenstrual dysphoric disorder (PMDD)
41, 50–1, 294–5, 325–6
premenstrual syndrome (PMS) 50, 294–5,
325–6
prenatal genetic screening 202
Prentice, Kristen 285, 287–99
primary healthcare 65–6, 81, 190–6,
237–8, 284–5, 301–12, 317–20,
323–33, 337–54, 407–18, 451–5,
458, 477–9, 500–5, 509–14, 535–7,
544–5
see also services
primary infertility, concepts 228–46
privatisations 451–2, 458, 475
Profile of Mood States (POMS) 530–1
progesterone 41, 51, 71–2, 262–3
prolactin 45, 71–2, 294–5, 345–7
prosecutions, intimate partner violence
391, 393, 399, 556
prostitution 144, 371–2, 375–6, 445,
453–4

protection orders, intimate partner
  violence 391, 392
PRSP *see* Poverty Reduction Strategy Paper
psychiatric disorders 1–8, 149–64,
    189–96, 227–46, 292–6, 317–20,
    345–54
  see also individual disorders; mental
    disorders
psychiatric morbidity, mother-infant
    relationships 194, 208, 210–14
psychiatric research, ethics 285, 287–96,
    338–40
psychodynamic therapy 43–4, 81, 88,
    212–13
psychoeducational therapy 88, 274–6
psychopharmacology 13, 282–3, 337–54
  see also psychotropic drugs
  clinical research 338–54
  concepts 282–3, 337–54
  ethics 338–40
  historical background 337–8
  lists of drugs 339, 344, 350
  reproduction issues 346–54
  sources/interpretation of data 340–1
  treatment response in women 345–6
psychosocial factors 74–81, 192, 194,
    206–8, 227–46, 259–76, 307–12,
    375–83, 412–13, 414–18, 434–8
psychosocial rehabilitation in women,
    findings 16, 25
psychotic disorders 6–7, 9–28, 106,
    198–200, 329, 338–54, 426, 466
  see also postpartum. . .; schizophrenia
psychotropic drugs
  see also antidepressants;
      antipsychotic. . .
  breastfeeding 282–3, 349–51
  concepts 13, 21–5, 338–54, 414–18,
    511–14, 544–5
  lists of drugs 339, 344, 350
  reproduction 346–51
  side effects 13, 21–5, 282–3,
    338–54
  women 343–51, 544–5
puberty 99, 191, 264, 318–20,
    518–22
public awareness programmes
  FGM 495–6
  intimate partner violence 365–6, 397,
    556
Puerto Rico 471

quality determinants, parents 541–2
quetiapine 25, 109, 339, 344
Quran 361, 433, 473, 475, 486–7, 492, 495

radiotherapy 243–6
Raja, Shoba 169–87
Rajkumar, Ravi Philip 65–95
randomised clinical trials, concepts 338–41
rapid cycling findings, BPD 18, 25
rational emotive therapy 273–6
reattribution therapy, somatisation 80
referrals to specialists 80
refugees 364–5, 371–2, 375, 406–18,
    466–8, 479
  see also asylum-seekers; migration
rehabilitation 16, 25, 83, 129–31, 509–14
relationships principle, gender-sensitive
    psychiatric care 327–8, 333
religion 76–7, 125, 175–6, 178–80, 192,
    229, 234, 267–70, 410–11, 413–18,
    433, 456–7, 464, 469, 473, 486–7,
    492–6, 549
RePEAT *see* Research Protocol Ethics
    Assessment Tool
reproductive health 189–96, 213–14,
    227–46, 292–6, 301–12, 345–54,
    535–7, 551–6
reproductive hormones 12, 41, 45, 51,
    54–5, 71–2, 99, 156, 204, 262–5,
    294–5, 345–54
research 145, 213–14, 287–96, 338–54
  ethics 285, 287–96, 338–40
  phases 341–2
Research Protocol Ethics Assessment Tool
    (RePEAT) 289–90
resilience 409–10, 469, 504
  see also coping
respectful relationships, gender-sensitive
    psychiatric care 333
Restorative Justice (RJ), intimate partner
    violence 396
restraint/seclusion uses, gender-sensitive
    psychiatric care 329, 331–2
Richter, Linda M. 505, 539–48
risky health behaviours 141–3, 262
risperidone 12–13, 25, 339, 344
Roberts, Laura 287–99
Rochat, Tamsen 505, 539–48
Rojas, Graciela 284–5, 301–15
role strain theory 434–8
Rondón, Marta B. 281–5, 323–36

Roszak, Theodore 7–8
Royal College of Nurses 328
Rwanda 371–2, 375

safe houses, intimate partner violence
    389–90, 398, 505, 553–6
safety issues, gender-sensitive psychiatric
    care 330–3
Salamoun, Mariana M. 149–68
Samoa 550
Sarabia, Silvana 282–3, 337–58
Sati 124–5
Satyanarayana, Veena A. 192, 227–57
Saudi Arabia 449, 476, 486–7
schizoaffective psychoses, concepts 25–6
schizophrenia
    see also psychotic disorders
    age at onset 12
    ageing women 16
    alcohol and substance abuse 12
    burden and stigma 14, 15, 16, 177–80
    caregivers 15, 16
    concepts 6–7, 9–28, 177–80, 187, 205,
        287–96, 338–54, 466, 500–1
    consumer voices 177–80, 187
    course 11
    depression 11, 13, 20
    epidemiology 10–11, 287–96, 466,
        500–1
    homelessness 14–15, 27, 178–9
    marriage 13–14, 27–8
    medications 12–13, 27
    menopause 287–96
    mortality 10–11, 13, 16, 127–9
    oestrogens 12
    outcomes 11
    parents 13–14, 27–8, 177–80
    psychopathology 11
    psychosocial rehabilitation 16, 25
    sexuality 27
    suicides 10–11, 13, 16, 127–9
    treatments 11, 12–13, 27, 177–80,
        338–54
schools 130–1, 398
science-based mental health services
    416–17
scientific advances, child development
    539–40
Scotland 230
screening, intimate partner violence
    interventions 388–9

Second World War 370–1
secondary infertility, concepts 228–46
Sector-Wide Approaches (SWAps) 508–14
secure infants 541–2
self-confidence 505, 519–22, 554–5
self-control 519–22
self-directed violence, trauma types 150–1,
    152
self-esteem 329–30, 399, 409, 411, 427,
    434, 453–4, 505, 517–22, 554–5
self-harm 6, 117–31, 152, 163, 198–200,
    329–33, 466, 470–1117
    see also suicides
    concepts 117–31, 152, 163, 198–200,
        329–33, 466, 470–1
    definitions 117–18
self-help 3, 44, 129–30, 399, 410–18, 469
self-referrals 413–18
Serbia 550
serotonin reuptake inhibitors (SSRIs)
    80–1, 343–5, 346, 350
serotonin system 45, 51, 72, 80–1, 127,
    156, 294–5, 343–6, 350
serotonin-norepinephrine reuptake
    inhibitors (SNRIs) 343–6
sertraline 42–4, 339, 344, 346, 353
services 65–6, 81, 190–6, 213–14, 237–8,
    245–6, 284–5, 287–96, 301–12,
    317–20, 323–33, 337–54, 383,
    388–99, 407–18, 451–5, 458,
    477–9, 496, 500–5, 509–14, 535–7,
    544–5
    see also primary healthcare
    barriers 319
    children and adolescents 283, 317–20,
        544–5
    Chile 284–5, 301–12
    cultural issues 477–9
    financing issues 416–17, 513–14
    gender-sensitive psychiatric care
        317–20, 323–33, 338–42, 458
    global policies 502–5, 509–14
    globalisation 451–5, 458
    intimate partner violence interventions
        388–99, 549–56
    knowledgeable staff 332–3
    legislation issues 415–16
    migration 407–18
    psychopharmacology 13, 337–54
    respectful relationships 333
    restraint/seclusion uses 329, 331–2

services (*continued*)
   safety issues 330–3
   sexual safety issues 330–3
severe mental illness (SMI) 6–7
   see also bipolar affective disorder;
     psychotic disorders
sex hormones 12, 41, 45, 51, 54–5, 71–2,
   99, 156, 204, 262–5, 294–6, 345–54
sexual coercion, intimate partner violence
   504, 549–56
sexual exploitation 27, 371–7, 444–58,
   509–14
sexual harassment, working women 430,
   438–9
sexual interest/functioning 13, 141–3,
   162–3, 191–6, 261–4, 267, 456–8
sexual safety issues, gender-sensitive
   psychiatric care 330–3
sexual satisfaction 192, 457
sexual violence 47–50, 152–3, 158,
   159–60, 162–4, 190–6, 199–200,
   240, 295–6, 320, 330–4, 365–6,
   371–7, 381, 387–99, 406–18, 430,
   438, 444–58, 463–79, 509–14,
   520–2, 549–56
sexuality 21, 27, 49
shame issues, menopause 267–8
shelter stays, intimate partner violence
   interventions 389–90, 398, 505,
   553–6
side effects, medications 13, 21–5, 282–3,
   338–54
SIDS *see* sudden infant death syndrome
Sierra Leone 371, 374, 493–4
Singapore 200–1, 209, 261, 470–1
single mothers 283, 310–12, 317–20, 443
slavery 444–6
sleep problems 260–5, 271–6, 425
SMI *see* severe mental illness
smoking 139–42, 201–2, 260, 269, 271,
   339, 345, 522
SNRIs *see* serotonin-norepinephrine
   reuptake inhibitors
social anxiety disorder 37–55
   see also anxiety...
social factors, depression and anxiety
   disorders 46–50, 414–18
social implications, globalisation 451–3
social inclusion issues, migration 407–18
social learning theory 519
social mobility factors, infertility 233–4

social support 16, 25, 53, 130–1, 156,
   158–9, 200–2, 206–14, 243–6,
   266–76, 389–90, 409–18, 430–3,
   469–71, 504, 543–5, 552–3
socio-economic status 46, 259–60,
   265–70, 302–12, 323–33, 362, 374,
   406–18, 434–9, 445–6, 449–51,
   470–1, 501–5, 541–2, 544–5
socio-political contexts
   differences between countries 505,
     507–14
   promotion of mental health 500–5
Somalia 49, 364–5, 375, 408–9, 488, 493
somatisation
   biological factors 3, 70–4
   causes 66–8, 70–81, 163, 238–9,
     365–6, 388–99, 425–6, 468
   classification systems 68–9
   clinical features 66–9, 76–7, 78–9, 82
   comorbidities 65–6, 81
   concepts 2–3, 47, 65–88, 163, 191,
     238–40, 261–4, 305–12, 365–6,
     370–1, 388–99, 425–6, 468,
     500–1
   cultural variations 67–8, 76–7, 78–9
   definitions 66–7, 68
   diagnosis 68–9
   epidemiology 77–8, 81–2, 305–12,
     500–1
   gynaecological infections 238–9
   lifespan changes 77
   medications 80–1
   personality disorders 75–6
   psychosocial factors 74–81
   symptoms 66–8, 76–7, 78–9
   terminology 66–9
   trauma responses in women 74–8
   treatments 69, 79–81
   violence impacts 47, 163, 388–99
somatoform dissociation, concepts 87,
   425–6
sons, cultural preferences 202–3, 208–14,
   505, 517–22
South Africa 41–2, 141, 390, 453–4, 542
South Asia
   see also individual countries
   cultural impacts 473–4
Soviet Union 126, 128, 377, 448–9
Spain 209, 436
spina bifida 22, 24, 349
spirit possessions 4, 66, 68–9, 76–8, 86

Sri Lanka 474
SSRIs *see* serotonin reuptake inhibitors
'stay-at-home' mothers 536–7
stereotypes 202–3, 208–14, 500–1, 505,
    517–22, 535–7
stigma 7, 14, 15, 16, 140–1, 143, 145,
    169–87, 192, 228–46, 325, 329–33,
    432, 518–22
still births, trauma types 151, 153, 202
stoning of women 361, 475
stress 2–3, 65–88, 231–2, 241–6, 264–76,
    364–5, 369–83, 406–18, 424–39,
    450–8, 466–79, 550–6
    see also dissociation; somatisation
stress-diathesis model 3
strokes 263, 418
sub-Saharan Africa 41–2, 50–1, 142–4,
    228, 263, 320, 488
subpopulation effects, suicides 123–4
substance abuse *see* alcohol and substance
    abuse
Sudan, female circumcision 49, 487, 488,
    491–3
sudden infant death syndrome (SIDS)
    533–4
suicides 6, 10–11, 13, 18–19, 45, 117–31,
    152, 163, 198–200, 318–20, 418,
    451, 454, 470–1, 520–1, 551–2, 553
    alcohol and substance abuse 122–3,
        126, 127–9, 131, 199
    anxiety disorders 127–9, 318–20,
        470–1, 551–2
    biological factors 126–7, 553
    BPD 18–19
    causes 126–9, 198–200, 470–1, 520–1,
        551–2, 553
    children and adolescents 318–20
    comorbidities 127–9, 163, 551–2
    cultures 117, 125–6, 470–1
    definitions 117–18
    depression 18–19, 122–3, 127–9, 182,
        198–200, 318–20, 451, 454,
        470–1, 551–2, 553
    ecological fallacy 6, 123–4
    EDs 111, 128
    epidemiology 118–24, 163, 454, 470–1
    gender paradox 6, 121–2
    gender ratios 118–31, 470–1
    globalisation 451, 454
    infertility 192
    methods 122–3, 130, 152

modernisation effects 125–6
postpartum period 198–200
pregnancy 125, 128–9, 198–200
prevention programmes 6, 117, 129–31
schizophrenia 10–11, 13, 16, 127–9
schools 130–1
subpopulation effects 123–4
transitional countries 125–6
understanding female behaviour 6,
    122–3
surrogate mothers 195
SWAps *see* Sector-Wide Approaches
Sweden 195, 209, 229, 231, 267, 408,
    413–18, 423–4, 426, 429, 431, 436,
    468, 472
Swedish International Development
    Agency 328
Switzerland 274
sympathoadrenomedullary system 44–5
Syria 448–9

Taiwan 17, 38, 212
Tanzania 550
TCAs *see* tricyclic antidepressants
Telstra 185–6
temazepam 350
temperament 127, 157–8
temperament and character inventory
    (TCI) 157–8
'tend-be-friend' responses, trauma 156
teratogen, definition 348
terrorism 2, 370–83
Thailand 550
Thara, R. 9–35
therapy, gender-specific issues 3
thyroid 41
tiagabine 23–4
Tigrayan society 412
tobacco 139–42, 201–2, 260, 269, 271, 339,
    345
tokenism, working women 431
topiramate 23–4, 350
trance 66, 68–9, 86, 87–8
transitional countries
    see also cultures
    suicides 117, 125–6, 470–1
transitional housing programme (TSH),
    intimate partner violence
    interventions 390
trauma 2–6, 37–55, 65–88, 141, 145–64,
    193–4, 197–214, 273–6, 287–96,

trauma (*continued*)
  330–3, 364–5, 369–83, 388–99,
    407–18, 450–8, 466–79, 490–4,
    509–14, 520–2, 544–5, 549–56
  see also dissociation; post-traumatic. . .;
    somatisation
  epidemiology 150–4, 330–3, 466
  FGM 363–4, 490–4
  future directions 164
  genetics 155–6
  global policies 502–5, 509–14
  immediate emotional responses 154–5
  'inability to forget' problems 157
  interventions 164, 212–14
  mental disorders 156–64, 450–8, 466,
    509–14
  neurobiological responses 155–6, 505,
    553–4
  physiological factors 157
  psychiatric consequences 5, 149–64
  psychological factors 157–8
  responses 154–6
  risk factors 156–9, 213–14, 408–9
  sociocultural factors 158–9, 463–79
  types 149–54, 159–64, 295–6,
    408–18
trauma re-enactment syndrome 163
treatments 11, 12–13, 21–5, 27, 42–4, 69,
    79–81, 82–3, 84–5, 87–8, 104–11,
    169–87, 200–2, 212–14, 237–8,
    271–6, 282–3, 292–6, 306–12,
    329–33, 337–54, 379–83, 414–18,
    438–9, 477–9, 501, 543–5
  see also medications
  definition 105
  management contrasts 105
triazolam 350
tricyclic antidepressants (TCAs) 80–1,
    338–54
trihexiphenidyl 350
Trinidad 470–1
tsunami of 2004 377–8
Tunisia 49, 55, 423–4, 428–9, 432, 433,
    437, 487
Turkey 85, 198, 229, 235, 377, 448, 472,
    542
Tutsis 371

UDHR *see* Universal Declaration of
  Human Rights
Uganda 141, 143–4, 472, 544

UK 105–8, 110, 120–9, 141, 209, 230–1,
    236, 242–4, 264–5, 426, 435, 451–2,
    472, 488, 531–2
unipolar depression
  see also depression
  concepts 37–55, 466
United Arab Emirates 486, 488
United Nations 371–2, 406–7, 426, 429,
    447–8, 458, 471, 476, 502–5,
    508–14
  see also Convention. . .
  Declaration on the Elimination of
    Violence Against Women (1993)
    512
  Declaration of Human Rights 418
  Development Program (UNDP) 426,
    429, 458
  education 447–8
  global policies 502–5, 508–14
  High Commission for Refugees
    (UNHCR) 371–2, 406–7
  (International) Children's Fund
    (UNICEF) 371–2
  MDGs 508, 512–14
  Population Fund (UNFPA) strategic
    plan 2008–2011 512
Universal Declaration of Human Rights
  (UDHR) 508
unpaid workload of motherhood
  concepts 504, 505, 525–37, 539–45
  recognition factors 505, 531–7
urbanisation, globalisation 453–4
USA 120, 122, 129, 151–2, 203, 205, 230,
    236–8, 259–61, 264–8, 271–2,
    288–9, 291, 293, 310–11, 393–9,
    408, 412, 426, 431, 435–6, 449, 470,
    472, 488, 491–2, 520–1
uterine body cancer 242–6
uterus 227–8, 235–8, 242–6

VA *see* Veterans Administration
Vaddiparti, Krishna 365–6, 387–403
vagina 48–50, 242, 260–7, 361, 363–4,
    475, 485–96
Valium 339, 414–18
valproic acid 22–4, 339, 344, 347, 349, 350
Varma, Deepthi S. 365–6, 387–403
Veterans Administration (VA) 295
victim-focused interventions, intimate
    partner violence 388–91
Vietnam 200, 207, 209, 372

violence 3, 7, 47–50, 131, 139–40, 144–64,
190–200, 203, 228–9, 262–4,
272–3, 275–6, 283, 317–20,
329–33, 359–68, 371–7, 387–99,
406–18, 430, 444–58, 463–79, 504,
509–22, 543, 549–56
see also intimate partner violence;
trauma
alcohol and substance abuse 7, 131,
139–40, 144, 146, 162–4, 262,
471–2, 552–6
combat experiences 150–3, 159–64,
191–2, 295–6, 362–3, 369–83,
406–18, 444–58
definition 465
depression and anxiety disorders
47–50, 160–4, 272–3, 450–8,
463–79, 519–22, 543–5, 549–56
menopause 262, 272–3, 275
migration 408–18, 479
pregnancy 193, 203
somatisation 47, 163
virginity tests 475
vitamins 24
voluntary decisions, informed consent 283,
290–1, 340
vulva, cancers 242

Wanjiru, Faith 173–7
wars 2, 150–3, 159–64, 191–2, 295–6,
369–83, 406–18, 444–58
Wasserman, Danuta 6, 117–37
wellbeing 267–70, 323–4, 329–33,
338–40, 364–5, 382–3, 405–18,
434–9, 465, 469, 501–2, 505,
508–14, 525–37, 539–45
see also mental health
widows of war 375
Winnicott, Donald 543
Wolfensohn, James D. 447–8
woman-centred counselling, menopause
272–6
Women, Gender and Equity Knowledge
Network of the CSDH 324, 503–4

women's mental health, World Health
report (1998) 9
work-life balance 435–9
'working mothers' 536–7
working women
see also employment status; job burnout
concepts 360–1, 362, 423–39, 445,
446–58, 521, 525–37, 544–5
discrimination 430–3, 445, 464, 504
family-friendly work policies 435,
438–9
Islam 433
management issues 438–9
research 434–9
role strain theory 434–8
sexual harassment 430, 438–9
socio-economic status 362, 434–9,
501–4, 544–5
tokenism 431
unpaid workload of motherhood 504,
505, 525–37, 539–45
workload of motherhood 504, 505,
525–37, 539–45
World Bank 423, 447–8, 513–14
World Conference on Disaster Recovery
(WCDR) 380–2
World Health Organization (WHO) 9,
77–8, 118–21, 150, 198, 204, 228,
259, 283, 302–3, 323–4, 362–3,
365–6, 370–1, 376, 388, 405–6,
425–6, 465–6, 470, 477–8, 487,
501–2, 504, 508–9, 512, 549–50,
551
World Health report (1998) (WHO) 9, 443
World Medical Association 331
World Psychiatric Association (WPA) 331

Yemen 476, 486, 488
yoga 233
Yugoslavia 371–2

Zimbabwe 42
ziprasidone 13, 339, 344
Zulfawu, Ibrahim 169–72

Index compiled by Terry Halliday